The Organization and Development of a Medical Group Practice

Center for Research in Ambulatory Health Care Administration

The Organization and Development of a Medical Group Practice

[1976]

The preparation of this text
was assisted by a grant from
The Robert Wood Johnson Foundation,
Princeton, New Jersey,
and with the cooperation of
the *Medical Group Management Association,*
Denver, Colorado.

The opinions, conclusions, and proposals in the text are those of the authors and do not necessarily represent the views of either *The Robert Wood Johnson Foundation* or the *Medical Group Management Association.*

Ballinger Publishing Company • Cambridge, Massachusetts
A Subsidiary of J.B. Lippincott Company

This book is printed on recycled paper.

International Standard Book Number: 0-88410-143-6

Library of Congress Catalog Card Number: 76-26953

Printed in the United States of America

Library of Congress Cataloging in Publication Data
Main entry under title:

The Organization and development of a medical group practice.

1. Group medical practice. I. Medical Group Management Association. II. Center for Research in Ambulatory Health Care Administration.
R729.5.G607 362.1'04'25 76-26953
ISBN 0-88410-143-6

Contents

List of Figures

List of Tables

Preface

The need to collect and organize information essential to the formation and development of a medical group practice has provided the stimulus for this text. *The Organization and Development of a Medical Group Practice* represents one consolidated reference source encompassing the various steps and decisions necessary for group practice formation. In order to present a comprehensive, unbiased overview of the subject, the text does not endorse any one legal type of group practice organization, nor does it recommend any one method of operation.

Because numerous goals and objectives can be identified in newly emerging groups, and because each group exists in its own microcosm of pressures and influences, it is not possible to formulate any single, universally applicable model of group practice organization. For this reason, both the editors and the authors of this text have attempted to capture the commonalities of medical group practice which exist independently from varying operational or organizational characteristics. Throughout the text, the group practice prototype upon which generalizations are based consists of three to ten physicians who represent more than one specialty, and who maintain basic ancillary services, i.e., laboratory and radiology as a minimum, within their practice. Within this framework, a primary purpose of the text is to present clearly and concisely the *basic alternatives* to be considered by individuals interested in forming a group practice. Such alternatives will enable them to make knowledgeable, effective decisions in their particular circumstances.

In addition to the exploration of those common elements uniting all group practices, the text also considers more specifically the impact of varying operational modes on the formation and development of a medical group. The goals of the individuals involved as well as the stated mission of the group may be considerably different when variables such as free-standing or hospital-based, and fee-for-service or prepaid are combined in unique configurations.

Finally, the text is designed not only for students in the administrative and professional segments of the health care field, but also for attorneys, insurers, architects, bankers, government officials, and, in general, any individual or organization interested in exploring the various facets of the organization and development of a medical group practice.

Acknowledgments

Project staff who have been responsible for the editing and preparation of this text includes:

John McCormick, M.H.A., Project Director
Mary Alice Krill, Ph.D., Assistant Project Director
Jane Grant, M.A., Research Assistant

Primary Editorial Consultants:

Louis E. Glorfeld, Ph.D., Publications Consultant
Tom E. Kakonis, Ph.D., Editorial Consultant

The project staff gratefully acknowledges the assistance of:

Mr. David Cusic and Mr. Frank Karel of The Robert Wood Johnson Foundation, the Center for Research in Ambulatory Health Care Administration Staff, the Medical Group Management Association Staff and its Library Reference Service, The Robert Wood Johnson Foundation Project National Steering Committee, and the American College of Medical Group Administrators.

In addition, the project staff wishes to recognize the contributions of:

AUTHORS

Lawrence M. Butler, Vice President, Institutional Strategy Associates, Inc., Cambridge, Massachusetts

Robert L. Doctor, M.H.A., Consultant, Denver, Colorado

C. Robert Fox, Assistant Administrative Director, Geisinger Medical Center, Danville, Pennsylvania

Jane Grant, M.A., Research Assistant, Center for Research in Ambulatory Health Care Administration, Denver, Colorado

Edward Hume, Hume, Mansfield, and Silber, Ltd., Chicago, Illinois

Phillip A. Kieburtz, President, Phillip A. Kieburtz and Associates, Bellevue, Washington

Mary Alice Krill, Ph.D., Assistant Project Director, Center for Research in Ambulatory Health Care Administration, Denver, Colorado

Bruce P. Larson, Associate, Ellerbe Architects, Inc., Bloomington, Minnesota

James W. Loy, M.H.A., F.A.C.M.G.A., Administrator, Chickasha Clinic Inc., Chickasha, Oklahoma

John McCormick, M.H.A., Project Director, Center for Research in Ambulatory Health Care Administration, Denver, Colorado

Richard Montanari, Instructor, School of Business, University of Colorado, Boulder, Colorado

Leon Rabe, Mayo Clinic, Rochester, Minnesota

Ronald L. Rushing, C.P.A., Director of Fiscal Services, Kelsey-Seybold Clinic, Houston, Texas

John E. Schneider, Graduate Student, Health Services Administration, University of Arizona, Tucson, Arizona

Carol Shearer and William Shearer, Consultants in Prepaid Medical Care, Los Angeles, California

Mark Silber, Ph.D., Hume, Mansfield, and Silber, Ltd., Chicago, Illinois

Stephen J. Sletta, Senior Law Student, School of Law, University of Colorado, Boulder, Colorado

Donald Starr, F.A.C.M.G.A., Business Manager, Tucson Clinic, Tucson, Arizona

Roger H. Stinson, Consultant, Chicago, Illinois

A.J. Wilwerding, President, Setter, Leach, and Lindstrom Architects, Inc., Minneapolis, Minnesota

STEERING COMMITTEE MEMBERS

Austin Ross, Chairman-Administrator, Virginia Mason Medical Center, Seattle, Washington

F. Kenneth Ackerman, Jr., Administrator, Geisinger Medical Center, Danville, Pennsylvania

W. Grayburn Davis, M.D., Executive Director, American Group Practice Association, Alexandria, Virginia

Seth Goldsmith, Sc.D., Columbia University, New York, New York

Clyde T. Hardy, Associate Dean, Bowman Gray School of Medicine, Winston-Salem, North Carolina

B. Jon Jaeger, Ph.D., Duke University, Durham, North Carolina

L. Russell Jordan, President, Alton Ochsner Medical Foundation, Ochsner Clinic, New Orleans, Louisiana

Donald Madison, M.D., University of North Carolina, Chapel Hill, North Carolina

Maurice Mitchell, Chancellor, University of Denver, Denver, Colorado

Frank Newman, M.D., Group Health Cooperative of Puget Sound, Seattle, Washington

Marshall Rozzi, The Robert Wood Johnson Foundation, Rochester, New York

Louis J. Segadelli, Executive Director, Group Health Association, Inc., Washington, D.C.

Jesse L. Steinfeld, M.D., Chief of Medical Services, Veterans Administration Hospital, Long Beach, California

ADVISORS TO THE PROJECT

David E. Allison
Everett A. Boring
Bryan Charles
Homer H. Clark
Richard W. Cleeremans
J. Charles Dickson, M.D.
James M. Ensign
Robert K. Garrity
Clyde C. Gelwick
Peter C. Guthery
Stanley A. Hager
Jule Hannaford
Roger Hauch
Regina Herzlinger
Henry Hood, M.D.
John T. Lenane
Dr. Robert E. Lenberg
John S. McDonald
Robert B. McLauthlin
Chester L. Meador
David J. Ottensmeyer, M.D.
Robert J. Pelletier
William W. Phillips
Fred Rochlin
Jim Skarstad
John G. Smillie, M.D.
John V. Therrell
Vernon Tock
Dudley P. Towne
M.H. Weinberg
Charles Westcott
Dr. William Wilsted
A.J. Wilwerding

SUPPORT PERSONNEL

Jane Arnold
Barbara Hanna
Ron Hedstrom
Von Jansma
Melody Sowa
Sheila Swan

The Center for Research in Ambulatory Health Care Administration (CRAHCA) is a Section 501(c)3 tax exempt charitable organization as defined by the Internal Revenue Code. Founded in 1974, the purpose of CRAHCA is to improve ambulatory health care in general and group practice in particular through better administration by developing new and innovative educational, research, and demonstration programs. CRAHCA is an affiliate organization of the Medical Group Management Association (MGMA) which is a Section 501(c)6 tax exempt trade association. Founded in 1926, today MGMA is the oldest and largest membership organization representing group practice administration. The American College of Medical Group Administrators (ACMGA) is another affiliate organization which is also a Section 501(c)6 corporation. ACMGA was founded in 1956 to provide recognition for and to promote professional advancement among group practice administrators. Through various combinations of governing boards and staff, activities and programs are developed and implemented by MGMA/CRAHCA/ACMGA. The chief administrative staff for these organizations includes Richard V. Grant, Ph.D., Fred E. Graham II, Ph.D., and J. Douglas Patterson, M.H.A.

Introduction: Group Practice Defined

Because ambulatory medical care accounts for the majority of provider/patient contacts in our health care delivery system, most individuals seeking medical attention pass through the portals of the physician's office where key decisions are made concerning the further utilization of the health care system's various components. Today, there is widespread concern, on the part of both health care providers and the public, that the ambulatory health care system, whether found in urban or rural America, may not be as well organized to deliver primary care or as closely integrated into the total health care system as desired. Further concern exists regarding the degree of emphasis placed upon inpatient services as opposed to ambulatory modes of health care organization and delivery. Interest in alleviating this situation is manifested in publicly supported efforts to reach target populations through, for example, neighborhood health centers and migrant health centers; the public and private development of health maintenance organizations; the reorganization of hospital outpatient clinics and emergency rooms; the use of various types of new physician surrogates; an increase in the number of physicians practicing in a common facility often close to a hospital; and, finally, the growth of medical group practice.

In response to the growing complexity of the health care delivery system, group practice as an operational model can provide an organizational means for improving the accessibility, continuity, quality, and efficiency of medical care for the public. Within the group practice setting, physicians are able to carry on their professional work in contiguous offices with certain shared facilities such as examination and/or consultation rooms, laboratory and radiographic equipment, reception areas, and a business office. A single medical record can be maintained for each center patient and, while each patient may identify primarily with one physician, the physicians as a group can coordinate coverage for professional services, including referral, consultation, and peer review.

While the exact composition of physician and allied health personnel in the center will vary, the group should be capable of providing primary care on a continuous basis to a broad spectrum of the public; provisions can be made for specialty and inpatient care to the extent such care is not available within the group itself. Compensation for services provided by physicians in the center may be on a predetermined formula, and administrative functions including personnel, finance, procedures, and planning can be vested in an administrative staff.

Thus, the ambulatory health center or group practice can be defined generally as a medical service system involving the cooperative practice of medicine and/or surgery by physicians for the purpose of pooling experience and skill, facilities and equipment, technical and other personnel, as well as operating expenses and, possibly, earnings. Such a pooling of resources not only establishes a convenient and efficient means for physicians to practice medicine, but also provides a similar convenience to patients in the form of centralized service.

Representatives of national group practice organizations and national physicians' organizations describe group practice in various ways. The American Group Practice Association (Alexandria, Virginia) defines a medical group as: "Any group of seven or more full-time physicians maintaining a private organization for purposes of providing general medical care of high quality. Such group or clinic shall have on their full-time staff at least five physicians in different major specialties, two of which specialties shall be internal medicine and general surgery." The Council on Medical Service of the American Medical Association offers the following definition: "Group medical practice is the application of medical service by three or more physicians formally organized to provide medical care, consultation, diagnosis or treatment, through the joint use of equipment and personnel, and with income from medical practice distributed in accordance with methods previously determined by members of the group." A third organization, Medical Group Management Association (Denver, Colorado), includes the clinic manager when it defines group practice as: "An organized medical group of three or more doctors of medicine, sharing common facilities, actively engaged in the practice of medicine, and employing a person or persons in the active supervision of their business affairs." The Council on Medical Service, consisting of the American Medical Association, Medical Group Management Association, and the American Group Practice Association, currently is attempting to agree upon a standard definition of group practice. The following revised definition of group practice was proposed on July 30, 1974: "Medical group practice is the provision of health care services by a group of at least three licensed physicians engaged full-time in a formally organized and legally recognized entity; sharing the group's income and expenses in a systematic manner; and sharing equipment, facilities, common records, and personnel involved in both patient care and business management."

While many other definitions of an ambulatory health center or group practice exist, the above descriptions include those of major national organizations and are important in the initial formulation of a concept of the ambulatory health care center. Depending upon the perspective of the definition, various criteria emerge as the basis for identifying the nature of group practice. Throughout this text, however, all of the definitions presented here will be considered applicable.

Group practices may operate under a variety of legal forms and as either public or private organizations. Professional services may be rendered through either fee-for-service or prepayment financial arrangements, and the group may affiliate itself in varying degrees with other health care delivery organizations.

In order to provide a means of ensuring accuracy of communication and to facilitate an understanding of the material discussed in the following chapters, a short taxonomy of the principal organizational and operational modes of group practice is presented here. The definitions should not be construed as exhaustive or universally applicable, but rather as a generic means of classifying any possible types of group practice for more precise comparisons.

In providing health care services to patients, a group practice may adopt any one or a combination of practice types and methods of payment. *Free standing group practice* represents the traditional role of group practice in this country's health care delivery system and involves: (1) the grouping together of physicians within varying legal forms, such as a medical partnership or a professional corporation; (2) the acquisition of joint office space, usually in close proximity to a hospital; and (3) the establishment of a fee schedule or a per capita rate from which charges are covered for services rendered by the group practice. A free standing group practice is not linked contractually or organizationally to any other organization.

The second practice type includes group practices which are *affiliated* with or derive some *authority* from a hospital. This type of practice generally is referred to as *hospital-based*; however, the actual degree of involvement of the hospital may vary considerably from practice to practice. Although closely paralleling the free standing medical group, the hospital-based practice usually is located within or adjacent to the hospital, but may have only a minimal association with the hospital involving merely a tenant-leasor relationship. Due to state statutes as well as to the organizational and tax structures of most hospitals, hospital-based group practices are emerging with varying organizational configurations and may be linked contractually (other than for teaching) and organizationally to the hospital. At one end of the continuum, this affiliation may consist of hospital *sponsorship* in which the group practice is allowed to maintain its autonomy. At the opposite end, the hospital administration exercises administrative *control* and the physicians are employees of the hospital. With national emphasis shifting from inpatient services to outpatient services, hospital-based group practice has received considerable attention and is viewed by many as a means of maintaining hospital census.

Group practices also vary in their methods of payment. The *fee-for-service* method, usually found in free standing groups, entails establishing a fee schedule from which patients are billed charges. *Prepayment*, the other main category of payment mechanism, has received much emphasis in recent years, yet the development of new prepaid plans has been slow because of two prerequisites for the establishment of any prepaid center: (1) the introduction and establishment of prepaid criteria and systems, and (2) the establishment of a group practice. As in the fee-for-service group, the prepaid group practice may be either free standing or hospital-based, and it involves a guarantee of services offered

Figure I-1. Paradigm of Practice Types and Payment Modes

Type / *Payment*	*Free Standing*	*Hospital-based, Sponsored, Controlled, or Affiliated*
Fee-for-service	The Denver Clinic and the Mayo Clinic	The Ochsner Clinic and the Virginia Mason Clinic
Combination—prepaid and fee-for-service	The Marshfield Clinic, the Kelsey-Seybold Clinic, and the Wichita Clinic	The Geisinger Medical Center
Prepaid*	Group Health Association, Inc. and Ross-Loos Medical Group	Kaiser-Permanente and the Group Health Cooperative of Puget Sound

*Contractual services represent a variation of prepaid services, although in some instances contractual services can assume fee-for-service characteristics in both free standing and hospital-based group types.

by the plan to a group of enrolled individuals in exchange for a prepaid, per capita fee. Such an arrangement places responsibility for the maintenance of the health of the patients being served in the hands of the group practice. Because continued costly and marginally necessary hospital confinement for prepaid patients would jeopardize the financial solvency of the prepaid plan, the physicians in the group have the added incentive of maintaining the health of patients enrolled in the plan through increased outpatient and preventive services. Also gaining prominence is the *combination* of fee-for-service and prepayment within a single medical group practice.

Figure I–1 illustrates the different possible combinations of the types of practice and the modes of payment and includes actual group examples which may be helpful in defining the group's mode of operation—practice type plus method of payment.

The definitions in figure I–1 are practical, operating definitions and capture quite accurately the nature of group practice in its various forms. For example, if a hospital-based professional corporation elects to establish a satellite group practice across town on an experimental, prepaid basis, the operational mode of the satellite may be defined as a *prepaid, hospital-affiliated group practice corporation* whose facilities are free standing. In this instance, the label applied to the group practice accurately describes the nature of the group's operational as well as organizational form.

In this text, the formation and development of a medical group will be discussed from the perspective of a free standing, fee-for-service group. Areas in which differences may occur as a result of varying payment mechanisms will be considered when appropriate.

SCOPE OF THE TEXT

There exists today only a minimal amount of information to assist individuals interested in planning and operating a medical group practice. The knowledge which has been generated by the practitioners, academicians, government agencies and private organizations on various aspects of group practice varies widely in scope and quality. Certain information which could be of great assistance in the complex process of initially organizing and developing a group practice is not available even in rudimentary form. Furthermore, available information often is difficult to retrieve or understand and may be presented in a disorderly and severely fragmented fashion. *The Organization and Development of a Medical Group Practice* attempts to remedy this situation by presenting in four major parts a comprehensive compilation of information: The Formation and Development of Group Practice; Organizational Planning; Medical Group Systems Development; and Facility Design, Construction, and Financing. The sequential order of the parts is intended to reflect as accurately as possible the logical progression of decision-making involved in the formation of a group practice, from its inception to its actual operation.

Part I, "The Formation and Development of Group Practice," investigates the concept of group practice through a presentation of both its history and current status, as well as through an examination of anticipated future trends in the field. An understanding of this concept is further refined through a discussion of both internal and external factors influencing the group formation process. A synthesis of the group practice concept with the various goals of individuals involved in the formation of the group results in strategies necessary to implement specific group objectives. Part I culminates with a description of the first important step in the planning process: the determination of a unified mission or goal, followed by the selection of strategies necessary for the realization of that goal.

The planning process necessary for determining strategy represents the basic thrust of Part II. After the initial decision concerning mission has been validated through a detailed consideration of such planning criteria as community demography, geographic distribution of presently available services, and general costs and projected cash flow, the alternatives available in legal organization, management structure, financial systems, and staff compensation are presented. A discussion of administrative, professional, and patient care policy planning then concludes the section.

The first two parts of the text describe the process by which a medical group practice progresses from its inception as a nebulous idea needing concrete formulation, to a well planned organizational entity having a clearly defined mission and purpose. Parts III and IV are devoted to aspects of planning associated with day-to-day operations of the medical practice, and with the design, construction, and financing of the group practice facility.

Part III, "Medical Group Systems Development," incorporates the planning and development of operating systems including communications; patient registration; patient appointments, scheduling and referral; medical records; charges, billing, and insurance processing; and purchasing and inventory systems. In addition to a consideration of alternative operating methods for each system, policy considerations in each area are presented. To further demonstrate the alternatives available in the area of operating systems planning, Part III concludes with an exploration of systems automation, focusing on electronic data processing and statistical analysis.

Finally, Part IV offers information and guidelines concerning not only the planning and construction of a new facility, but also the renovation or remodeling of an existing or leased facility. Interim and long-term financing, design and construction procedures, and center equipment requirements are some of the broad categories treated in this final section.

REPRESENTATION AND RESOURCE ASSISTANCE

Newly forming groups interested in pursuing further the subject matter discussed in this text may contact any one of the national organizations listed below. These organizations represent various segments of medical group practice and can offer valuable assistance in the organization, development, and operation of group practice by providing newly forming medical groups with resource material and technical expertise.

Medical Group Management Association (MGMA), founded in 1926, was formerly known as the National Association of Clinic Managers. The purpose of MGMA is "to improve business administration in medical groups in order to better serve the members of the Association, the medical groups they represent, and medical group practice." Administrators and managers of medical group practices throughout the United States and Canada comprise the membership of MGMA.

The Association hosts an annual national conference in addition to four annual sectional organization meetings and sponsors a number of educational programs on various topics. The programs are offered in many locations, and the resulting educational materials are published regularly. The organization and business functions of medical groups are under continual study by both national and regional committees concerned with accounting procedures; clinic, public, and professional relations; clinic business procedures; clinic organization; credit control; personnel; research; publications; and purchasing and maintenance. The Association publishes numerous pamphlets and books which explore various aspects of group practice operations and management. *Medical Group Management*, the Association's bimonthly journal, contains material presented at various Association conferences, as well as editorials, articles, and other information pertinent to the needs of group practice administrators.

To qualified member clinics and to clinic managers, the Association offers a Placement Service which is administered through the executive office in Denver, Colorado. The Association also offers a consultation service designed to provide information, suggestions, and problem analysis to both well-established and newly-formed clinics. In 1956, members of Medical Group Management Association established the American College of Clinic Managers in order to coordinate and improve educational standards and opportunities in the field of group practice administration, to provide both incentive and recognition for excellence in the field, and to lend added stature to the profession of clinic administration.

MGMA's Library Reference Service offers one of the most complete collections of ambulatory care information available in the nation. The library was established to assist those involved in or desiring to learn more about the management of medical group practices, health maintenance organizations, and other recently emerging forms of medical care delivery organized according to the group practice model. Library materials cover all aspects of medical group practice management and development, excluding only the clinical aspects of medical practice. In assisting management decision making by providing needed information from various sources, the Library Reference Service emphasizes:

1. the *selection* and *collection* of pertinent information and material from the various journals, reports, books, monographs, and other resources in the health care field;
2. the *organization* of material within the library for ease in retrieval;
3. the *generation* of information resources, both primary and secondary, to augment the existing literature; and
4. the *dissemination* of information on group practice and health maintenance organization administration.

The executive office of Medical Group Management Association is located at 4101 E. Louisiana Avenue, Denver, Colorado 80222.

The *Center for Research in Ambulatory Health Care Administration* (CRAHCA), a nonprofit organization affiliated with Medical Group Management Association, was founded in 1973. CRAHCA's activities closely parallel those of MGMA and the Center serves as the research arm of the Association. Among the Center's activities are projects such as the compilation of this text, which was sponsored through a research grant from The Robert Wood Johnson Foundation. The primary purposes of the Center are:

1. to conduct comprehensive research on the development of a national strategy to improve ambulatory health care for all segments of the general public, to develop programs appropriate to this goal, and to publish related materials;
2. to centralize and coordinate attempts by governmental agencies, educational and health institutions, professional associations, ambulatory health care managers, and the general public to solve the problems of inequitable availability of quality medical care;
3. to organize and centralize information pertinent to ambulatory health care management for use by all segments of the public; and
4. to develop appropriate educational programs and publish related materials.

The address for the Center for Research in Ambulatory Health Care Administration is 4101 E. Louisiana Avenue, Denver, Colorado 80222.

The *American Group Practice Association* (AGPA), a national organization representing physicians in group practice, was known originally as the American Association of Medical Clinics. Its principal objectives are to evaluate the standards of medical practice in clinics, to improve graduate medical education and research in clinic practice, and to disseminate scientific findings relating to group practice. More recently, AGPA has moved into the mainstream of current health care problems and has concerned itself with the organizational patterns by which health care professionals attempt to improve the delivery of health care in their own communities. The Association also has been active in the continuing process of communicating to national health planners the contributions of group practice physicians to the improvement of community health care delivery.

The Association's annual meeting provides a forum for the exchange of ideas on a nationwide level and is augmented by five regional meetings designed for discussion of methods of improving efficiency in the delivery of ambulatory health care. To encourage further discussion and planning on a year-round basis, AGPA maintains committees on ancillary services, automated systems, education of paramedical personnel, finance, graduate medical education, legislation, plans and policies, prepaid medical care, and professional standards.

AGPA's monthly journal, *Group Practice*, is the Association's official medium for communicating group practice news, information, positions and policies, and for exploring the physician's role in today's society. *Group Practice* also includes a classified advertising service. In addition, the Association operates a Placement Service, both for physicians seeking clinic affiliation and for clinics seeking personnel to fill vacancies. Its highly specialized consulting service is available upon request from a group practice clinic. An AGPA representative will visit the clinic in order to study its facilities, systems, or personnel, and will compile a written report and evaluation outlining the study results. The Accreditation Commission of AGPA, established in 1968, is concerned with the quality of medical practice in group practice clinics. Physician and administrator members of the accreditation Survey Teams periodically perform on-site evaluations in order to certify a clinic as a comprehensive medical and diagnostic center.

The executive office of the American Group Practice Association is located in Alexandria, Virginia, 22313, 20 South Quaker Lane, P.O. Box 949.

The Accreditation Council for Ambulatory Health Care was formed only recently and represents a unified effort of the Joint Commission on Accreditation of Hospitals, American Group Practice Association, American Hospital Association, American Medical Association, Group Health Association of America, and Medical Group Management Association to administer an ambulatory health care accreditation program. On January 1, 1976, the Accreditation Council program absorbed AGPA's accreditation program.

Group Health Association of America (GHAA), a national nonprofit organization of prepaid group practice plans, came into existence in 1959 when the Group Health Federation of America and American Labor Health Association merged.

The major activities undertaken by GHAA on behalf of both its membership and group practice in general are:

1. assistance in the organization of new prepaid plans and the expansion of existing plans through technical and professional consultation and support, public relations activities, and the resources of a national center for information and research;
2. representation of the legislative interests of its members both nationally and on a state level;
3. representation in the various administrative governmental agencies concerned with prepaid group practice;
4. development and maintenance of standards for the operation of prepaid group practice plans through a system of inspection and follow-up monitoring;
5. development, publication, and dissemination of educational materials through the Group Health Foundation and Library and Group Health Institute.

Group Health and Welfare News, GHAA's monthly newsletter, reports developments and trends in the medical care and prepaid group practice fields. It also includes information on the operation, problems, and progress of specific plans; reviews of books and publications; and more general articles on people and issues important in the field. The published *Proceedings* of the annual Group Health Institute offer more in-depth information on the state of health care as it relates to prepaid group practice.

The executive office of Group Health Association of America is located at 1717 Massachusetts Avenue, N.W., Washington, D.C., 20036.

Part I

The Formation and Development of Group Practice

Chapter 1

Historical Perspectives, Current Status, and Future Trends

HISTORICAL INFLUENCES

Many readers will not be familiar with health care delivery in the group practice form. For this reason and for purposes of descriptive consistency, acceptable definitions of group practice have been set forth in the Introduction to this text; however, such statements clarify only the physical attributes of this practice form. In an effort to create an awareness of the philosophies, aspirations, and roles of the principal figures in group practice, the first two text chapters will provide a short description of the early beginnings of group practice in the United States as well as a profile of the typical group practice administrator, medical director, and member physician.

Early Groups

At the beginning of the twentieth century, the dominant medical mode, particularly on the populous East Coast, was solo practice in the traditional framework imported from Europe. As a result of a scarcity of physicians in remote areas, one of the first group practice arrangements in the country was organized in 1883 by the Northern Pacific Railroad to provide medical care to the labor force building the trans-continental railroad.[1] Evidence of even earlier development does exist; an industrially owned group sponsored by the Homestake Mining Company established a medical group in the 1870s to serve its employees in its more isolated South Dakota mining operations. These early beginnings were probably somewhat less significant in the overall development of group practice than was the momentum gained through the successes of the Mayo Clinic in Rochester, Minnesota, which was organized in 1887 as a single-specialty practice by the Mayo family. This clinic became the prototype for subsequent group practices and eventually embodied the concepts of multi-specialty and hospitalization and served as a training base for many physicians throughout the Midwest who, upon returning to their local communities, established group practices patterned after that of the Mayo Clinic. In 1931, a study of seventy-seven private group practices revealed that forty-one were located in the states of Minnesota, Wisconsin, Iowa, South Dakota, North Dakota, Texas, and Illinois.[2] Nearly every group studied included at least one physician who at some point either in his training or his practice was associated with the Mayo Clinic.

While most early private group clinics were located throughout the Midwest, several diagnostic clinics did develop in the East. The International Ladies Garment Workers Union organized "The Union Health Center" as early as 1913. The Benjamin Franklin Diagnostic Clinic in Philadelphia and the Mount Sinai Diagnostic Clinic in New York were two early forerunners of specialized diagnostic group practices. By 1930, the number of private group clinics throughout the United States had increased to about 150, in which nearly 2,000 physicians were practicing.[3] About this time the concept of group practice received major stimulation with the publication of the *Report of the Committee on the Cost of Medical Care* (1932). This committee possessed the foresight to recommend that medical service, both preventive and therapeutic, be furnished largely by organized groups; such groups be organized around a hospital for the rendering of complete home, office, and hospital care; and the costs of medical care be placed on a group payment basis, through the use of insurance, taxation, or both.

Medical Specialization

Simultaneous with the population shift westward was a proliferation of scientific knowledge growing out of the Industrial Revolution. Efficiencies of specialization, division of labor, and sophisticated technology in American industry became forces to contend with in the health care industry as well. Physicians found coping with the complexities of modern medical science increasingly difficult. The capital investment required became prohibitive for the individual practitioner. The accumulation of more explicit knowledge together with advanced technology led to the specialization of medical practice and reliance upon joint and cooperative efforts. Patterns of referral and consultation resulted from this specialization and directly influenced the development of a variety of group practice arrangements. Today, medical specialization has progressed to such a degree that it now is accepted as the obvious course for medical students to pursue. Of 280,000 active physicians in the United States in 1967, 69,000 were in general practice. The list below indicates the ten largest medical specialties in the United States as of 1967 and further demonstrates the degree to which the trend from general to specialized practice of medicine has developed.[4]

Specialty	*Number*
General Practice	69,000
Internal Medicine	39,000
General Surgery	28,000
Psychiatry	18,000

Specialty	*Number*
Obstetrics/Gynecology	17,000
Pediatrics	16,000
Radiology	10,000
Anesthesiology	8,900
Pathology	8,800
Ophthalmology	8,600

As specialization became more popular, physicians found it necessary to learn more about particular areas of medicine. Early departures from standard general practice represented an effort to exploit this extended knowledge. Diagnostic clinics and the separation of surgical practice from general practice, as epitomized by the Mayo group, are examples of this trend. The relative abundance of medical practitioners in the United States at the turn of the century further facilitated the specialized practice of surgery. The United States probably was better supplied with physicians in 1900 than any other country in the world at any time in previous history.[5] Thus, it was possible for large numbers of physicians to develop surgical skills without reducing the availability of general practitioners.

With the advent of more highly trained surgical specialists and the introduction of new equipment, consumer expenditures began to rise. The need to economize and to render more efficient care became apparent and resulted in a preferential status for larger group practices due to their economies of scale. Immense growth in the need for scientific expertise associated with new medical technology, as well as progressively increasing demands for services, led to a proliferation in both the number and types of allied health workers. Currently, the distribution of allied health workers in group practice is reported to be 25 percent in nursing, 25 percent in other technical professions, and 50 percent in clerical or bookkeeping occupations.[6] In 1967, the American Medical Association's Congress on Socio-Economics projected a requirement for a 20 percent increase in allied health manpower to meet immediate needs.[7] The National Advisory Commission on Health Manpower states that the question of delegation and use of allied health manpower is the critical issue to be resolved if the health manpower supply is to be used effectively and productively.[8] As an outgrowth of medical specialization, allied health personnel working in a group environment play a vital role in productivity and in the delivery of comprehensive health services, especially when physicians are scarce.

In addition, an increasing reliance upon new diagnostic and laboratory equipment and the personnel who operate such equipment, as well as the need to share and consult with other medical specialists, has created a major shift in the medical practice environment. The hospital, an institution with a large number of medical resources concentrated in one area, has begun to replace the home or office as the focal point of quality medical care. This trend toward institutional care has fostered further growth of group practice and, as a result, many groups have established their office practices adjacent to or near a hospital.

Shifting Medical Education Emphasis

The same forces working toward change in the mode of medical practice have contributed to change in the educational methodology for training physicians. The shift away from apprenticeships and toward formal training in a university occurred at approximately the same time that medical care became institutionalized, and for many of the same reasons. With the creation in 1889 of a laboratory for research at Johns Hopkins Medical School, medical education began to shift from a primarily humanistic to a combined humanistic-scientific approach.[9] It is of interest to note that the Johns Hopkins Medical School was the foremost example of group practice arrangements organized by medical faculties. At the time, such an organizational change represented a radical departure from the more traditional, individualistic structure previously embodied by schools of medicine. In 1967, the National Conference on Group Practice recommended the formation of group practice arrangements by medical school faculties to provide a model for medical students.[10] Gradually, greater attention has been paid to the care rendered in outpatient departments of medical schools as a result of upgrading the status of faculty members assigned to those departments, and such steps have heightened the awareness of the student toward the importance of ambulatory care.

Over the past fifty years, the time a physician must spend pursuing his medical education has increased markedly. In the past, four years of medical school marked the end of a student's formal training, but today's medical student faces additional years of training consisting of an internship and specialty residency, as well as the possibility of a year or two of sponsored practice in his specialty before specialty boards regard his education as complete. The *Millis Report on Graduate Medical Education* suggests that no physician can rely solely upon what he learned in school and that the education of the physician must continue as long as he chooses to practice medicine.[11] Thus, continuing education appears to be a requirement for the responsible practitioner, and this trend has encouraged young physicians to practice in group arrangements where time can be allocated for such activity.

Impact of Consumer, Labor, and Industrially Sponsored Groups

Physician owned and sponsored groups, compensated on a fee-for-service basis, have dominated the field since the inception of group practice. More recently, a concern for the availability of quality, comprehensive medical service at reasonable costs has prompted a variety of other agencies to participate in group practice sponsorship. The earliest examples of this type of group were industrially sponsored and developed out of a need to provide medical services to employees. The previously cited Homestake Mining Company and the Northern Pacific Railroad groups are typical examples. While often credited with initiating a wide spectrum of coverage for their members, industrially sponsored groups have found it increasingly difficult to finance and administer modern health care delivery, and few such groups remain as sponsors. Labor sponsored groups also tend to be few in number, but nonetheless are significant. The retail-wholesale and department store unions in St. Louis, Missouri, were instrumental in obtaining one of the first comprehensive care plans through a group practice.[12] The Community Health Association of Detroit is a large, prepaid group practice plan sponsored by the United Auto Workers Union. Probably of greater significance than actual sponsorship is organized labor's effort to purchase medical services for union members through established group arrangements.

The impetus for prepayment types of group practice came largely from outside the medical profession. Immediately following World War II in 1947, the Kaiser Foundation Health Plan, the Group Health Cooperative of Puget Sound (Seattle), and the Health Insurance Plan of New York (HIP)—currently the three largest prepaid plans—were organized. Kaiser evolved from an industrial plan organized to serve shipyard and other employees of the Kaiser Corporation; Puget Sound resulted from a merger of cooperatively minded consumers and physicians; and HIP was created when Fiorello LaGuardia, then mayor of New York City, determined that city employees needed comprehensive medical care coverage and subsequently contracted with HIP for all city employees and their dependents.

Growth of prepayment was slow, due in part to hostility from organized medicine, lack of visibility to the general public, and more general acceptance of indemnity fee-for-service insurance. By 1970, only twenty-five to thirty prepaid plans were in existence, covering four million people. When medical care costs began to rise sharply in 1965, prepayment came to the attention of government officials and third party payors. At their best, prepaid plans provided a complete medical system which took responsibility for all the patient's medical needs. Total out-of-pocket cost to plan members was lower than to those who used indemnity insurance coverage. These factors gradually won the bipartisan political support which resulted in passage of the HMO Act in 1973.

Military Experience in Group Practice

Historical events such as World Wars I and II exposed large numbers of physicians to the type of group practice found in the armed forces and thereby stimulated this system of health care. Of thirty clinics studied in 1930, all but four were organized shortly following World War I.[13] These events, coupled with population upheavals resulting from transplanting drafted physicians to other sections of the country, fostered the acceptance of group practice as a viable alternative to traditional medical practice. In addition, the utilization of numerous allied health professionals to assist the physician is standard practice in military medicine. Drafted physicians, practicing in the military environment, came to rely upon the competence of these trained, nonphysician health workers and tended to perpetuate this reliance in the civilian setting.

Influence of Organized Medicine

While events happening outside the field of medicine served to foster growth of the group practice ideal, there were additional influences arising within the profession itself. Acceptance of the group practice concept by organized medicine has been slow and, initially, group practice physicians did not enjoy the status granted colleagues in individual practice. In a 1932 issue of the *Journal of the American Medical Association* existing group practices were referred to as "medical Soviets."[14] The denial of hospital privileges to group physicians was one means employed to restrict medical group endeavors. While reluctance on the part of organized medicine to embrace the group practice of medicine has slowed its progress, the challenge has served to strengthen the group ideal through modification and innovation for the good of all concerned. A basic concern of those in medicine has been the preservation of rugged individualism among practitioners and the maintenance of the personal physician-patient relationship. Organized medicine views its obligation to the health needs of the nation best being served if it retains control of the destiny of the nation's health care, and it is fearful that group practice might open the door to the intervention of government agencies and other nonmedical professionals. Finally, the politics of economic competition between group practices and solo practitioners has been a realistic concern to the American Medical Association (AMA) which predominately represents the solo practitioner.

In recent years, however, there has been a lessening of this opposition. The Committee on the Costs of Medical Care, formed at the time of the annual meeting of the American Medical Association in 1927, is of historical significance, not from the standpoint of any endorsement of its actions by organized medicine, but rather due to its insight into the health problems of the nation, many of which we still face today. In 1958, the AMA Commission on Medical Care Plans extended recognition to group practice forms of health care delivery and urged greater tolerance of this form of practice.[15] At the First National Congress on the Socio-Economics of Health Care sponsored by the AMA in 1967, the efficiencies of group practice and the quality of health care rendered in a group setting were specifically recounted.[16]

Influence of the Federal Government

The involvement of the federal government in the health affairs of its citizenry has escalated from one of minimal participation in the early 1900s to one of partnership with health professionals today. A major event in the development of this relationship was the economic depression of the early 1930s when it became impossible for private and state agencies to provide for the socioeconomic needs of large masses of the population. Federal programs were initiated to provide a number of needed services, culminating in the passage of the Social Security Act in 1935 which marked the beginning of federal assistance on behalf of the citizens. Although attempts to include health provisions in the original act were defeated, the seeds of cooperation were nonetheless sown. Government influence on a number of fronts has increased steadily. The early 1960s were especially crucial when, during a span of only three years, over twenty pieces of health legislation were enacted by the Congress. In 1965, Medicare legislation was enacted and for the first time the government became a major purchaser of health care services. Previously, the federal government's role had been confined mainly to the financing of medical research efforts.

Group practice, as an alternative operational mode, has not escaped the scrutiny of federal agencies seeking more efficient and economical means of providing purchased services. Beginning in 1932 with a Senate subcommittee recommendation that group practice be encouraged for reasons of economy, subsequent commissions and conferences have continued to encourage the development of group arrangements. For example, the National Conference on Group Practice, held in October 1967 and sponsored by the Department of Health, Education and Welfare, was called specifically to explore ways to stimulate the growth of group practice in the United States. Federal involvement can be credited with governmental contributions which have stimulated the growth of individual health expectations and the resultant demand for increased services. Furthermore, the institutionalization of care and an increased need for health care personnel are in part a result of federal programs. Of great significance is the creation of a public attitude that the federal government will provide for health care needs. This state of mind induces the public to seek recourse through legislative bodies which, in turn, tends to encourage an even greater level of government involvement.[17]

Impact of Health Care Legislation

A number of health related measures have been enacted by the Congress in recent years. Acts providing for Medicare, Health Maintenance Organizations, Professional Standards Review Organizations, and the National Health Planning and Resources Development acts have had particular impact on group practice formation and are deserving of special mention.

Medicare and Medicaid. The Medicare Bill (Public Law 89-97) was signed into law on July 30, 1965, and became effective July 1, 1966. Its two major provisions, Title IVIII Medicare and Title XIX Medicaid, have as their primary purpose the accessibility of health care to those over the age of sixty-five as well as to those on poverty level incomes. Heralded as one of the most significant pieces of social legislation in the history of American medicine, this act places the government in the position of being the major purchaser of health care in the nation. Medicare provides coverage to over twenty million beneficiaries while Medicaid potentially covers forty million additional persons. Sixty million citizens, or 30 percent of the total population, now have greater access to health care, and the government has acquired a vested interest in the cost and quality of the services it is purchasing. Aside from administrative burdens, the impact of Medicare legislation on prepaid group practice appears to be largely favorable. The Kaiser Foundation Health Plan reports that Medicare beneficiaries receive expanded health care options, that the burden of subsidizing care for the age sixty-five group has shifted away from members under the age of sixty-five and toward a broader base, and that the service providers have felt little or no impact.[18] The DHEW National Conference on Group Practice (1967) recommended that the government encourage the use of group practice under Medicare and Medicaid as a means of providing quality control.

Health Maintenance Organizations. The Federal Health Maintenance Organization (HMO) Act (Public Law 93-222) of December, 1973, was of particular significance to advocates of prepaid group practice. This legislation represents federal endorsement of an organized system of care currently operative in various parts of the country. Indeed, the act stands as a tribute to the proponents of this concept. Under the law, funds are provided for HMO development with fairly rigid stipulations that such organizations accept the responsibility of delivering prepaid, comprehensive health care services to a voluntarily enrolled group of beneficiaries. One of its major features, the dual-choice provision, affords many individuals the opportunity of choosing a provider for needed health services. HMO size as well as organizational structure appears as diverse as local innovation allows. HMOs have grown in numbers from 37 in the pre-1970 era to 183 in thirty-two states at the beginning of 1975. Coverage currently is provided to 5.5 million member beneficiaries. Table 1-1 below depicts the growth of HMOs during the period 1970 to 1975.[19]

Table 1-1. HMOs by Operational Years

Operational Year	*Number of HMOs*
Pre-1970	37
1970	41
1971	52
1972	79
1973	133
1974	183

HMO development to date has been largely centered in urban areas with the majority of plans and enrollment located in the state of California. The interfacing of Medicare, Medicaid, and HMOs is being encouraged by the federal government with a view toward eventually channeling Medicare and Medicaid payments through an HMO for quality control purposes. A survey conducted in 1974 offers evidence that such interfacing is occurring. Again, while largely a California phenomenon at this time, 58 percent of the HMOs outside of California do report having Medicare and Medicaid recipients as plan members. In California, however, 78 percent of the Medicaid recipients who responded in the survey reported being enrolled in an HMO.[20]

Professional Standards Review Organizations. Professional Standards Review Organizations (PSROs) were created by congressional action (Public Law 92-603) in October 1972, with the intention of establishing a professional standards review system throughout the nation for recipients of Social Security medical payments. Their express purpose is to promote the effective, efficient, and economical delivery of quality services to beneficiaries and to ensure that acceptable standards of practice are followed before compensation is made by the government. The law calls for the establishment of designated PSRO areas throughout the nation and the formation of PSROs to accomplish the goals of the system. Area PSROs will be able to utilize and accept the decisions of any established peer and utilization review mechanism existing among the area's health providers as long as such mechanisms demonstrate the capacity for working in concert toward the stated aims of the PSRO.

National Health Planning and Resources Development Act of 1974. Public Law 93-641 contains two new titles to the Public Service Act and represents a major step toward the implementation of a federally controlled national health care policy. Title XV, National Health Planning and Resources Development, establishes regulatory mechanisms for new health facilities services centrally controlled by the Office of the Secretary of Health, Education and Welfare. The Title provides for the creation of health service areas throughout the nation, the establishment of Health Systems Agencies (HSA) responsible for establishing and annually reviewing a health systems plan, and the yearly implementation of grant applications dealing with the provision of health services. The law requires consumer participation in health planning and makes it mandatory that HSA governing boards consist of a majority of consumers (up to 60 percent) with at least one-third of them direct providers. Title XV establishes an organizational structure, which includes the Secretary of HEW; the

National Council on Health Planning and Development; the State Health Planning and Development Agencies; the Statewide Health Coordinating Councils (SHCC); and the Health Systems Agencies (HSA) for planning, implementing, and reviewing programs.

Title XVI, Health Facilities Construction, essentially is designed to replace the Hill-Burton Program. Under the provisions of this title, a state plan establishing priorities for construction of new health facilities would be developed by a state agency and approved by a statewide health coordinating council, which is appointed by the state governor as the representative of the local HSA. This law specifies that no more than 20 percent of the annual funds may be obligated for new inpatient facilities in those areas experiencing rapid population growth and not less than 25 percent is to be obligated for outpatient facilities serving medically underserved populations. The Congress, through enactment of this legislation, has set into motion programs aimed at accomplishing predetermined national health care goals and having as their stated priority the development of medical group practices.[21]

GROUP PRACTICE AS IT EXISTS TODAY

An inquiry into group practice logically begins with an analysis of why particular groups exist, what services they provide, and what function they perform. Groups may be classified as therapeutic, consultative, diagnostic, or some combination of these, depending upon their primary function. A practice offering general medical services to a continuing patient clientele is considered to be a *therapeutic group*. Within this classification are the diagnostic and consultative functions usually required in the examination and treatment of patients. Eighty-three percent of all groups surveyed by the American Medical Association (AMA) in 1969 reported activities related to these functions.[22] A significantly larger proportion of multispecialty groups are therapeutic than are single specialty groups. *Consultation groups* usually are found within single specialty practices and function primarily on a referral basis offering the benefit of specialized opinion or treatment for specific and limited disorders. Upon termination of the referred service, the patient resumes general care from his primary physician. Less than 1 percent of the groups surveyed in 1969 regarded their services as either strictly consultative or diagnostic. A third classification of group by function is *diagnostic*. These organizations limit the scope of their activities to the rendering of examination and diagnostic services and refer patients to their primary physicians for follow-up management. Although constituting only a small percentage of all groups, the AMA survey identified approximately fifty groups throughout the United States who classify themselves solely as diagnostic clinics. Surveyors found difficulty in classifying such groups who specialize in radiology, pathology, and anesthesiology because their functions can be perceived as overlapping and interchangeable. Accordingly, a residual category was created for such groups and they comprise 12 percent of all the groups surveyed in 1969.

A second means of classifying groups is according to type of services rendered. These categorizations are related directly to the previous functional classifications. As an outgrowth of specialization, *single specialty groups* are composed of practitioners representing only one of the variety of medical specialties.

Usually consultative or diagnostic, single specialty groups constitute approximately 54 percent of all groups and include 35 percent of all group physicians, based on a 1975 AMA survey of group practices. Such groups tend to be small (three to five physicians) and are popular practice settings for anesthesiology, orthopedics, pathology, and radiology. The *multispecialty group* includes two or more medical specialties. The majority of these function as therapeutic groups embracing the concepts of primary care with built-in internal mechanisms for specialty consultation. The 1975 AMA survey indicated that 35 percent of the groups and 59 percent of all group physicians operated in this environment. Multispecialty groups tend to be larger than other group types, averaging thirteen physicians per group. The *general practice group* is composed solely of general medical practitioners and, as such, resembles a single specialty group. It functions, however, primarily as a therapeutic group and in that way resembles the multispecialty group. Such groups usually are small—three or four physicians. They comprise 11 percent of the total number of groups and include 6 percent of the physicians. Table 1-2 below indicates the number and percentage of group physicians as of 1975.[23]

It must be recognized that no one type of group practice is the answer to health care delivery in the nation today. While the DHEW National Conference on Group Practice (1967) has endorsed the concept of multispecialty practice because of its broader, more comprehensive approach, it also recognizes the need for flexibility in meeting local demands. The following quotation captures the philosophy of that assembly: "It is extremely important to note that a well trained physician, strongly motivated to conform to the purpose of the group is the *sine qua non* of a good group practice."[24]

Yet a third method of categorizing groups is by mode of operation which may be any combination of organizational affiliation (free standing or hospital-based) with method of payment (fee-for-service, prepaid, combination of fee-for-service and prepaid, or contractual). (The reader interested in precise definitions

Table 1-2. Total Groups and Full-Time and Part-Time Group Physicians by Type of Group

Type of Group	*Groups*	*Group Physicians* *Total*	*Full-Time*	*Part-Time*	*Unknown Time*
			Number		
Total	8,483	66,842	53,556	6,975	6,311
Single Specialty	4,601	23,572	21,255	1,351	966
General Family Practice	906	3,959	3,478	184	297
Multispecialty	2,976	39,311	28,823	5,440	5,048
			Percentage		
Total	100.0	100.0	100.0	100.0	100.0
Single Specialty	54.2	35.3	39.7	19.4	15.3
General Family Practice	10.7	5.9	6.5	2.6	4.7
Multispecialty	35.1	58.8	53.8	78.0	80.0

of these terms is referred to the Introduction.) The *free standing group* has been the most dominant method of operation among group practices. Typical of this mode is the group of physicians who band together formally to form a practice, deliver services, and bill their patients for these services, usually on a fee-for-service basis. The free standing group is an independent entity operating with its own organizational resources. This mode has been the traditional method employed by physicians in both solo and group practice for the delivery of health services in this country.

Whereas the free standing group is an independent entity, the *hospital-based group* operates under an agreement between the group physicians and the hospital from which the physicians practice. Office space for such groups usually is located within the hospital itself or on the hospital grounds. Occasionally, such offices are provided free of charge. Certain specialty groups such as anesthesiology, pathology, and radiology are particularly well suited for a hospital-based operation. With increasing emphasis on outpatient care and centralization of resources in established health care institutions there should be added impetus for establishing hospital-based modes of group practice in the future.

Classically, *prepayment* involves enrollment in a health plan for a fixed, pre-established fee levied as payment for future required health services. Data provided by the AMA in 1975 identified 713 groups, 8.4 percent of all groups, who derived income in full or in part from prepaid mechanisms. Analysis of table 1-3 indicates that in 1975, 40.2 percent of all groups with prepayment mechanisms had less than 5 percent of their patient care volume related to prepaid activity.[25] The 1973 passage of HMO legislation indicates the potential for sizable future expansion of the prepaid mode within both free standing and hospital-based group practice settings.

Group Organization

Existing groups have assumed a wide variety of organizational forms and methods of governing. Organizational forms generally fall into the categories of sole proprietorship, partnership, corporation, or association. *Sole proprietorship* implies that the legal ownership of the group rests with one individual. Under this form, the sole proprietor employs additional physicians on a salary basis to assist him in his practice. This form of organization is used less frequently than are other forms and, in the AMA's 1975 survey, represented only 1.6 percent of all groups. A *partnership*, as an organizational form, is the most traditional and currently the second most frequently employed method of organization. Of the total number of groups surveyed in 1975, 27.2 percent were partnerships. Essentially, a partnership is a legal agreement between two or more physicians who are co-owners of a business. Partners agree to pool resources and to share, by some predetermined formula, in the profits and losses of that business. All co-owners in the partnership usually share unlimited liability and are legally liable for acts committed by any of the partners in the conduct of the partnership's business. The *corporation*, as a form of medical organization, has increased in use among group practices and was the method chosen by 15.6 percent of the groups surveyed in 1969 and by 61.0 percent in 1975. Economics, the growth of the practice, malpractice litigation, removal of restrictions from state laws of professional incorporation, and taxation have influenced this trend. The corporation is a legal entity unto itself and, as such,

Table 1-3. Groups with Prepayment Plans by Percentage of Prepaid Activity by Type of Group

Percentage of Prepaid Activity	*Total*	*Type of Group*		
		Gen./Fam. Practice	*Single Specialty*	*Multi-Specialty*
		Number		
	662*	72	215	375
Less than 5	266	33	103	130
5–14	144	21	59	64
15–24	58	4	24	30
25–49	52	5	12	35
50–74	41	6	11	24
75–99	78	3	4	71
100	23	0	2	21
		Percentage		
	100.0	100.0	100.0	100.0
Less than 5	40.2	45.8	47.9	34.7
5–14	21.8	29.2	27.4	17.1
15–24	8.8	5.6	11.2	8.0
25–49	7.9	6.9	5.6	9.3
50–74	6.2	8.3	5.1	6.4
75–99	11.8	4.2	1.9	18.9
100	3.5	0.0	0.9	5.6

Total percentages may not add to 100.0% due to rounding.
*Total excludes 51 nonrespondents to the question.

is subject to taxation on the income of the practice. Corporation laws generally provide for limited liability of shareholder physicians with respect to the acts of other shareholders but retain unlimited liability provisions for the shareholder's own acts toward his patients. The *association* form of organization was preferred by 6.4 percent of the groups surveyed in 1975. This type of organization includes some of the benefits of the corporation while excluding the unlimited liability feature of the partnership. The association may become the preferred method of organization in those states prohibiting professional corporations. Table 1-4 summarizes the percentage distribution of groups by form of organization and type of group according to the AMA's survey of 1975.[26] A detailed discussion of these alternatives can be found in Chapter 5.

Types of Governance

The business and professional policies of group practices generally are governed by a medical director, a partnership, a board of directors, or an executive committee. The governance of a group is closely associated with its organizational form and ownership; a detailed discussion of governance follows the chapter on legal organization (Chapter 6). Within a group practice, the *medical director* usually serves as chief executive and usually is charged with the responsibility of overall clinic management. Regardless of whether the position is appointed, elected, or assumed, the medical director retains ultimate responsibility for policy development and implementation. Governance by a *partnership* involves the sharing of overall management responsibility between two or more partners

Table 1-4. Total Groups by Form of Organization and Type of Group

Form of Organization	*Total*	*Type of Group*		
		General Practice	*Single Specialty*	*Multi-Specialty*
		Number		
Total	7,547*	828	4,041	2,678
Sole Proprietorship	119	13	32	74
Partnership	2,053	364	889	800
Professional Corporation	4,606	373	2,801	1,432
Association	484	58	235	191
Foundation	33	0	7	26
Other	252	20	77	155
		Percent		
Total	100.0	100.0	100.0	100.0
Sole Proprietorship	1.6	1.6	0.8	2.8
Partnership	27.2	44.0	22.0	29.9
Professional Corporation	61.0	45.1	69.3	53.5
Association	6.4	7.0	5.8	7.1
Foundation	0.4	0.0	0.2	1.0
Other	3.3	2.4	1.9	5.8

Total percentages may not add to 100.0% due to rounding.
*Total excludes 936 nonrespondents to the question.

in the group. Partners may act jointly on policy decisions or may delegate specific areas of responsibility among themselves. A *board of directors* may be composed of members of the group, sponsors of the group, or some combination of these. Although the board may appoint a medical director to recommend professional policies and/or may employ an administrator to implement policies and procedures, the board itself retains ultimate responsibility for overall management. Finally, the *executive committee*, although similar in many respects to a board of directors, does vary, in that management responsibility and accountability are vested in a body elected solely from the owners or partners of the practice. It is usual for an executive committee to operate through a medical director and/or administrator, as in the case of a board of directors. In the 1969 AMA survey a group administrator was employed in 33.6 percent of all clinics, in 53.6 percent of all multispecialty groups, in 28.2 percent of all general practice groups, and in 19.8 percent of all the single specialty groups.

Composition of Groups

Data from the 1975 AMA survey indicate an average group size of 7.7 physicians. Multispecialty groups with an average 13.0 physicians tend to be larger than single specialty groups (5.1 physicians) or general practice groups (4.4 physicians. The National Advisory Commission on Health Manpower compiled physicians. The National Advisory Commission of Health Manpower compiled information on the primary specialty of physicians in groups practices in 1967. In table 1-5 physicians in group and in nongroup practices are compared by

Table 1-5. Physicians in Group (Nongroup) Practice Arranged by Primary Specialty

	Active							
Primary Specialty	*Group Practice*	*Nongroup Practice*	*Intern-Resident*	*Total*	*Inactive*	*Overseas*	*Address Unknown*	*Total*
I. Active:								
A. General Practice	6,105	62,199	668	68,882	0	1,808	0	70,690
B. Medical Specialties:								
Allergy	88	814	32	934	0	11	0	945
Cardiovascular disease	157	1,532	330	2,019	0	49	0	2,068
Dermatology	264	2,876	473	3,613	0	82	0	3,695
Gastroenterology	76	485	127	688	0	19	0	707
Internal Medicine	4,768	27,294	7,478	39,540	0	1,013	0	40,553
Pediatrics	2,056	11,311	2,951	16,318	0	465	0	16,783
Pulmonary diseases	28	1,117	65	1,210	0	37	0	1,247
Subtotal	7,437	45,429	11,456	64,332	0	1,676	0	65,998
C. Surgical Specialties:								
Anesthesiology	2,114	5,687	1,187	8,988	0	153	0	9,141
Colon and rectal surgery	48	583	14	645	0	4	0	649
General surgery	2,952	18,488	6,695	28,135	0	931	0	29,066
Neurological surgery	263	1,412	482	2,157	0	56	0	2,213
Obstetrics and gynecology	2,375	12,110	2,598	17,083	0	466	0	17,549
Ophthalmology	731	6,706	1,172	8,609	0	171	0	8,780
Orthopedic surgery	1,349	5,048	1,433	7,830	0	190	0	8,020
Otolaryngology	580	4,046	733	5,359	0	89	0	5,448
Plastic surgery	70	931	196	1,197	0	20	0	1,217
Thoracic surgery	179	1,195	229	1,603	0	42	0	1,645
Urology	665	3,673	818	5,156	0	94	0	5,250
Subtotal	11,326	59,879	15,557	86,762	0	2,216	0	88,978
D. Psychiatry and Neurology:								
Child psychiatry	18	681	248	947	0	16	0	963
Neurology	174	1,510	568	2,252	0	67	0	2,319
Psychiatry	535	14,561	3,558	18,654	0	292	0	18,946
Subtotal	727	16,752	4,374	21,853	0	375	0	22,228
E. Other Specialties:								
Aviation medicine	4	576	79	659	0	153	0	812
General preventive medicine	6	897	38	941	0	95	0	1,036
Occupational medicine	81	1,617	16	1,714	0	19	0	1,733
Pathology	698	5,975	2,160	8,833	0	186	0	9,019
Physical medicine and rehabilitation	46	855	214	1,115	0	30	0	1,145
Public health	4	1,582	33	1,619	0	96	0	1,715
Radiology	2,315	5,957	1,759	10,031	0	202	0	10,233
Subtotal	3,254	17,459	4,299	24,912	0	781	0	25,693
F. Unspecified/Other	67	5,313	8,204	13,584	13,395	668	1,306	28,953
II. Total	28,726	207,031	44,558	280,315	13,395	7,524	1,306	302,540

primary specialty. A review of these data reveal the specialties of internal medicine, general surgery, and obstetrics and gynecology to be the three largest in terms of numbers of specialists in group practice. Group physicians having completed specialty board examinations are listed in Table 1-6.[27] Internal medicine, surgery, and radiology comprise the three specialties having the greatest numbers of board certified practitioners in group practice. The majority of allied health personnel employed in group settings in 1969 were categorized as clerical employees. As table 1-7 indicates, the average number of allied health personnel per physician totals 2.51.[28]

Growth of Group Practice

From the late 1800s to the present there has been a steady increase in the number of practicing groups. Precise measurements of this growth are difficult to assemble due to the lack of a common definition of a medical group. Major surveys were conducted by the Public Health Service (PHS) in 1946 and in 1959, and by the AMA in 1965 and in 1969. It was estimated that the number of group practices had grown from two in 1890 to 150 by 1930.[29] The *Final Report of the Committee on the Costs of Medical Care*, published in 1932, projected the increase to a total of approximately 200.[30] Results of the first PHS survey indicated a growth to 368 multispecialty and general practice groups in 1946 and to 1,154 by the 1959 survey.[31] In 1965 an AMA study revealed an annual average percentage gain of 18.5 percent in the total number of groups between the years 1959 and 1965 to a total number of 4,289 groups. Data from both the 1969 and 1975 AMA surveys were adjusted to assist in drawing comparisons with previous surveys. These adjusted figures demonstrated an average annual increase of 9.5 percent in number of groups between the years 1965 and 1969 and growth to a total number of 7,733 group practices.[32] The 1975 AMA survey indicated a further decrease in the annual growth of the number of group practices to 3.9 percent for a total of 7,733 (adjusted) but a continued increase in the percentage of physicians practicing in groups. Table 1-8 summarizes the data for the years 1959 to 1975. Despite difficulties in measurement, there remains little doubt of the steady growth both in the total number of group practices and in the number of physicians practicing in group environments over the past eighty years.

According to a 1930 study, the existence of a group clinic in the eastern states was so rare that it was the exception. Despite its midwestern origin, group clinics are now diffused throughout all the states. Only two states in the AMA study of 1969 had fewer than ten groups each.[33] From recent 1975 data reflected in Table 1-9, the New England census division has the fewest total number of groups. The largest number of groups was located in the West North Central division.

Status of Accreditation of Clinics

Increasing pressure from consumers and government to ensure the delivery of quality services and to do so efficiently and economically has elevated the issue of quality control. In response to these needs, the American Group Practice Association (AGPA) formed the Accreditation Commission of AGPA in November 1968, thereby launching a program to accredit its member clinics. The express goals of this accreditation were to certify the delivery of excellent

Table 1-6. Physicians in Group (Nongroup) Practice Arranged by Specialty Boards

	Active							
Specialty Boards	*Group Practice*	*Nongroup Practice*	*Intern-Resident*	*Total*	*Inactive*	*Overseas*	*Address Unknown*	*Total*
Anesthesiology	1,216	2,379	15	3,610	48	43	4	3,705
Colon and Rectal Surgery	34	255	0	289	13	4	0	306
Dermatolgy	213	1,868	5	2,086	65	36	3	2,190
Internal Medicine	2,915	12,155	72	15,142	377	142	8	15,669
Neurological Surgery	226	860	3	1,089	14	18	2	1,123
Obstetrics and Gynecology	1,541	6,078	14	7,633	184	94	5	7,916
Ophthalmology	570	4,239	9	4,818	151	49	4	5,022
Orthopedic Surgery	1,038	3,069	4	4,111	65	49	2	4,227
Otolaryngology	512	3,146	10	3,668	244	32	2	3,946
Pathology	627	4,427	28	5,082	130	9	12	5,314
Pediatrics	1,575	7,312	228	9,115	235	155	20	9,525
Physical Medicine and Rehabilitation	23	403	2	428	11	11	1	451
Plastic Surgery	58	572	2	632	15	5	0	652
Preventive Medicine	28	1,502	14	1,544	200	87	9	1,840
Psychiatry and Neurology	440	7,070	13	7,523	248	59	18	7,848
Radiology	2,113	4,653	20	6,786	224	84	5	7,099
Surgery	2,165	10,895	170	13,230	245	291	20	13,786
Thoracic Surgery	280	1,413	10	1,703	17	41	1	1,762
Urology	500	2,207	3	2,710	120	32	3	2,865
Subtotal	16,074	74,503	622	91,199	2,606	1,322	119	95,246
Those having no board	13,046	134,919	43,947	191,912	10,871	6,249	1,189	210,221
Total	29,120	209,422	44,569	283,111	13,477	7,571	1,308	305,467

Table 1-7. Allied Health Personnel per Physician in Group Practice

Type of Group	*Total (N= 102, 126)*	*Reg-istered Nurses*	*Licensed Practical Nurses and Nurse's Aides*	*Lab-oratory and X-ray Techni-cians*	*Clerical*	*Other*
All groups	2.51	.40	.31	.52	.95	.33
Single specialty	2.26	.31	.15	.60	.92	.28
General practice	2.78	.52	.57	.40	1.07	.22
Multispecialty	2.73	.46	.44	.45	.95	.43

Table 1-8. Group Practice Growth, 1959-1975

	1959	*1965*	*1969**	*1975**
Total Number of Groups	1,546	4,289	6,162	7,733
Total Number of Physicians	13,009	28,381	38,834	59,809
Percentage of Physicians Practicing in Groups	8.0	15.6	17.6	18.5

*Data is as adjusted by the AMA to provide comparable information.

health care; to ensure that the clinic is maximizing the possible benefits of group practice; to ensure that the clinic is delivering health care with cost effectiveness; and to identify substandard practices and assist in their upgrading. The AGPA Commission has recently been replaced by the Accreditation Council for Ambulatory Health Care, which was formed as part of the Joint Commission on the Accreditation of Hospitals. The founding organizations of the new council are the American Group Practice Association, the American Hospital Association, the American Medical Association, the Group Health Association of America, Inc., and the Medical Group Management Association.

FUTURE TRENDS IN GROUP PRACTICE

Events of the past century have contributed to major changes in the health care system of the United States. The practice of medicine has relied increasingly upon a scientific base, and the sole practitioner has found himself surrounded by a variety of formal and informal associations of interdependent practitioners. Specialization in medicine brought with it an inherent need to refer and to consult. Institutions have replaced homes and offices as hubs of medical activity, and improved lines of communication and transportation have rendered these institutions more accessible. The education of health care providers has changed and new types of providers are being relied upon to assist the physicians. Innovative organizational systems have been developed to meet local health needs, and the financing of health care has changed from self-financing to support by agencies such as employers and government. Gradually the federal government has become involved in the health affairs of the nation, thus moving from

Table 1-9. Number of Groups by Census Division, 1946-1975

	1946	*1959*	*1965*	*1969 (Actual)*	*1969 (Adjusted)*	*1975 (Actual)*	*1975 (Adjusted)*	*Average Annual Rate of Growth 1946-1975 (%)*
Total	368	1,546	4,289	6,371	6,162	8,483	7,733	11.1
New England	8	24	148	249	241	476	445	14.9
Middle Atlantic	17	81	412	690	665	1,064	974	15.0
South Atlantic	21	182	542	892	869	1,277	1,211	15.0
East North Central	75	254	848	1,190	1,140	1,613	1,315	10.4
East South Central	19	98	258	406	398	507	481	11.8
West North Central	87	359	585	792	774	930	884	6.3
West South Central	57	234	511	703	689	755	719	9.1
Moutain	40	113	241	358	348	481	435	8.6
Pacific	44	201	740	1,077	1,027	1,358	1,255	12.2
Possessions	0	0	4	14	11	22	14	13.3

Source: Center for Health Services Research and Development, American Medical Association, Chicago, Ill. 1976 *Special tabulations*

private sponsorship and control toward public regulation. Future trends in group practice will be heavily influenced by such events.

Consumer Expectations

The knowledge explosion that has created sweeping changes in medical practice has affected the general population as well. The consumer of health services today is more aware, more enlightened, and more demanding. He views good health as a precious asset and considers it a basic right. Accordingly, consumers are demanding a voice in what services will be delivered and how. They want comprehensiveness as well as continuity in medical care while jealously guarding the personal relationship between patient and physician. The multispecialty group provides the framework in which to respond to these consumer needs. Groups in the future can anticipate greater involvement in community health and can expect consumer input into the planning of services. The formation of new groups will be required to accommodate an increased demand, and effective mechanisms for the assurance of quality control will become an even greater need.

Cost of Health Care

As specialization increases and technological sophistication expands, pressures for cost control will increase. Recent escalation of awards in malpractice suits and the ensuing rise in insurance premiums have added to the public's expenses for medical care. The mandate is cost control. Theoretically, the multispecialty group offers the environment within which this mandate may be answered. Modern equipment requires capital investment beyond the resources of most individual physicians; thus, the pooling and sharing of resources are effective cost control methods. By delegating appropriate tasks to allied health professionals, physician productivity and professional talent and time may be used more economically. Administrative costs generated by the necessity to comply with new governmental and insurance programs tax the capacity of providers to the maximum and result in increased expenditures for administrative activities. Improved management systems are within the capabilities of the group and have the potential of reducing administrative costs over the long term. Future groups can expect the development of practices designed to effectively reduce the expense of current malpractice litigation. Resolutions in this area will aid in reducing costs attributable to the practice of defensive medicine. In addition, hospitals with established facilities, equipment, and manpower will receive increased use as hospital-based groups seek ways to overcome capital investment costs.

Reimbursement Patterns

Future groups will possess an important advantage if they have the ability to provide required services and hence are able to negotiate with major purchasers of medical care. Consumers today are seeking ways to budget for health care expenditures. The private health insurance industry, prepayment, and government plans gradually are increasing their coverages to include more comprehensive benefits. Future groups can expect that a substantial portion of a patient's medical bill will be covered by insurance programs or prepaid plans. Groups can look for heightened interest in the prepaid mode of group practice stimulated in large part by HMO legislation. Eventual passage of a national health insurance law most certainly will influence future group operations through marked increase in demand for services along with associated administrative burdens. One study of national health insurance implications forecasts up to a 75 percent increase in outpatient services under a full coverage bill and states that unless the final bill contains a realistic deductible provision the demand for outpatient services will far exceed the capacity of the current health care system.[34] Future groups also can anticipate greater involvement of all third-party payors in the planning, organizing, and controlling of their purchased services. Group practice will continue to flourish as long as the primary objective remains the delivery of high quality medical services.[35] The need for a text such as this is testimony to the fact that group practice has evolved into a viable organizational structure for dealing with the complexities of modern health care.

Chapter 2

Considerations for Medical Group Formation

RATIONALE FOR GROUP PRACTICE

With increasing acceptance by medical societies, government, and consumers, medical group practice as a mechanism for health care delivery is more popular than ever before. The discussion of events and factors contributing to its growth (Chapter 1) provided the reader with a clearer understanding of the organizational concept of group practice. The factors attracting physicians to such practices will be examined in the following presentation, but first it is necessary to make some assumptions about physicians as people.

Physicians have long been considered to be dedicated, unselfish, self-sacrificing individuals. It is more realistic, however, to view today's physicians as no less dedicated but subject to the same personal, social, family, and economic pressures affecting other members of contemporary society. They too raise families, require vacations, pursue hobbies, send children to college, participate in community life, and enjoy leisure time. Physicians, as do other professionals, take pride in and appreciate recognition evidenced through advancement. Viewing physicians from this perspective makes it possible to examine some of the more salient factors attracting physicians toward group practice.

An optimum working environment is of significance to any professional. Important to the achievement of this optimum is the creation of opportunities for intellectual and professional stimulation which a group setting can effectively provide. Daily interaction with his professional peers and access to immediate consultation resources not only offer the intellectual challenges necessary for personal growth but result in better patient care. The immediate availability of knowledgeable colleagues greatly facilitates the confirmation of diagnoses and the prescription of appropriate treatment, and serves as a professional review system through which the physician may be subjected to peer scrutiny and constructive criticism. The consultation process within the group environment is not limited solely to physicians—other health professionals working in group settings can contribute toward shared group goals. Daily contact and personal communication between physicians and paramedical personnel can reduce the risk of error or delay and can enhance both the appropriateness and timeliness of the care.

In general, a group practice can offer a wider range of services than are available through a solo practitioner. Group practice physicians are able to take full advantage of specialization and, through referrals within their own group, can offer patients the best available care. Referrals can be accomplished with a degree of confidence not readily attainable in nongroup settings; because of personal knowledge of a colleague's capabilities, a group physician can be assured of the quality of patient care and follow-up without risking the loss of his patient to an outside physician. (See Chapter 13 for a full discussion of the internal and external referral process).

Although contributions to improving medical technology have advanced the science of medicine tremendously in recent years, the capital expenditures necessary for equipment acquisition often are prohibitive for individual practitioners. Group practice provides an opportunity for pooling the financial resources necessary to acquire late models of sophisticated equipment. Once acquired, such equipment may be expensive to operate, often requiring the services of specially trained ancillary personnel. Contracting professional services from allied health professionals also can be expensive, especially for an individual in single practice. Sharing in overhead expenses enables the group to provide allied health services in the interest of comprehensive care. Economic conditions necessitate the efficient utilization of both equipment and services.

In addition, third party financing of health care has added to the billing and administrative burdens plaguing providers today. The AMA survey of group practices in 1969 indicates that at that time one-third of the allied health workers in groups held clerical positions.[1] Today, as a result of computer technology, electronic data processing has rendered some clerical positions unnecessary. A survey conducted in 1970 by the Medical Group Management Association indicates that one-fourth of the smaller clinics and as many as 89 percent of the larger clinics in its Western Section use some form of electronic data processing.[2] Specialization also has infiltrated the business activities related to medical practice with the advent of specialists in insurance, medical records, government regulations, and bookkeeping. A group environment makes possible the sharing of operational and investment expenditures to the benefit of all parties concerned.

For many in solo practice, daily around-the-clock coverage for patients is a very real problem. The group environment facilitates preplanned scheduled recess from the practice and offers group physicians the opportunity to participate in more normal life styles. Through the rotation of on-call rosters and the establishment of time-off policies, the physician is much better able to plan his daily schedule, barring emergencies, and can be assured of freedom from call at regular intervals. The group physician can plan to attend meetings and to take vacations knowing this his group practice colleagues will be able to give attention to his patients, that his patients' records are accessible, that his patients will know to whom to turn in a time of crisis, and that he is not running the risk of losing patients or income. Physicians working in the group environment also are better able to fulfill desires directed toward attaining increased competence in specialized fields of medicine. Patients, in turn, will benefit from the resulting medical care provided by highly motivated and knowledgeable practitioners. In addition to pursuing areas of direct clinical interest, some physicians may wish to participate in research projects, to publish results of clinical investigations, to teach clinical medicine, or perhaps to assume roles of leadership within local medical societies. Personal goals such as these require a certain freedom from routine as well as a spirit of cooperation and encouragement among individuals with similar goals. Ongoing educational opportunities, such as in-service meetings or journal club sessions, are more easily attainable in a group environment; some groups allow for sabbatical leaves without loss of income in order that physicians can pursue post-graduate training.

The subject of physician productivity in a group setting often is a topic for debate and is the focus of those concerned with the total quantity of services provided. It has been estimated that a 4 percent increase in physician productivity would be the equivalent of graduating 11,200 more doctors and would make available presently needed physicians.[3] In a formal sense, productivity is the relationship of the quantity of input to its resultant output—that is, how many patient visits or services result from the number of hours a physician spends seeing patients. Theories that purport to explain alleged increased productivity in the group setting can be summarized as follows:[4]

1. Division of labor, or specialization, results in greater skill in a smaller range of tasks.
2. Acquired skills should be applied to appropriate tasks.
3. A large organization has the potential for more efficient equipment utilization.
4. In larger organizations, the chances of equipment and personnel being idle are reduced.

In general, physician productivity has been increasing. The National Advisory Commission on Health Manpower reports that between the years 1955 and 1965 physician productivity increased at an average annual rate of between 3.5 percent and 4.2 percent per year and that in order to fulfill projected needs it will be necessary to continue at such a rate in the future by using paramedical personnel to a greater degree, by expanding the scope of services provided under the direction and guidance of the physician, and by upgrading the quality of services, especially through increased specialization.[5] When productivity within the field of medicine is discussed, the impact of the quality of services provided is frequently overlooked by those responsible for the planning of more efficient operations. It would appear that public demands for total, comprehensive services that require physicians to manage 100 percent of the problems and public demands for 100 percent efficient care are sometimes incompatible. In a theoretical sense, however, a group practice offers the framework within which significant increases in productivity can be realized, both quantitatively and qualitatively. In a group setting, specialization among physicians and allied health professionals is fostered and delegation of responsibility appropriate to levels of competence is made easier through close working relationships. The organized pooling of resources, both human and material, creates an opportunity to capitalize upon more cost-effective delivery.

The business side of medical practice frequently is burdensome to many practitioners who may have little inclination toward or training in that aspect of medical practice. Such physicians may be attracted to group settings because there they can rely on outside experts to manage the nonmedical portion of the practice and can share with other physicians the associated overhead expenses of hiring them. The 1969 group survey by the AMA indicated that, of 6,233 respondents, 27 percent of the four-physician groups, 70.4 percent of the eight to fifteen-physician groups, and over 90 percent of all groups with more than fifteen physicians employed a manager.[6]

Most certainly, there are additional factors contributing to the rationale for practicing medicine in group settings. The opportunity for young physicians to join an established practice, to become immediately productive, and to enjoy the benefits of predictable income will motivate some. Income itself and the security of that income through periods of illness, disability, and retirement may be a reason for joining a particular group. The provision of insurance and the ready availability of organizational and emotional support in the event of malpractice litigation is yet another potential impetus for selecting the group practice environment.

In the final analysis, if group practice is to flourish as expected, the delivery of services in this setting must be beneficial to the patient; quality rather than quantity of care is more likely to be a criterion for group success. Within the group setting, especially within the multispecialty type, patients have direct access to one source for a full range of integrated and comprehensive services, including twenty-four hour coverage, emergency service in response to crisis situations, and shared coverage in the absence of a patient's primary physician. It is possible to facilitate the continuity of patient care even when the patient's original physician temporarily or permanently leaves the group. By maintaining a continuous medical history record permanently on file, the patient only need choose another primary physician from within the group. Referral from one physician to another within a group has been cited on occasion as a restriction of the patient's freedom to choose a physician. Within the multispecialty group environment, however, the patient has the advantage of knowing that the group physicians themselves have already made a responsible choice concerning the professionals who practice within the group and that the group is concerned with maintaining high professional standards of practice.[7] By virtue of being organized entities, therefore, groups offer ideal frameworks from which consumer participation and interests can be served. Proponents of the prepaid mode of group practice maintain that their members receive more appropriate treatment through lower utilization of unnecessary services. Subscribers to such plans are able to budget their medical care expenditures, resulting in a major advantage to many.

The various rationales presented here for medical group practice may be largely philosophical. Many of the advantages lack documented evidence and, where evidence does exist, certain advantages appear unrealized to the extent theoretically possible. Nevertheless, what evidence is available generally supports group practice as a form of medical care organization which is more advantageous than is solo practice in terms of accessibility, quality, continuity, and efficiency.[8]

PROFILE OF THE GROUP PRACTICE PHYSICIAN

An underlying motivational drive for most physicians is an inherent desire to aid their fellow men. A physician usually is people-oriented and people-interested and is able to appreciate the vast array of preventive, diagnostic, therapeutic, rehabilitative, and health education requirements of the population he serves and able to arrange for their delivery. The group practice physicians who have banded together to better serve their community endeavor to offer patients the best available care in a setting designed to reduce both costs and inconvenience to the patient. To work effectively within a group, the physician must be willing to subject himself and his work to the scrutiny and evaluation of his professional colleagues. As an educational mechanism, such a review reflects the group's overall concern for maintaining high standards of performance in the interest of its clientele. The willingness to be evaluated requires special maturity and an overriding conviction that the patient should receive the best treatment available. The physician who insists on absolute independence and on total freedom to carry on his professional practice in the manner he personally feels is best probably will not be happy or productive within a medical group environment.

Group practice implies a team effort toward a common, predetermined set of objectives and, in deference to the overall welfare of the group, necessitates certain sacrifices of the individual physician's personal goals. The physician's actions or his failure to act reflect not only upon himself but upon the group as a whole. The successful group physician is willing to integrate his personal goals with those of the medical group, to compromise in the best interests of the group, and to exercise tolerance when other group members' personal goals become issues for the group. He can ill-afford to adhere rigidly to preconceived personal opinions, but rather must adopt a more flexible posture when issues concerning the welfare of the group arise. The group physician accepts and respects the fact that other members have personal prejudices concerning the policies and direction of the group. Differences among members in age, levels of training, professional specialties, work ethics, political orientations, geographic origins, and family status are but a few of the myriad of factors influencing goal orientation. Group physicians who work well together are able to express their views openly, even though such views may be in opposition, without fear of being ostracized. These physicians are secure in the knowledge that others who do the same do so with the express intent of strengthening the group.

Certain professional and business decisions often must be reached by group consent. Within the group, especially the partnership, decision-making is viewed as a democratic process in which all aspects of an issue are raised and all individuals concerned are allowed to participate. After issues are raised and viewpoints are expressed, the will of the majority is exercised. Cooperative participation in decision making, respect for varying viewpoints and the individuals who raise them, and the resultant bonding of group members leads to a heightened commitment to the express goals of the group and to a strengthening of group resolve.[9] The group physician recognizes the importance of his participation and input to the group and consequently assigns a high priority to such participation.

In the area of group leadership, the group physician occupies a unique position. Depending upon the organizational structure of the particular group, a physician may be owner, employer, or employee. He may assume a combination of these roles, or he may assume all three at the same time. It is little wonder that during the conduct of the practice difficulties may arise as a result of role conflict. Whether by seniority, election, or rotation, clearly defined leadership within a group practice is absolutely essential for its continued growth. The group physician should accept this fact and be willing to assume his appropriate or designated role regardless of its level of visibility within the organization. A spirit of cooperative effort is necessary, for in many groups leadership roles change from time to time so that different individuals have the opportunity to direct the course of the group. Assuming this vantage point exposes the individual physician to a broadened perspective of group practice and ultimately can lead to sympathetic cooperation at all organizational levels. The ideal leader is *not* one who regards the group as merely an extension of himself. Anyone who assumes responsibility for leadership must be capable of directing without dominating, must encourage full discussion of issues, and must strive for consensus while maintaining a strong determination to attain the long-range goals of the group. An abrasive, opinionated, intolerant individual in a leadership position can cause irreparable damage to a group. Compatibility among members is directly related to the value system each physician brings with him into the group.[10] An individual physician's personal values and the importance he attaches to them in relation to the group's goals will determine whether the physician will be compatible with the group. The insightful group physician closely examines those factors he deems important to the practice of his profession, the goals and practice orientation of the group itself, and the values of his professional colleagues and subsequently elects to practice medicine in a setting conducive to fulfilling his own needs.

ROLE OF THE GROUP PRACTICE PHYSICIAN

Associated with membership in a group practice are a variety of roles and unique professional relationships which a physician may assume in his practice of medicine. Individual physicians involved in group practice are responsible not only to themselves for their actions; on the contrary, they are accountable to the group of which they are a part. The group physician has the responsibilities of regarding the objectives of the group as foremost in importance and of allowing such objectives to guide his actions at all times. Concern for professional competence, reputation, attitudes, and goodwill is implicit in the realization of the objectives of the organization. Group members are expected to assume roles of leadership or to participate in planning and policy meetings and committees when the affairs of the group are decided. Dedicated physicians in both solo and group practice pursue their profession within a strict set of ethical guidelines as established by local and national societies representing organized medicine. In this endeavor the group's professional stature, reputation, and liability are the responsibilities of each member.

A group's professional responsibility to the patient can never be of secondary priority. In the final analysis, the patient is the group physician's primary responsibility and is the *raison d'être* of the group. Physicians alert and responsive to the health needs of their clientele must remain responsible for professional competence and for the maintenance of a current knowledge of the field. Currently, health is viewed by consumers as a state of mind.[11] Preventive care, health education, and continuity of care from the acute stage to the home stage contribute to ameliorating this state of mind. Consequently, physicians are being held increasingly accountable for the public's health and are expected to adopt a broader approach to health care. The effecting of quality control through mechanisms for peer review and professional audit can serve to measure the quality of care delivered within the group. Group physicians can assume the responsibility for rendering such reviews and issuing constructive criticism on behalf of the patient and members of the group.

As a part of the health delivery system for an entire community, group physicians operate within a larger body of practitioners. While the group may have been formed to meet specific needs of a particular patient population, it is unlikely that a single group, especially in the early organizational stage, can provide for its total health care needs. Other groups and solo practitioners, as well as various medical facilities and agencies, have come into being to fulfill health needs within the community. A group physician, therefore, cannot isolate himself if he is to discharge effectively his patient care responsibilities. Group physicians must assess the resources and the capabilities of the group, identify outside sources that can provide any required services, and establish policies for both intragroup and extragroup referral of patients. They also must establish appropriate channels for interaction with extragroup providers. With the welfare of the patient foremost in mind, group physicians must maintain a close liaison with other local physicians to ensure that the group's patients are receiving an adequate standard of care. For such a system to be effective, group physicians must be responsive and responsible to outside sources who may choose to utilize the resources of the group in providing services. Group physicians should see that referred patients are afforded the best available care and that the referring physician is kept advised of his patient's status. Through such liaison and reciprocity mechanisms, group physicians offer a wider array of comprehensive services and are better able to discharge their responsibilities to the patient.

During the early years of group practice, group physicians were sometimes denied hospital privileges in an attempt by organized medical societies to thwart the development of this type of medical practice. Today, even non-hospital-based medical groups receive very little opposition in attaining hospital privileges. Group physicians must be able to rely upon ready access to inpatient facilities for many of their patients. Once privileged to use the hospital, the group physician incurs certain responsibilities to that hospital over and above those he maintains with his group. Most often these entail adherence to hospital rules and policy, contribution of time toward teaching, grand rounds or emergency room coverage, participation on hospital committees, and timely dictation of reports and medical record completion. He also is subject to participation in, and critique by, hospital board peer review and utilization review committees similar to those within his own medical group. The establishment of a sound professional rapport with local community hospitals does much to enhance the stature of the entire group in the eyes of community practitioners and is essential for the extension of services offered by those groups with no hospital facilities of their own. As members of a hospital staff, group physicians must discharge their hospital responsibilities diligently in order to avoid negligent practices resulting in adverse publicity for both the hospital and the medical group.

During the course of his practice, a group physician will have many contacts with the administrator of his group practice, if such an individual is employed by the group, as well as with the hospital administrator. In the case of the physician/group administrator, the relationship usually is one of employer to employee concerning matters of overall center operations, personnel policies, staffing, business affairs, or liaison with other health agencies. It has been said that group physicians should expect their manager to be proficient in personnel management, finance, credit and collections, accounting, law, and insurance—in that order of importance.[12] Daily contact is necessary for a smooth and efficiently managed practice. Obviously, no one set of guidelines can be adopted as the standard for such relations; situations, personalities, and philosophies are subject to great variance. In a general sense, this relationship is a mutually supportive one: each individual contributes in his own way to group goals; each exercises authority over predetermined areas of responsibility; each remains mindful and respectful of the unique contributions of the other; and each contributes input to group decisions.

Unless the physician becomes involved in active participation on hospital committees, group physician relations with the hospital administrator are more indirect. Daily contact for purposes of rendering management or policy decisions concerning hospital business operations is nonessential. When issues are raised between the group practice and the hospital, the group physician usually voices his opinions indirectly through the group administrator. Items of professional concern are, as a rule, channeled from the group physician to an appropriate hospital committee or to the chief of the medical staff of the hospital. This indirect relationship tends to exist even within those group practices that are hospital-based.

PROFILE OF THE GROUP PRACTICE ADMINISTRATOR

A great diversity in educational background, level of training, and managerial philosophy, as well as the size and mode of practice which he serves, make it difficult to develop a profile of the medical group administrator. The field of health care administration has become increasingly comprehensive to accommodate the financial and business needs of health care facilities, groups, and agencies. The medical group administrator, now an allied health professional in his own right, offers a special degree of competence for contributing to the growth and development of group practice. The orientation of professional health managers can be characterized as follows:

> He is problem-oriented. He seeks to take action rather than sit back and discuss academic problems. His mind is also policy-oriented, thinking ahead, thinking about the best way to meet future problems and events that arise. The managerial mind learns from experience. It is objective and realistic in decision making. It is committed to getting results.[13]

Medical group administrators possess a wide variety of credentials and experiences. Historically, the emergence of their roles paralleled those developed in hospital administration. At the beginning of the twentieth century, hospitals began to be concerned over financial matters and at this time hospital business managers gradually began to assume the role of hospital administrators. Previous administrators—physicians, nurses, and pharmacists—had been medically oriented. Today, however, training an administrator specifically in hospital administration is a predominant trend, although any given hospital has practicing executives who are the products of previous developmental phases. The profile of group practice administrators also is undergoing change. Initially, the business, financial, and managerial functions of the medical practice were handled by the physician(s). As group practices grew in size and complexity and the emphasis on quality professional care increased, physicians began to delegate managerial duties to others better trained to carry them out. Thus, during this second phase of development, with no formal academic preparatory program upon which to draw, group practice administration was assumed by individuals from a variety of academic disciplines. Administrators having backgrounds in accounting, bookkeeping, business administration, banking, nursing, pharmacy, office management, teaching, and occasionally hospital or other health care administration can be found filling the role of group practice administrators today. In smaller groups, managerial responsibilities are less complex and first line supervision as well as a high degree of technical competence in the business affairs of the practice are required of the administrator. In larger groups, the administrator's role changes from that of technical specialist to generalist. In these situations, the administrator's profile is one of a manager at an executive level, motivating others and relying upon them for expertise in specialized areas to accomplish the mission of the group. Over the years various titles have been attached to group practice administrators—clinic manager, business manager, or superintendent. As groups grew larger in size and their organization began to resemble corporate structures, titles such as director, administrative director, or executive director were attached to the administrative executive of the practice. Today, the descriptive title of group practice administrator is used universally.

Phase three in the evolution of the administrative profile is in its infancy. Graduate education in the specific field of group practice administration is almost nonexistent at present. The need to stimulate the development of academic programs leading to formal training and advanced degrees in group practice administration has been recognized by many as a first step toward the attainment of its full recognition as a health care profession. As a move in this direction, tutorial or preceptorship training of graduates in health care or hospital administration has been initiated in several of the larger group practices. The ultimate objective of a project sponsored by the Center for Research in Ambulatory Health Care Administration is the establishment of a preceptorship program for on-site orientation and training in group practice management. The trend is toward formal academic education for future group practice administrators and toward the establishment of continuing education programs to upgrade and maintain the skills of practicing administrators.

The administrator is the group's emissary to the community at large. Any profile of the group administrator should include his role as a representative of and spokesman for the group to a variety of individuals and agencies. As the group's representative, the administrator can keep abreast of the activities of the community as a whole through contacts with business, educational and consumer groups. The integration and coordination of health services available through the group to other health agencies is optimized through a close liaison between the group's administrator and the administrators of other health institutions and agencies. Such liaison serves to keep the group informed of current developments and provides a source of input for the group's position on health related issues. Representation in the planning of health services by new federally created planning agencies is another means of alerting the group to current trends and new health programs within its area. Negotiations with third party payors, consumer groups, labor representatives, and building contractors are additional responsibilities assumed by group administrators.

ROLE OF THE GROUP PRACTICE ADMINISTRATOR

For years it has been common for large health care institutions such as hospitals to employ an administrator to manage complex activities. The role of administrator has evolved from a necessity to meet changing needs. Early hospitals were formed under the auspices of the church and were managed by parish priests. As the growth of hospitals continued the task of administration gradually became the responsibility of the professional employees. Finally, as hospital financial affairs became more complex, the role of the manager trained in hospital administration emerged. Similarly, as group practices have grown in size and importance, a new role for the group practice administrator has evolved. Physicians working in the group environment and intent on practicing the medical skills for which they have been specifically trained often have looked toward an administrator to relieve them of the more burdensome and/or unfamiliar aspects of medical practice that interfere with the full-time pursuit of their art. Administrating a group practice is one of the most delicate and difficult occupations in the health care industry.

Both physicians and administrators should realize the precise reason for employing an administrator—to manage the nonmedical aspects of the group's business. To perform this task adequately and for the benefit of all group members, the administrator requires the same degree of freedom and latitude to operate as that required by the physicians in the discharge of their patient care responsibilities. The administrator should be regarded as a specialist in his own right and should be accorded commensurate authority. Physicians also must recognize the scope of the administrator's nonmedical responsibilities. Whereas a physician has one primary responsibility—the care of his patients—the administrator has a multitude of business responsibilities. An administrator may be involved in a variety of personnel actions affecting physicians and employees of the group, including recruitment, hiring, training, staffing, motivating, evaluating, supervising, firing, scheduling, and paying. He becomes occupied with advising and counseling and must zealously maintain a neutral posture with respect to all employees if he is to sustain credibility. The administrator is looked to for expertise in the management of the fiscal affairs of the group and is almost solely responsible for accounts receivable, billing, collections and related procedures. He must maintain current knowledge of tax law, third party payments, state and federal government regulations, and medical accounting and bookkeeping procedures, and he is responsible to the group for the acquisition, maintenance, storage, and security of supplies and medical equipment. He is the primary source to contact on matters related to the facility itself; adequate parking spaces, appropriate waiting rooms, traffic flow, cleanliness, maintenance, physician's offices, and the number of examination and treatment rooms are his responsibilities.

The administrator is charged with the management of all nonmedical activities and must plan, organize, direct, staff, and control these activities. Limitation by the group of his authority to carry out these functions can cause major difficulties.[14] With policy emanating from the physician directors and implementation delegated to the administrator, he must possess considerable diplomacy to carry out the desires of the group. This role often places the administrator in an awkward and defensive position. Physicians should recognize the value of endorsing the administrator's participation in long range planning and policy making, since his unique position affords him an excellent vantage point from which to monitor the organization's viability. His input into the formation of plans, policy, and procedures can prevent many unproductive decisions. In return for appropriate recognition and authority, an administrator is challenged to perform competently in managing the group's business affairs.

The group practice administrator has responsibilities and relationships to the medical director, the physicians, and the ancillary workers employed by the group. The role of the manager in the group setting is one of leadership, boundary mediation, systems regulation and innovation, and service.[15] As a leader, the administrator attempts to have all parties involved working together in a cooperative effort toward the common objectives of the group. As boundary mediator the administrator must arbitrate disputes between individuals or groups concerning issues and points of view. The roles of regulator and innovator are related to planning, coordinating, and scheduling so that professional employees can do what each does best and in the most efficient manner. Finally, the role of the manager is one of service and as administrator he is employed solely to ensure the successful delivery of medical service.

The group administrator often is responsible to the medical director for carrying out the latter's decisions on medical policy and procedure. Through the various mechanisms previously described, the administrator implements decisions and sees that they are carried out. The administrator reports to the director, identifying problems or potential problem areas, presenting solutions, and informing him of administrative activities.

Physician owners of a group practice, after formulating policy and procedural guidelines, become the major source of group revenue and recipients of the restraints they have initiated. Difficulties may develop when the employer policy setter breaks a policy that the employee administrator must enforce. Consequently, an administrator must be characterized by impartiality and must be concerned primarily with the long range welfare of the group. It is his responsibility to create an environment—facility, staff, and procedures—which allows the physicians to work productively.

The administrator is the coordinator of ancillary services on behalf of the physician employers. He is responsible for the recruitment, training, assignment, promotion, and dismissal of employees, and he must discharge these responsibilities equitably. In being alert to the needs of the employees, he is responsible for voicing their concerns before the governing body of the group. In the attempt to create a favorable work environment for ancillary as well as physician personnel, the administrator should utilize consistent management practices. He must be careful to avoid the tendency to become authoritarian in his work relationships with ancillary employees. His responsibilities are those of leading, mediating, regulating, innovating, and molding a variety of personalities and expertise into a united effort toward the realization of the group's common goals. The following chapter will examine how these goals are embodied in a statement of group mission.

Chapter 3

Establishment of Group Mission

ASSESSING MISSION IMPLICATIONS

Regardless of the basic operational mode selected by the founders of a group practice—be it free standing, hospital-based, or prepaid in combination with either—the group inevitably will adopt certain missions and, consciously or otherwise, will pursue some objectives while ignoring others. The mission or missions adopted by a group practice define its reason for being and have profound implications for the range of activities in which the group may engage, such as ownership and utilization of facilities, sharing of revenues and costs, and responsibility for patient care. In addition, the kind of physician best suited to membership in a particular group, in terms of both specialization and philosophy of medical practice, is dictated to a large degree by that group's mission. Missions adopted by a group also can determine how complex formal decision making mechanisms must be and what kinds of internal systems and controls are required. Finally, a group's missions can determine the ways it relates to its external environment, including the patient population, other health care providers, community groups, and government agencies.

Those setting out to establish a new group practice should be aware of the range of mission possibilities available and of the implications of each mission for the long-term operational and philosophical character of the group. By confronting these issues at the outset, the group can anticipate difficulties and build into the mission mechanisms for resolving them, or can revise the mission statement to avoid creating problems for the group's current and future members.

Missions typically fall within the four broad categories of personal convenience, practice economics, professional development, and medical service.

Each category contains a spectrum of mission possibilities; however, neither the missions within a category nor the categories themselves are mutually exclusive. A group practice may pursue several missions simultaneously or sequentially, and may assign priorities to any subset of missions. Established missions often change with time. In this chapter, several of the more common missions within each of these categories will be discussed and some of the more important internal and external considerations suggested by their adoption will be considered.

Personal Convenience

Although it is not often acknowledged, personal convenience is a purpose underlying many group practices. The life of the solo practitioner can be difficult, particularly if he practices in a medically isolated location or is in a medical specialty that imposes heavy and unpredictable demands upon his time. A frequently encountered rationale for the formation of a group practice is the opportunity which this kind of organization provides for patient coverage and for regularizing schedules and office hours. Patient coverage is an ever-present need in the traditional solo practice and the qualifications and capabilities of a particular back-up physician must be acceptable to the solo practitioner. In the group practice setting, physicians providing coverage for one another must be, at least on the professional level, mutually compatible. Patients dealing with a group tend to view the physicians within that group as being more interchangeable than physicians in solo practice. This attitude contributes to a greater need for making professional standards explicit. The larger the group, the greater the need.

Establishing a set of professional behavioral norms is more than a philosophical issue. The number of medical malpractice suits and the size of awards resulting from such suits have skyrocketed in recent years; so, also, has the cost of insurance premiums. As one seeks to limit exposure in this area it becomes critical to consider the qualifications and standards of conduct of current and prospective group members. In solo practice, a physician usually must be concerned with only his professional conduct. Working within a group setting, however, he may become liable for the actions of others.

This liability implies establishing a mechanism for screening and selecting member physicians. While it need not be formalized or rigid, there should be mutually understood criteria of professional competence. Similarly, if the conduct of a member physician jeopardizes the well-being of the patients, the group should have some procedure for terminating his membership. The conduct in question might relate directly to his professional performance or might affect indirectly his medical judgment or patients' confidence in the group. The necessity of consensus concerning decisions on terminating the membership of an individual physician highlights a larger issue in the group practice setting—the need for developing a sense of group cohesion that enables the membership to resolve differences concerning medical practice, ethics, and personal matters. Unless these problems can be dealt with amicably, experience has shown that they inevitably cause dissolution of the group.[1]

Another important consideration involved in a mission directed toward developing established hours through formalized coverage arrangements is the need for a system of scheduling patients and assigning them to individual group members. Patient appointments and scheduling always have been part of the practice of medicine, whatever its organizational form. Assigning or referring patients to individual members within a group poses special problems and requires careful planning so that each group member will be satisfied that he is being treated fairly, with respect both to the use of his time and to the appropriateness of particular patients to his areas of clinical interest. Chapter 13 includes a detailed discussion of patient appointments, scheduling, and referral systems.

When more than one group member treats a patient, a uniform medical records system, including a standard encounter or charge form, should be used to ensure continuity of care. A group of physicians housed in the same building or sharing a common business office, but having no mission involving shared responsibility for patient care, can continue effectively with each member using his own medical records system. Surprisingly, however, this arrangement exists even in groups whose missions go beyond the simple sharing of physical facilities. One of the most difficult issues on which to develop consensus appears to be medical record-keeping. Those contemplating the establishment of a group practice would do well to devote much thought early in the planning process to the development of a medical records system compatible with the needs of each of the group's members (see Chapter 14).

Another frequently encountered rationale for the establishment of a group practice is the acquisition of office space near resources required for the effective and efficient practice of medicine. Should the basic rationale for locating close to specific medical resources be the convenience of the physicians, the group should assess the appropriateness of that location to serving the patient population. The convenience of the physician and the convenience of the patient may conflict; however, in most instances involving locations close to support services, physicians' convenience is really synonymous with the provision of quality medical care. When a group practice is combined with a prepayment plan and it becomes necessary to sell enrollments to a defined population, the question of practice location becomes extremely important and patient convenience must be assessed. In addition, it must be determined if the capacity of these resources is sufficient to accommodate the current and future needs of the group.

The convenience rationale for group practice formation also may extend to educational resources. It is not uncommon for physicians who serve part-time as medical school faculty to form group practices located near the medical school or the teaching hospitals in which they practice. Locating the group practice close to the homes of the individual member physicians is yet another convenience factor, but it is important that the group review the appropriateness of such a location for serving the desired patient population.

Practice Economics

Many group practices are established under the assumption that the net operating incomes of the group's members will be increased through reduced costs and/or increased revenue. Group practice can facilitate the sharing of fixed cost resources and provide advantages of scale in the volume purchasing of equipment and supplies. Fixed cost items, such as exotic laboratory and diagnostic test equipment, can be shared by an entire group membership, thereby reducing effective cost on a per-member basis, and a group may generate a purchasing volume large enough to avail itself of a volume discount on both supplies and equipment. By reducing individual operating costs, the group practice should increase net operating income for the member physicians.

Financial benefits of this sort have an impact on the cost effectiveness of patient care. Increased net income can be reinvested to enhance professional development, reduce future costs, procure special or improved equipment, expand the physical plant, recruit staff, mount outreach or marketing programs, and reduce future fees or prepaid charges. Since each of these investments reflects an underlying mission of the group, and each investment decision has an impact on the financial returns of the group practice to its members, consensus is necessary before any action can be taken.

In adopting a predominantly economic mission, a group needs to feel comfortable with the underlying business rationale. To benefit fully from the cost reduction potential inherent in group practice, the members should be willing to engage in budgeting, productivity monitoring, and control processes.[2] Some physicians find such management techniques difficult to accept and regard them as intrusions on their professional conduct; however, if the group is to minimize costs by sharing fixed cost resources, it must determine on a regular basis whether each member is utilizing such resources at the appropriate rate, given the scale of that individual's practice. To do otherwise would be to admit that, although the stated goal of the group is to minimize costs to the benefit of all, the members of the group are not willing to ensure that the goal is achieved. Part of a willingness to accept management techniques appropriate to an economic mission is an initial recognition of the management function's value in a group practice. This is particularly important in group practices in which an individual is charged specifically with administrative responsibilities. Unless that person—be he one of the physicians or a professional administrator—is seen as more than simply a business office manager, the group may never achieve its cost containment or revenue realization potentials.

Group practices can achieve cost savings in other ways. One that has received a great deal of publicity recently is the use of paraprofessional or allied health personnel in routine medical services. Whereas the solo practitioner may be limited in this area by insufficient volume or supervisory capacity, the group practice frequently can employ nurse practitioners, physician's assistants, or other allied health professionals. If such personnel are to contribute to minimizing the overall cost of group practice operation, the group needs a program either for training or for hiring well-trained paraprofessionals, a program of supervision and monitoring after hiring, and perhaps most importantly, consensus on the use of paraprofessionals in the rendering of quality, economical medical care. It is essential, however, that the group be aware of possible constraints on cost reduction in the group practice setting. Several federal laws enacted in recent years—notably, those dealing with Fair Labor Practices, Equal Employment Opportunity and the Occupational Safety and Health Act—may limit the group's flexibility with respect to wage levels, hire/fire policies, and working conditions.

In addition to taking steps that yield cost savings, a group may expand the overall revenue base of the practice. If a proper mix of specialties is represented, the group can function as a self-contained referral system. Even if it relies heavily upon external referrals, as an organization in a position to negotiate contractual relationships with other providers, a group may expand a referral network or guarantee that a basic referral pattern is protected. In either case, the group seeks to enhance its referral capabilities beyond those of an individual physician. Further discussion on establishing a referral system can be found in Chapter 13.

Another revenue expansion possibility lies in the pooling of professional fees. In itself, the pooling of fees does not necessarily expand the total revenue available. Should the group be structured so that senior members are compensated more than junior members, however, expanding the base of junior members could increase the total compensation of those in senior positions beyond what they could otherwise generate on their own. The income to all members might be increased should the group decide to use paraprofessionals and thereby increase the capacity of the physicians to generate professional fee income. The pooling of fees requires the establishment of fee schedules so that each member of the group charges at levels agreed upon by all. A patient allocation system is needed so that no one physician is unfairly burdened with patients. To further ensure equality, the group may want to institute central billing and accounts receivable management systems and an income distribution plan.

A group practice can attempt to expand its revenue producing potential in ways beyond the generation of additional professional fees. For example, it may realize income from the lease of jointly owned facilities, such as space in excess of the group's needs, or group members may share in the proceeds from capital gains on the sale of physical resources which they own jointly.

Within the general mission of practice economics there may be objectives other than the expansion of net operating income. Often, physicians are concerned about stabilizing their income stream. The physician who becomes ill or goes on vacation may find that his income fluctuates widely during the course of the year if he derives the bulk of that income from service fees. In a group practice which pools the professional fees of its members, a physician is assured of greater income stability. Supplemental income generation offers additional stability to the base income of the group. Under a prepayment method of charging, in which the physicians are compensated on a capitation arrangement, the group usually finds that its income stream is more stable and more predictable—particularly after it has gained experience in marketing its services on a prepaid basis. Prepayment and its implications for the organization and delivery of health services are considered in more detail below when missions related to the provision of medical services are discussed. Suffice it to say here that to the extent prepayment is selected as a means of stabilizing an income stream, one must consider a variety of influences relating to the attractiveness of the services package, the accessibility of the group practice to the enrollee population, the potential effects of competing prepayment plans, and the impact of prevailing health insurance coverage and of federal and state legislation concerning Health Maintenance Organizations.

Professional Development

Many physicians consider the enhancement of their professional qualifications and capabilities a primary goal. The group practice setting can contribute to this process by providing a framework for a formal program of continuing education. At its simplest, this might involve establishing a good medical library. The group also might consider subsidizing trips by members to conferences, seminars, and scheduled programs of medical societies and other professional organizations. Because the group provides backup coverage, an individual is able to take part in such programs without concern that his patients will be neglected or that his income will be affected adversely. Some group practices may make it a condition of membership that each member satisfy recertification requirements in his specialty. For example, one group of primary care physicians recently required that all of its members take the family practice board examinations so that they would be certified in this new specialty. With an accelerating trend toward compulsory recertification in many specialty areas, many physicians need convenient means to participate in continuing education programs that better enable them to satisfy such requirements.

The recent Professional Standards Review Organization legislation is also likely to have a strong impact in this area. As PSROs evolve, the standards of professional performance that they promulgate may be incorporated in the content of continuing education programs. The group practice desiring to ensure that its overall performance falls within such guidelines may want to consider formal participation in these programs, or even the development of a program of its own. As continuing education activities move from simple subsidies for participation in outside programs to the actual development of programs, it will become increasingly necessary to budget time and costs and to assign responsibility for program development and scheduling.

The group mission of professional development can assume forms other than continuing education per se. One is active participation in teaching and research, particularly when a group is based at a teaching hospital. As the trend toward decentralized medical education increases and more and more community hospitals either provide residency rotations or become affiliated with medical schools, physicians in communities served by these hospitals find themselves attracted toward teaching. Thus, some group practices may be formed with a clear direction to enabling their members to engage in teaching and research.

In some cases, physician groups have provided educational opportunities within their own practices for allied health professionals, medical school undergraduates, and residents. This situation, however, usually is limited to fairly large groups which concentrate in a single medical specialty and have a patient population of requisite teaching value. Whatever the level of involvement group members wish to have, a commitment to the areas of teaching and research requires consideration of various issues, such as:

1. The development of a system for monitoring the proportion of each member's time devoted to patient care, teaching, and research.
2. The development of mutually agreed upon levels of effort in each of these areas, in order that other group goals are met.
3. The negotiation of faculty appointments and titles.
4. In the case of group practices involved in residency rotations and other training programs, the development of an internal consensus concerning the

presence of undergraduates and/or residents within the facility and their effect on patient attitudes.

5. The development of didactic and clinical experiences with educational value for those being trained.

The conduct of research requires the group to establish a regular process of grant seeking, monitoring, and control, a system of designating responsibility for the process, and a policy of internal review to guarantee that research projects undertaken are compatible with the professional interests of the group as a whole.

Group practice, by its very nature, affords yet another vehicle for professional development, the opportunity for regular peer contact and review. As in several other mission areas, intensity of effort in this area will vary. At a minimum, even in a group setting in which each physician has his own distinct set of patients, an atmosphere conducive to seeking out a colleague's advice should develop. This process of informal consultation can be refined into a peer review system. As interaction becomes more structured, however, the group requires more formalized systems involving the adoption of specific performance standards and sanctions. Medical group practices may need a committee or an individual to keep abreast of such standards and to translate them into decision rules or guidelines for the group. For example, groups having the most informal of peer consultation and review procedures need a uniform medical records system. Unless each member of the group can understand and interpret the decision making processes of the others, peer review will be ineffective. A group practice structured as a health maintenance organization or using a similar, multidisciplinary team approach to patient care, will find some form of peer review system even more important. In organizations marked by shared responsibility, it is often difficult to promote a sense of individual responsibility without a well-conceived system of individual performance standards and sanctions endorsed by the group.

Another aspect of the professional development mission relates to practice economics. To the extent that a group is in a financial position to utilize more advanced equipment and techniques, the group's overall practice of medicine will be upgraded. Thus, an appropriate mission for a group practice would be making access to more sophisticated hardware economically feasible for each member of the group. This mission will necessitate a decision making mechanism for determining equipment needs and a procedure for determining the extent of the financial investment required to procure such equipment. In addition, the amount of investment must be compared with the group's income objectives. After the equipment is in place, a system for allocating its use among the group members also is required.

Medical Service

The fourth major mission area concerns the establishment of medical group practices for purposes of upgrading or introducing specific medical services to a particular community. This mission, similar to the others, can take many forms and can be expressed in many ways. A frequently pursued medical service mission is the recruiting of needed medical manpower. The existence of a group practice in a community may attract other physicians to that community. Clearly, for the new physician arriving in town, the opportunity to join an established group and thereby step into an existing referral system has great appeal. A group practice, therefore, may become a valuable recruiting device for the community in acquiring physicians to practice in shortage specialties. The present members of the group practice or its founders, however, must agree on the growth objectives of the group, its eventual size in terms of numbers of physicians, and its eventual configuration in the range of specialties represented. Ultimately, total size will be determined by the size of the population that can be reasonably and effectively served and the general availability of physicians in the area. The group will want to give careful consideration to its recruiting efforts and will want to determine how much of an individual member's time should be spent on identifying potential new members and assessing their qualifications.

An appropriate budget for the recruiting program also must be developed. The availability of space and equipment should be taken into account when determining whether the group can accommodate additional members. The group may want to retain some flexibility here, and to this end may want to consider ownership of its facilities. The lease versus buy decision is treated in greater detail in Part IV.

The group may want to include a variety of incentives in its recruitment package—for example, some sort of income subsidy while the new physician is building his practice, or perhaps the assurance of housing in a desirable area. Another possibility is for the group to develop linkages between its medical service mission of attracting needed physicians to the community and a professional development mission of teaching residents on rotation. This relationship might result in a period of educational apprenticeship, perhaps in the form of a fellowship, for a physician who would then join the group either for a defined period of time or on a permanent basis. For any kind of physician recruitment strategy to be successful, it is important that the group have as complete an understanding as possible of the current distribution of medical specialties within the community and the region. In a very pragmatic sense, it is important to determine what the competition is, and to not overlook the fact that other communities also may be engaged in their own physician recruitment efforts. Knowing what they are doing may be critical to the success of the group's own program.

Another common medical service mission is the provision of a set of specific services to a given population. Implicit in a decision to pursue such a mission is the assumption that the services in question are in fact needed—an assumption that should be tested by analyzing the current availability of such services in the area, their cost, accessibility, and utilization by the population. The group also should consider the plans of other groups or institutions in the area to offer the same or similar services, and in determining whether the services contemplated actually can be introduced, should try to anticipate possible constraints imposed by existing and evolving regulatory legislation. In addition, the group should be aware of the relevant certificate of need and zoning laws that may apply in its jurisdiction.[3] Health Systems Agencies (HSAs) may play an important role in determining whether the facilities and services planned by the group unnecessarily duplicate other resources within the community. Depending upon whether the objective is to meet the needs of a specific target population on a comprehensive basis or, rather, to provide a limited range of services to as broad a group of consumers as possible, it will be necessary to determine the adequacy of the group practice's location, of the fees charged, and of the outreach mechanisms. It may be helpful to involve consumer organizations in the area as well as institutions such as hospitals and neighborhood health centers in the process of specifying community needs and, perhaps more importantly, in assisting the group in attaining patient utilization after the services are in operation.

A group practice can go beyond a simple medical service mission and can provide a total health plan as well as health services to a population. By providing a comprehensive set of medical services to a patient population on a prepaid basis, the group assumes a share in the medical risk of that population and, in effect, becomes a health maintenance organization. This further elaboration of a medical service mission is really a difference in kind rather than degree. Considerable literature is now available on areas that a group of physicians or any other potential sponsor of a health maintenance program should give careful attention to before embarking on a mission that anticipates both the financing as well as the delivery of medical care. Recent experience has revealed a very high failure rate for newly formed prepaid group practices, and the problems which they have encountered run a broad gamut from strictly managerial to environmental.[4] Despite the support which prepaid group practice is now receiving from the federal government, this style of practice traditionally has met with a great deal of resistance from state insurance commissioners as well as from medical societies throughout the country. Indeed, such resistance has been one of the major forces preventing the growth and establishment of prepaid group practice in many areas.[5]

Current health maintenance organization legislation and subsequent regulations and guidelines should be studied to determine whether the prospective prepaid group practice can qualify as an HMO and, by virtue of such qualification, can enjoy the benefits available to it by federal statute. Sponsors of the group should analyze carefully the prevailing health insurance coverage and financial capacity of the population to be served. They will need to develop written contractual arrangements with hospitals and other nongroup providers who will provide continuity of care and complement the group's services in such a way that a comprehensive program of health care—primary, secondary, and tertiary—can be made part of the service plan. Formal arrangements with appropriate private third party payors—such as Blue Cross and commercial insurance companies—with regard to the marketing of a health maintenance plan option also may be required. Similar agreements may be made with public payors, such as Medicare and Medicaid, as well as with major employers and unions.

All of the considerations discussed earlier in reference to a medical service mission within a group utilizing fee-for-service charging will apply in the prepaid setting. It will be necessary to analyze the availability and utilization of medical services in the area and to ascertain whether the proposed services are needed. In a sense, the group contemplating a prepaid comprehensive approach has an even greater obligation to engage in this kind of analysis. In most cases the group will be seeking to change existing medical care relationships within a population, not merely to supplement those existing relationships with services that either are not currently available or are not available in sufficient quantity or quality. An important part of the rationale behind the prepayment/comprehensive benefit concept is that by its nature this form of practice promotes health maintenance, and hence better quality health care. Higher quality care, however, may or may not result in actual practice; much depends upon the quality of care already being delivered, the morbidity and behavioral characteristics of the population, and the capabilities and performance of the group practice itself.

Regardless of its payment mechanism or range of services, therefore, a medical group practice that establishes as its mission the provision of high quality or better quality care, is setting for itself a goal that may be so difficult to define and measure that it is not likely to offer much in the way of tangible guidance to the group. For this reason, the foregoing mission possibilities have been stated at a somewhat lower level of abstraction. Each mission possibility contributes in its own way to a quality of care mission. Even the practice economics missions, given an enlightened reallocation of the net income resulting from enhanced revenue realization and/or cost reduction, can have a positive effect on the quality of medical care and the cost of that care to the patient population.

In figure 3-1, personal convenience, practice economics, professional development, and medical service are displayed as the four categories into which the more common missions fall. Each mission's implications for both internal operations and external relationships also are indicated. As the reader considers the adoption of a particular mission or set of missions, he may want to use this matrix along with the text to develop a better understanding of what each mission may entail.

Testing Missions for Internal Consistency

While any one mission may be well suited to the philosophy of the physician group and may be entirely feasible, certain combinations of missions may be unworkable, both at the philosophical and operational levels. Problems posed by some of the more obvious mission combinations concern potential inconsistencies. For example, a personal convenience mission as well as a practice economics mission may imply locating the group practice near particular medical resources. Should the same group also desire to pursue a medical service mission which requires that it be geographically accessible to a particular patient population, a conflict may develop. If perceived at the outset of the planning process—before major commitments are made and the cost of program revision becomes prohibitive—such conflicts need not be insoluble.

Typically, conflicts among missions manifest themselves in relation to certain basic characteristics of the group, such as:

1. The *number* of member physicians;
2. The range of *specialties* represented;
3. The *location* of medical care delivery points;
4. The total amount of physician *time* available;
5. The total amount of *money* available—both in the form of investment and operating income.

Considerations	Missions: Personal Convenience		Practice Economics		Professional Development				Medical Service		
	Est. Hours Coverage	Proxim. to Resources Residences	Increasing Net Oper. Income	Stabilizing Income Stream	Cont. Education	Teaching and Research	Peer Contact Review	Shared use of Advanced Equip.	Recruiting Medical Manpower	Providing Medical Services	Providing Prepaid Services
External											
1. Appropriateness of practice location for patient access		X									
2. Projection of service utilization and capacity requirements		X							X	X	
3. Review of plans of other groups and institutions		X								X	X
4. Legal and governmental controls and guidelines											
a. Service/Facilities – Comprehensive Health Planning – Certificate of Need – Zoning								X		X	
b. Professional Standards Review Organizations							X				
c. Prepayment – Health Maintenance Organizations – National Health Insurance – Medicare/Medicaid – Insurance commissions – Attorneys General											X
d. Personnel – Fair labor practices – Occupational Health and Safety Act – Equal employment opportunity			X	X							
5. Professional organizations											
a. Recertification trends					X						
b. Attitudes toward prepayment											X
6. Physician distribution in region									X		
7. Availability, utilization and cost of services in region										X	
8. Health status and morbidity characteristics of the population										X	
9. Prevailing health insurance coverage and financial capacity of population											X
10. Contractural arrangements with providers and payors			X	X					X		X

Considerations	Missions: Personal Convenience — Est. Hours Coverage	Personal Convenience — Proxim. to Resources Residences	Practice Economics — Increasing Net Oper. Income	Practice Economics — Stabilizing Income Stream	Professional Development — Cont. Education	Professional Development — Teaching and Research	Professional Development — Peer Contact Review	Professional Development — Shared use of Advanced Equip.	Medical Service — Recruiting Medical Manpower	Medical Service — Providing Medical Services	Medical Service — Providing Prepaid Services
Internal											
1. Screening and selecting member physicians	X								X		
2. Professional performance standards	X				X		X				X
3. Procedure for physician termination	X										
4. Patient scheduling	X										
5. Medical records systems	X						X				
6. Budgeting			X						X		
7. Productivity monitoring and control			X			X					
8. Recognition and strengthening of management function			X								
9. Hiring, training, supervision of allied health professionals			X								
10. Fee schedules				X							
11. Patient Allocation among members				X							
12. Billing and receivables management				X							
13. Income distribution plan				X							
14. Investment policies			X	X				X			
15. Curriculum development					X	X					
16. Research review process						X					
17. Equipment, manpower allocation among members								X			
18. Growth objectives									X		
19. Recruitment program design									X		
20. Buying vs. leasing equipment, space									X		

Figure 3–1 cont'd

To illustrate how these factors can become the focal point of a conflict between missions consider the following examples:

1. *Personal Convenience/Practice Economics:* The need to have multiple members in the same specialty in order to provide patient coverage may conflict with the need to have multiple specialties in order to establish an effective internal referral mechanism. Location of the practice dictated by an interest in having ready access to medical or other resources may not be consistent with what would be an optimal location for attracting patients under fee-for-service or for building enrollments under prepayment. Given a concern about the amount of time they must devote to the practice, the group's physicians may not be comfortable with the time commitments required to implement good internal cost control systems.
2. *Personal Convenience/Professional Development:* If there is a substantial allocation of physician time to formal programs of continuing education, teaching, and research, it may not be possible to provide adequate patient care coverage. Professional development activities may imply a practice location inconsistent with the personal convenience of the physician—near a medical school or a teaching hospital.
3. *Personal Convenience/Medical Service:* The medical service needs of the population within the group's service area may not be capable of supporting the number of physicians in a particular specialty that would be necessary to achieve the desired workload and, hence, level of personal convenience.
4. *Practice Economics/Professional Development:* The cost of participation in or development of programs in continuing education, teaching, or research, as well as the planning and on-going costs associated with a formalized peer review system, may be insupportable given the group's financial objectives.
5. *Practice Economics/Medical Service:* Potential demand for the medical services to be provided by the group may not generate sufficient revenue to satisfy the group's minimum financial requirements or sufficient utilization to produce the desired economies of scale. A mission to operate on a prepaid basis may necessitate the inclusion of services that cannot pay their own way and, therefore, contribute to unanticipated deficits.
6. *Professional Development/Medical Service:* The capacity, in terms of time availability, of the physician group to render care at a desired rate may be eroded by extensive involvement in professional development programs.

The attempt to resolve potential conflicts among missions is the essence of strategic planning. The group practice must be viewed as a system in which a change in any one component can cause change in others. The existence of Mission A, therefore, can make it difficult to pursue Mission B. Missions A and B must be translated into operational terms which are compatible with one another, so that it is possible to pursue both missions with a reasonable expectation that both can be achieved.

Translating Missions into Objectives and Strategies

The terms which enable the group to resolve apparent conflicts in missions which it intends to pursue are the objectives and strategies the group adopts in its everyday operations. Until they are expressed in terms of objectives that exist in the real world, missions will not receive a high degree of concerted effort toward their attainment. Objectives are *concrete* statements of what the group intends to accomplish in pursuit of a particular mission. They reflect what is possible given the particular set of circumstances facing the group at a particular time. Over the years, missions may remain constant, while the objectives set in support of these missions vary. For example, each of the various levels of effort that might be subsumed within a professional development mission could be expressed in terms of the following objectives:

1. A peer review committee will be established and will meet regularly.
2. Each member of the group will participate in approved continuing education programs.
3. Each member of the group will be board certified in family practice.

Each group will want to approach the establishment of objectives in its own way. Having at least tentatively adopted missions, the process of translating them into objectives should not be difficult. A useful discussion of this process is contained in *Self-Analysis Manual for Maternity and Infant Care Projects*, developed in part by Case Western Reserve University School of Medicine.[6] In this discussion a distinction is drawn between prime objectives, sub-objectives, and criteria. These are illustrated in table 3-1 in the form of a prime objective drawn from that text. This objective might fall within an overall medical service mission of providing comprehensive prepaid services to an enrollee population. Criteria—indices that are used to measure whether objectives are being achieved—are discussed in greater detail in Chapter 19.

Strategies

A strategy describes the way multiple objectives are balanced to create an internally consistent plan of action. Moreover, strategies take into account those external forces which could adversely affect accomplishment of the group's objectives. A plan that simply relates one objective to another in a closed system without regard to the characteristics of the population to be served and of other providers of care to that population is not strategic. It is vulnerable to environmental changes because it does not anticipate those changes. Assume that a group of physicians decides to start a group practice and that one of its major missions is the personal convenience of locating the group in a physician's office building near the community hospital. In thinking strategically about its medical service mission this group might consider the kinds of issues shown in table 3-2.[7] As a starting point, a primary mission orientation is adopted. In this case, it is locational. In another situation, the primary group mission may dictate a particular population, a set of services, or a financing mechanism (fee-for-service or prepaid). Even when it is unclear which mission, if any, is primary, it is useful to select one tentatively to begin the strategic planning process.

In this example, with the primary mission to establish the program in a certain location, the sequence of strategic issues is given as: *g, a, c, i, e*. The group must answer these questions:

Table 3–1. Examples of Objectives and Criteria

Prime Objective	*Subobjectives*	*Criteria*
To reach and enroll the greatest number of eligible patients that can be effectively served.	1. Outreach To establish and maintain contact with each patient within the clinic's catchment area who is eligible for our services.	a. Number of new residents who learned of clinic through clinic-initiated measures (data source: initial interview). b. Effectiveness of case finding activity by various referral sources (from referral services records). c. Ratio of total number of patients enrolled in clinic to estimated target-at-risk (from clinic records). d. No-show rate for initial registration and initial screening exam (from appointment records). e. Accessibility of clinic to population-at-risk (from geographic survey).
	2. Coverage To maximize the number of patient contacts the clinic provides within available resources (to include increased number of registrants and more timely reassessment of present patients).	a. Present clinic enrollment. b. Clinic patient load per day (quarterly average). c. Patients per physician ratio (using patients on the active rolls and number of equivalent full-time physicians). d. Number of months clinic is delinquent in providing appointments for routine screenings (from a sampling of patient records).

g. What population would most likely be drawn from this location?
a. What are the medical and support service needs of this population?
c. What financing mechanism would best fit the economic and behavioral characteristics of this population?
i. What services would be most appropriately supported by this financing mechanism?
e. What location would be most appropriate for the delivery of these services?

If the answer to question *i* does not agree with the answer to question *a* (that is, the services best supported by the most appropriate financing mechanism are not the same as those needed by the population), the group has uncovered an internal inconsistency that eventually could lead to problems in generating demand and must rethink the locational rationale that led to the need to service this population in the first place. Similarly, if the answer to question *e* (the location most appropriate for the delivery of the services) does not agree with the primary mission orientation as to location, the very basis of the mission must be reevaluated. For example, if the original orientation was to base the practice at a health center in the neighborhood, and if

Table 3-2. Sequence of Strategic Issues

	Primary Mission Orientation			
Strategic Issue	*Population*	*Services*	*Location*	*Financing*
a. What are the medical and support service needs of this population?	1		2	5
b. What is the most appropriate location for delivering services to this population?	2	5		
c. What financing mechanism would best fit the economic and behavioral characteristics of this population?	3			
d. What population would be most in need of these services?		1		
e. What location would be most appropriate for the delivery of these services?	5	2	5	3
f. What financing mechanism would best support these services?		3		
g. What population would most likely be drawn from this location?			1	4
h. What population would most likely use this financing mechanism?		4		1
i. What services would be most appropriately supported by this financing mechanism?	4		4	2

analysis indicates that X-ray therapy, available only at a hospital, is a significant service need of the neighborhood population, an inconsistency appears. Perhaps the problem can be overcome by introducing transportation capability, rather than by changing the location of the group itself. Without early strategic planning, this inconsistency might not emerge until later, when a less desirable option had to be chosen because of inadequate funds or other constraints. The development of a well-conceived, internally consistent strategy is a process of successive refinement. Regardless of the primary mission orientation (and it could be chosen arbitrarily), all of the group objectives must be considered and adjusted until they become mutually supportive.

The test of whether the group can achieve its objectives and fulfill its missions is performance. In order to anticipate that performance, the founders should develop a *detailed operating plan.* Such a plan will require the establishment of planning criteria, the selection of an appropriate legal organizational form and governance structure, the development of a financial plan and staff compensation program and, finally, the development of major operating policies. Each of these components of the planning process will be discussed in Part II.

Part II

Organizational Planning

Chapter 4

Establishment of Planning Criteria

OVERVIEW OF THE PLANNING PROCESS

The planning process is an attempt to establish indicators of successful performance before dollars and time are irretrievably committed. For medical group practice development, planning involves knowing when and if strategies are being carried out successfully, objectives met, and missions achieved. The purpose of this chapter is to discuss ways in which such indicators of success—that is, planning criteria—can be established. As noted earlier, a group practice may pursue a variety of missions not related directly to medical service. Still, the group's *medical service program* is its central activity, and this program must succeed before other missions can be pursued. Throughout this chapter the word "program" will refer strictly to the *medical service program* in order to distinguish that sphere of medical service from the professional development, practice economics, and personal convenience activities previously described. After group missions have been balanced and integrated, and after a sound medical service strategy has been developed, program planning can be initiated with the assurance that the group practice will fulfill its missions successfully, barring any insurmountable obstacles.

The planning process can be divided into three phases: demand, capacity, and cash flow. Each is concerned with the quantification and projection of performance against a set of planning criteria.[1] The group begins with forecasts of program utilization—the projected *demand* for services. Ordinarily, these forecasts are expressed as *encounters* or *patient contacts* per month. An encounter or patient contact may be self-initiated or scheduled by the group or its staff. It may involve personal contact with the staff and one of the groups' available services, or it may involve only telephone contact. For simplicity, in this book the term "encounter" will be used throughout to designate patient utilization of group services. Encounter forecasts are fundamental to the planning process because they are based on assumptions concerning the nature of the user population and its need for the group's services. On the basis of this forecast of monthly encounters the group is able to estimate the program's *capacity*. This process involves decisions regarding the scale of the facility, equipment, manpower, and other resource needs appropriate to the projected demand pattern.

Once the capacity requirements are determined, they can be converted into projections of *cash* disbursements, which in turn can be timed to the pattern of acquisition and retention of resources required to meet projected demands. Essentially, the projection of cash outflows is a quantification of needed funds. For the program to meet its financial obligations over the given time period, there must be cash inflow generally equal to the projected outflow, both in duration and magnitude. After the cash receipts forecast is netted against the disbursement forecast, there will likely be a cash deficit, which may be financed via grants, contributions, invested capital, or loans. If the group practice sponsors cannot agree on a means of financing the projected deficit, the plan must be modified.

The first step in modifying the plan is to adjust the cash flow analysis projections. If this adjustment does not improve the pattern of needed funds, the next step is to adjust the resource availability projections of the capacity analysis. If these adjustments are inadequate, then the encounter projections of the demand analysis must be modified. Changes in the level or timing of anticipated demand impinge on the underlying strategic assumptions about the existing need for and probable use of the program's services; consequently, a modification in the demand analysis amounts to a revision of the strategic plan itself, and inevitably jeopardizes the mission statement. In such a case, the group must return to the strategic planning process described in the preceding chapter. Figure 4-1 illustrates schematically the sequence of tasks in the overall planning process and their relationship to the three major phases: demand, capacity, and cash flow.

Planning is critically important and should not be the vague responsibility of a group or committee. Such bodies may be established to monitor the planning process, make strategic planning decisions, and review and contribute to the planning process results; but only one individual should have primary responsibility for producing the plan. Moreover, he should have enough money and time to produce as thoughtful and well-founded a plan as possible. Many group practices will not initially have planning capabilities, and so it may be necessary to contract for that expertise. Nevertheless, the forming group should have a basic understanding of the planning process to better communicate with the contracted planner. That basic understanding will help to establish an initial mission and identify those strategic planning decisions requiring the group's involvement.

Because so much depends on the availability and quality of data, it is difficult to specify an appropriate planning budget. In terms of time, however, an initial plan should be produced in a minimum of four and a maximum of six to nine months. In reality, planning is not a one-time exercise. Rather, it is a necessary, ongoing activity, important throughout the life of the group practice.

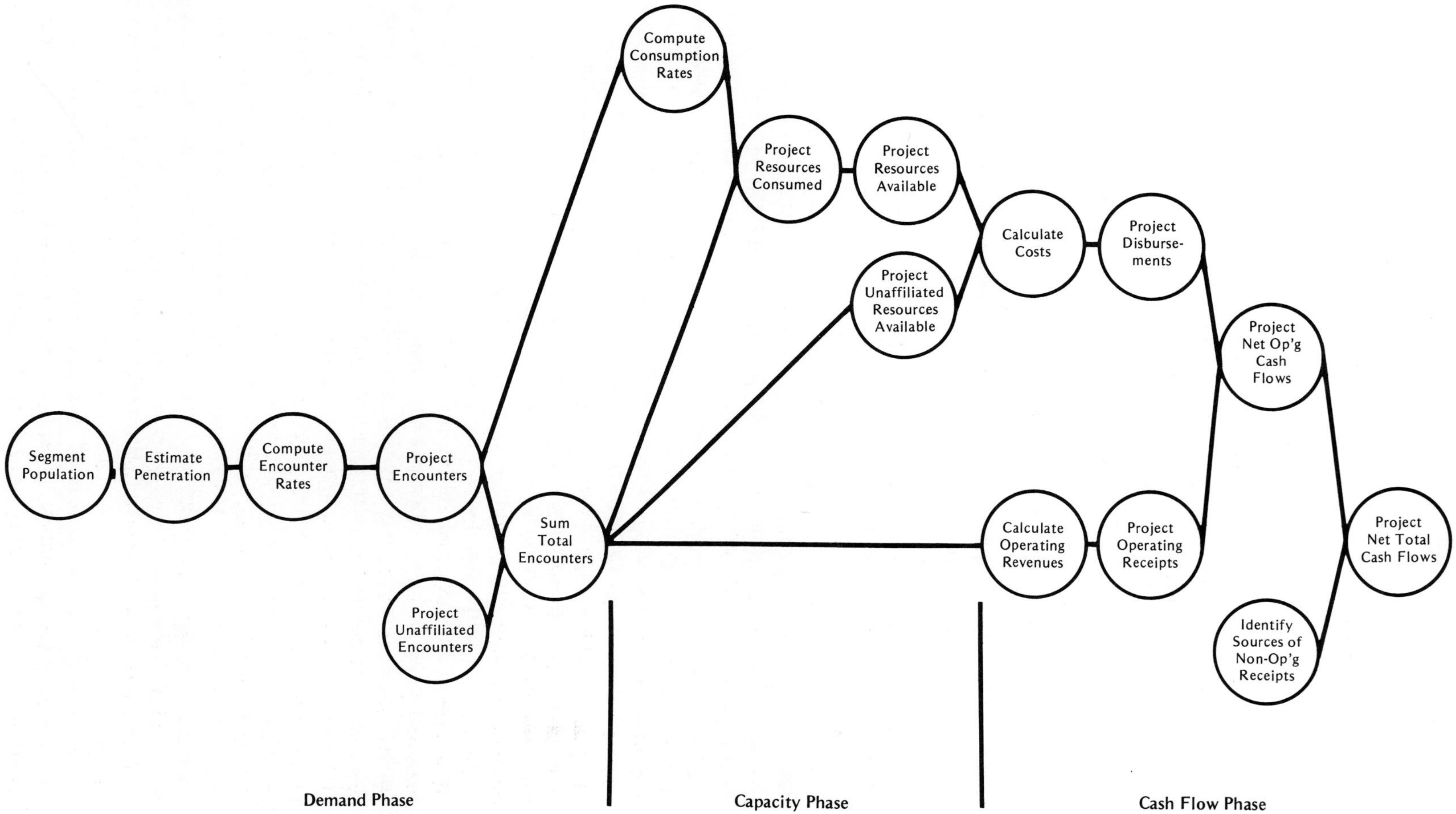

Figure 4-1. Planning Sequence

As internal and external factors change, there will be a need to assess the impact on missions, strategies, and program. The planning process provides the framework for such assessment.

DEMAND PHASE

The group cannot assume that there will be a demand for its particular services by the target population defined in the strategic plan; the extent of the plan must be quantified. Patient utilization may be defined as broadly as is appropriate to account for the range of services offered by the group. Then, the number and the timing of each relevant type of encounter must be anticipated for the foreseeable future. Consequently, the need for physical, manpower, and financial resources over the planning period may be better assessed. Indeed, the pattern of projected costs and revenues emerges from these utilization assumptions. Depending upon whether or not these patterns are acceptable, the assumptions and/or the marketing policies intended to stimulate utilization may be revised.

Segmenting the Population

There is a practical need to divide potential users into discrete segments; it is easier to plan for fairly uniform populations than for diverse masses or individuals. Segmentation is also of considerable strategic value. It is, in fact, essential for the program designed to deliver medical care on a prepaid basis to all or some of its users (that is, to underwrite as well as provide care). Implicit in segmentation is an awareness of those medical, socioeconomic, demographic, and/or behavioral characteristics which distinguish one segment from another and which may influence utilization patterns. Without such an awareness, no marketing strategy can be effective.

Even for the program not intended to operate on a prepaid basis, the identification of population segments can have a significant value beyond simplifying the planning task. A program whose mission is to ameliorate the health condition of a particular population group (the aged, the ghetto resident, etc.) must develop the same familiarity with that group's salient characteristics as that required of the program selling a form of insurance along with the delivery of medical care. But regardless of the financing mechanism, there will be identifiable population segments with certain characteristics in common that enable the group to consider their aggregate utilization of the program. Key issues are whether the individuals in a given population segment have similar needs for services, and whether they are likely to respond to the program's or some other party's efforts to translate those needs into a fairly predictable utilization pattern. The "other party" may be an employer, union, professional organization, educational institution, school system, or any other body with which members of that segment are associated. The segments that will be most appropriate for one program may be entirely irrelevant for another. It is important to remember that the goal of segmentation is to improve planning, not to establish different classes of patient care. The following are possible bases for the segmentation of a target population; obviously, they can be combined in various ways:

1. age, sex, or other demographic variables;
2. employer or union affiliation;
3. residence within particular census tracts or housing projects;
4. third party payor representation, such as Blue Cross/Blue Shield, commercial insurance, Medicare, or Medicaid; and
5. ethnic, racial, or language characteristics.

Estimating Penetration

Once the population segments are defined, the degree to which each will be "penetrated" by the program should be determined. Penetration means how many persons out of the total number in each segment are likely to use the program at least once during the planning period. Numerous factors may influence the extent of penetration within segments:

1. medical risk profile;
2. perception of need for program services;
3. awareness of the availability of program services;
4. predisposition to utilize the services after becoming aware of them;
5. range of benefits reimbursed by prevailing insurance coverage;
6. accessibility of the program's facilities both in terms of geographic and transportation convenience;
7. current patterns of utilization of other facilities for receipt of services which are the same as those being offered by the program; and
8. degree of satisfaction with care received in other facilities.

Any or all of these factors may be important in determining how many persons in a particular segment will use the program, either by enrolling, registering, or simply walking in. The group will need to gather information on these factors for each segment, and information sources will vary with the segment definition. If it is an employee group, census data and any available utilization records of other community institutions may be analyzed. One group successfully surveyed its target population through a detailed analysis of nearby hospitals' emergency ward records. The records were sorted by census tract to select those who lived within the defined target area, and then by family membership, using last names and addresses. The record of visits for each family was analyzed by number. Those making more than one or two visits to an emergency ward were assumed to be using it for primary care and were considered potential users of the new program.

Computing Encounter Rates

The next step in planning is to estimate the number of encounters to be generated by each segment, using the anticipated penetration level. This can be expressed in terms of encounter rates, or the number of encounters per 1,000, or some other convenient base number of potential users. Consider the following example:

Total population of segment 10,000
Penetration % estimate 75%

Total number of users 7,500
Average encounters per user 6.0
Total patient contacts 45,000
Encounter rate per 1,000 users 6,000

Regardless of whether the total number of encounters in a segment is estimated as an average number per week or as an absolute number per some base aggregation of users, that total should incorporate the notion of repeat as well as first-time encounters. For example, 300 pediatric visits per 1,000 may represent 150 first time and 150 repeat visits. The same rate could represent 250 first time visits and only 50 repeat visits. Estimates must be as precise as possible because all subsequent planning will hinge upon them.

A determination of the types of encounter appropriate in classifying program utilization by the members of each population segment is largely discretionary. Usually such determination depends upon the types of services available by the program. Each type of encounter should have either a distinct *pattern* or a significantly different *level* of resource utilization. There have been various attempts to quantify, in terms of relative value, the degree of effort involved in different types of physician office visits. One such attempt is the Identifiable Medical Procedure (IMP) system. The number of IMP units assigned an office visit is a function of the training and type of personnel providing the service, as well as the health status of the patient. Table 4-1 is a list of major types of ambulatory medical procedures as defined by the IMP and indexed according to the California Relative Value Schedule (CRVS).[2] These particular values were generated in specific settings at specific times. Nevertheless, for planning purposes the list does serve as a useful starting point in categorizing types of encounter.

In addition to physician's office visits, the group may want to distinguish among other categories of nonphysician encounters, such as psychiatric counseling, family planning counseling, and drug rehabilitation. For most types of encounter, the group will be able to base rate estimates on the experience of other programs or institutions in the same geographic area. Such data can be obtained either directly from their administrators, indirectly from the applicable Health Systems Agencies, or from third party payors such as Blue Cross/Blue Shield, Medicare, Medicaid, state welfare, and commercial carriers.

Projecting Encounters

At this point, the group has estimated total numbers of encounters to be generated from each segment. Now these encounters must be extended over the planning period. Scheduling is possible for some types of encounters, such as registration visits and new patient physical examinations. For others, however, such as emergency minor surgery, scheduling is not possible and occurrence is a function of the overall medical risk of the population. For this type of visit, the group must rely on estimates based primarily on the experience of other institutions and programs serving the population segment and, if necessary, on the general experience of a population in other settings. A reasonable sequence of steps involves first projecting the monthly encounters that cannot be scheduled by the program. Then, based on the resulting pattern of demand

Table 4-1. Possible Ambulatory Encounter Types

Type of Encounter	*CRVS Unit Rating*
Physical examination, adult, presenting illness	3.5
Nonroutine radiologic test	3.4
Other diagnostic test	3.2
Physical examination, child, presenting illness	3.2
Physical examination, adult, no presenting illness	3.0
Serious accidental injury	3.0
Minor surgery	3.0
Physical examination, child, no presenting illness	2.9
Specialist consulation	2.8
Home visit	2.5
Routine radiologic test	2.4
Complex laboratory test	1.8
Acute or chronic condition, initial visit	1.8
Mild accidental injury, follow-up visit	1.8
Minor surgery, follow-up visit	1.7
Mild accidental injury, initial visit	1.6
Acute or chronic condition, follow-up visit	1.4
Therapeutic service	1.0
Simple laboratory test	0.8
Telephone call	0.5
Administration of allergy antigen	0.15
Nurse visit	0.1
Administration of injection or immunization	0.07

that cannot be controlled, the group can distribute the encounters that lend themselves to scheduling or to other forms of program control.

An example of this strategy is the purposeful delay of marketing or outreach activity toward a particular population segment until a certain time after the program has commenced. After marketing has begun, one would anticipate that the bulk of new enrollments, registrations, and walk-ins from that segment would occur. The program then can exert yet another form of control. For new enrollees or registrants, the date of their first visit (which usually consists of a medical and personal history interview and, perhaps, a complete physical examination) can be set, thus contributing to a smooth rate of growth in utilization. In projecting the monthly encounters by type and segment, the group should watch for ways of distributing utilization growth and should try to avoid subjecting the program to a peak utilization load in the early months, followed by a precipitous drop-off thereafter.

The consequences of this whip-saw pattern can be disastrous. Initially, a far larger staff and facility may be needed than are either available or can be justified on the basis of continuing cash inflow (either from external sources or from enrollment/fee-for-service revenues). Unless standby resources of external funds, manpower, and equipment are available, the group may be faced with some agonizing choices. It may elect to service the peak load inadequately, with perhaps irreversible damage to its reputation. It may choose to assume an inordinately high startup deficit which, if it can be financed at all, may be at an intolerably high cost. Finally, it may be obliged simply to turn potential users away after they had been led to believe they could be served. Then, after the peak period has passed, the group may be forced to reduce staff, thus causing both organizational and community problems, particularly the latter if significant numbers of persons from the community had been hired to provide support services. Any resulting excess of capacity in facilities may not be reduced easily. Costs may have to be borne by the program, thus increasing the deficit, need for, and cost of external financing. If those costs are passed on to the program users in the form of higher fees or prepayment charges, future growth in demand will obviously be affected adversely.

Projecting Unaffiliated Encounters

Generally, even a program specifically directed toward developing encounters within well-defined segments can expect a certain number of unaffiliated encounters. Such encounters may be generated by persons who are enrollees, registrants, or walk-ins, but it is their unaffiliated nature that is consequential. They cannot be forecast with the same insight as encounters derived from segments with readily definable characteristics—medical, demographic, and behavioral. For unaffiliated encounters, the group often will have to rely on the best estimates available. One simple technique for making such estimates is to draw on a map a series of concentric circles around the program facility's location. It may be assumed that census tracts within the innermost circles will yield the greatest number of encounters, both segmentable and unaffiliated. This assumption, of course, must take into account known characteristics of the transportation system (cost, convenience, route structure, and trip time) and of geographical barriers that may reduce accessibility.

Summing Total Encounters

The final step in the demand phase is to combine projections of encounters derived from the various population segments with those of unaffiliated encounters. The result is a month by month "snapshot" of anticipated program utilization by type of encounter for the period under consideration. This projection is the foundation of all that follows. It is based upon a specific concept of the population to be served (as expressed in the definition of types of encounters, and of the marketing program to be employed (as expressed in the penetration levels and time phasing of encounters). Thus, the projection is both a tangible description and a test of the validity of the program's strategic design.

CAPACITY PHASE

In the capacity phase, the group must determine the program's requirements in order to handle the volume and pattern of encounters projected. The size of the physical plant, the number of staff members and their skills, the amounts and types of equipment and supplies, the scale of administrative staff, and other elements of overhead must be determined. In short, the group must establish the capacity of the program in terms of the physical and human resources that must be committed to service the projected demand. Additionally, the extent to which marketing efforts are envisioned and the resources that must be committed to stimulate the projected demand must be determined.

Computing Consumption Rates

A set of *resources* can be defined and related to encounter types through the use of *consumption rates*, much as a set of encounter *types* is defined and then related to population segments through the use of *encounter rates*. For each type of encounter identified, the group should ask what *resources* will be consumed and in what quantity for one encounter. Each question will be answered in turn.

Resources. Each type of encounter will require a certain constellation of staff, facilities, equipment, and supplies. It is the task of the group to describe, in whatever detail is convenient and meaningful, the set of resources required for each type of encounter. Resources may be categorized at a general level, even if the encounter type itself is specific. For example, a laboratory test visit could be viewed as consuming a certain amount of staff resources with no differentiation by staff type. The eventual goal of this analysis is the development of cost and cash outflow forecasts; specific definition of resources will make those forecasts much more accurate. It is also true, however, that the forecasts can be developed on the basis of aggregate resource definitions, and in some cases the group may find that more detailed estimates are only rough guesses, lending the semblance but not the substance of increased accuracy.

The group does have some flexibility in determining just how specifically resources will be described and in the degree of encounter-relatedness that can be imputed to them. In the final analysis, all program resources can be allocated to encounters, but not all should be. The purpose of this exercise in capacity planning is to derive a sense of the scale of resource need from an estimate of demand. Consequently, only those resources that can be related meaningfully to some type of encounter should be identified. Figure 4-2 presents a list of resources defined at a specificity level that should serve most planning purposes.[3] Of course, the group may break down these resources to an even more detailed level. Also indicated are which resources will have to be forecast frequently on an unaffiliated basis and which can be related to encounters.

Quantity. In order to quantify the amount of each encounter-related resource consumed by an average encounter, the group must identify first a unit of consumption for each resource, and, second, the number of such units to be consumed. As a rule, personnel resources are estimated most easily by the number of man-hours consumed. Machine hours is a convenient unit of consumption for many types of fixed equipment, and the square foot of floor space is a convenient unit for estimating building space consumption. For supplies, the unit of consumption may be either one item of a particular type or perhaps a minimum order lot size such as a dozen. The most appropriate unit of consumption for a particular resource usually will be self-evident. The consumption rate itself is similar to the encounter rate discussed earlier; that is, it can be developed either as the number of units consumed per encounter or per 100, 1,000, or some other base aggregation of encounters. If developed the latter way, the rate should be restated on a per encounter basis.

PERSONNEL
- Physicians and Dentists
- Psychologists and Other Independent Professionals
- Nurses (PHN, RN and LPN)
- Dental Hygienists and Other Formally Trained Technicians
- Paramedical and Outreach Personnel*
- Administrative, Clerical, and All Other*

OUTSIDE SERVICES*
- Consultants – In Program
- Consultants – Outside Program
- Contractual Services – In Program
- Contractual Services – Outside Program
- Data Processing

TRAVEL*
- Local Travel
- Out-of-town Travel

SPACE AND RENTALS
- Rental of Space
- Utilities*
- Other*

CONSUMABLE SUPPLIES

EQUIPMENT
- Buildings and Fixed Equipment
- Office Furniture
- Vehicles*
- Other Equipment
- Rental of Equipment

OTHER*
- Insurance and Bonding
- Publications, Printing, and Subscriptions
- Repairs and Other Services
- Overhead
- Telephone, Telegraph, and Postage

EMPLOYEE BENEFITS*
- FICA Employer's Share
- Insurance
- Retirement Plan Contributions
- Hospitalization
- Other

*Probable "unaffiliated" resources.

Figure 4–2. Possible Resource Categories

Projecting Resources Consumed and Resources Available

Resource consumption rates will yield a monthly forecast of consumption when they are applied to the forecasts of encounter by type, which resulted from earlier calculations of demand. Because the ultimate goal is to estimate the cash flow implications of these resource requirements, the pattern of resource units consumed must be translated into a pattern of dollars spent. For most resources, however, it is not sufficient to measure consumption alone; availability must be measured as well, for it will indicate the scale of resource acquisition, and it is the acquisition pattern that determines the cash flow.

Resources are typically acquired in increments larger than a single unit. The group must decide whether underutilization calls for a reduction in capacity through the *elimination* of an entire increment of resource, or whether over-utilization calls for an increase in capacity through the *addition* of an entire increment. Such decisions are not always easy. A premature reduction in capacity may hamper the program's ability to service higher utilization levels in the future. On the other hand, a premature increase in capacity may impose excessive operating costs if the anticipated levels of higher utilization do not materialize. Fortunately, options are available which will permit the delay in capacity reduction or addition until such time as utilization trends become established. For example, personnel can be hired part time or can work overtime; facilities can be rented on a monthly basis; equipment can be shared with other institutions; excess floor space can be leased out to other tenants; marketing efforts can be scaled up or down. Because the group must consider such basic issues as operating hours, staff recruitment efforts, size of recruitable manpower pool, and the existence of other community facilities to be shared, the translation of consumption into availability—in short, capacity planning—is a highly critical exercise. It is as important to the overall planning process as the forecast of demand on which it is based. In forecasting demand through the projection of encounters, the planner incorporated assumptions about the nature of the population to be served and the effectiveness of the program in generating utilization. In the same way, he must take into account external factors in forecasting capacity. He must develop explicit assumptions about the nature of the labor force and the facilities pool available to the program. Moreover, he must evaluate the effectiveness of the program in acquiring labor to serve the user population.

Projecting Unaffiliated Resources Available

At times, somewhat arbitrary allocation formulae must be applied to resources indirectly related to service during specific types of encounters. Obviously, the program could not function without heat, light, and power resources. It is possible to allocate units of consumption for these resources, for various types of encounters in proportion to the square footage of floor space used during those encounters. This allocation process is clearly a tedious one and finally not very useful, inasmuch as the same total number of resource units is likely to be consumed whether or not the encounters occur. Resource consumption is determined largely by the overall established scale of the facility, not by that facility's actual utilization. In a sense, these unaffiliated (or program-related) resources indirectly reflect utilization in that the scale of the facility is itself based upon some projected level of demand. Such resources and administrative, clerical, and outreach personnel are even more difficult to relate to encounters, for they too exist to support the program.

The most straightforward approach to forecasting the program's unaffiliated resource capacity is to time the introduction of such resources in increments appropriate to the overall level of program utilization. The notion of resource consumption can be generalized quite simply. Rather than estimating the number of resource units to be *consumed* by a given type of encounter, the group estimates the number of resource increments that should be *available* for consumption by the entire program to support a given level of demand, as defined by the total number of encounters. For example, at a certain level of demand at least one assistant administrator and two secretaries will be needed. Implicit in this is the notion that a particular level of program utilization could not be efficiently achieved without these resources in these increments. If the forming group elects to develop resource capacities which will not meet the level of projected demand, the impact of demand exceeding supply must be considered.

CASH FLOW PHASE

In this phase of planning, resource requirements may be reduced to a common denominator—dollars; that is, the amount of money needed to purchase various resources and to operate at the planned capacity levels. Cash outflow and disbursements must be financed through a combination of internally and externally derived funds. Initially, the group may assess the extent to which internally derived funds will cover cash outflow by a monthly netting of the cash receipts generated through operating revenues, against the cash disbursements. Any residual inflow (or surplus) could be available to reduce future deficits, to reinvest in the program, or possibly to increase the level of staff compensation over a period of time. Any residual outflow (or deficit) would have to be financed through external funds.

Calculating Costs

The forecast of cash outflow consists of two steps:

1. calculating a dollar value—or cost—represented by all units of resource available each month; and
2. determing the timing of cash payments—or disbursements—in recognition of these costs.

To calculate the cost of available resources, a cost per resource unit can be determined and multiplied by the total number of those units to be made available during the planning period. For some units, such as the cost per square foot of fixed facility floor space, the unit cost can be determined directly. In estimating the total cost of building or renting a facility, it may be helpful to think in contractors' terms of cost per square foot. Personnel resources may or may not be costed out in man-hours, man-days, or some other time-related measure. Part-time clerical personnel or consulting specialists who are compensated in relation to time worked would have a specific dollar cost associated with a unit of time. Since the month is the basic planning period, salaried personnel and other resources purchased for longer periods of time typically will have a cost defined in terms of that longer period. That cost can be broken down to a monthly figure which can then be applied to the monthly forecasts of units available. Whether the cost per unit is determined directly, because it is the prevailing method of pricing the resource, or indirectly, because the total cost is broken down to a monthly figure, the end result should be the same: a month by month forecast of the dollar value of the resource to be made available.

Projecting Disbursements

The development of a medical group practice from the initial program concept through the operation at capacity involves several categories of resources. Staff must be employed at appropriate times so that the program develops as demand warrants. Supplies must be maintained and carried in inventory. A wide variety of ongoing operating costs must be met regardless of demand fluctuation. The most significant cash outflow is reflected in disbursements for facilities, equipment, and staff. Ordinarily, there will be considerable activity prior to the first month of program operation. Planning, construction or renovation, the procurement of some equipment, and various salary costs will occur before the first patient is seen. There will be yet a further delay between the time patients are seen and their reimbursements are received. To ensure the continuing solvency of the program, it is vital that the timing of cash disbursements be estimated precisely. Funds must be obtained to cover those disbursements, and appropriate sources must be identified.

Facilities and Equipment. Establishing a new program involves either construction of a new facility or rental and probable alteration of an existing structure. Since either approach may represent major expenditures, it will be useful to test the alternatives in terms of cash flow; that way, each may be evaluated on the basis of preoperational or postoperational fund requirements. Construction costs may be met by progress payments, a lump sum payment, or periodic mortgage payments after an initial down payment. If a mortgage is required, local bankers should be consulted to determine the applicable down payments, interest rates, and security conditions. Purchase and modification of existing facilities may involve similar payment options. The possibility of borrowing to finance the work also may be explored. Rental simply involves equal payments over the lifetime of the lease, with an estimated accommodation for rent adjustments if the lease must be renewed before the end of the initial period. At this stage in the planning process, it also may be well to assess the pattern of cash disbursements involved in the modular construction or expansion of the facilities. In certain circumstances, it may be possible under either the purchase or rental alternative to plan for facility expansion as demand increases. Leasing versus construction is discussed in greater detail in Chapter 7 and Part IV.

The program's equipment requirements should be described in cash outflow terms, similarly to the analysis of structural requirements. Lease or buy decisions have pertinent implications for cash flows which should also be analyzed. Some or all departments may wish to add equipment on a modular basis as demand increases. Chapter 27 offers a more detailed discussion of equipment requirements for a new group practice.

Staffing. Because the timing of cash disbursements to support program staff is so much a function of the prevailing level of staffing, and because precipitous increases and reductions in staff generally are undesirable, a smooth staff build-up paralleling actual demand growth is critical. If negative cash flow is to be kept at a tolerable level during the development of the program, advance and initial staffing should be sufficient to serve the early user population but substantially below that needed at ultimate program capacity. The rate at which staff is phased in will depend upon planned demand build-up and actual observed demand. Furthermore, some services initially purchased outside as part of a comprehensive prepaid program may be added as the program matures and demand increases.

Alternative disbursement patterns can accompany given levels of staffing, just as they can support given levels of facility and equipment availability. Salaries typically are paid weekly or monthly, but professional staff need not be on a salary payment basis. There are a variety of compensation options which can affect both the timing and the magnitude of disbursements. Some of these options are:

1. *Fees based on services rendered.* Staff physicians may be compensated on essentially the same basis as they would be in solo practice, with their respective fees flowing through to them in direct proportion to their provision of service.
2. *Capitation payments.* Staff physicians may receive a single payment per individual covering a specific time period, typically a year, regardless of the amount of service rendered during that period. The capitation payment to the physician could be disbursed in monthly installments or in sums paralleling the receipt of the enrollee's prepayments to the program.
3. *Case payments.* Staff physicians may receive a fee covering a package of services related to the assumption of a "case" or defined problem. Unlike the fee-for-service, the case charge is not directly tied to the utilization of specific services; but unlike the capitation payment, there can be multiple case charges per individual patient.
4. *Income shares.* Staff physicians may receive a share of the program's net income allocated in accordance with some formula based on factors such as seniority, patient load, area of specialization, etc.

These compensation arrangements may exist in isolation or in combination with each other and with a base salary. A common approach is the base salary plus a bonus contingent upon an income surplus.

The group should explore the cash flow implication of alternative disbursement patterns associated with various staff compensation options and with methods of facility, equipment, supply, and other resource acquisition. With the selection of a pattern of disbursements for each resource, the group can formalize a monthly statement of anticipated cash outflow and, therefore, a statement of cash need.

Calculating Operating Revenue

After determining how many dollars are needed, the group must ascertain how they are to be generated. Early in the planning period, an objective should be set to reach cash flow equilibrium within a given time after the program has commenced, usually three to five years. By the end of that time, cash receipts from operations should at least equal cash disbursements. The level of operating receipts will be determined by the prices established for the services rendered. In the ambulatory setting, however, greater user discretion and lower insurance coverage increase the impact of pricing on utilization. If an improperly set price level can have a negative impact on demand in a fee-for-service program, it is all the more likely to have the same effect in a prepaid program. The prepaid enrollee is asked to invest a predictable number of payments, analogous to insurance premiums, each of which may be higher than the price of an encounter in a fee-for-service program. In return, he is entitled to a package of services which he may or may not use. Consequently, the group will need to test the pricing structure for effectiveness in meeting costs *and* the expectations of the population to be served. In doing so, the following steps may be employed:

1. Select a time interval during which the pattern of month to month resource availability is expected to have stabilized.
2. Calculate total program costs estimated to be incurred during the period.
3. Identify the types of encounters that will generate revenues.
4. Determine the relative cost of each of these types of encounters.
5. Allocate total program costs, based on the number of encounters of each type projected for the period, to identified encounter types in proportion to their relative costs to arrive at base revenue per encounter figures.
6. Factor into each revenue per encounter figure an allowance for bad debt loss.
7. Compare the revenue per encounter figures with analogous figures prevailing in the community and make necessary adjustments.

Once the group is satisfied that the revenue per encounter figures meet the objectives of *cost* coverage and marketability, the problem of pricing specific services so their combined effect produces the overall revenue per encounter figures may be considered. Chapter 15 explores the pricing and charge system in greater detail.

At this point the group has developed a set of revenue figures per encounter or per enrollment. By applying them to the forecast of encounters or initial enrollment visits, the revenue stream may be projected.

Projecting Operating Receipts

Accurate revenue calculations will contribute to the generation of sufficient cash to finance the ongoing cash need defined by the disbursement forecast. Given a forecast of operating revenues, the flow of cash receipts must be anticipated. There are likely to be multiple sources of cash receipts. Not only may the patient be responsible for payment of all or a portion of the charges for particular types of encounters, a third party acting in his behalf may be responsible as well. Such third parties include the traditional health care insurers—Medicare, Medicaid, Blue Cross/Blue Shield, commercial carriers, and workmen's compensation. In addition, employers, unions, or other intermediaries may be responsible for fee payments for services rendered or for the prepayment of capitation charges. The mix of payors appropriate to the planned program should be defined carefully, not only for marketing purposes but also because each of these payors is a source of cash receipts and each will have a characteristic pattern of reimbursement. In accounting terms, there will be differing receivable periods. In combination, these reimbursement patterns will determine the flow of cash into the program.

The group's goal will be to speed up the flow of cash receipts. A good policy in dealing with third party payors is to strive for prepayment even if fee-for-service care is provided. Under such a policy a final settlement may be required at year's end; over-reimbursement stemming from too high interim payments can be corrected by a refund to the payors or by a credit carried forward to the next year. Nevertheless, simply having the funds on a predictable and, preferably, before-the-fact basis is of great value to the program. Any interest earnings that may accrue from this pool of cash could help offset losses that are bound to occur in the course of operations. The group also should consider building into its operating receipts forecast an allowance for bad debt losses. One approach is to reduce the projected revenue at the outset by a certain percentage, perhaps between 5 percent and 15 percent, selected on the basis of the experience of other health care providers in the community. To be more precise, the group may establish bad debt allowances by payor and by encounter type, on the assumption that certain types of encounters are less likely than others to be paid in full.

Projecting Net Operating Cash Flow

By matching the monthly disbursements forecast against the monthly operating receipts forecast, the group can compute the net monthly cash flow from operations. Then, by summing these monthly figures, which include positive balances or surpluses as well as negative balances or deficits, the group can calculate the cumulative net cash flow from operations. Should this cumulative amount be a surplus (which is unlikely if the planning period covers the months prior to and immediately following program startup) the group need only be concerned with the disposition of that surplus, and that disposition would depend greatly on the group's organizational form, as discussed in the next chapter. The surplus could be disposed of in any or all of the following ways:

1. carry the surplus forward as cash to be used to defray deficits that may occur in months subsequent to this planning period;
2. invest the surplus in the program through the acquisition of additional resources to serve a broader population of users, to provide a broader range of services to the existing population, or to enhance the quality of service or the professional development of the member physicians;
3. eliminate the surplus by reducing the price of services via the lessening of individual fees or prepayment premiums; and
4. use the surplus to increase the compensation to program staff either through higher salaries or bonuses.

Identifying Sources of Nonoperating Receipts

In addition to receipts from program operations (e.g., receipts derived from fee-for-service and/or enrollment revenues) the program will most likely receive funds from nonoperating sources. *Grant* funds, whether derived from public or private sources, are typically categorical; that is, they can be used to finance certain program operations and not others. Some grants are earmarked for planning, others for construction or the provision of specific types of service. Still others may be available to defray the startup deficit through the first year or two, regardless of the causes of that deficit. To qualify for grant financing, the program will have to have a certain orientation toward services provided and/or population to be served.

In-kind contributions consist of services, facilities, or equipment donated in lieu of cash. Such donations can be treated on a cash basis so they can be offset against the cash outflow projected for these resources during the financial planning process. *Donations* of cash from philanthropic and other sources may be unrestricted, and their significance for a particular program will depend on the fund-raising efforts contemplated. Cash received from *equity financing* is a category of non-operating receipts particularly relevant to the professional corporation, and *debt* financing will impose not only the usual debt-servicing costs—interest payments—but also the obligation of repayment of the loan.

Projecting Net Total Cash Flows

The precision of the group's nonoperating receipts forecast will depend upon when financial planning is undertaken and the extent of preliminary contacts with external financing sources. If it is undertaken prior to contact with external funds sources, the forecast of net operating cash flows represents a statement of cash need that will *not* reflect known infusions of external funds. On the other hand, if the planning is undertaken after some external funds (such as those cited above) have been committed or received, the group is in quite a different position and may then proceed with the allocation of known dollar amounts to each month of the planning period, in accordance with established schedules. In this case, the group is testing whether or not the pattern of available nonoperating receipts will be sufficient to cover projected operating costs. When the total negative cash flow is allocated to the potential funds sources already identified, and in compliance with any restrictions tied to the receipt of those funds, the group may find that a negative cash balance remains at the end of the planning period. Faced with this situation, the amount of nonoperating receipts may be increased or the operating deficit reduced. These actions are not mutually exclusive; both can be done.

In increasing the amount of nonoperating receipts, the group's first obligation is to assess the possibility of obtaining additional noninterest-bearing, nonrepayable funds from some of the sources already identified. In figure 4-3 the key variables of the planning process are displayed, along with the upward or downward adjustments in relation to each variable that would reduce the operating deficit. These processes are presented in the preferable order of consideration. Moving from adjustments in the cash flow forecast to the capacity forecast and finally to the demand forecast, the group comes closer to changing the program's basic strategy.

Cash Flow. To ensure that an action has the desired effect of reducing the operating deficit without at the same time reducing the effectiveness of the

	Direction of Change
CASH FLOW	
Revenue per encounter	↑
Cost per unit	↓
CAPACITY	
Increments available	↓
Units per increment	↑
Consumption rates	↓
DEMAND*	
Encounter rates	↓
Types of encounter	↓
Penetration %	↑
Segments	↑

*Not applicable to the fee-for-service program.

Figure 4–3. Adjustments in Key Variables to Reduce Operating Deficits

program, the group should consider the following alternatives in the area of cash flow:

1. *Increase the revenue per encounter.* This approach involves increasing the prices for program services. The fee-for-service program would increase its fees; the prepayment program would increase its enrollment charges. The group should assess the price sensitivity of the user population and of the third parties paying on its behalf. An increase in prices may cause decrease in demand, reflected either in a drop-off in utilization or in rate of enrollment. There may be certain services, or types of encounter, toward which the user is less price-sensitive than he is toward others.

2. *Decrease the cost per unit.* The cost per unit of resources available for consumption may be reduced in a variety of ways. Better terms may be negotiated with suppliers by seeking quantity discounts or package deals. Competitive bidding may be introduced in appropriate cases. Job qualifications may be revised downward, and persons with lesser qualifications could be hired at a lower starting salary and trained on the job. Excess facility or equipment capacity could be leased out at a fee, thereby defraying effective cost. The group should, of course, assess the effects any decrease in performance standards associated with the acquisition of lower cost resources might have on the quality of care rendered.

Capacity. Various alternatives also are available in the area of capacity:

1. *Decrease the increments available.* The number of increments of an available resource could be cut back. For example, even though the cost per man-hour of a physician's time may not be reduced, fewer physicians may be hired. Similarly, fewer items of equipment or a smaller facility may be acquired. Assuming the level of encounters remains constant and hence the

consumption of resource units is undiminished, a decrease in available resources would be accompanied by the greater risk of exceeding the program's capacity. The group should assess the feasibility of servicing the projected demand with fewer increments of resource. Peak loads and higher than projected levels of demand must be anticipated. In addition, the likelihood of adding/eliminating increments of particular resources on a month to month basis without incurring additional phase-in/phase-out costs must be assessed.

2. *Increase the units per increment.* The number of resource units (man-hours) that could be derived from one resource increment (physician) also is amenable to adjustment. By lengthening the duration of resource availability, such as through longer work days and the use of equipment at night, it may be possible to achieve a higher degree of productivity from any one particular increment than had been originally anticipated. Improvements in operating efficiency through systems changes, work flow simplifications, use of paramedical personnel, and sharing of common resources also could lead to greater efficiency and could reduce the number of resource increments needed to make available the same number of resource units.

The group should assess the degree to which significant one-time costs may accompany the effort to gain greater productivity from particular resources. Efficiency studies may be required. More paramedical staff than expected may have to be hired. Careful attention also should be given to the higher maintenance costs associated with greater productivity. In the case of machines these costs may be more easily quantified than in the case of staff. A higher rate of staff turnover may result from the expectation of higher rates of productivity.

3. *Decrease the consumption rates.* The number of resource units that must be consumed in the course of particular types of encounter or on behalf of the program as a whole could be reduced. Conceivably, the same quality of care could be rendered with the commitment of less time on the part of the more expensive staff, or in smaller offices, or with a smaller administrative component. Over time, the consumption rates of specific resources might be expected to decrease gradually, as the overall health of the user population improves and as normal learning curve efficiencies take hold. The group should gauge carefully the possible consequences of revisions in the resource consumption rates for the quality of care rendered. The substitution of nonprofessional for professional staff time may result in less adequate care or in care perceived as less satisfactory by patients. The use of less building space or other resources not directly involved in the delivery of care may have the long-range effect of making the program less attractive to patients and, hence, may lessen demand.

Demand. The group must be even more careful in making adjustments in demand as a means of reducing the program's operating deficit; any modification in factors affecting demand constitutes a direct modification of the strategic rationale and mission of the program. Typically, the prepaid program, through its marketing efforts, has a broader range of options than does the fee-for-service program in terms of influencing demand. It can take steps to increase the enrollment and the revenue base. Because costs and revenues are not directly linked, both actions can be taken with much greater assurance that their combined effect will be the reduction of a projected operating deficit.

The following are some suggested measures that may be undertaken:

1. *Decrease the encounter rates.* In the prepaid setting, certain types of encounters increase program costs each time they occur. To service these encounters, the program must make resources available as they are consumed; direct and not fixed costs are involved. Hospitalization is such an encounter type. Clearly, the fewer hospitalizations and the shorter their durations, the less cost is borne by the program. The group also may try to lower the encounter rates for all types involving the consumption of high fixed cost resources beyond their optimum capacity. Avoiding the need to add another resource increment may contribute to significant cost savings. Again, the group should assess the consequences of limiting the incidence of high cost encounters, and to do this probably will have to build into its projections the more frequent incidence of lower cost encounters. By providing more routine preventive medicine, for example, the health of the enrollee population may be maintained at a level high enough to diminish the incidence and duration of hospitalization encounters. Certainly, the provision of many common diagnostic and therapy services in the lower cost outpatient setting would limit the use of higher cost hospital facilities.

One way, therefore, to justify an encounter rate reduction is to assume a greater degree of efficacy by the program staff in providing preventive medical care. Another way is to shift the marketing focus away from those population segments that have inherently higher encounter rates for expensive encounter types and toward segments with lower rates. This shift, however, constitutes an important strategic change. In essence, the program would be attempting to select better medical risks as enrollees. In addition, such individuals may be the most difficult prospects to sell on the prepayment concept. The group could postpone the marketing effort directed at the higher risk segments until after an adequate revenue base has been established with enrollments from the lower risk segments. In this way, the program's ability to provide expensive services to the high risk enrollees is not hampered by a lack of funds.

One further alternative involves limiting the enrollment period to a particular month during the year or to some other interval. In this way the program can target all segments, high as well as low risk, at the same time; however, because a fixed enrollment period leads to a more random enrollment base, the high risk potential enrollee is prevented from selecting himself into the program at his discretion.

2. *Decrease the types of encounters.* Especially high-cost encounter types could be eliminated altogether by dropping them from the program's service package. The program might, for example, no longer provide dental services, thus reducing this type of encounter rate to zero for all segments. Once again, the group should assess the impact that such an important change in services would have on the marketability of the overall program. Before actually eliminating a major service from the program, consideration should be given to postponing the availability of that service until after an adequate revenue base has been established through the sale of a less comprehensive package; however, as noted in connection with the elimination or postponement of marketing to high risk populations, the less comprehensive package may be the most difficult to sell. The group should anticipate both greater marketing

costs and a longer period before the program reaches its target enrollment level.

3. *Increase the penetration percentage.* If the objective is simply one of increasing revenues and not reducing costs, the group may consider increasing the penetration of any one segment already targeted by the program. Greater penetration of a segment may be possible both for prepaid and fee-for-service groups if additional marketing efforts are directed toward the population segment and/or modifications are made in the services offered so that the program becomes more marketable. The group should evaluate the cost implications of either of these actions.

4. *Increase the number of segments.* Finally, there is the possibility of identifying additional population segments to be served. In terms of high versus low risk population segments, however, the group will want to be sure that any new segments added will yield revenues at least equal to costs; otherwise, any potential for containing the deficit would be lost.

Numerous combinations of these actions could have the effect of reducing the projected operating deficit. That action or combination of actions which brings the operating receipts and disbursements into line without a major strategic change should be selected. If a strategic change involving modifications in the population to be served or the services to be rendered is needed, all of the issues raised in Chapter 3 should be reconsidered and, if necessary, the planning process repeated. After the forming medical group practice has established its mission and validated or modified that mission through the planning process, it is faced with choosing a legal organization form. In the following chapter alternate legal forms will be reviewed.

Chapter 5

Legal Organization

Due to rapid developments in the legal area, it should not be assumed that the following material is complete or reflects the most current law. This information is designed to help physicians and other health care providers in the planning of efficiently organized group practices which have as an ultimate goal the delivery of low cost, yet quality primary medical care.

LEGAL OPTIONS FOR MEDICAL GROUP ORGANIZATIONAL FORM

In Chapter 4 the discussion centered on the establishment of planning criteria as they relate to fulfilling the consumer demand and projecting medical group resources. Usually, the next decision following the planning phase is to determine the legal organizational type(s) under which the group physicians will practice medicine and own property. Unfortunately, the legal aspects of the practice are often difficult to understand and this step can be quite a sobering experience for individuals who are unaware of the ramifications posed by various legal requirements.

Group practices are characterized by a number of legal organizational forms presumably chosen because of differences in tax benefits, personal liability, and retirement fund. The partnership form is the second most preferred; 27.2 percent of all groups surveyed in a 1975 American Medical Association study were legally organized as partnerships. Historically, the evolution from sole proprietorship has been largely a function of regulations endorsed by the Internal Revenue Service, the issue being whether such groups are entitled to be taxed as corporations.

As illustrated by the Pelton case in 1936, the IRS initially levied taxes against groups of professionals as though they were, in fact, corporations, even though incorporation by professionals was illegal under most state laws. The IRS traditionally took the view that most bona fide partnerships possessed more corporate than partnership characteristics. As partnerships became large, however, their large management structure often became unwieldy and decision-making slow. At a time when incorporation was still prohibited by state law, many physician groups reorganized into unincorporated associations under which they were able to centralize management authority in a board of directors. Furthermore, continuity of life for the association was still possible in spite of the death or resignation of one of the group members. This organizational form also provided the possibility for fringe benefits in the form of insurance and pension plans for employees. This arrangement continued to be desirable as long as the IRS taxed partnerships and associations as corporations; however, in the late 1940s the IRS reversed its attitude and challenged the right of such organizations to be taxed as corporations. Consequently, many existing professional organizations moved toward the corporate form, if it was legal under the laws of their state.

In 1960 the IRS initiated a new set of regulations making it extremely difficult for partnerships and associations to be taxed as corporations. These regulations contained provisions which recognized the authority of local statutes regarding corporations and as a consequence a number of states adopted laws making professional corporations legal entities. In 1965 still another set of IRS regulations made it clear that the IRS was not obligated to abide by state statutes regarding professional corporations.

Clearly, the impetus for preferences in organizational form has been influenced by a number of factors, not the least of which has been the IRS. Fulfilling the need for centralized management, continuity of life, limited liability, tax advantages, and pension and retirement funds has stimulated the progressive movement of group practice to the corporate legal organization. The detailed discussion of each legal type of organization which follows will be presented in an historical sequence beginning with the partnership and concluding with the professional corporation.

The basic alternatives for the legal structure and organization of the group practice are few, and each can be modified to fit the particular needs of a group. It is important, therefore, to understand the nature and purpose of this discussion; the material presented here is designed to orient the physician or the medical group administrator to the legal organizational alternatives of group practice. It is not intended to provide the group with information sufficient for the forming of an organization and the initiating of medical practice without additional assistance. Rather, it is designed to give the reader a working understanding of the concepts involved so that he may profit from time spent with attorneys or other advisors. The information is intended as a framework; further advice should be sought from attorneys, accountants, and other consultants whose expertise is essential to the successful organization of a medical practice. The alternative legal forms considered in this chapter include the sole proprietorship, partnership, unincorporated association, nonprofit organization, and professional corporation.

SOLE PROPRIETORSHIP

Sole ownership, the simplest form of group practice organization, usually is represented by a temporary arrangement that results when a successful sole practitioner can no longer meet the needs of the community. Consequently, the physician hires associates on salary, but as sole proprietor he remains responsible for management, policy determination, and financial matters. The essential legal relationship between the sole proprietor and his associates is that of employer/employee; this relationship commences when both the employer and the employee reach agreement upon the employment contract.

The employer physician, as the individual proprietor, has total and final authority in the administration of the organization. The sole owner may or may not wish the employed physicians to share in the decision-making process or in any surplus practice income. On the other hand, he must supply the initial capital and is responsible for all the financial obligations. With only a single source of capital, expansion of the group practice may be limited; this single feature could represent a major disadvantage of this form of organization.

Employed Physicians

The sole proprietorship becomes a group practice upon completion of the employment agreement. It is not necessary that the contract be written; it may be oral or it may be implied from the conduct of the parties. Oral contracts, however, do present difficulty when the participants attempt to substantiate the agreements contained in the contract. It appears in the best interest of both the employer and employee, therefore, to draw up a written agreement containing at least all of the conditions and obligations of the employment that are deemed to be unusual.

An employee is the agent of his employer; unlike a partner, however, the employee is not responsible for the obligations or negligence of the employer. As the extension of the employer, the employee can act for him in any business affair; however, in order not to be held personally liable for his actions as an agent, it is essential that he inform all those who deal with the practice of his employee status and of his authority to act on behalf of his employer.

The employed physician's wages are subject to social security withholdings, unemployment deductions, taxes, and workmen's compensation, and therefore the employed physician is able to participate in pension plans, group insurance, and social security benefits. In addition, employment can supply such intangible benefits as experience, stability, and a predictable source of income. The owner of a sole proprietorship can set up an HR 10 plan (Self-Employed Individuals Retirement Act—Keogh Regulation) for the benefit of himself as well as his employees, and thereby becomes subject to social security taxes on his earned income.

Obligations of the Employer

The individual proprietor usually makes all of the decisions and establishes all of the practice's policies; he alone is responsible for all capital, and his personal assets are vulnerable in the event that business creditors claim the money invested in the practice. There is no separation between the property of the medical group and the property of the sole owner.

As an employer, the sole proprietor is required to pay social security taxes and state and federal disability, as well as to make unemployment contributions and, according to law, bear the expenses generated by these withholdings. The sole owner pays personal tax only on taxable income, including business profits, at the current individual tax rate.

Termination of the Sole Proprietorship

The group is only as permanent as its sole owner. If the owner is competent to select and retain capable key personnel to help him in the operation of all aspects of the business, the group usually will succeed. If, however, the sole owner is unable to provide effective management, the group probably will suffer. The group's ownership, as well as its operation, can be transferred at the will of the owner if he simply sells the practice to others. Unless the owner has made provision for the group to reorganize upon his death or retirement, the group could face liquidation at any time.

The primary advantages of sole ownership include simplicity of operation and ease of decision-making. Employee status for the physician in a sole proprietorship, however, does prevent his participation in decision-making for the group and may stifle his professional growth. As a result, the sole proprietorship group may experience high turnover. One major advantage of the sole proprietorship form is that it provides a means of testing the group's abilities to work together prior to a commitment to a more complex legal organization.

PARTNERSHIP

The partnership offers an alternative organizational structure for those physicians seeking professional and financial development within a group setting while sharing equally in liabilities, decision-making, and profits. A partnership is regarded as the traditional legal form of medical group practice; compared to the sole proprietorship, however, it can be exceedingly complex and requires a great deal of careful planning.

A partnership is defined as: "A legal relationship which is created by an oral or written agreement between two or more persons who combine their capital and labor to engage in business or the practice of a profession."[1] *The Uniform Partnership Act* offers an alternative definition: "A partnership is an association of two or more persons to carry on as *co-owners* of a business *for profit*" (*UPA* § 6; emphasis added).[2] The *UPA* definition indicates that the partnership has a community of interest and a sharing of profits. Unlike the sole proprietorship, the partners are neither employees nor employers, but rather are co-owners. The partnership, however, may employ nonpartner physicians. The sharing of profits indicates one important limitation of a partnership—it is an association for profit and cannot be formed for nonprofit purposes.

A Practical Look at the Advantages and Disadvantages of the Partnership

In considering the partnership as a legal organizational alternative, the physician must evaluate not only his own personal needs and goals, but those of his potential associates as well. Choosing a partner is a major decision because some individuals do not work well in a group. The physician also must determine whether his specialty has a long-term role in the group practice. Any number of physicians can participate in a partnership; in general, however, combinations of twos or threes of the same specialty are typical. More than one physician in a specialty within the partnership has resulted not only because of opportunities for professional development, but also because of the need to cover vacations and other absences occuring within the department or partnership. Ultimately, size of a partnership also is regulated by the medical needs of the community served by the practice.

Although friendship and personal compatibility are important elements of a successful partnership, the physician must also view his partners as professional associates with whom he can learn, as well as work. The physician just beginning the practice of medicine usually is wise to seek an association with a more experienced practitioner before forming a partnership with his friends.

Some of the advantages and disadvantages of partnership practice are presented in table 5-1.

Partnership Trial Arrangements

Before entering into a partnership arrangement, the group may want to work together in a trial arrangement. Several methods are available, including the sole proprietorship plan discussed earlier. Other possible, widely used alternatives, include expense sharing, office sharing, and the employing of an associate.

Under the expense sharing plan, the physicians continue their individual practices but share the costs of operation, while maintaining strict, separate accounts for their respective assets, income, and liabilities. Usually, a joint operating fund is established and the participating physicians reimburse the fund each month. Depending upon the arrangement, one physician may contribute more funds than his expenses justify. The expense sharing trial arrangement offers a measure of independence, while providing the opportunity for some savings of costs and for informal consultation which, hopefully, will reduce any inequities.

Nonetheless, the expense sharing arrangement should be written and signed by all participants to avoid confusion over the intent and terms of the agreement. Although expense sharing may be considered to be a temporary relationship, many physicians have subsequently abandoned plans for further development into a partnership and have retained only the expense arrangement for their professional practice. It is very important for the expense sharing physicians to inform both their creditors and their patients of the nature of their relationship so that no one is led to believe he is dealing with a partnership.

Office sharing is a trial arrangement more closely resembling the group practice setting than does the expense sharing relationship. With this plan, the physicians not only share expenses but also practice in the same office, purchase common equipment, and employ common medical and clerical assistants. Income, patients, and patient records, however, remain with separate physicians. This arrangement, along with the expense sharing, is a common approach for established practitioners experimenting with group practice. As with the arrangements discussed earlier, any unusual terms of the office sharing arrangement should be written because of possible common ownership of equipment and property, or common holding of an office lease. Division of property, retention of the common office, staff placement, and other consequences of

Table 5-1. Advantages and Disadvantages of Partnership Practice

Advantages	*Disadvantages*
Partnership with an established and reputable practitioner is an aid in obtaining hospital privileges and acquiring status in medical organizations.	Interference of spouses in partnership affairs, or bickerings between them, may lead to friction.
Combining different talents improves the capacity to render service and stimulates patient confidence.	The close relationship involved may lead to personality conflicts.
Continuous coverage is assured during vacations, convention trips, days off, and illness.	Independence and individuality must be restricted for the sake of partnership harmony.
Informal consultation is always available on difficult cases.	Partners share responsibility for the professional and business mistakes of each other.
Partners can more easily devote themselves to the areas of practice in which they are particularly qualified or interested.	Partners are legally liable for each other's actions within the scope of partnership—malpractice, contracts for purchase of equipment, etc.
Most partners are able to take time off to improve their skills through postgraduate training.	If the partnership practice includes more than one specialty, other physicians may be reluctant to refer patients.
By pooling their funds, partners can enjoy the benefits, comfortable office space, special equipment, and trained personnel, which may be beyond the reach of the sole practitioner.	The potentially high-earning specialist may not realize as large an income in partnership as he would in solo practice.
Sharing overhead usually increases the percentage of net income.	If income is not divided equally, or if a partner does not bear his share of the patient load, disagreements over the division of income may arise.
The "starvation" period of practice-building is eliminated for the new physician in partnership with an established practitioner.	A partner may sometimes find it necessary to share in expenses from which he derives no benefit.
Partnership can provide relief for the overworked doctor.	Partners acquire each other's enemies as well as friends.
Partnership stabilizes the income of the older doctor during the later years of practice when income normally tends to drop.	Joint ownership of equipment may result in loss if it becomes necessary to dissolve the partnership.
If a partner dies, the survivor, by prior agreement, may purchase his interest.	

Source: B. D. Hirsch, *Business Management of a Medical Practice* (St. Louis: C. V. Moseby Company, 1964), p. 30.

termination of the arrangement also should be included in the agreement. Because a group of physicians in close proximity may appear to be organized as a partnership, they should take special care to inform the persons they deal with of the nature of their arrangement. The appearance of a partnership may lead to each associate's liability for the obligations of the other physicians.

When an established physician seeks to enter into practice with other physicians, a trial plan commonly used involves hiring an associate. Because this alternative resembles the sole proprietorship, it requires only brief discussion here. One physician hires another with the understanding that a partnership will result if the trial plan proves satisfactory. The employer/employee arrangement usually works best when the incoming associate is much younger than the employer physician; when the associate has adequate professional qualifications, but is lacking adequate finances; or when the associate is new in the community. In the past it was considered generally acceptable for the employer physician to include in the employment contract a provision or covenant prohibiting the employed physician from leaving and starting a competing practice after he became established in the community; alternatively, the contract clause also could require payment of an agreed upon sum of money to serve as "liquidated damages" should the employed physician breach the agreement not to compete.[3] The Pension Reform Act (1974) prohibits provisions in qualified retirement plans which stipulate that an employee who quits and goes into competition forfeits all benefits under the retirement plan.

Creating the Partnership

The partnership is a voluntary association of two or more persons, and it is essential that the relationship be based on an agreement freely entered into. A contract, implied or expressed, is central to the formation of the partnership. An expressed agreement is created by the expressed desire of the physicians to become partners and may be either written or oral; an implied contract for a partnership is inferred from the actions of the partners. If two individuals act as partners, and if certain criteria apply, an implied partnership agreement exists between them. Any person having the capacity to contract, as determined by local law, has the capacity to become a partner; however, most states have special medical practice statutes which require that all partners in a medical group practice be licensed doctors of medicine.

The Written Agreement. In addition to the practical advantages of having the conditional terms of the partnership expressed in writing, the law requires that certain partnership agreements be committed to writing.[a] The first of these is a partnership agreement that by its terms cannot be executed within the period of one year (i.e., a partnership for two years or a partnership formed for a particular purpose which cannot be completed within one year). This type of partnership agreement usually falls within the requirements of a state's Statute of Frauds, and the agreement cannot be enforced unless there is tangible evidence, such as a written document. In addition, a written agreement is required if the partnership contract confers authority between the partners to deal in real property. The failure to have such authority reduced to writing does not affect the rights of partners between themselves to deal in real property, but whenever a third person attempts to challenge a contract made by the partnership, some courts hold that the authority of the partner executing the property contract must be evidenced in writing.

The Contents of the Agreement. It is important that the written agreement be followed closely and be reviewed periodically; a written agreement that is a

[a]Partnership law, as well as other legal aspects of group practice discussed in this chapter, is determined by each state and can be quite localized. This chapter relates only to general principles and the reader must consult his local attorney to determine the law in his state.

mere formality is useless. The partners should understand fully and should determine concretely the various obligations and rights involved in their partnership. They might consider some of the following provisions for their agreement:

1. *Date of Formation.* The partnership agreement must indicate the date the physicians are to be considered as partners.

2. *Names of the Participating Physicians.*

3. *Statement of an Agreement to Act as Partners.* An essential criterion for establishing a partnership is the determination of the intent of the physicians involved.

4. *Specific Nature and Purpose of the Professional Enterprise.*

5. *Duration.* A partnership's duration can be determined by the passage of a specific period of time, the completion of a specific task, or the will of the partners.

6. *Name of the Organization.* Usually, local or state laws require that the firm name include the names of some or all of the professionals involved; however, some states do allow a clinic name as long as it is not misleading.

7. *Contribution of Capital.* Generally, a professional partnership needs little capital because the partners themselves are the chief assets; capital, however, may be used as a means of arranging each partner's share of the partnership. The established physician may contribute his accounts receivable as capital and continue to amortize until his capital account equals that of other partners.[4] For a partnership consisting entirely of established physicians, capital contributions could be made in equal amounts of cash. The contributions provision may also stipulate what is and is not considered contributed capital, such as loans and leases to the partnership by one partner.

8. *Withdrawals for Expenses and Salaries.* Partners receive a share of the profits and do not receive a salary in the technical sense. If desired, provisions could be made for the partners to receive monthly or quarterly advances to be deducted from the year-end profits. Formulae devised for determination of cost and profit distribution are discussed in detail in Chapter 9.

9. *Keeping Financial Accounts.*

10. *Duties of Partner-Physicians.* Provisions could be made for the internal relations between the partners as to the designation of call duty, hospital duty, vacation time, sick leave, educational leave, and other areas of possible conflicts. The policy-making and business decisions process may be delegated to various governing units such as an executive or professional committee. Depending upon the ownership arrangement, the partner who "owns" the greatest interest in the practice may control the business policy decisions, and this arrangement may continue even after equality among the partners is achieved. Some expenditures, however, may require agreement among all of the partners.

11. *Distribution of Profits and Sharing of Losses.* The agreement can provide a detailed arrangement for the distribution of profits, or it can stipulate that the distribution be in accordance with a plan adopted by the partners at a later date. Many partnership agreements provide for distribution plans to be enforced, even if approved by a less than unanimous vote of partners. The unanimous vote of the partners, for any change in the distribution arrangement, usually is very difficult to obtain.

12. *Restraints on the Individual Practice of the Physicians.* Often, partnership agreements include the obligation of the partner to devote his efforts full time to the group practice and disallow outside work. Also included may be restraints not to compete, which are similar to such covenants in employment agreements and are intended to protect the partnership if a partner withdraws from the group practice.

13. *Changes in the Professional Staff.* The departure of any partner acts as a a dissolution of the partnership (UPA § 29). Dissolution is the point at which the partnership can no longer legally operate as an ongoing organization, and the partners must either form a new partnership or wind up the old partnership. To overcome the effect of dissolution, the agreement should provide for the continuation of the partnership when a partner withdraws or a new partner is added. The agreement also may control the treatment and obligations of a withdrawing partner.

14. *Termination of the Partnership.* Since a partnership may fail to survive an event, thus causing dissolution, provision should be included in the agreement that will govern the procedures for winding up the partnership's affairs, including distribution of assets, possession of medical records, and continuation of patient care.

15. *Miscellaneous.* In addition to the above considerations, the partnership agreement may include several other provisions required by the partners to meet future contingencies. Each of the prospective partners may compile a list of the reasons why other partnerships have dissolved. The partners then would be prepared for those difficulties and could make provisions for the necessary solutions in the agreement. They also may want to include provisions for the arbitration of future disputes. The partnership agreement may be considered an exercise designed to test the partners' ability to agree on certain obligations or policies. If major disagreement results, the physicians should seriously reconsider the partnership intention.

Criteria for Determining the Existence of a Partnership. Many partnerships exist very informally and without any expressed agreements; therefore, disputes may arise concerning whether there is a partnership agreement or whether the relationship between parties is, in fact, a partnership. In making such determinations, the following criteria have been applied by both the courts and the *Uniform Partnership Act.*

1. *Parties Designation.* Although the parties' designation of the relationship as a partnership or as any other business form deserves some consideration, it is not unquestionable. Conversely, parties cannot avoid partnership liabilities even by an expressed stipulation disavowing a partnership.

2. *Contributions of Capital.* The contribution of capital to a practice does not in itself establish a partnership.

3. *Sharing of Gross Income.* The sharing of gross returns does not in itself establish a partnership, regardless of whether or not the persons sharing such returns have a joint interest in any property from which the income or return is derived (*UPA* § 7 (3)).

4. *Joint Ownership of Property.* A partnership is not established by common or joint ownership of the property by the parties. The same is true regard-

less of whether such owners do or do not share in any profits made by the use of such property (*UPA* § 7 (2)).

5. *Sharing of the Profits of the Business.* The receipt by a person of a share of the profits of the practice is *prima facie* evidence of a partnership. Naturally, the share of profits includes by definition the sharing of operating expenses. The inference, however, will not be made where alternative business reasons for the share exist, such as a bonus or wages to an employee, rent to a landlord, payment to a creditor, payment for a sale of an asset, including goodwill, or an annuity to a widow (*UPA* § 7 (4)).

6. *Business Purpose and Conduct.* A crucial test for determining the partnership relation is whether or not the parties actually are attempting to carry on business together for profit. The partnership arrangement should indicate that the parties have contemplated joint participation in the management and operation of the practice.

Partner by Estoppel. The partnership relation carries with it partnership liability for each of the partner physicians. In general, partnership liability means that all partners will be liable for the debts and actions of the partnership; for example, if Dr. Jones and Dr. Smith were partners, and Dr. Smith negligently performed an operation on Mr. Wilson, then Dr. Jones could be held negligently liable and could be required to satisfy the claims of Mr. Wilson.

The partner by estoppel is a legal doctrine available to a third person to prevent or estop an individual from denying that another is his partner. No actual partnership exists, however, solely by the use of the doctrine of estoppel. Nevertheless, the physician who is practicing with others in a relationship, such as an employer/employee setting, office sharing, or expense sharing, must take particular care to avoid the circumstances that give rise to the use of the doctrine of partner by estoppel.

The doctrine of partner by estoppel is available to third persons to use against a physician if the physician, either by expression or by implication, portrays himself to be a partner, or expressly or passively consents to another's representations of him as a partner. The physician then becomes liable to any person who, in good faith, reasonably relies upon the partnership representation, and thereby suffers detrimental consequences (*UPA* § 16). This is based upon the rationale of equitable estoppel; after the representation has led to liabilities for him, it would be inequitable for a physician to then deny that his colleague is a partner. For example, Dr. Williams and Dr. Johnson are practicing under an office sharing arrangement, and either by Dr. Johnson's representation or by the appearance of the office facilities, a patient reasonably concludes that Dr. Williams is the partner of Dr. Johnson. Dr. Williams, by failing to inform the patient of the actual nature of the physicians' relationship before the patient has relied upon that impression to his own detriment, could be prevented or estopped by that patient from later claiming not to be the partner of Dr. Johnson.

The doctrine of estoppel also may be employed when one person, who may or may not be a member of a partnership, represents another person as his partner. The physician thereby confers upon the actual nonpartner the authority to bind the physician to third persons, just as if the physicians were, in fact, partners (*UPA* § 16). The third person, seeking relief for a claim from the representing physician, must have reasonably, and in good faith, relied upon the partnership representation and subsequently have been affected detrimentally. For example, Dr. Brown represents to his patients or creditors that Dr. Green is a partner. If Dr. Green negligently treats a patient on behalf of Dr. Brown's medical practice, then Dr. Brown also may be liable for any injuries suffered by the patient.

The liability created by the doctrine of estoppel is only applicable to the person making the representation; therefore, in the example concerning Dr. Brown's practice, a third physician, who indeed was in partnership with Dr. Brown and yet had made no representation concerning Dr. Green's role in the partnership, would not be liable to anyone who had dealt with Dr. Green.

Relations of the Partners to One Another

The partnership relation involves the practice of medicine as a group and includes the operation of a business as a group. Because the physicians also will be acting as businessmen, each with a different specialty, statutes establish various rights, obligations, and assumptions that are attributed to each partner. To some extent, these incidents of partner status may be expanded upon or limited by the partnership agreement. Some incidents, however, are implied in the partnership relation and cannot be altered.

Partner as a Fiduciary. *Fiduciary* is a legal term denoting a position of trust or confidence. Partners are considered to be fiduciaries of one another and owe to one another the same duties and obligations as a trustee owes to a beneficiary. The obligations of a fiduciary require that every act or contract entered into by the partner on behalf of the partnership be performed in good faith. The partner must place the interests of the partnership above any personal ambitions and must be professional in conduct and manner. Partnership business has priority and a partner does not have the right, without the consent of all other partners, to engage in any other business which may be in competition with or detrimental to the practice. The partner is bound to this restriction even in the absence of a specific obligation in the agreement.

The partner, as a fiduciary, must account to the partnership for any profits or benefits personally acquired by him without the consent of the other partners in any transactions connected with the formation, conduct, or termination of the partnership, or from the use of the partnership's property (*UPA* § 21). If a partner purchases or holds partnership assets in his own name, then he is a trustee of those assets for the partnership and can be compelled to account to the partnership for the assets themselves or for the value of the assets. Furthermore, these fiduciary obligations may continue even after the physician becomes separated from the partnership.

Rights and Duties Concerning Management. The one physician-one vote rule can apply in a medical partnership. All partners have equal rights in the management and conduct of the partnership business (*UPA* § 18 (c)). Unless the partnership agreement provides otherwise, this equality of control exists regardless of each partner's share of assets or the profits. This equality may be altered, however, to reflect each partner's contributed share of capital, years of experience, or other differentiating factors. Provisions may be made in the agreement whereby the management of the partnership is delegated to a smaller number of partners, such as an executive committee or a forum of a majority of the partners; however, no action may be taken or decision made by a smaller than unanimous number of the partners, if such action or decision would be contrary to any agreement made by all of the partners (*UPA* § 18 (h)). The basic principles of management should, therefore, be contained in the partnership agreement, thereby requiring the consent of all partners before any alteration can be made to the partnership agreement itself.

Partnership Books and Records. On demand, a partner must render to any other partner full and complete information on all matters affecting the partnership business (*UPA* § 20). This rule illustrates an important aspect of group practice; that is, the physician loses considerable privacy in the conduct of his practice. A partner may be required to disclose general information about his financial condition and his health, as well as any other information that might have even a remote effect upon the partnership business. The rationale behind this provision stems from the doctrine that each partner is an agent of the partnership. To supply notice or information to the partnership, one need only inform a partner-agent. If a partner has been given the information, the entire partnership is deemed by law to have been informed. This legal doctrine of imputed knowledge operates whether or not the information actually is conveyed to all partners; therefore, a partner should be made aware of his duty to inform the others and to facilitate actual disclosure. In addition to the rendering of information, each partner is entitled, at all times to have access to the partnership books and records which must be kept at the principal business office of the partnership (*UPA* § 19).

Capital Contributions and Reimbursement. Capital contribution is the amount that a partner agrees to place into partnership assets; the contribution may be in cash or in other forms of personal assets. Subject to agreement to the contrary, a partner is entitled, upon demand, to repayment with interest, of capital or other advances made to the partnership (*UPA* § 18 (a) (d)). When a partner withdraws from the partnership or merely wants his contribution back, he is entitled to it; however, payment of the contribution is subject to the claims of his creditors.

A partner must be reimbursed for all expenses paid or incurred by him in the ordinary conduct of the partnership business (*UPA* § 18 (b) (c)). For example, if a partner must advance a sum of money to a medical supply firm in order to purchase equipment, this advance is considered a loan to be paid back with interest. The partner cannot demand reimbursement, however, if the expense was incurred due to his own negligence, or if it was not incurred as a part of the partnership business.

Payment for Partners' Services. A partner is not an actual employee and, therefore, does not receive a salary as such. Rather, he receives a share of the profits of the business, which may or may not be determined according to his productivity. While a salary and a share of profits based upon production may appear as two sides of the same coin, two basic differences can be identified.

First, the remuneration paid to the physician based upon his share of partnership income is not a business expense and therefore is not tax deductible; secondly, the physician's income is not in exchange for work performed for an employer. The physician is the employer owner, and he cannot be a salaried employee of himself. As a result, no partner is entitled to remuneration of his services, on behalf of the partnership, except with the consent of all partners. The *Uniform Partnership Act*, however, does allow a partner, who is winding up the business after dissolution of the partnership, to receive salaried compensation for such services (*UPA* § 18 (f)). The doctrine regarding remuneration may be different in those states where *UPA* is not in effect. Because a partner does not receive a salary, he is entitled to such share of the profits of the partnership as is specified in the partnership agreement, and he must contribute toward the losses according to his share of the profits. In the absence of a partnership agreement to the contrary, the partners share profits and losses equally (*UPA* § 18 (a)). If the partners have not agreed to another formula, the more productive physician has no more right to a greater share of the practice's profits than does the less productive physician and he also shares equally in any loss.

The simplest arrangement in an agreement is to provide for equal share of the profits in combination with equal responsibility for the workload. Most partnerships, however, have special circumstances that justify an alteration of the equal share arrangement. These circumstances may be numerous and varied in nature, but usually involve a partner or partners who are more valuable to the practice's income than bookings reflect. Various arrangements available to the partners to include in the partnership agreement are discussed in detail in Chapter 9; however, listed below are a number of general considerations.

1. *Guaranteed Minimum to Founder.* For a medical group partnership that developed from the nucleus of one or a few established practitioners, the agreement may provide for a guaranteed minimum of the profits up to a certain amount with a 50-50 split for any profits over the stated amount. The agreement also could outline the terms of the founder's share of the profits and state the reasons for the arrangement. The minimum is usually a set dollar amount subject to change.

2. *Guaranteed Minimum to Newcomer.* A new physician may require special consideration in the profit distribution because of the time needed to establish his bookings. The usual solution to the newcomer's need for a stable income is to provide in the agreements for a minimum share of the profits for a certain period of time. The new partner would receive a certain amount, plus any amounts due him from his own bookings, if any. If the newcomer is an employee, the arrangement would be a salary and not part of profit distribution. The guaranteed minimums to newcomers usually are enforced for a very short time. Most existing practices, however, do not recruit partners. Rather, they usually recruit physicians to practice in the capacity of physicians employed by the partnership for a specified period prior to becoming eligible for partner status.

3. *Guarantees to All.* The guaranteed minimum approach can be modified to provide for guarantees to both the senior and junior partners in the practice. The typical arrangement involves an unequal percentage distribution up to a certain amount and equal percentage distribution of profits after that amount.

For example, for the first $40,000, the seniors would receive 75 percent and juniors would divide the remaining 25 percent, but any profits above $40,000 would be divided equally. By retaining this arrangement on a permanent basis, the partnership provides a monetary incentive to retain the experienced physician who has the ability for high income production.

4. *Equality and Production.* Another alternative involves the merger of an equal share system with one based upon actual bookings. The arrangement under this alternative could develop in the following manner. The physicians would share equally in the first one-half of income and distribute the second half based upon the percentage for each physician of total bookings. All physicians, therefore, would receive an equal floor amount, but those physicians who have a more productive practice would receive an amount reflecting their productivity. This arrangement has the advantage of providing incentive, but represents a disadvantage for those physicians whose specialty is not as busy as others; their share of profit will be permanently less.

5. *Every Man for Himself.* For various reasons, some physicians may prefer to distribute profits based exclusively upon the partner's actual production. The profits are divided according to the physician's percentage share of the partnership's total booking. Adjustments can be made for those specialties with a low volume but higher costs of care, or for those specialties which usually involve high patient charges. These alternatives, however, share the common perspective of keeping a partner's income completely tied to his actual production.[5]

6. *Point System.* Many partnerships have established remuneration systems based upon each physician's receiving a share of the profits according to the number of points he has accumulated. In drawing up point systems, the following factors may be used to establish points: seniority, group value, number of patients referred to other partners, productivity, publications and research, and administrative activity. Conversely, points may be deducted to reflect the costs to the partnership of a particular specialty. A point system may provide incentive for a well-rounded physician who is interested in his work, in further training, and in writing and research. On the other hand, the point system is difficult to establish and can cause friction if hard-to-define factors such as group value or professional standing play a prominent role in point assignment or deduction. The need to constantly review and modify as necessary the point assignment is critical to its proper functioning.[6]

The chart below reflects the operation of a point system for a partnership in which each physician had practiced for a different number of years. Dr. Kearney joined Dr. Francis shortly before they formed a partnership and Dr. Joseph was brought into the organization in 1964. Although this model represents a three-physician partnership, it could be adapted to a greater number of physicians.

An example—not to be adapted for actual use without legal advice—is the income clause below. Elsewhere it is specified that net income is what remains after partnership expenses have been paid out of the common kitty.

The monthly net income as defined in this agreement shall be shared among the partners proportionately to the points allotted each of them as follows, as of April 1 each year:

	1964	*1965*	*1966*	*1967*	*1968 on*
Theodore Francis, M.D.	20	20	20	20	20
Ralph Kearney, M.D.	12	16	20	20	20
Albert Joseph, M.D.	8	11	14	17	20
Total points	40	47	54	57	60

The distribution shall be made in the following manner: The net income for each month shall be divided by the total points of all the partners to determine the value of one point, and the share of each partner for that month shall be the value of one point multiplied by the number of points to which he is entitled. Distribution of monthly net income shall be made not later than the tenth day of the month following the month in which it is earned.[7]

Profit-Sharing and Pension Plan. Although pension and profit-sharing plans will be discussed more thoroughly later in this chapter, an introduction to the arrangements available to a partnership is presented here. In 1962, the KEOGH Regulation (HR–10 or Self-Employed Individuals Retirement Act) was enacted to enable self-employed professionals organized as sole owners or partners to establish a tax-deferred pension plan. Under this plan, the employer partner is allowed to contribute a designated portion of his income to a pension trust fund. Any pension or profit-sharing plan adopted, however, must be submitted to the Treasury Department for a qualification or approval, and it cannot discriminate in favor of owner-employees. In the case of a qualified pension plan, contributions of 15 percent of earned income or $1,500, whichever is the lesser, are deductible to the employer partner, and the earnings of the trust fund are not taxed to the trust. The partner or beneficiary must pay ordinary income tax on benefits when they are received; however, the recipient is usually in a lower tax bracket when he finally is taxed on the contribution.

The pension plan provides income upon retirement; retirement age usually is designated in the partnership agreement, with provisions for early or deferred retirement, as well as disability retirement. By removing the necessity for a physician to have to practice in his later years, a pattern can be set for keeping the activities of the organization in the hands of active personnel. Furthermore, a pension plan can help stabilize personnel and reduce turnover by fulfilling an obligation to individuals who have devoted a lifetime of service to the partnership practice.[8]

Taxation. Unlike a corporation, partnerships are not taxpayers and do not pay federal income tax on the income generated by the partnership business. Rather, each individual partner is taxed directly on his share of the partnership's taxable income. The partner also may include in his individual return any losses that the partnership may have suffered.[9] A partner's share of the tax liability is determined by either his share of the partnership's profits, gains, or losses as determined in the partnership agreement or by *Internal Revenue Code* provisions which operate in the absence of such an agreement.[10] In other words, the Internal Revenue Service does not consider the partnership as an entity with income, but considers its income to be the individual income of the participating partners. This approach presents desirable tax consequences for the individual partner since he is able to treat the partnership income in his tax return as having the same status as it would have for the partnership itself. For example, if the income was tax exempt, the partner need not include it, and partnership depreciation and business losses may be applied against the income of the individual partner.

A partner may not deduct as a business expense any earnings paid to himself, unless the remuneration occurs when he deals with the partnership in a nonpartner capacity, or unless guaranteed payments are made to a partner without regard to the profits of the partnership (i.e., special administrative work).

The general partnership is required to file an information return (currently Form #1065) indicating its profits and losses and showing the methods chosen for the computation of its taxes and the income attributed to the partners' individual returns.[11] The partnership return determines methods of accounting, computation of depreciation, and deduction of other expenses. A partner cannot alter any of the tax methods on accounting procedures from the manner in which such methods are stated in the partnership filing.

Relations of the Partners and the Partnership to Third Persons

The partnership's relations with its patients, creditors, and others are manifested through the conduct of each partner. The business is an aggregate of the common activity and conduct of all the partners, but in order to transact business with the partnership, an outsider often must deal with a single partner. Each partner, therefore, must have the authority from the partnership to speak and act for it.[12]

Partner as the Agent of the Partnership. "Every partner is the agent of the partnership for the purpose of its business, and the act of every partner, including the execution in the partnership name of any instrument, for apparently carrying on in the usual way the business of the partnership of which he is a member, binds the partnership, unless the partner so acting has in fact, no authority to act for the partnership for the particular matter, and the person with whom he is dealing has knowledge of the fact that he has no such authority" (*UPA* § 9 (1)).

While at first glance the above provision appears to be straightforward, it actually provides only for a general grant of authority conferred by law upon a partner which can be altered by agreement of the partners or by other limiting provisions of law.

The *Uniform Partnership Act* provisions specifically state that a partner is an agent. The concept of agency is defined as: "The fiduciary relation which results from the manifestation of consent by one person to another that the other shall act on his behalf and subject to his control, and consent to so act."[13] To conform properly with this definition of agency, the partnership agreement should contain a specific authorization for each partner to act on behalf of and with the consent of the partnership. With an agency provision, each partner is the expressed agent of the partnership and possesses the authority to act as such. The *UPA* provisions state, however, that this agency authority exists only if the partnership does not rescind it. According to law, the partner is the agent of the partnership, and the law assumes that the partnership relation contains the manifestation of authority regardless of an expressed authorization. By operational law, the authority of the partner to deal in partnership affairs (as this authority arises out of the partnership relation) is termed *apparent authority.*[14]

The apparent authority of the partner extends only to those acts that relate to the usual business of the partnership. For example, in order for a third person to hold the Gotham Clinic to an obligation made by Dr. Smith, that person must prove that the obligation is related to the clinic's usual business. The purpose of the law is to provide assurance to patients or creditors that by dealing with the partner they are, in fact, dealing with the partnership. An act that is obviously against the interests of the partnership, however, should be recognized as such by the third person and, as a result, is not binding upon the partnership.[15] An act that is against the interests of the partnership can bind the partnership only if the partners actually have authorized the act (*UPA* §9 (2)). For example, if Dr. Smith promises a patient that the partnership will treat the patient and his family free of charge for the rest of their lives, such a promise may seem outside and actually contrary to the business interests of the partnership. Of course, regardless of the nature of the act, if the third person knew, in fact, that the physician had no authority to make such agreements, then the act cannot bind the partnership (*UPA* §9 (4)). The members of some groups, however, may establish special center policies such as not requiring medicare patients to pay deductibles and co-insurance.

A partner, therefore, is deemed to have authority to bind the partnership in pursuance of its business. The partnership can rely upon the law to protect it against claims made by third persons based on acts obvious to a reasonable man to be outside normal partnership business. If, in order to provide for the safety of the group, the partnership has removed authority from a partner to act for the partnership in certain matters, it must inform the third person of these limitations to prevent being obligated by his acts. The following list includes actions and powers which are part of a partner's authority unless specifically restricted:

1. *Compromise and Pay Bonafide Debts.* A partner may pay debts that the practice owes, either with the partnership funds or by transferring partnership property.
2. *Release Claims Against the Partnership.* In addition to paying debts, partners have the power to settle with those who have claims against the partnership and to obtain releases for the partnership.
3. *Payment of Personal Debts with Partnership Funds.* If a partner uses partnership funds to pay his debts, he is required to account to the partnership for those funds. The partnership, however, cannot refuse to pay his creditor those funds, if the creditor has agreed, in good faith, to the payment.
4. *Obligating the Partnership for the Purchase or Acquisition of Property.* The physician has the authority to make pledges or obligate the partnership for any expense or purchase that is within the nature of the partnership's practice.
5. *Hiring and Firing Employees.*
6. *Execution of Contracts for the Use of the Personal Property of the Partnership.* For example, the physician may lease assets of the practice. If the

partner leases an asset essential to the carrying on of the practice, however, such an act will not bind the partnership.[16]

7. *Receipt of Information for the Partnership.* Any knowledge or notice given by a third person to a partner concerning matters which pertain to the partnership business is considered to have been given to all of the partners and is binding upon them. For example, if a patient notifies Dr. Jones that the patient cannot make his 2:00 P.M. appointment, then all the partners are thereby notified of the cancellation (*UPA* §12). Of course, if a partner is acting adversely to the interests of the partnership, then notice to him will not be imputed to the partnership.

Limitations on Authority. Those considering partnership practice should not become too alarmed by the apparent magnitude of partner powers just discussed. The authority of partners also has been limited by law to prevent certain activities that would tend to destroy or disrupt the ability of the partnership to carry on normal business (*UPA* §1 (3)). Unless the partnership business has been abandoned or the partnership has expressly authorized otherwise, a partner does not have authority to assign any partnership property for the benefit of creditors; to submit a partnership claim or liability to arbitration; or to acknowledge a claim against the partnership. A partner cannot dispose of the good will, reputation, or trade name of the partnership, nor can he bind the partnership assets for nonbusiness purposes, intermingle his own financial obligations with those of the partnership, or perform any act that would make it impossible to carry on the ordinary business of the partnership.[17]

The law assumes that the provisions of statutes and court decisions are known by all. Consequently, any third person dealing with a partner under the above limitations of authority cannot claim ignorance of the law if unauthorized action on the part of a partner is not honored by the partnership.

To avoid being bound by business actions of his partners, a physician may announce that his partners no longer have the authority to act for the partnership. Since the majority rules in a partnership, it is doubtful that a single partner, as a minority, can terminate the authority of any co-partner to bind him as a partner without dissolving the partnership prior to the act in question (*UPA* §18 (h)).

Partnership Liability. The partnership can become liable to third persons either by a contract entered into by a partner or by an injury or "tort" done to a third person by a partner.[b] "For those claims based upon breach of contract, the partners are *jointly* liable." A contract creditor must sue all of the partners to be entitled to damages from all partners (*UPA* § 15(b)). He cannot simply sue one partner and then take his court judgment to the other partners to be honored. For example, if Dr. Smith purchases machinery for the Gotham Medical Partnership from the ABC Company, ABC would have to sue all partners to recover the price for the equipment from all partners. A suit against only Dr. Smith would prevent ABC from later bringing action against other partners for any balance remaining after Dr. Smith's payments. Furthermore,

[b]A tort is a legal term for an injury incurred by a person to himself or his property for which he may seek damages in a court of law.

many states expand upon this joint liability by providing that, if a contract creditor has released a partner from an obligation, then all partners have been released. In many cases, a creditor may be able to avoid the need to join all partners by suing the partnership as an entity.

"All partners are *jointly* and *severally* liable for torts committed by a partner while he was engaged in partnership business" (*UPA* § 15(a)). Torts can include fraud in dealing with others, negligent treatment of a patient, deceit, and negligent conduct while pursuing partnership business. Joint and several liability means that a partner is not only responsible for torts committed by any copartner, but he is individually liable for all the damages, regardless of the failure of the injured party to sue him. In other words, as indicated above, a third person who is suing for a contract claim and fails to include one of the partners in his lawsuit, cannot later file another lawsuit to require the excluded partner to pay; however, if the third person is making a tort claim, he can bring a separate lawsuit against every partner until his claim is satisfied. For example, if Dr. Slow negligently treats Mr. Fast, Mr. Fast can then sue Dr. Slow or any of his partners and can continue to sue the partners until he is satisfied. In the case of joint and several liability, failure to sue all partners at the same time does not prevent Mr. Fast from suing different partners at another time. In the case of criminal acts committed by a partner, the state cannot extend criminal liability to the other partners, unless the criminal act was committed within the scope of the partnership business, or unless the other partners approved or took part in the act.

Remedies Available to Third Persons. Remedies are the award or judgment that a creditor or injured person receives should he be successful in a court suit against a partner or the partnership. For obligations on judgments against the partnership, the successful plaintiff can assume the partnership property, cash, or other assets; if partnership assets are not adequate, the partners are personally liable for the balance. This procedure, however, is available only for the satisfaction of partnership wrongs; the personal creditor of a partner seeking to satisfy his claims cannot reach the assets of the partnership. While the partnership, as a business, is secure from the claims of personal creditors of a partner, a personal creditor may reach a partner's interest in the partnership. By taking the partner's interest, a personal creditor may be the recipient of the partner's share of the profits, but the partner remains at his medical practice within the group.

Entering a medical group practice partnership requires the physician to choose carefully and to analyze the potential of his future associates. The physician will be working in close quarters and for long hours with several different people; he will have obligations towards them as well as rights of his own that others must respect. In his relations with the public, however, he will become part of a different entity. The partners will deal with third persons as a group. It is vital, therefore, for the physician to consider the responsibilities inherent in practicing medicine as a group partner. Any partner in the group has the authority to bind the partnership and all of the partners to contractual obligations (joint liability). Any partner's negligent act which occurs while pursuing the business of the partnership will make other partners responsible to the injured party (joint and several liability). The physician must realize that the debts of the partnership can result in the loss of the partnership's assets, and can render him obliged to personally cover those debts, if partnership assets are inadequate.

Partnership Property and the Property Interest of the Partners

The major assets of the medical partnership are the talents and skills of the physician partners. There is some property, however, such as the owned or leased office or office building and the medical and office equipment, which a medical partnership may need to provide care. The property or assets either may be owned by the medical partnership, or may be owned by another organization or individual and rented to the medical partnership.

Although some partnerships do own all of their equipment, the usual arrangement is for some or all of the partners to form a separate partnership or corporation to own the assets. Under this arrangement, the medical partnership's capital or property is essentially an established amount of cash. When a physician joins the partnership, he usually pays a stated amount; when he departs, he receives reimbursement for his partnership interests. Each physician usually is given an opportunity to buy into the physical assets of the organization. If the medical partnership owns all of its equipment, the amount needed by a new partner to buy in might be quite substantial; conversely, the partnership could be faced with an overwhelming obligation if a departing partner should demand immediate return of his contribution. When a separate organization is used to own the assets, however, a physician can withdraw from the medical partnership and still remain a partner in the asset organization. In addition, individuals other than medical partners can buy into the asset partnership or corporation.

Although the medical partnership can form a corporation to own the assets, the discussion here will be concerned only with the ownership of the assets by a separate partnership or by the medical partnership.

Real and Personal Property. A partnership may own both real and personal property. Real property is land and any attached improvements to that land. For example, if a medical partnership owns a lot, that land is considered its real property. Any structures or improvements on the land, such as a building, house, driveway, or vegetation, also are considered as part of the partnership's real property. Personal property includes all other assets, equipment, or devices, such as office equipment, automobiles, and furnishings. A lease for use of land also is considered to be personal property.

Prior to adoption of the *UPA*, a partnership was considered an aggregate of individuals and, therefore, was incapable of owning either the real or personal property in its own name. The current view, however, does provide that the partnership may hold, own, and transfer property in its own name (*UPA* §8 (3)).

Determination of Property Ownership. One of the most common areas of controversy involved in partnership law is the determination of whether a partnership asset belongs to the partnership or whether it is being used by the partnership and actually is owned by the individual partners. The mere use or possession of a particular piece of property does not make it partnership property.[18] The intentions of the partners will govern the determination of whether the property is to be considered as partnership property. In addition, any property brought into the partnership at its formation, through contribution, and any property subsequently purchased or otherwise acquired for or on account of the partnership, usually is considered to be partnership property (*UPA* §8 (1)). Unless a contrary intention is apparent, property acquired with partnership funds is partnership property (*UPA* §8 (2)). To help prevent possible confusion, the partnership records should designate clearly what property it owns and should treat other property as leased.

Property Interests of the Partners. Although partnership property does belong to the partnership, each partner has certain rights or interests in the property and in the business of the partnership, and these rights are considered by many physicians to be a primary concern in forming a partnership. The proper rights of a partner include his rights in specific property, his interest in the partnership, and his right to participate in the management of the partnership (*UPA* §24).

Partners' Rights in Specific Partnership Property. When an individual owns or has an interest in property, he is said to have a tenancy in that property. The concept of tenancy should not be confused with the concept of a leasing tenant; the former notion refers to a partner's actually owning rather than leasing property. The tenancy of the partner is not exclusive because he shares his ownership rights with other partners. A partner is, therefore, a tenant in partnership for each partnership asset he owns with his copartners (*UPA* §25 (1)). The rights and limitations of a partner's tenancy include:

1. In the absence of a contrary agreement, each partner has the equal right to the access and the use of the firm's property for partnership business.
2. A partner cannot assign or sell his interest in the property unless he does so with the agreement of all other partners.
3. A partner's interest in the specific property can be assumed only by creditors of the partnership.
4. The partner's spouse or family cannot acquire any of his rights in the property by virtue of marriage or birth.[19]

Ownership of the partnership property is dependent upon membership in the partnership. If a partner dies, his rights in the partnership remain with the partnership and the remaining partners; if he withdraws from the partnership, however, thereby causing dissolution, he will be entitled to his distributive share of the property.

Partners' Interest in the Business of the Partnership. A partner also has a "property right" in the business of the partnership; he has a right to receive a portion of the income generated by the partnership. The partners' interest in the firm is considered to be personal property, regardless of the ownership of any real property by the partnership. In the absence of an agreement to the contrary, a partner may assign, sell, or otherwise dispose of his interest in the partnership, and such an assignment or sale does *not* dissolve the partnership (*UPA* §27 (1)). The holder of a partner's interest is entitled to receive only the profits and capital to which the partner would be entitled. The holder is *not* a partner and does not have any right to interfere in the management of the partnership (*UPA* §27 (1)). Finally, the partner's spouse or heirs receive a right in the partner's interest in the partnership as a result of marriage or descent.

Unlike the partner's property right in the partnership property, his personal creditors are able to reach his interest in the partnership to satisfy their claims. The creditor must bring his claim to court and obtain a judgment in his favor. The creditor may then take his judgment to court again and obtain a charging order against the debtor partner. The charging order is presented to the partnership, and the partnership is obligated to pay to the creditor whatever share of the profits is due the partner until the judgment is paid off. The creditor is known as a charging creditor (*UPA* §28) and, in certain cases, can cause a dissolution of the partnership to satisfy his judgment (*UPA* §32 (f)(2)).

Although the physician may view a medical partnership as a service organization, it is also a business and as such does own property. The medical partnership can own real property (land) and personal property (equipment, supplies, etc.) in its own name, or the physicians can form another organization to own the assets. If a partnership form is chosen to own the assets, the property must be classified as to partnership ownership or merely partnership use. Only partners can have a tenancy in partnership property. The partner's property rights in the partnership enable him to have access to and use of the property for partnership business; however, his tenancy is limited by the presence of his partners' rights to use of the property. A partner also has an interest in the profits and surplus of the partnership business which is considered personal property; he may sell his interest and his creditors may obtain a court order to assume his interest.

Partnership Dissolution and Winding Up

Dissolution is an important consideration requiring clarification at the onset of the partnership. Hopefully, by understanding the essential points of dissolution, the prospective partners can provide and plan for such a contingency.

Because a partnership is essentially an agreement by all partners to practice together and pursue a profession, the partnership is composed of and peculiar to those physicians forming the group. If a physician dies, retires, or otherwise departs from the group, the remaining partners no longer comprise the same group that initially made mutual promises to pursue a medical practice. Of course, some of the group can immediately form a new partnership and continue the medical practice, but it is important to realize that the new partnership is a replacement, not a continuation of the old partnership.

Definitions. Dissolution can be understood by discussing the conditions under which it occurs. According to the *UPA*, the "dissolution of a partnership is the occurrence of some event which causes any partner to be unable to participate in the carrying on of the partnership business" (*UPA* §29). Dissolution does mark a point at which the ability of the partners to carry on new business ends, and they must re-form into a new group or disband. The dissolution, however, does not mean that the partnership is terminated; it must fulfill its obligations and complete, or wind up, its current business (*UPA* §29). Although the capability to be an ongoing business ends by dissolution, the partnership relations, including the duties, rights, and obligations of the partners, continue until the winding up of the partnership affairs is completed (*UPA* §30). The process for winding up the partnership is dependent upon whether some or all of the remaining partners continue to practice as a new group, or whether the partners go their separate ways. If the practice continues, winding up may require only the transfer of the old partnership's assets, accounts, and obligations to the new partnership. Disbursal, however, will require liquidation of assets and distribution of patients and records.

Cause of Dissolution. The partnership agreement can provide additional circumstances under which the partnership dissolves. The partnership is dissolved by law, however, under the following circumstances:

1. *Expiration of the Term of the Partnership or the Completion of its Purpose.* If the partnership agreement states a term or a purpose, then according to the terms so stated, the partnership expires (*UPA* §31 (1)a). If the partners want to continue to practice after the term, then they will become partners at will. Under the new partnership at will, the rights and duties of the partners remain the same as before, unless this is inconsistent with the will of any partner (*UPA* §23).

2. *Express Will of a Partner.* No one can be forced to remain a partner. Although an individual physician may be responsible for losses caused to his partners, they cannot prevent him from leaving. In order to affect a dissolution, therefore, a partner must give his intent to discontinue the existing partnership relation. If a partner causes dissolution in violation of an agreement, he has breached his promises to his partners and may owe them damages (*UPA* §31 (2)). If the partnership depends upon the continuous will of the partners, then the intention to dissolve follows the terms of the agreement, and no legal injury can occur to the other partners (*UPA* §31 (1) b).

3. *Withdrawal or Admission of a Partner.* Legally, the partnership is changed if a new person enters it or an existing partner withdraws. Because of this change, a new agreement must be made. Partnership agreements, however, can be drafted to allow for admission of new partners and the continuation of the agreement by having the new physician sign the old agreement. The agreement itself contains the expressed will of the partners to carry on when a partner joins or withdraws (*UPA* §31 (1) c).

4. *Expulsion of a Partner.* Dissolution is caused whenever a partner is expelled from the business. If the expulsion is in good faith and pursuant to the agreement, the agreement is not breached and the remaining partners are not liable to the expelled partner. If the expulsion is not made in good faith or without power conferred by the agreement, the expelled partner is entitled to damages; however, he cannot force a restoration of the partnership (*UPA* §31 (1) d).

5. *Illegality.* The partnership is dissolved by any event which makes it un-

lawful for the business of the partnership to be carried on, or for the members to carry on as a partnership (*UPA* §31 (3)). The partners, however, may be able to continue by changing the partnership purpose.

6. *Death of Any Partner* (*UPA* §31 (4)).

7. *Bankruptcy of Any Partner.* Since a partner's ability to guarantee the debts of the partnership is essential, the bankruptcy of a partner causes dissolution (*UPA* §31 (5)).

8. *Decree of a Court.* A court may order a partnership to dissolve as a result of certain circumstances that are discussed below (*UPA* §31 (6)).

The above list indicates the events which by law can independently terminate the partnership; other events, however, require judicial action to cause dissolution. A partner, or any other person who owns a partner's interest, may bring an application to the court based upon one of the criteria set forth below. The proceeding for dissolution is one of equity because the court is being asked to order that the partnership be dissolved. In an equity proceeding, the court usually considers all the facts, circumstances, and possible consequences in deciding the order to dissolve. The dissolution action is accompanied by an action for accounting which requires the court, if the court orders dissolution, to determine the share of profits or losses for each partner upon distribution of assets.

The following list includes the circumstances under which the court shall order a dissolution:

1. *Insanity.* The dissolution will be ordered if the court finds any partner to be insane (*UPA* §32 (1) a).
2. *Incapability to Perform Contract Obligations.* If a partner has become permanently incapable of performing the obligations he agreed to in the partnership agreement, a court shall order dissolution (*UPA* §32 (1) b).
3. *Prejudicial Conduct.* The partnership shall be dissolved whenever a court finds that a partner has been conducting himself in such a way that tends to prejudicially affect the carrying on of the business, including: (1) breach of the partnership agreement, (2) pursuing self-interests, (3) criminal activity, or (4) any activity that would not make it reasonable for the partnership to carry on with him (*UPA* §32 (1) c, d).
4. *Inevitable Loss.* The dissolution will be ordered if the business of the partnership can only be carried on at a loss (*UPA* §32 (1) e).
5. *Other Equitable Circumstances* (*UPA* §32 (1) f).
6. *Request of a Holder of a Partner's Interest.* When a holder of a partner's interest in the partnership requests, the court will grant dissolution if the partnership term has expired (*UPA* §32 (2)).

It should be noted that the court is required, by the use of the word *shall* in the law, to order a dissolution if it finds that one of the above circumstances is satisfied.

Effect of Dissolution. Except for the winding up of the affairs of the partnership, dissolution terminates all authority of any partner to act for the partnership (*UPA* §§33,34). If the partnership is dissolved by a definite and foreseeable cause, such as expiration of a term or court order, then all partners should be aware of the dissolution. In some cases, however, dissolution can occur without the knowledge of a partner (*UPA* §34). For example, if Dr. Smythe is out of town purchasing equipment for the partnership when his partner dies, then the partnership and partners will remain liable for the purchase, provided that Dr. Smythe is unaware of the dissolution. An act performed by a partner after dissolution will bind the partnership to the third person if the third person either knew of the partnership before or had dealt with it before, and if the third person did not know of the dissolution (*UPA* §35). In no case, however, will the partnership be bound by an act occurring after dissolution, if the dissolution was caused because it would be illegal to carry on the business, or if the partner performing the act became bankrupt (*UPA* §35 (3)).

Although dissolution does terminate authority, it does not terminate the liability of the partners for partnership debts or claims made by the partnership prior to dissolution (*UPA* §36). The partners, however, can agree among themselves who will continue to be responsible for the debts. The partners whose obligations have been assumed are released if the creditors agree to the assumption. Agreement to discharge a partner from liability can be expressed or can be implied from the creditor's conduct (*UPA* §36 (2, 3)).

If the business of the partnership is carried on after dissolution by the remaining partners, alone or with the addition of new partners, the new partnership remains liable for all of the debts of the previous partnership. The new partnership has, by law, assumed the debts of the old partnership and remains liable to its creditors (*UPA* §41). Those partners who did not continue in the new partnership usually will be paid their interest or share in the partnership just as if it actually had been liquidated. Each partner's distributive share is that portion left over after payment of creditors; therefore, the remaining partners must calculate what would have been received and then account to the partner. If the business is continued without accounting to a noncontinuing partner, he may demand his share at any time, with interest, or he may demand any profits derived from the use of his right in the property of the dissolved partnership (*UPA* §42).

If a partnership composed of Dr. Smythe and three pediatricians dissolves because Dr. Smythe retires, then Dr. Smythe and his former partners usually will liquidate the business and distribute the profits. Conversely, let us assume that the three pediatricians have decided to stay in the same office, keep the records, and continue to practice. The new practice becomes a replacement business and may account to Dr. Smythe for his interest in the old partnership. The form chosen to terminate Dr. Smythe's partnership interest can have serious tax impacts. Dr. Smythe can be paid his determined interest or arrangements can be made for extended payment of Dr. Smythe's interest. In some cases, however, the pediatricians could decide to continue and not account to Dr. Smythe. If they do so, he may demand payment of his share, plus interest, or in lieu of interest, Dr. Smythe can require payment of any profits attributable to the use of his rights in the property of the old practice. Dr. Smythe is not liable for the debts of the new group if he informs those people who deal with the partnership of his departure (*UPA* §35 (1)).

Winding Up. Unless otherwise agreed, upon dissolution any partner who is not responsible for dissolution due to contravention of the agreement or by his unlawful conduct has the right to wind up the partnership affairs and in this capacity has the authority to bind the partnership and the partners (*UPA* §37). As the agent of the partnership, the remaining partner(s) must act in good faith and is entitled to compensation for his services in winding up (*UPA* §18 (f)).

When dissolution occurs, except in violation of the partnership agreement, each partner is entitled to have partnership property applied to discharge the liabilities of the partnership and to have the surplus applied to pay in cash the net distributive share owed to each respective partner (*UPA* §38 (1)). In addition, if dissolution was caused by the violation of the agreement by a partner, the nonviolating partners may seek damages from the violating partner for breach of the agreement and are entitled to continue the practice possessing the partnership property for the duration of its term (*UPA* §38 (a) II). The violating partner is entitled to have his interest paid to him if the practice is carried on and he is released by his former partners from all existing liability (*UPA* §38 (c) II). For example, if Drs. Smith, Green, and Brown have been partners in the Hill Top Clinic for a term of six years, and after three years Dr. Brown tells his partners that he is quitting the practice to take up cattle raising, then Dr. Brown has wrongfully caused dissolution of the partnership in violation of the agreement. Dr. Smith and Dr. Green cannot prevent Dr. Brown from leaving and must account to Dr. Brown for the net amount owed to him. The remaining partners, however, can deduct from Dr. Brown's share any losses that the practice suffers due to Dr. Brown's departure. Dr. Green and Dr. Smith can continue in possession of the property and continue the practice until the end of the term. In order to continue, however, Dr. Green and Dr. Smith must release Dr. Brown from any existing liability; this release operates only as a promise between the partners, and unless the creditors agree to it, Dr. Brown is still liable to them.

Distribution of Assets. After dissolution and the termination of the rights of the partners, the partnership accounts must be settled. Subject to some alterations in an agreement, the distribution of the partnership's assets is accomplished in the following order:

1. *Creditors.* Payment of the liabilities of the partnership owed to its creditors (*UPA* §40 (b) I).
2. *Creditor Partners.* Payment of loans, advances, or any other liabilities owed to a partner, except for capital contribution or shares of profit (*UPA* §40 (b) II).
3. *Capital.* Return of whatever remains of the capital initially contributed to the partnership by the partners (*UPA* §40(b) III).
4. *Profits.* Distribution of profits to the partners according to their respective share (*UPA* §40 (b) IV).

If the liabilities exhaust the assets of the partnership, the partners will be required to satisfy the creditors personally. Each partner's share of loss contribution will be determined in the same manner as was his respective share of profits.

Agreement Provisions for Dissolution. A group may lose a partner at any time through resignation or death. Unless there is a clause in the partnership agreement which stipulates that such an occurrence does not cause immediate dissolution of the partnership, the physician partner must be prepared for the expense and activities involved, as well as the absence from his practice, that dissolution can cause. At the inception of the partnership, cooperation among the partners usually is strong. At this time, agreement on dissolution affairs may be more readily obtained than at a later date, and it may be expedient to provide a non-dissolution clause in the partnership contract. In the absence of such a clause, however, the following aspects of dissolution should be considered for inclusion in the partnership agreement:

1. *Notices*: Where the partnership is dependent upon the will of the partners, a provision for notice provides the partners with adequate time to prepare for separating or for the formation of a succeeding partnership. The use of a notice clause allows for the physicians to notify patients of any adverse effects the dissolution may have upon their care.[20]

2. *Providing for Death*: Although some deaths are predictable, many cannot be foreseen and specific arrangements are not possible. General provisions, however, such as the buy-out of the deceased partner's interest by the surviving partners, can be formulated in advance, and the obligation to sell can be made binding upon the deceased partner's representative or estate.[21] The partners may wish to provide that the buy-out occurring upon death, retirement, or disability, be made in installments to allow a constant source of income for the departing physician or for his family. The method of evaluating a departing partner's interest may be a gross cash figure, a percentage of current accounts receivable, or a settlement amount. The method should be established in the agreement in order to avoid confusion and later controversy.[22]

3. *Office.* Usually when the partners are unequal owners or when one partner has seniority, the majority or senior partner will remain in the office space and will be required to buy out the vacating partner's interest in the furniture and other property in the office. The price can be set in a variety of ways including: (1) original cost of the items minus depreciation, (2) independent appraisal, or (3) a preset formula. If the partners are equal owners or of equal experience, the need for prior agreement as to who remains is critical. The partners may consider requiring the premises to be vacated by all if agreement cannot be reached on who is to remain.[23]

4. *Disposition of Records.* As with the decision on the use of the office, medical records may remain with the senior partner or with the majority owner physician. If the departing partner is to leave the community, then the medical records should be distributed to the physicians who remain in the area.[24] The physician who first saw the patient may retain that patient's records, or the records can be apportioned according to the physicians' estimates of the patients' preferences. Wrong guesses can be remedied by provision for the delivery of the record to the doctor chosen by the patient directly. A final alternative is to photocopy the records and supply each physician with a copy.[25]

5. *Goodwill.* Essentially, goodwill is an intangible asset that represents the professional stature, general reputation, good name, etc. that a physician has contributed to the practice. If the remaining partners wish to continue the practice, they will have to buy from the departing partner not only his interest in the tangible assets of the practice, but also his interest in the reputation, trade, and custom of the practice. For example, since Dr. Smith founded the

Prestige Medical Clinic several years ago, due to its reputation, patient following, or stature, that name has come to represent a definite business advantage to anyone practicing under it. When Dr. Smith departs, therefore, the remaining partners must pay for the continued use of the name. Dr. Smith should be paid for his efforts in establishing the Prestige Clinic as a recognized medical practice. Some agreements specifically exclude goodwill as an asset and refuse to allow it to be considered upon dissolution. If it is recognized as an asset, however, provisions should be made for its evaluation. It should also be remembered that if the goodwill is transferred to the partners pro rata and if the IRS is able to establish that the goodwill has a substantial value, the partners receiving it may face large tax liabilities. It is for this reason that it may be wise to provide in partnership agreements that the resignation or death of a partner does not terminate the partnership.

6. *Accounts Receivable.* Accounts receivable represent the past services of the partners and a future source of income. For the partnership that is liquidating, the usual arrangement is to continue the winding up procedure until all of the collectible accounts receivable have been paid. If the business is to be continued, which usually is the case, provisions must be made to ensure that the departing partner will receive either his share of the income from accounts receivable or a fair settlement for his share. There are three alternative methods for handling a departing partner's share of the accounts:

a. *Limited Time Method.* The departing partner receives his full share of accounts receivable, less business and collection expenses, but only for a limited amount of time, such as six months or a year.[26]

b. *Bargain Sale.* The remaining partners are required to pay the departing physician a certain amount in settlement of his right to receive his share of the accounts receivable. By accepting payment of the settlement price, the departing partner loses all rights to receive any share of the accounts receivable. The payment can be a set amount of cash or can be based upon a percentage of the partner's share of accounts.[27]

c. *Sale by Formula.* This alternative is similar to the bargain sale, but the determination of the amount involves a more complicated formula. The departing partner receives an amount equal to "R–V–L–C" multiplied by "S" where:

where:

R = the total amount of accounts receivable

V = the amount that is deemed uncollectible

L = the normal collection losses

C = the estimated booking costs of forwarding the money to the departed partner

S = the departing partner's percentage interest in the partnership income at the time of his departure

$$\text{Share} = S(R - V - L - C).$$

In other words, the partner receives his estimated share of accounts receivable after collection costs. Usually, the payment of gross amounts for accounts receivable is paid on an installment basis to provide a constant source of income for the departing partner and to ease the burden on the cash flow of the continuing business.[28]

UNINCORPORATED ASSOCIATIONS

The sole proprietorship, partnership, and corporate organizational models represent the basic legal alternatives available for medical group practice. There are, however, several variations of these basic models, including the unincorporated association and the nonprofit organization.

Despite recent activity in state legislatures to enact laws allowing physicians and other professionals to incorporate their practices, some legal barriers may arise that could lead either to restricting the use of professional corporations or preventing a group of physicians from incorporating their practice. As a response to any restrictions placed upon a professional corporation, a group of physicians may consider the adoption of an unincorporated association as a form of practice. The unincorporated association offers many of the same benefits as a corporation and usually is authorized in most states. While in some states specific statutes exist for the regulation and operation of unincorporated associations, in many other states the use of the unincorporated association model is controlled only loosely by the common law.[c]

Unincorporated Association: Definition

An "unincorporated association" is an organization formed without a charter or process of incorporation for the pursuit of some specific purpose.[29] The association is formed according to a document, usually referred to as the articles of association, which is signed by the original associates and subsequently acknowledged by future members. If the interests of ownership are represented by transferable shares, the association usually is considered as a joint-stock company.[30]

The unincorporated association may be viewed as a hybrid between a partnership and a professional corporation. It has many of the attributes of the corporation such as centralized management, continuity of organization, and transferability of interests, but as in a partnership, each member of an unincorporated association is personally liable for both the professional and business obligations of the association.[31] Furthermore, unlike a corporation, the association is not considered a separate legal entity distinct from the members. Usually, its property cannot be held in the name of the association and the members must join together in pursuing any legal action for the association.

Organization

The association is created by the execution of the articles of association through the original members. State law may require that the articles be filed with a supervising agency, and other statutes may regulate some of the provi-

[c]The *common law*, as frequently defined, includes those principles, usages, and rules of law which do not rest for their authority upon any express statute or written declaration, but upon statements of principles found in the decisions of the courts. As distinguished from statutory or written law, it embraces unwritten law founded upon general custom, usage, or common consent and is based upon natural justice or reason.

sions of the articles. The articles of association bear the same relation to the association as the charter bears to the corporation. The document establishes the governing board and the duties of the officers, the relations of the members of the practice among themselves and the capital contributions of the members, as well as the duration of the practice and the specific professional service to be rendered by the association.[32]

Management and Operation of the Unincorporated Association

Unless the articles of association establish otherwise, each member has a direct voice in the management of the association. Depending upon the size and particular preferences of the group, the association may develop a centralized management which will limit a member's direct control and make most of the day-to-day management duties of the practice the responsibilities of a smaller body.[33] The laws of many states require that all associates be physicians, thereby preventing the interference of nonprofessionals in the operation of the practice.

Due to the unlimited liability of the members, the articles of association usually carefully define the ownership interests of the members. In many states, a physician in an unincorporated association may have to reach into his personal assets to cover the misconduct of an associate if the association's assets are not adequate. Unlimited liability, therefore, necessitates the careful screening of prospective associates on both the shareholder and employee levels. The articles also usually include restrictions on the transfer or sale of ownership interests, similar to the buy-sell or right-of-first-refusal arrangements found in the corporate structure.

Medical Practice in an Association

In some states, because of legal or other considerations, incorporation of a professional practice is not a feasible alternative for the forming group. Under such circumstances, the unincorporated association can offer many of the advantages of corporate practice. The proper drafting of the articles of association can settle traditional partnership problems such as centralized management, establishment of the physician's duties and rights, and designation of the "business" responsibilities of the practice. The association also facilitates better planning for the settlement of an associate's interest at death, retirement, or withdrawal.[34] The ownership interests in the property of the practice and the professional's share of accounts receivable may be reduced to a dollar value prior to an associate's death. In this way, for estate and inheritance tax purposes, the value of the physician's interest can be reflected more accurately than under a partnership arrangement.[35]

The management and operation of an association may be influenced by the Internal Revenue Service's possible classification of an association as another form of corporation for taxation purposes. Often, the more the association resembles a corporation, the higher the likelihood it will be subject to both corporate tax liabilities and benefits. Due to an increase in the value of his "shares," the association form may enable the physician to recover part of his professional income as capital gain. An association practice may be able to utilize compensation benefits similar to those available to corporate employees, such as participation in retirement plans and group insurance, and reasonable salaries paid to an associate-employee, which are usually considered to be a deductible business expense.[36]

As a universal rule, state statutes authorizing professional corporations preserve the personal liability and responsibility of the professional employee. With respect to liabilities arising out of the business of the practice or the negligence of fellow professionals, the corporate shareholder's liability is usually limited to his contribution. The associate, however, may be personally liable for all obligations, both business and professional, incurred by the association while he is a member. Articles of association may contain provisions which limit an associate's liability to the amount of contribution, but in many states these provisions are usually ineffective against third parties, unless those third parties have had previous knowledge of the restrictions.[37]

Apart from the combination of the characteristics of a professional corporation and a partnership, the unincorporated association does contain many unique attributes. It offers the use of centralized management, perpetual duration, and freedom of sale of the "ownership interests"; however, the associates usually will be personally liable for both the professional and business obligations and liabilities of the group practice. The articles of association, similar to the articles of incorporation for a professional corporation, constitute a means by which to establish the framework for the structure of the practice. Unlike a corporation, however, the association is not a separate and distinct entity from its members. For the purposes of the income taxation regulations and its companion benefits, the unincorporated association is taxed as a corporation.

Since the recent enactment of professional corporate statutes in most states, the use of unincorporated associations for a group practice has diminished. For a variety of reasons, however, including the personal desires of the group, the laws of the appropriate state, or various professional considerations, the group may not be able to form a professional corporation. Under these circumstances, the group may want to consider using an unincorporated association model.

NONPROFIT ORGANIZATIONS

This discussion of the legal alternatives for medical group practice has been based on the notion of a practice organized for profit. Because most businesses, including group practices, are organized to make a profit, it would be unrealistic to avoid discussion of the financial aspects of a practice; however, the medical group practice may be organized for nonprofit purposes as well. Traditionally, the quest for profit has been the motivating force in the capitalistic economic system. Parallel to the profit motive, however, has been a composite of many other motives, all of which can be referred to as nonprofit. These motives include religious and moral concepts, resentment of needless emotional and physical suffering, and the desire to help the needy.[38] The physician considering group practice may feel that he owes it to himself and to society to consider providing all or some of his medical services through a nonprofit organization.

Definition of Nonprofit

A nonprofit organization is one that is "not intended to produce monetary gain for its members or professionals, except as salaries for services rendered to the organization." Profit means the excess of income over expenses in an enterprise during a given period. The Internal Revenue Service provides that organizations formed and operated for religious, charitable, scientific, educational, social welfare, and many other purposes will not be taxed on their income surplus and, therefore, by implication defines these organizations as nonprofit.[39]

Other than through the above mentioned general definitions, the precise meaning or characteristics of a nonprofit organization is difficult to capture. Most state laws do not make any serious effort to define nonprofit, both because of the personalized nature of the term "nonprofit," and because an exact definition of terms may aid those who, in attempting to avoid the spirit of the law, will seek "loopholes" to avoid income taxes.[40] As a result, the reader must carefully consider the treatment given the nonprofit organization in his own state. With the help of his attorney, he can decide whether the purposes he has in mind for his medical practice conform to those allowed by the state for a nonprofit organization. Perhaps the only universally applicable guide is motive; when ethical, moral, or social motives are clearly the dominant forces behind medical group practice formation, that practice can be considered nonprofit.[41]

Forms of Nonprofit Organization

The sole proprietorship, partnership, and professional corporation can be formed as nonprofit organizations.

Sole Proprietorship. The recipient of the profits for a sole proprietorship is usually the owner or founder of the practice, and the practice's profits are taxed to him through his individual tax returns. The sole proprietor may contribute some or all of the profits, less his remuneration, to a charitable cause, and through this indirect process, a sole proprietorship may serve nonprofit purposes. Charity or other good deeds performed by individuals usually are encouraged by the community and this encouragement may take the form of approbation and esteem. In addition, the government encourages individual enterprise by allowing charitable contributions, within certain limits, to be tax-deductible. Generally, tax deductions are allowed for gifts to formally organized entities such as corporations, trusts, or associations. Other than the tax relief, however, there is little governmental support for individual philanthropic activity.

Partnership and Association. A partnership is an association of two or more persons who as co-owners conduct a business for profit. A partnership for nonprofit, therefore, actually is a contradiction in terms. Similar to the sole proprietor the partner may donate his profits, less any remuneration, and then deduct the amount donated; however, the partner will face the same regulations on individual philanthropy as does the sole proprietor.

If the profit element of a partnership is eliminated, the result is an association of two or more co-owners to carry on certain activities.[42] In other words, we are left with an unincorporated association. The reader should recall that an association is similar to a corporation and may provide in its articles of association that all profits and property of the association shall be used for nonprofit or charitable purposes. For a professional practice, the association has few advantages over a partnership or corporation, but most of the disadvantages of both. Because of its unique status under the law and because of other disadvantages, the unincorporated association is seldom utilized for a nonprofit medical practice.

Corporation. A nonprofit corporation is usually a nonstock, nonprofit corporation organized under state law for charitable, scientific, philanthropic, religious, or educational purposes. In most states, nonprofit corporation statutes closely resemble or are a definite part of the state's general or professional corporation statutes. The nonprofit corporation, therefore, usually will be subject to all the procedural and substantive requirements discussed next in the professional corporation section.

In most states there must be at least three incorporators to file and acknowledge the articles of incorporation. The articles will describe the framework of the nonprofit corporation, providing for its board of directors, its term of existence, its members, and other basic provisions. The board of directors or trustees, as they may be called, should be chosen carefully and in some states need not be limited to clinic associates or professionals. Because a nonprofit group practice operates for the benefit of the public, it may be desirable to provide for public representation on the board if allowable under local laws.[d]

While the corporation is strictly nonprofit, and no part of the property or income can ever accrue to the benefit of the organizers, trustees, or physicians, in many cases the corporation is not precluded from making money and accumulating capital as long as these assets are used strictly for the stated purpose or purposes as shown in the original articles of incorporation. The Internal Revenue Service and other governmental agencies, both state and federal, have placed limits upon the accumulation of funds and the scope of permissible activities available to the nonprofit corporation. A nonprofit corporation usually has no fixed capital created by the issuance of shares of stock. Reserves usually are established, however, in the same manner as in other corporations, and permissible investments can be made out of the capital assets. The board of directors can establish a fixed capital and provide for it never to be impaired, and it can establish working capital for the ongoing investments of the corporation.

A nonprofit corporation usually may accept outside gifts. This increases the availability of tax-free capital to carry out the functions of the corporation. It provides opportunities for medical progress and research to help strengthen the medical group and achieve its community or professional goals. Because of the acceptance of gifts and the maintenance of other capital, a carefully planned budget must be followed to ensure the tax-free status, and advice from a competent accountant or attorney is essential.

There can be no distribution of corporate income to the physician except

[d]Since none of the profits or proceeds of a nonprofit corporation may accrue to the benefit of any individual professional, the nonprofit corporation cannot have shareholders. The corporation, however, may have *members* which, for voting and other purposes, correspond to shareholders. The public representation, however, should be limited to nonprofessional matters to avoid the ethical problems previously discussed.

as salaried employees of the corporation, or for services of a professional nature to the corporation pursuant to its purposes. Because the physicians are employees, however, they may be eligible for participation in a pension or retirement plan coverage, and care should be exercised so that the tax exempt status is not lost. The Internal Revenue Service might maintain, for instance, that a pension plan resulted in making earnings of the corporation available to individuals. It is also necessary to ensure that salaries are considered reasonable by the Internal Revenue Service. Ordinarily, the attorney for the nonprofit corporation will request from the Commissioner of Internal Revenue a ruling as to the organization's tax exempt status. The articles, bylaws, and any other relevant material must be examined in order to determine qualification for the exempt status.

Foundation. The foundation is a form of the nonprofit corporation which provides an organization capable of administrating an endowment gift from a grantor. The act of incorporation or endowment is the foundation. The grantor (an individual or organization) who provides the funds or property and specifies the purposes for which the funds or property are to be used is the founder. The organization that is established may be referred to as the trustee or the foundation.[43] After establishment of the organization, the board of directors or the trustees usually are charged with the exclusive management of the endowment within the framework laid down by the founder.

Some foundations are established in a charitable trust form. The grantor, by a deed of trust, conveys money or property to the trust or trustees (usually a nonprofit corporation) in order to benefit members of a specified group, class of people, or the public in general.[44] The corporation may administer the trust property for the benefit of the specified group or for its purposes.

Most medical group practices are organized for motives other than nonprofit, religious, or charitable. The most popular and effective alternative available to the group for a nonprofit practice is the corporation. Unlike a partnership or a sole proprietorship, both the corporation and association may be organized exclusively for nonprofit and may be directly exempt from taxation. The nonprofit status of a sole proprietorship or partnership is dependent upon the individual or collective activity of the owners in contributing their share of the practice's income to approved charitable institutions.

Before concluding the section on nonprofit medical organizations, it may be wise to offer a word of caution to groups anticipating this choice. The previous discussion of nonprofit organizational forms may be a somewhat overly optimistic appraisal of possibilities available under the present Internal Revenue Service structure. Unless a group practice is to operate as a Health Maintenance Organization (HMO), it may have an extremely difficult time securing a nonprofit exemption under Section 501 C3. In order to attain the nonprofit status, the group would have to show that it could generate sufficient revenue that would be used for charitable or educational purposes.

In the past some groups have owned through a nonprofit corporate structure the facility in which they practice. The IRS has been critical of many of these arrangements and has questioned the high rental rates paid to the nonprofit corporation. To alleviate this problem, groups have been forced to merge the professional corporation for the practice of medicine into the nonprofit corporation. This merger created yet another problem. The American Medical Association has stipulated that individuals who are not physicians cannot be members of such a corporation. The IRS, on the other hand, requires that a number of the corporation directors be outsiders in order for the corporation to qualify as nonprofit under the 501 C3 regulation.

Other groups who have made tax deductible contributions to nonprofit corporations formed for philanthropic purposes found themselves to be classified as foundations and subject to the disadvantages of the 1961 tax law. In order to avoid this status a group can be merged into a nonprofit corporation. The examples mentioned above are among the very few nonprofit options for medical group practice which currently would be recognized by the IRS. Other than HMOs, those groups presently operating under a nonprofit status probably do so as a result of the 1969 tax reforms.

The decision to practice as a nonprofit organization does require a great deal of forethought and advance planning by the physicians and their attorney, accountant, and administrator. The property, earnings, and surplus of the organization must be managed carefully in order to establish and maintain the nonprofit status; however, they must also be managed aggressively in order to ensure that the organization remains solvent. The physicians should be assured that the nonprofit practice will not result in any foreseeable dissent among the physicians over their individual financial concerns.

PROFESSIONAL CORPORATION

The dominant legal form of medical group practice traditionally has been the partnership; recently, however, physicians have been adopting the corporate form for professional practice. The professional corporation offers the advantages of both the sole proprietorship and the partnership forms because the physician is at once an owner of shares of corporation stock and an employee of the corporation as well. A partnership, by definition and operation, is established for profit. The corporation, however, can provide a framework for nonprofit practice for those physicians who, because of humanitarian, ethical, or tax considerations, want to establish their practice as a nonprofit organization. For the formation of a professional corporation there is no statutory framework similar to the *Uniform Partnership Act.* Each state has its own statutes governing the professional corporation and the generalizations presented here must be compared with the appropriate individual state laws before any decision is made about forming a professional corporation.[e]

This chapter discussion is designed to familiarize the reader with the structure of professional corporations so that when deciding among the organizational forms and seeking advice from his own attorney, he will be aware of the salient points of the corporate form and can devote his attention to seeking answers to specific questions.

Definition

The greatest difficulty in discussing any legal concept is defining that concept briefly and concisely, and while a corporation is too complex for simple

[e]See Appendix 5B for a listing of citations to state professional incorporation regulations.

definition, nevertheless the reader must be presented a framework for reference. According to *Webster's Dictionary*, a corporation is: "a body formed and authorized by law to act as a single person although constituted by one or more persons and legally endowed with various rights and duties." This definition, however, does not fully capture the concept of a corporation; the reader may find the following definition, offered by United States Supreme Court Chief Justice Marshall, to be more descriptive: "A corporation is an artificial being, invisible, intangible, and existing in contemplation of law. Being the mere creature of law it possesses only those properties (i.e., powers or characteristics) which the charter of its creation confers upon it."[45]

General Description. A commercial or professional corporation is created by a group of individuals called incorporators. These incorporators develop the articles of incorporation or charter, which is an instrument containing the basic provisions of the organization of the corporation, including the name of the corporation, the term of its existence, its powers and purposes, its capital stock structure, its management structure, its registered office and agent, and its method of amendment.[f] The articles of incorporation must be signed by the incorporators, filed with the state government (usually with the secretary of state's office), and the appropriate fees must be paid. After the articles are accepted as in order by the state, the corporation's existence usually begins. Some states issue charters representing the state's authorization of the existence of the corporation; other states simply designate the articles as a charter. Some state laws, however, require that articles of incorporation related to the practice of medicine be referred by the secretary of state to the State Board of Medical Examiners for review and approval prior to the issuance of the charter.

As Chief Justice Marshall has indicated, a corporation is an artificial being whose abilities, powers, and purposes are defined exclusively by its charter or articles, together with state law. The corporation cannot perform any act or pursue any course of business unless it is so authorized by its charter. In addition to the articles of incorporation, the shareholders or members of the corporation adopt bylaws outlining the operating principles of the corporation and providing additional detail about the corporation's organization. The procedures, powers, and purposes of the corporation as presented in the articles of incorporation and the bylaws dictate the operation of the business aspects of a medical group practice. The physician occupies a dual position in the professional corporation because he can both own corporation stock and be an employee of the corporation. Subject to agreement among the shareholders or according to state law, a physician can transfer or sell his interest in the practice simply by selling his shares of stock; the physician, however, is bound by the terms of his employment contract and if he withdraws from the employment of the corporation, or otherwise violates these contract provisions, he can become liable for breach of contract.

The professional corporation may or may not issue stock. When the corporation is formed to issue stock to represent corporate ownership, those owners are referred to as stockholders or shareholders, and the corporation operates

[f]Since a corporation is capable of bringing suit in court and being sued, the corporation must designate a person and place where judicial as well as other legal papers can be served or presented to the corporation.

for a profit. If the corporation is nonprofit, stock is not issued, and individual physicians are referred to as members. In this discussion of the professional corporation, it will be assumed that stock is issued to reflect ownership. The salient features of the nonprofit corporation have been discussed previously.

Ethical Considerations. The corporate form of practice for a shareholder physician involves reconciling the corporate attribute of limited liability for an owner-physician and the professional standard of the physician's accountability to his patient. The close personal relationship between a doctor and his patient requires that the physician be directly accountable to the recipient of his services. The professional corporation laws have attempted to preserve this doctor-patient relationship by providing that:

1. Professional service can be rendered by the corporation only through authorized physicians.
2. All professional employees and the corporation are subject to the standards of the medical profession and subject to disciplinary action if the standards are breached.
3. Any professional person who is a shareholder, employee, or connected with the corporation must terminate his connection with the corporation if he becomes disqualified to practice medicine.
4. The relationship between the physician and his patient is not in any way affected by the corporation, and the physician is liable for any services he renders.

Direct professional accountability has been preserved by eliminating the limited liability of the corporate employee or shareholder furnishing the service. In matters not connected with the professional aspects of the practice, however, the limited liability of the shareholder or employee is preserved. For example, if Dr. Smith were engaged as an employee-shareholder of the Smith and Jones Professional Corporation, he would be personally liable for any claim of malpractice against him. Dr. Jones would be liable if he had participated in the action leading to the malpractice suit. If, however, the corporation were sued for a nonprofessional act such as a breach of contract, both Dr. Smith and Dr. Jones would be liable up to the amount that each physician paid for his stock.[46]

Medical ethics also require that there be no intervention into the physician-patient relationship by a nonprofessional agency.[47] The American Medical Association has provided that a corporation is not a nonprofessional intervening agency if the ownership and management of its affairs remain in the hands of licensed physicians.[48] State laws require, therefore, that the ownership of the corporation be held by the physicians and that ownership by a nonprofessional can cause dissolution or termination of the corporation.

One of the major issues in the creation of professional corporations has been the Internal Revenue Service's challenge of the use of pension plans by physicians and other professionals in the corporation. A single pension plan covering both lay employees and professionals traditionally has prohibited the members of a particular profession from splitting their fees with nonmembers of the profession. The pension plan involves a contribution from the employer and the employees to a retirement fund intended for return of a pension at a later date, and the investments of the professional corporation's pension plan may result in fee splitting. Initially, the AMA maintained that its members could not adopt a single plan including both lay people and physicians. Through its judicial council, however, the AMA has reversed this ruling, and physicians are now free to adopt a pension plan which includes lay employees if the plan meets with Internal Revenue Service approval.[49] A profit-sharing plan, however, cannot include lay employees except when the plan is considered a qualified retirement plan under the *Internal Revenue Code.*[50]

State Laws Affecting Professional Corporations

In addition to the medical profession and the Internal Revenue Service, the various states have adopted special laws containing provisions for professional corporations. The state's control over the corporation lies in its ability to reject the corporation's articles. Composing the articles of incorporation, therefore, is a technical legal skill that must combine the applicable state laws with the needs and desires of the particular physicians. The state laws vary greatly and the following similarities suggest only the basic components of usual state incorporation laws:

1. All the provisions and requirements of a state's corporate laws apply to the professional corporation.
2. Professionals must change their status from that of a partner or sole proprietor to an employee of the corporation.
3. Individuals may incorporate to form a professional entity to render the *same* professional service which the individuals may perform as partners or individual practitioners.
4. The professional corporation may not issue stock to anyone who is not a duly authorized member of the same profession as the corporation.
5. The professional corporation may be organized to render only one type of professional service and the mixing of various professions in one corporate entity is prohibited (i.e., types of professions are medicine, legal, accounting, etc.).
6. The corporate name of the professional corporation must contain such words as "professional association," "professional corporation," or the abbreviations of such words. A number of states require that the corporate name include the last name of one or more of its shareholders unless the profession's ethics committee authorizes the use of the corporate name without the surname of any professional.
7. A shareholder of a professional corporation may sell or transfer his shares only to a licensed person of the same profession. The sale or transfer usually requires the approval of a majority or all of the shareholders.
8. The professional corporation cannot render professional services except through those persons who are licensed within the state to render the same professional service. Furthermore, the corporation's shareholders, directors, or officers must also be licensed to practice the profession. Some professional corporation statutes specifically provide an exemption from this provision for the secretary and the treasurer.
9. The professional corporation cannot alter the relationship or the liability between the professional and his patient.

10. An officer, shareholder, agent, or employee remains personally and fully liable for any negligent, wrongful acts, or misconduct committed by him or by any person under his direct supervision who performs professional services.

11. Clerks, secretaries, lay administrators, and other employees are not classified as "employees" and are not usually considered, by custom and practice, to be rendering professional service to the public for which a license or other professional authorization is required.

12. In most states, a professional corporation may invest its funds in real estate, mortgages, stocks, bonds, or other types of investments and may own real or personal property necessary or appropriate for rendering its service.

13. The requirements of state professional corporation statutes shall not alter, restrict, or otherwise modify the state's other laws applicable to the relation between the professional and his patient, or the standard of conduct applicable to the professional.[51]

Advantages and Disadvantages of the Professional Corporation

The complexities of forming a professional corporation are quickly overcome when one becomes involved in the corporate operation. The corporate form has both advantages and disadvantages that should be thoroughly weighed before the final selection of an organizational framework for group practice is made.

General Advantages. Formerly, one of the major advantages of professional incorporation for the physician was the availability of tax deferrals allowed through the use of the corporate pension and profit-sharing plans. The advantages of incorporation, however, have been greatly diminished by the pension reform act which allows more generous contributions to HR 10 plans and subjects both corporate and HR 10 plans to the same ceilings on benefits. In spite of this legislation, there are other, nontax advantages to be considered as well. For example, in a corporation the management of the practice is centralized in a board of directors or similar governing group which is charged with all the duties, responsibilities, and liabilities of management. While initially these board members are usually the incorporators, later board members can be elected by the shareholders. Only through their election of the directors do the shareholders have a hand in the management of the affairs of the corporation. The board of directors, or the officers chosen by it, relieve the physician of the decision-making emanating from the business management of his practice.[52] Furthermore, the corporate medical group is assured that the responsibilities of constant management are held by a specific person.

Incorporation also allows a professional to be insulated from nonprofessional negligence or wrongdoing involved in the operation of business. For example, it is possible that in a medical group's waiting room, a patient might slip on the floor which was negligently left slick, and as a result might file a law suit for injuries against the group physicians. In such a suit, a shareholder is liable only to the extent of his investment in the corporation; were he a partner, however, he would be fully responsible and required to pay for all injuries. State statutes regarding incorporation are carefully worded to ensure that the personal and singular relationship between physician and patient is retained, and some of the statutes may be interpreted in such a way as to insulate a particular shareholder physician from any legal proceedings against his colleague(s).[53]

A partnership is dissolved by law when a partner retires, dies, or otherwise can no longer serve as a partner, whereas a corporation, is a legal entity and its life is determined by its articles regardless of any change in ownership. This attribute of "immortality" is especially desirable for the corporation developed for a one man practice. The files, accounts, and property of the medical practice remain in the possession of the corporation upon the death of the physician, and are not involved in the settling of his estate after his death. In addition, the ownership interests of a professional corporation can be transferred easily to new physicians simply by the sale of the physician's shares of stock to another physician. Furthermore, with ownership of the assets placed into the corporation, sale or transfer of any asset is a simple matter. Even among medical groups that utilize the partnership for the delivery of medical services, the corporation is a common method of owning the assets or property necessary for the medical practice. In such instances, the corporation leases to the partnership the necessary equipment and in some cases employs all nonprofessional personnel such as receptionists or secretaries. Such asset corporations are considered to be commercial organizations and are not subject to restrictions imposed upon professional corporations.

A further advantage of the professional corporation is that its operation may be more formalized than, for instance, the partnership or unincorporated association. The articles of incorporation and the bylaws specifically outline the purposes and powers of the corporation. Physicians practicing within other organizational forms, however, can avoid the problem of colleagues' distractions or whims interrupting the delivery of health care, by exercising care in drawing up initial agreements.

Tax Advantages. The professional corporation, whether formed for profit or nonprofit, offers the individual physician a more advantageous tax arrangement than does the partnership. While the tax rate of a sole proprietor or partner can be as high as 50 percent of his earned taxable net income (gross earned income less all allowable deductions), the *corporate tax rate* is 20 percent for its first $25,000 of adjusted gross income (gross income less all business expenses and capital depreciation); the tax rate on the next $25,000 is 22 percent. Income in excess of $25,000 per year is exceedingly rare for most professional corporations because most of the income is paid out in salaries.[54]

The *business expenses* of the corporation, such as physicians' salaries, personnel wages, maintenance, etc., can be deducted from the corporation's income as expenses. A partnership does not allow deduction of the physician's salary. As a result, if the physician pays his individual tax rate on his salary and if the corporation pays the tax on the remainder at a corporate tax rate the total tax is generally less, when compared to the individual partner who must pay the tax on the entire amount. A self-employed individual or partner may use his automobile for business purposes and may deduct his automobile expenses, but these costs must be justified if he takes a tax deduction for more than 12¢ per mile for the first 15,000 miles, and for 9¢ per mile over 15,000 miles. The corporation, however, may reimburse an employee for automobile expenses on corporation business for up to 15¢ per mile without requiring the employee to account for his actual costs.[55]

A corporation can obtain *group life insurance* for its employees, and the premiums are tax deductible to the corporation if paid for benefits up to $50,000 for each employee. The premiums are not taxed to the employee and the benefits received as a result of death are not taxed to the employee's beneficiary. It is possible that in the future in order to obtain a tax-free insurance plan, the corporation will have to include all employees, but will be able to make distinctions based on categories acceptable to the insurance company and reflective of the differences in employee compensation. The physician or administrator should keep in mind that group insurance not only involves tax benefits, but also can be purchased at a cost which is significantly lower than the cost of individual policies.

Most physicians carry *disability insurance* so that they will have some income in the event of any accident or illness that would prevent them from working. If the professional purchased the insurance, the premiums would not be deductible; however, a portion of the proceeds from the policy would be tax-free income. The professional corporation can purchase the disability insurance for some or all of its employees and the premiums may be deducted as a business expense. The value of the premiums is not taxable income to the employee, but any proceeds over $100 per week are taxable to the employee at his regular rate. Although some physicians or administrators would rather secure their own disability policies and receive benefits tax free, most physicians believe that the tax deduction would be more helpful while they are working and that the income received due to disability would not involve a high tax rate.[56]

The professional corporation can establish *medical reimbursement plans* for employees relating to medical expenses incurred by themselves or their families. Without a medical reimbursement plan, and if income tax deductions are itemized, the taxpayer can deduct only one-half of his medical health insurance up to $150, and only his medical expenses that exceed 3 percent of his adjusted gross income. The standard deduction does not allow any medical deduction, but is determined to reflect some medical expenses. For the highly paid professional or corporate employee, therefore, there is little chance of a medical expense deduction. The corporation, however, may reimburse medical expenses for its professionals and employees. Such reimbursements are not considered part of the professional's or employee's taxable income and do not affect the use of the standard deduction.[57] The reimbursed employee who itemizes, however, can not take a medical deduction in addition to reimbursement.

For the employer-corporation the medical reimbursements are tax deductible business expenses. The reimbursement plan, unlike pension plans, may differentiate between employees entitled to receive the benefits, and usually covers only key or permanent employees. The employees or professionals covered under the reimbursement plan should be fulltime employees with qualifications not based upon shareholder status. The purpose of a medical reimbursement plan is not to provide free benefits to physicians or employees, but rather to serve various business purposes including the improvement of employee morale, as well as employee health, tenure, and stability.

When an employee of the corporation dies, the corporation may pay a $5,000 *death benefit* to the employee's beneficiary(s). The benefit is a deductible expense for the corporation and is not considered as taxable income to the beneficiary. Any similar payments made to a self-employed individual's beneficiary are taxable. The death benefit usually is used in connection with payment of a deceased employee's pension share to his beneficiary.[58]

One of the major benefits resulting from professional incorporation is the opportunity for a professional to utilize a *qualified retirement* plan, the advantages of which include: (1) the corporation can take a tax deduction at the time of pension plan contributions to a retirement fund, trust fund, or insurance policy; (2) the employee-beneficiaries are not taxed on the contributions; and (3) the earnings of the fund are tax free until distribution. When the benefits of the plan are distributed to the employees, the amount contributed by the employer is averaged over ten years and taxed to the employee as ordinary income. For the ten year averaging provision to apply, the employee must have been a plan participant for five years. Capital gains rules will apply only for employer contributions prior to 1973, and the amount received by the employer which is attributable to the plan's earnings is taxed at the lower capital gains rate. If the employee dies before receiving all retirement benefits, his designated beneficiary will receive the benefits free of federal and, usually, state estate taxes.[59]

The corporation can administer the investments of the fund itself or it can utilize the services of a bank, trustee, insurance company, or other investment counselor. Formerly, it was not uncommon for a group to invest 50 percent of the plan's funds into insurance policies and 50 percent into property, stocks, or other securities. The freedom of investment offers the professional corporation employee some discretion as to the funds that are vested to him and those he can designate as certain investments for his retirement fund. Many medical groups have sold their clinic building or assets to the pension or profit-sharing plan for ownership. In the future, however, this arrangement may not be possible because under the Pension Reform Act there is a question as to whether or not qualified retirement plans may continue to own such facilities.

General Disadvantages. The professional corporation offers substantial advantages in the taxation, business, and medical aspects of group practice, but also involves several disadvantages that should be considered carefully when selecting an organizational form for medical group practice.

The physician's loss of independence in the management of the business and financial affairs of the practice may be greater in the professional incorporation than in the partnership. The physician is no longer free to take time off whenever he pleases; he must make arrangements with the other physicians and the management of the coporation for his vacation, study, or relaxation time. The professional is usually an employee under contract and must honor the obligations and duties contained in the employment agreement. Should he violate his employment agreement, he will be liable to the corporation and may be required to pay damages to the corporation or risk termination. In addition, incorporation will result in the physician's losing some of his investment freedom if the corporation adopts a pension plan. The pension plan requires contributions from those physicians who wish to participate in the retirement plan. The surplus that a physician may wish to place into other forms of investment is channeled into the corporation plan and becomes subject to management by the plan.[60]

A professional corporation is a formally structured organization whose purposes and powers are established in its bylaws and articles of incorporation, and whose operation cannot be formally altered without amendment to those instruments. The established methods of decision-making and bookkeeping, as well as the nature of directors' meetings, shareholders' meetings, officers' duties and other established policies must be honored by the physician.

Further disadvantages arise from the fact that the taxation and liability consequences of professional incorporation usually stimulate close regulation and scrutiny from state and federal governments. The physician may find himself faced with the task of additional reporting in the operation of the corporation. In addition, private business may treat the corporation differently. For example, although the physician remains personally liable for his professional negligence, in some cases the premiums for medical malpractice insurance coverage will dramatically increase for the incorporated medical practice.[61]

Continuous legal services are required for the professional corporation to safeguard its taxation status and its efficiency of operation. Some physicians may not work well with lawyers and the necessity for additional legal consultations may detract greatly from their estimation of the benefits of professional incorporation. Any form of group practice, however, will involve considerable need for legal services and, aside from some special attention to regular corporation needs, a corporation actually may not need the services of a lawyer more often than do either the partnership or sole proprietorship.

Tax Disadvantages. Unfortunately, the professional corporation does involve substantial tax disadvantages for the physician, including some mandatory financial burdens as well as the risk of additional tax liabilities.

As a shareholder, the professional is entitled to receive dividends which comprise his distributional share of the corporation's earnings. Dividends are paid to shareholders when the board of directors decides to declare a dividend payment, but can be paid only out of the corporation's taxable profits. Any dividend received by a shareholder is taxable income to him and not deductible by the corporation. Therefore, the profits of the corporation are actually taxed twice, and this additional taxation may amount to a substantial burden since dividends may be taxed to the shareholder physician with a high income at a rate above 50 percent. The Internal Revenue Service does allow smaller corporations to avoid the double taxation of earnings by electing to be taxed under Sub-chapter S of the amended *Internal Revenue Code of 1954* (see below, p. 130). The use of Sub-chapter S, however, does involve various restrictions on pension plan use that may outweigh its helpfulness in alleviation of the double taxation of profits.[62]

The double taxation results only when dividends are paid out or if the corporation has a profit. Many professional corporations retain their earnings to redeem a departing shareholder's stock, to finance center expansion, to use in acquiring new equipment, or for other capital expenditures. As a result, the physician-shareholder usually will never receive a dividend. In some cases, when the corporation's earnings are equal to its business expenses, including the physician's salary, the corporation will not have any profits to be taxed or to be distributed to shareholders.

Upon incorporation the physician will become an employee and his salary will be subject to the various withholdings imposed by law on all corporate employees. Income tax withholding results in lower net salary for the physician, and necessitates monthly income tax payments rather than quarterly deposits on estimated taxes paid by the self-employed; the physician, therefore, will lose the short-term interest that his savings designated for the quarterly payments might have earned.[63] Professional employees' salaries also are subject to social security, FICA contributions. The FICA tax withheld from the employee's pay is 5.85 percent of the first $13,200 of earned income. This percentage is matched by the employer, thus making a total contribution of 11.7 percent of $13,200 per year. The employer's matching contribution is a tax deductible business expense. The self-employed professional also must make FICA contributions; however, the rate for a self-employed professional is only 7.9 percent on the first $14,100. Future acceleration in the cost of living as well as congressional action may result in a steady increase in both the percentage rates and the base compensation amounts.[64]

In a partnership, a share of the profits represents each partner's remuneration for his services. This remuneration is not a tax deductible business expense, and there are no limits placed upon any amount received by the partners. For the corporate employer, however, Section 61 of the *Internal Revenue Code* allows reasonable compensation to be deducted as a business expense. If the compensation is determined to be unreasonable by the Internal Revenue Service, the unreasonable portion may be considered as a dividend distribution; the deduction may be disallowed and the disallowed portion will be subject to corporation and employee tax liability. Until recently, the assumption of the IRS was that compensation not exceeding the professional's precorporation income or 100 percent of his total billings would be considered reasonable and fully deductible. According to recent Internal Revenue opinions and court cases, however, a payment deemed reasonable under the above criteria will not be allowed as a deduction if it is in reality a distribution of corporate earnings and not compensation for services. The apparent rationale behind considering a dividend payment as a reasonable compensation is that part of the professional's earnings is based upon the goodwill that he brought with him into the professional corporation. Although the forced dividend payment remains an unsettled doctrine, the physician or administrator should be aware of this possibility when establishing the corporate salaries.

When retaining earnings in order to avoid paying out dividends, the accumulated earnings tax on retained profits must be considered. Section 351 of the *Internal Revenue Code* imposes a penalty tax on earnings accumulated by corporations, rather than distributed to shareholders, for the purpose of avoiding the income tax on dividends. Every corporation is permitted to accumulate a maximum of $150,000. An accumulation in excess of that amount may be interpreted as an attempt to avoid taxation; the corporation must disprove this presumption by demonstrating a reasonable business need for an accumulation in excess of the $150,000 maximum.

As an example, there are other items which, while not considered to be deductible business expenses, can be used to reduce an unreasonable accumulation. A medical corporation might need to accumulate earnings for an investment in additional equipment or a new building expansion. Group insurance premiums for benefits in excess of $50,000 are not deductible but may be used to reduce the unreasonable accumulations. Additional contributions to qualified pension and profit-sharing plans are nondeductible but can reduce the unreasonable accumulation, thereby bringing it within the $150,000 maximum.[65]

A professional medical corporation may be considered as a personal holding company under Section 531 of the *Internal Revenue Code.* The corporation will be treated as a personal holding company if more than 50 percent of its stock is held by five or fewer individuals and if 60 percent or more of its gross income derives from personal service contract income, that is, income received under a contract for personal services rendered by the corporation, with some person other than the corporation having the right to designate the employee who is to perform the service. In other words, any income from services rendered by the physician of a patient's choice may be subject to a 70 percent penalty tax. Furthermore, personal service income may result if an employee who is to perform the service is designated in the contract and if at some time in the year that employee is an owner of 25 percent or more of the corporation's stock.[66] Service designation, however, may not be possible without a written contract, and designation within the terms of the regulation probably cannot result from a mere expectation by the patient.[67]

The personal holding company tax can be avoided by several alternative corporate adjustments. The tax is imposed upon undistributed income and can be avoided simply by paying out all corporate earnings as dividends. This will produce taxation, but the double tax usually will be less than 70 percent. To avoid personal service contracts, the corporation should reserve the exclusive right in the contract to designate which employee will perform the services.[68] (This feature may be significant to many forming groups which anticipate more than 60 percent of their services being rendered through prepaid contracts.)

The 25 percent or more owner-employee creates a special problem for the one-man corporation. Obviously, in a one-man professional corporation it is only practical for the provider of the service to be designated in every contract. A complete distribution of a one-man corporation's earnings will avoid a personal holding tax, but may lead the IRS to believe that the corporation is only a sham, designed and maintained to avoid taxes. For the one-man corporation, therefore, the best solution to the personal service taxation dilemma is to carefully plan corporate expenses so that after distributing the income just enough to pay taxes remains.[69] Even if earnings are not retained, it also is advisable to utilize a written contract reserving for the corporation the right of service designation.

Section 482 of the *Internal Revenue Code* is employed by the IRS to allocate income and deductions among different trades or businesses owned by the same interests, if such allocation is necessary to prevent evasion of taxes or to clearly reflect the income of the different trades or businesses.[70] For a professional corporation the primary inquiry involves determining whether the shareholder-employee has an independent trade or business by virtue of his status as an employee, thereby warranting a reallocation of income. In other words, Section 482 will prevent a corporation from receiving income that was not earned by it, but rather by a physician on his own behalf. To avoid the occurrence of a Section 482 reallocation, the corporation must be recognized as earning income and must indicate that it is providing the medical services through its employees. An employee's only business or practice is in the employ of the corporation and his employment contract contains provisions against outside practice and competition after his departure.[71] The professional corporation, not the shareholders of the corporation, must keep the books and records, bill for services rendered, account for the receipts, pay the bills, and attend to all of the other everyday functions of the practice.

The advantages and disadvantages discussed in this section represent only a few of the key issues involved in the formation of a professional corporation. For a more complete survey of the benefits of corporate practice, physicians or administrators may wish to consult with colleagues who have practiced in a corporation. Above all, the physician should decide for himself whether practice in a corporate setting will satisfy his professional and personal goals.

Organizing the Corporation

The initial steps towards creation of the corporation are determining who the promoters or incorporators are to be, and the drafting of the articles of incorporation according to the requirements for incorporation as determined by state law. Only generalizations have been presented here; for more specific information the reader is advised to refer to the laws of his particular state.

Qualifications and Obligations of the Incorporators and Promoters. Generally, the incorporators of a professional corporation must meet both the requirements set forth in the state's general corporation laws as well as the additional requirements of the professional corporation laws. These requirements stipulate that the incorporator must have reached the age of capacity to contract (usually eighteen years old), and must have the mental capacity to contract. A specific requirement for the professional corporation is that the incorporator be licensed or otherwise authorized to practice the profession for which the projected corporation will be established. Many states, however, recently have eliminated this particular requirement from their professional incorporation acts. For example, in the formation of most corporations, lawyers act as the incorporators but perform only routine acts. In addition, state statutes usually require that there be one to three incorporators to sign the articles of incorporation.[72]

Incorporators or promoters have various duties to the public, the prospective corporation, and each other which reach beyond technical qualifications.[g] During the corporate formation the promoters are regarded by law as temporary partners and, therefore, owe to one another the duties of full disclosure and

[g]Promoters include not only the incorporators but also anyone who participates in the corporation's formation, capitalization, and initial business activities.

fair dealing in all matters concerning the corporation. A promoter's misconduct or breach of the partnership duties could result in his liability. Promoters also are considered by law to owe to the prospective corporation a fiduciary duty requiring the promoter to act fairly and openly in all dealings with the corporation. This usually applies when a promoter sells or otherwise transfers property to the corporation. In complying with the fiduciary duty, the promoter must disclose his interest in the property, his expected profit from its sale, and any other material factors that may affect the corporation's decision to purchase the property. Disclosure must be made to an independent board of directors or to all known and contemplated shareholders. For breach of the fiduciary duty a corporation can cancel or rescind the sale and request damages or a return of the excess profit made by the promoters on the sale.

Although payment by the corporation for a promoter's property may be in cash or other property, in most cases the promoter will receive shares of stock in the corporation.[h] In accordance with his fiduciary duty the promoter must receive stock valued at an amount equal to the value of the property transferred; for example, if a physician sells to the corporation he is promoting a city lot valued at $10,000, he must receive stock with stated value of no more than $10,000. After the sale, the corporation's worth would be increased by $10,000 and, therefore, must be accounted for by $10,000 worth of stock. The taking of stock valued higher than the property transferred can result in the perpetration of a fraud upon the public by the promoter who deals with the corporation. The misrepresentation caused by overvaluation of stock is usually referred to as "watered stock," and creditors of the corporation may bring a personal action against the promoter for recovery of the amount by which their stock has been "watered." The personal fiduciary obligation of the promoter to the corporation, and consequently to its creditors, exists regardless of the general rule of limited liability of a corporate shareholder.

Achievement of Corporate Status. The corporation must fulfill both statutory and traditional criteria to be considered as a validly established and professionally operating corporation. If the articles of incorporation are not drawn and filed properly, problems may arise when a defect or irregularity occurs. To deal with liabilities resulting from a defective corporation, the law has developed two concepts, *de jure corporation* and *de facto corporation.* A de jure corporation is one that has been organized in compliance with all mandatory requirements or in substantial compliance with all important requirements of incorporation. The corporate status of a de jure corporation cannot be challenged by anyone including the state in an action to forfeit the corporation's charter. A corporation which has failed to pay in full the filing fees, but has nevertheless obtained a charter, is an example of a de jure corporation.

A de facto corporation occurs when the organization has failed to fulfill the steps necessary to obtain de jure status. The de facto corporation can defend itself against challenges made by third persons towards its corporate status, but

[h] A corporation may be owned by several people and the mode of ownership involves the purchasing of shares of stock, each share representing the amount of proportioned ownership that the shareholder has in the assets of the corporation.

it cannot resist challenges made by the state. To obtain de facto status the following circumstances are necessary:

1. There must be some general law or legal method available in the state by which an organization can be validly incorporated.
2. There must have been an effort made in good faith to comply with the incorporative process.
3. There must be a user, in good faith, of the corporation.

De facto classification enables an organization to resist challenges to its corporate status; however, if the organization cannot comply with the de facto requirements, its corporate status can be challenged by anyone. If the challenge is successful, the corporation's organizers or shareholders can be personally responsible.

In some cases the organization may be able to resist challenges to its corporate status despite its lack of compliance with the corporate requirements of state law. If a third party deals with the organization as if it were a valid corporation and subsequently attempts unjustly to harm the organization by challenging its corporation status, for the particular transaction involving that particular person, the organization will be treated by the law as if it were validly formed. This doctrine represents a variation of estoppel and prevents a third party from denying the existence of a valid corporation.

In order to be taxed as a corporation, an organization must establish its corporate status with the Internal Revenue Service. Essentially, the IRS relies upon two doctrines for the determination of an organization's corporate status: *label theory* and *corporateness criteria.* Both doctrines are the result of a long, complex and confusing series of court decisions and IRS regulations. The *label theory* provides that if a state has a valid professional association or incorporation enabling statute, and if the organization has been formed in accordance with that statute, then for income tax purposes the organization has the status of corporation.[73] If, however, the state does not have a valid professional corporation or association enabling statute, or if the organization was not properly formed under such a statute, then the organization must meet a majority of the following "tests":

1. *Centralized Management.* The management of the organization must be delegated to a body similar to a board of directors and management must be divorced from the ownership of the organization.
2. *Continuity of Life.* The existence of the corporation must be able to withstand a change in ownership or the death of one or all of its shareholders.
3. *Free Transferability of Interest.* The ownership interests of the corporation must be able to be freely transferred without interruption of the existence or operation of the corporation.
4. *Limited Liability.* The owners of the organization must not be personally liable for the obligations of the organization.
5. *Separate Legal Entity.* The existence of a separate legal entity is the logical conclusion if the previous four criteria are met; the corporation, however, is differentiated from a very sophisticated partnership. Obviously, a professional corporation adhering to state and ethical restrictions would not be

able to fully satisfy the free transferability and limited liability criteria. Current views, however, require only that the organization meet at least half of the above tests; the organizational structure must contain more corporate characteristics than noncorporate characteristics to achieve a corporation tax status.[74]

Corporate Conversion. Physicians who establish a professional corporation may have already been in practice under some other legal form such as a sole proprietorship or a partnership, and usually desire to transfer accounts receivable, assets, and obligations from the previous form of practice to the corporation. Unfortunately, the transfer can create taxation and fiscal problems which must be overcome by prior planning. For convenience, in this section conversion from a partnership to a professional corporation will be used as an illustration.

Usually the assets of a partnership consist of its equipment and property, together with its accounts receivable. The equipment and property have a definite market value which may have been adjusted by the partnership to reflect depreciation. On the other hand, the accounts receivable usually are not assigned any value prior to collection, and income from these accounts will not be recognized until it is received. In converting the practice, the physicians will usually transfer the property and accounts receivable to the new corporation in exchange for stock. This exchange will result in a taxable event; any gain made as a result of the transfer will be taxable at that time, regardless of whether or not money was actually received. If the exchange is in compliance with Section 351 of the *Internal Revenue Code*, however, the transfer may not be considered a taxable event. This section provides that if the assets were transferred solely in exchange for stock or securities of the corporation and if the transferors owned at least 80 percent of the stock of the corporation after the transfer, then the transfer is considered as merely a continuation of the practice and as a nontaxable event.[75]

The use of Section 351 allows the corporation to be taxed on the income generated by the payment of accounts receivable, instead of requiring that the partners, who actually earned the income, be taxed. Ordinarily, an individual cannot avoid paying taxes on income he earned simply by giving to another person the right to receive the income; the IRS will use *IRC* §482 to reallocate the income back to the person who earned it and will require him to pay the taxes. As a result, unless the transfer distorts the income, transfer of accounts receivable to the corporation will also transfer the tax liability for that income to the corporation.[76]

The financial obligations or accounts payable of the partnership are usually transferred to the professional corporation along with the transfer of accounts receivable. Accounts payable are considered business expenses and, therefore, fully deductible; when transferred to the corporation, however, the accounts payable may be considered only as a capital expenditure and must be depreciated over several years rather than immediately deducted. An example of an account payable would be the obligation to pay a retired partner a pension. While the partnership may have been able to consider pension payments as salary, and therefore tax deductible as a business expense, for the assuming corporation the pension payment obligation may be considered only as a capital expenditure. Presently, the IRS maintains that the policy behind Section 351 is that transferred liabilities are deductible as a business expense to the corporation only if the liability also would be deductible to the partnership.[77]

The transfer of both the assets and the liabilities of the previous practice raises the possibility that the corporation will receive less assets than liabilities and as a result the transferor will be relieved of some possible net indebtedness. An individual is considered to have received income if he has been relieved by another of an obligation to pay money. Section 357 of the IRC provides that the transferor of the liabilities to the corporation will be taxed for any amount of liability assumed by the corporation that exceeds his basis in the assets and accounts receivable transferred.[i] If, therefore, a promoter transfers property with a tax basis (original cost less depreciation if any) of $10,000 and debts amounting to $20,000, the Internal Revenue Service would consider him to have received $10,000 of taxable income under the provisions of Section 357.[78]

Obviously, the transfer of assets (accounts receivable and property) that are not liabilities to a professional corporation, in exchange for shares of stock, does present the possibility of unwanted taxation, and the physician or administrator should anticipate this problem in the creation of the corporation. To help resolve the confusion generated by a transfer, the Internal Revenue Service has indicated that a corporation can obtain from the IRS a "closing agreement," which is a ruling in advance determining whether there will be any tax liability involved in the transfer of assets and liabilities to the corporation.[79]

Individual taxpayers are required to use the calendar year as opposed to a fiscal year for the calculation of their income and tax obligations. One of the problems in forming a professional corporation can be the "bunching of income" that can result if the partnership, operating on a fiscal year basis, wishes to transfer its assets to the professional corporation. With the dissolution and winding up of the partnership and the usual simultaneous commencement of the corporation's operation, the physician could be taxed on as much as twenty-three months of income in one year, although he received only half that much. For example, if a medical partnership with a fiscal year of February 1 to January 31 incorporates on February 1, 1975, the distributive share of the partnership's income from February 1, 1974, to January 31, 1975, will be included in his 1975 tax return along with his corporate salary for 1975. If the assets are transferred to the corporation, however, the physician actually will have received only his twelve month salary.

The bunching problem cannot be avoided completely, but there are limited alternatives available to relieve the burden to some degree. The payment of low salaries for the first year would reduce the amount of taxable income the physician would receive, and hopefully during this time wage controls would not be instituted. This method of payment can be implemented in several ways: payment of the professional employee's salary once a year on January 2 for the previous year's work; quarterly payment of salaries on the first day of the next succeeding quarter; or spacing the payment of salaries accrued in

[i]The reader should note that accounts receivable have no value until received and, therefore, the transferor's basis in accounts receivable is zero. Any transfer of assets involving accounts receivable will result in taxable income equal to the amount of liabilities assumed.

the first year over a period of several succeeding years.[80] While this system helps to avoid income bunching, it also reduces the amount of actual income from which the physician pays his taxes attributable to the distributed profit of the partnership.

The continuation of the partnership to receive the amounts due from accounts receivable, pay due obligations, and distribute the profits to the physician may offer the most advantageous solution to income bunching. The physician is paid a low salary by the corporation but receives a "normal salary" from the partnership until the partnership is terminated. After termination the physician's salary is increased to his usual income rate.[81] The retention of the partnership to pay partnership liabilities also may alleviate problems involved in the transfer of assets and liabilities to the corporation. The reduced salary and the partnership continuation method do have at least two key disadvantages that must be kept in mind: The corporation will have very little cash flow or income during the first year, and the dramatic increase in salary for the years following incorporation could result in objections by the Internal Revenue Service concerning the reasonableness of the increase. Furthermore, if restrictions similar to the recent Economic Stabilization program were placed on salary increases, the physician could be forced to receive a low salary for several years.

Articles of Incorporation. The organization of the corporate entity is determined by its articles of incorporation, which usually are restricted to the formulation of basic operating principles and characteristics. The articles must state the *name* of the corporation. The name of a corporation cannot mislead the public concerning the nature or purposes of the corporation, and the name cannot be similar to those of other corporations. The choice of name for a professional corporation is complicated by both state regulation and ethical considerations. The restrictions on a corporate name usually include the requirement that the corporate name contain an indication of its nature such as Professional Corporation, Professional Association, P.C., Ltd., or Chartered, and that the name include the last name of (at least) one of its current or past shareholders. If, according to statute or ethics, a fictitious name is allowed, in most cases it must be registered with the state.[82]

An important criterion for determining the corporate status of an organization is that its existence be independent of the death or departure of any shareholder. A corporation's duration either can be limited for a specific term of years or can be perpetual in duration. A provision such as "neither the death, insanity, bankruptcy, retirement, resignation, or expulsion of a member (shareholder) shall cause a dissolution of the corporation," is not usually required to establish duration.

A corporation's expressed powers and purposes are defined by the state's laws and the provisions of the articles of incorporation; a corporation's implied powers are those which are reasonably necessary to carry out its expressed powers. The rendering of professional service is a primary purpose of a professional corporation. In most states, a corporation also can specify in its articles that it possesses the powers required to render those professional services.[83] For taxation reasons, various additional purposes for incorporation, as stated in the articles of incorporation, include the need to attract new physicians, the need to expand, the desire to avoid partnership dissolution problems, and the desire to prevent the financial instability of a partnership.[84]

A share of stock, as a portion of ownership, is the tangible property interest that the shareholder has in the corporation. Two major classes of stock may be sold by the corporation. Common stock, the ordinary stock of the corporation, does not ensure the shareholder any guaranteed rate of return or dividend payment. Common stock holders usually have the right to participate in management. Preferred stock, while somewhat preferable in terms of the payment of dividends or distribution of assets, usually does not entitle the stockholder to any right to participate in the management of the corporation. Of course, there can be many subclasses of both common and preferred stock.

Most states restrict by law the ownership and transfer of the stock of a professional corporation. State laws uniformly require that all shareholders of a professional corporation be licensed or otherwise qualified to engage in the same profession for which the corporation was formed. Unfortunately, occasions do arise in which ownership by nonprofessionals cannot be avoided, such as through death and inheritance of shares, incompetency, or bankruptcy. To provide for these situations most states authorize ownership of shares by nonprofessionals for only the limited amount of time necessary to transfer ownership to another professional. If the temporary ownership continues beyond a reasonable time the state either can authorize the state's attorney general to dissolve, can prescribe a penalty according to administrative discretion, or can change the status of the professional corporation to that of a business corporation. In order to prepare for nonprofessional ownership and to avoid the threat of dissolution, the corporation can provide in the articles that any nonprofessional owner of shares is entitled to receive only dividends and is not entitled to participate in the management of the practice.

The formal structure of many corporations contains various clauses, independent of state requirements, which restrict the transfer of shares without a number of other shareholders approving, without first offering to sell to the shareholders, or without first offering to sell the shares back to the corporation at the outside offered price. These restrictions usually require authorization in the articles or in the bylaws, and then are expanded upon either in the bylaws or in a separate agreement among the shareholders.

A dividend is any distribution of cash, property, or additional shares paid to a shareholder in proportion to his share of ownership. As a general rule, dividends can be paid lawfully only out of a corporation's current profits or earned surplus. In most states, the decision to pay dividends is limited by two general restrictions: payment of any dividend is restricted if the payment would endanger the preference accorded to preferred shares of stock, and a corporation cannot declare a dividend if the corporation is insolvent or if the payment would cause insolvency. In addition to the general limitations and characteristics of the dividend payment, the articles also may contain additional procedures or regulations.

Although as a general rule shareholders do not have any right to exercise direct control or management over the affairs of the corporation, the shareholders do have the right to vote for the election or removal of directors, to amend the articles and bylaws, to institute dissolution, and to request access to the corporation books. The right to vote gives the shareholder an indirect control of the affairs of the professional corporation and the vote requires that the directors of the corporation be responsive to needs of the shareholders.

The shareholders usually are required to meet at least once annually to elect the board of directors and to consider any other action required to be brought before them by the articles or the bylaws. Procedures for special shareholder meetings which may be called at any time by an officer or a percentage number of shareholders, also are outlined in the articles or bylaws along with notice procedures, meeting places and dates, quorum (usually a majority), and any other procedures necessary to ensure fair and efficient shareholder meetings.

Because of its importance for the shareholders during formation of the corporation, the method of shareholder voting is usually outlined in the articles of incorporation. For decisions other than the election of directors, each share is entitled to a certain specified number of votes. Many professional corporations assign one vote for one share; if different classes of voting stock are used, however, a certain class may be entitled to more than one vote per share. Usually, a majority vote is required for approval of shareholder actions; however, the articles may specify that certain actions, such as amendment of the articles or bylaws or removal of a director, require a two-thirds or three-fourths vote for approval.

For the election of directors many corporations use a cumulative voting system. When a straight voting system is used for directors, unless state law or the articles require a greater number for election, a majority of 51 percent of the shareholders can control the election of all directors. Cumulative voting, however, will allow a minority of shareholders some representation on the board because each share is allowed one vote for each director to be elected. For example, if there are three directors to be elected and a particular shareholder has ten shares, then his total number of available votes is thirty. He can cast all of his available votes for one candidate or he may distribute the votes as he pleases. The result of cumulative voting is that a shareholder or group of shareholders who cannot command a majority of the votes will be able to elect at least one of the directors. Cumulative voting can be adapted according to the desires of the individual corporation, but in some states cumulative voting is mandatory. In many partnerships utilizing a "share system" of electing the central management committee, a cumulative system of voting also may be used.

Most states require that the management of the corporation be placed into the hands of a *board of directors* or a similar body.[j] The board, as a governing body, is distinct from the ownership of the corporation. This can create ethical problems, because unless the directors of the professional corporation are themselves qualified professionals, the operation of the corporation will be in violation of most statutory or ethical regulations. The articles of incorporation, therefore, should require that directors be professionals qualified to practice the profession for which the corporation has been established.[85] Al-

[j]Some states provide special rules for closely held corporations in which the ownership of shares is very small and limited. In the closely held corporation, there is usually a substantial identity between shareholders and directors; therefore, the statutes amend the limited management rights of a shareholder to resemble those of a director and do away with many of the formalities of the corporation. The use of a close corporation, however, may cause the Internal Revenue Service to conclude that the professional corporation is in reality a partnership and, therefore, may subject the practice to partnership taxation treatment.

though a director should be a qualified professional, unless the articles or state statutes so require, a director of the professional corporation need not be a shareholder in the corporation as well.

Usually, the initial board of directors is designated in the articles and holds office until the replacement directors are appointed or elected by the shareholders. Most states require at least three directors, and the articles of incorporation usually specify additional directors as they become needed. According to many state regulations, the usual term of a director is one year; however, the length of term can be altered by the articles and, to ensure continuity of management, a system of staggered terms for directors may be adopted. If the articles so provide, a director may resign at any time or may be removed at any time by a vote of the shareholders.

The directors are elected to the board by the vote of the shareholders. Some states, however, allow the articles to specify alternative procedures for selection of the board of a professional corporation. The articles can require that all candidates be approved by a "qualifications" or nominating committee, or that the present board of directors designate future nominees, subject to the approval of the shareholders. In addition, the shareholders can agree among themselves to specify certain individuals to serve as a part, or all, of the board of directors.[86]

The powers of management are exercised under the authority of the board of directors, when acting as a board in a properly called meeting at which a quorum is present. While the articles of incorporation may include special provisions authorizing the exercise of management powers outside of the meeting setting, this action usually requires the eventual approval of all of the directors. Each director occupies a fiduciary relation to the corporation and, therefore, must act in the utmost good faith and with reasonable care in all matters affecting the management of the corporation. According to the provisions of the articles of incorporation or the bylaws, the directors may or may not receive compensation. The duties of a director are nondelegable and he cannot appoint another to exercise his vote at a directors' meeting. The exercise of the vote of a director must not be hampered, and any advance agreement between directors concerning how they will vote usually is either specifically or by implication prohibited by state law.

The *officers* of the professional corporation are appointed or elected by the board of directors and usually hold office at the discretion of the board. Official positions commonly filled are that of president, vice president (one or more), secretary, and treasurer, as well as other positions particular to a professional corporation such as that of medical director, specialty director, or lay administrator. For ethical and statutory reasons, if an officer's duties involve professional decision-making or action, he should be a qualified professional.

Officers are considered to be agents of the corporation and possess the expressed authority given them by the articles, bylaws, and state statutes. In addition, the president or administrator has the implied authority to conduct the day-to-day business affairs of the corporation. The corporation is bound by any act or contract performed by any officer in accordance with his authority; therefore, officers, in addition to directors, are required to exercise reasonable care and loyalty in the performance of their duties. Such loyalty requires that the officer or director put corporate interests above his own concerning those activities or transactions related to the corporation's business or purposes.

Provisions of the articles of incorporation are drafted prior to the creation of the corporation; provisions other than those discussed earlier should be included only if they are vital to the operation or organization of the corporation. All article provisions should be clear, concise, and simple, with clarification or refinement relegated to the bylaws or the operating policies of the corporation. Provisions concerning amendment of the articles, arbitration of disputes, and liquidation of the corporation may be included in the articles. The incorporators, however, together with their legal counsel, may include any additional article provisions that are deemed necessary due to the specific needs or circumstances of the medical group.

Bylaws. After the articles of incorporation have been filed and the existence of the corporation has begun, the shareholders or initial directors of the corporation usually hold an organizational meeting to develop the bylaws of the corporation. Other actions that may be taken at the organizational meetings include the delegation of powers and duties to officers, the determination of the form of stock certificates, and the adoption of a corporate seal.[k] It is essential that detailed minutes be kept of corporate meetings, including the organization meeting, because in most court cases dealing with the corporate status of a professional corporation, the court decisions usually mention the existence of the minutes of such meetings as they are maintained in corporate minute books.[87]

The internal structure of the corporation is established in its bylaws, which usually expand or refine the provisions of the articles of incorporation. The bylaws typically may include provisions concerning the formalities of both shareholder and directors' meetings, voting procedures, the duties and authority of each corporate officer, the principal place of business for the corporation, the maintenance of corporate records, the issuance and transfer of the shares of stock, and the determination of the corporation's fiscal year.

To expand upon the possible corporate status requirement of centralized management, the bylaws may contain clauses which provide that control of the professional employees and their work be governed by the board of directors, who may in turn delegate authority to officers of the group practice. Such authority could include the assignment of patients, the determination of work deadlines and work hours; the establishment of quality review, the determination of patient fees as well as employee salaries and bonuses, the termination of employees; and the selection or rejection of patients.[88]

In most instances the spirit of cooperation is quite high during the formation of an organization, and a number of miscellaneous operating policies may be agreed upon more readily in the drafting of the bylaws from the mission statement. The specific content of the bylaws must be determined by the individual group shareholders or directors; the following strategies, however, may be provided for in the bylaws:

1. *Reduction and Admission of Professional Staff.* The basic procedures

[k]The certificate is an instrument issued to each shareholder designating his ownership of shares and represents the corporation's recognition of share ownership.

for admittance of additional physicians, trial employment, supervisory professionals for the new physician, and requirements for the purchase of corporate stock may be formalized in the bylaws. In addition, procedures for the expulsion of a physician usually are found in the bylaws.

2. *Financial Policies.* The bylaws may indicate the various accounting methods to be used by the corporation, such as cash basis or accrual basis. The cash method does not acknowledge income or obligations for accounting purposes until the money is received or transferred. The accrual method of accounting acknowledges the income or obligation when it accrues.

3. *Power to Deal in Property.* The corporation may give its directors, through the bylaws, the power to determine and direct the purchase, lease, and sale of both real property and personal property in the corporate name.

4. *Vacation and Leave for Physicians.* The availability of paid vacations, academic leave, or sick leave usually is determined in the bylaws together with any arrangements for compensation due the physicians during a particular leave of absence or vacation.

5. *Shareholder Voting and Stock Purchase Agreements.* The bylaws of many professional corporations will outline various requirements and limitations applicable to such agreements and will not allow the corporation to be a party to any agreement containing a prohibited provision.

6. *Insurance.* The bylaws may authorize the corporation to insure itself for any liability that is not a part of the liability of the shareholder/employee in his professional capacity.[89]

7. *Taxation.* The bylaws must indicate whether the corporation has elected to be taxed in a special way, such as through the use of *Internal Revenue Code* §1244 or Sub-chapter S income taxation methods.

The physician or administrator should consider the possibility that the professional corporation may not be a financial success. In establishing the capital structure of the corporation the incorporators may either issue shares of stock or obtain loans or bonds from individuals or shareholders, and if the corporation is not a success, the shareholder or bondholder probably will lose some or all of his investment. In most instances, however, any loss attributable to the bond will be tax deductible at the short-term capital gains rates if the bond is sold. The regulation for such losses allows the deduction of a loss for each year either up to $1,000 of the taxable income that year, or in the amount of capital loss over capital gain, whichever is less. On the other hand, under Section 1244 of the *Internal Revenue Code*, for a loss attributable to worthless shares of stock the physician may take an ordinary loss deduction. If the bond is held, and if the professional corporation goes bankrupt, the full amount can be deducted against ordinary income if it can be shown that the bond is worthless. Section 1244 is available only for common stock issued in exchange for cash or other property, but only includes stock and securities issued by a small corporation—that is, a corporation that has, after the issuance of the stock, an equity worth less than $500,000. The corporation's minutes or bylaws should contain a statement of intention or a plan for the use of Section 1244 treatment. The existence of a second class of stock or the partnership's receipt of stock as an original owner may bar the use of Section 1244 by the corporation. The use of Section 1244 allows a taxpayer to take up to $25,000 ($50,000 for a joint return) per year in ordinary loss deductions for stock losses. For most physicians the use of Section 1244 is a valuable business planning tool and offers opportunity for financial recovery if needed.[90]

Sub-chapter S provides a method through which the shareholders and the professional corporation can elect to be treated as a partnership for the profits and losses of the practice. Sub-chapter S is a section of the *Internal Revenue Code* which allows small corporations having only one class of stock and no more than ten shareholders to elect to be taxed as a partnership; the income of the corporation then is taxed to the shareholders as if they were partners. With the use of Sub-chapter S, the physician can make direct use of any losses that the corporation incurs and he can avoid corporate tax disadvantages such as unreasonable compensation.[91] Furthermore, the possibility of double taxation of the corporation's profits is eliminated by the direct assignment of the corporation's profits to the individual shareholders.

The use of Sub-chapter S by the professional corporation does impose two important limitations upon the corporation's use of a retirement plan. Any contributions made by the corporation for the retirement fund of an employee, who owns more than 5 percent of the corporation's stock, that are above the levels allowed for self-employed or partnership plans, will result in the employee's being taxed on the excess amount as additional compensation; and any employee contributions forfeited by an employee due to an early departure cannot accrue to the benefit of any other employee who holds more than 5 percent of the corporation's stock.[92] The pension reform act also may disqualify the retirement plan and add a 6 percent penalty for excess contributions. While the pension and profit-sharing restrictions do reduce the desirability of electing Sub-chapter S treatment, nevertheless, all of the benefits of general incorporation remain for a Sub-chapter S user. The professional group wanting other fringe benefits and not desiring to implement immediately a strong pension or profit-sharing plan, may find Sub-chapter S a convenient tax method. The election of Sub-chapter S is usually required in the bylaws or at an early meeting of the shareholders, and can be retracted at any time.

The forming group must realize that the use of Section 1244 stock or Sub-chapter S is an important and critical decision affecting the taxation of the professional corporation. Because the corporation must remain eligible in terms of the size and the capital limitations requirements of the respective IRC sections, continuous counseling from the corporation's attorney and accountant is a necessity. Furthermore, as with the other provisions of the articles of incorporation and the bylaws, there should be agreement among a substantial number of the group's physicians when any tax planning alternatives are adopted.

Restrictions on the Transfer of Shares. The legal and ethical considerations discussed earlier indicate that the shares of a professional corporation must be owned only by persons licensed to practice the profession represented by the corporation. In light of this restriction, some states require that the shareholders of the corporation approve any sale of the stock shares, and the high degree of personal and professional trust necessary among members of a professional corporation demands that the present shareholders approve the admission of new shareholders.[93] As a result, many professionals adopt a formal agreement which regulates the transfer of shares to new shareholders.

These restrictions may be included in the corporation's articles or in its bylaws, or may be developed in a separate shareholders' agreement which is ordinarily authorized by the articles or bylaws. The problems encountered in any drafting agreement dealing with restrictions on the sale of shares usually include the determination of the method of restriction, the selling price of the shares, and the method of payment.

In most states, any restriction on the transfer of shares of stock must be reasonable to be valid. Because the right to sell is fundamental to the ownership of property, an absolute or substantial restriction upon the professional's right to sell his shares in the medical corporation usually will not be allowed by state law. Within the framework of this reasonableness doctrine, most restriction arrangements involve either the use of a stock repurchase agreement by the corporation, or the use of a right-of-first-refusal agreement between the shareholders and corporation.

The corporation may obligate itself at the time of the original sale of the shares to repurchase the shares either when the physician/shareholder desires to withdraw from the group, or upon the death of a shareholder. The obligation to purchase may be absolutely binding upon the shareholder and corporation or may be optional according to the incorporators' desires. The repurchase agreement usually is valid if it is provided for in the articles or in the bylaws, and if there is a legal source of available funds from which the corporation can draw to repurchase the shares. In most states the funds must come only from the retained earned surplus of the corporation. To protect the rights of creditors and remaining shareholders, the corporation must not use any of the capital paid into the corporation for the repurchase. Many corporations, therefore, will establish a capital accumulations fund or will purchase insurance on the lives of the shareholders in order to help finance a stock repurchase. A considerable number of states, however, have stricken this provision from their professional incorporation acts and the model professional corporation act being prepared by the American Bar Association does not contain any such provision. Furthermore, a repurchase cannot be made if it would leave the corporation insolvent or unable to cover its debts.

The other frequently used method of retaining control in a small corporation is to have each shareholder agree at an early date that he will not sell or transfer his shares to a third party without first offering them to the other shareholders or the corporation. If the other shareholders or the corporation fail to purchase the shares under the conditions of the agreement, then the departing shareholder may sell his shares to a qualified third person. A right-of-first-refusal or cross-purchase, as this arrangement is usually called, ordinarily represents a reasonable restraint and can be enforced by the remaining shareholders or by the corporation. In small corporations the cross-purchase or right-of-first-refusal agreement is most workable; when there are large numbers of shareholders, however, the acceptability of a cross-purchase agreement may be diminished due to too many details and too much confusion.[94]

Regardless of the alternative method used, state law requires that in order to be enforceable, restrictions on the transfer must appear upon the face of the stock certificate. If the restriction does appear, and it is reasonable, the corporation has the legal ability to refuse to recognize the transfer. If the transfer is not recognized, the corporation can continue to treat the transferring shareholder as a current shareholder including the continuation of his right to vote and his participation in the medical practice.

The price of the shares may be represented in a number of ways, including a predetermined price, an outside offer, an arbitrated price, or book value. The predetermined price may be settled upon in the agreement, or it may be the value of the shares at the time of their original issuance by the corporation. The remaining shareholders or the corporation may be required to match the offered price of an outsider for the shares of the medical corporation; or an arbitrated price, selected upon the recommendation of an outside arbitrator, may be used by the shareholders or the corporation if other methods fail. Finally, the book value is calculated by dividing the net worth of the corporation (assets less liabilities) by the number of shares, in order to determine current value of the shares.

The determination of the book value involves special problems in calculating the worth of assets such as a library, furniture, or equipment, as opposed to, for example, the accounts receivable. There are two approaches to this problem: to provide for a purchase price on the book value of the equipment and property assets only, which usually is minimal for a medical service corporation, and to distribute receivables in the form of deferred compensation; or to include an estimated, collected accounts receivable amount in the buy-out price, and subsequently allow the corporation or remaining shareholders to purchase the stock from the departing shareholder physician. The choice of approach is determined by whether the remaining shareholders and the corporation or the departed shareholder will be responsible for the tax on the accounts receivable.[95] The deferred compensation method for accounts receivable requires the terminating shareholder or his estate to pay the tax on income from the accounts; if the shareholder receives his share of accounts receivable as a part of the stock valuation, the income will be taxed to him under the lower capital gains rates.[96]

Regardless of whether the corporation or the shareholders pay the departing shareholder, the terms or method of payment is determined either in the buy-out agreement or in a set of authorized alternative methods. The departing shareholder's ownership may be paid for in total or in installments. The needed funds for a payment in full can place a considerable burden upon the corporation or shareholders. Insurance obtained by the corporation or shareholders on the lives of principal shareholders will help supply the necessary funds for a buy-out, should one of the shareholders die, or for a lump cash sum to be paid to a retiring shareholder or his heirs.

If payment in full is not desirable, the deferred compensation approach can be used and the payments, including imputed interest, may be made in installments over a period of time. The installment method, however, does have disadvantages; the retired shareholder or the survivors of the departed shareholder may not want to tie future security to the success of the professional corporation, and for the remaining shareholders, long-term obligations may hamper capital acquisition, growth of the corporation, and recruiting activities. For example, a new professional entering the corporation may feel that he does not want part of his earnings paid to a retired shareholder.[97]

Costs of Incorporation. Those physicians seeking to incorporate their practice will discover that legal fees may vary greatly, from a few hundred to several thousand dollars. The variation depends upon a number of factors, including whether the attorney requires a flat fee or charges by the amount of professional time spent on the project, whether filing fees are included, and whether the fee includes the maintenance operations of an attorney. Although the method of computing the legal fees will be important, the group should attempt to screen the attorney to determine his qualifications. The attorney who is inexperienced in the area of professional incorporation may provide a lower fee, but may cost the group considerably more when he must correct an incomplete incorporation at a later date. The experienced attorney may recognize more easily the unique circumstances involved in the particular group's practice and will be able to provide a properly tailored arrangement. The group physicians may wish to ask their colleagues or other professionals who have worked with a prospective attorney about his skills and experience in professional incorporation.[98]

Ultimately, the costs of incorporation may depend upon what the group receives from the attorney in the way of advice and carefully drawn up documents for the corporation. For example, the reader may assume he must choose among three attorneys, Mr. White, Mr. Black, and Mr. Gray, each of whom has been well recommended by colleagues and seems to understand the problems of a medical group practice. Attorney White says the project will cost $500, attorney Black places the cost at $1,200, and attorney Gray requires $1,500. White explains that this fee includes $450 for the incorporation documents (articles and bylaws) and an additional $50 for the filing fees. White's fee is actually based upon an incomplete job. The stock certificates, minute books, and other necessary instruments of the corporation may cost an additional $100. Furthermore, the establishment of the pension or profit-sharing retirement plan may cost an additional $1,000. The maintenance services, including preparing the minutes of the annual meeting, and day-to-day counseling by White, may require an additional $600 per year. As a result, the actual cost of attorney White, based upon his item by item approach, may reach $2,200 instead of $500.[99]

Attorney Black requires $1,200, but his services include an orientation session, the actual incorporation, and a simple retirement plan; however, the filing fees, corporate-kit expenses as outlined above, and the various alternatives in the retirement plan may cause an additional estimated expense of $350. Furthermore, he may charge an estimated $250 per year for the continuous maintenance expenses. The total estimated cost of attorney Black may reach $1,900.

Attorney Gray's estimate includes the entire services as outlined for White and Black, including orientation, actual incorporation, pension plans and *reasonable* yearly maintenance duties. His quote of $1,500, therefore, which was originally the highest, actually may give the group the most service for its money.[100]

Although the selection of fee estimates is somewhat arbitrary, the physician must realize that ultimately the cost of legal services is based upon the amount of time the attorney must spend resolving differences or disputes among the physicians. If the physicians and administrator devote some effort and time to determining what they have in mind for their corporation, the time required of the attorney can be minimized.

The processes involved in organizing and creating a professional corporation are authorized and regulated strictly by state laws. The incorporators must be qualified according to ethical and legal standards and, in some cases, the corporation must reflect the personal, professional, and financial needs of each of the physician shareholders. All of these factors will have definite impact upon the drafting of eventual acknowledgements of the corporation's articles of incorporation, bylaws, and subsequent shareholder actions or agreements. Because these corporate instruments are not inflexible, but sometimes become difficult to alter or to understand, considerable care and thought must be exercised before any steps are taken to incorporate a medical practice. Confusion or mistakes in the drafting or filing of the corporation's documents can seriously frustrate the intentions of the physician founders and the mission of the organization.

Employment and Compensation

In addition to corporate documents that establish the operational structure of the professional corporate practice, the employment arrangements between the corporation and the physicians establish the physician's professional relationship with the corporation. The physician in corporate practice is an employee as well as a shareholder, and as such he must deal with the corporation as he would with any other employer.

Employment Contracts for Nonshareholder Physicians. A trial method of group practice can be the employment of one physician by another. Before adding a new shareholder physician to the practice, the professional corporation may wish to hire the new physician for a period of time in order to allow the corporation a chance to evaluate him. A trial employment relationship also gives the incoming physician an opportunity to evaluate whether the medical group will satisfy his professional needs and desires. Before engaging in any trial arrangement of physicians, however, the corporation should determine whether the state law allows employment of physicians who are not shareholders.

As with any contract of employment, the trial arrangement contract should contain all the aspects of the employment agreement. The contract may be written or oral; but, to help avoid confusion later over the terms of employment, and in accordance with any applicable state laws, it is preferable to have a written contract. Some general aspects of the employment of an incoming physician that might be represented in the employment contract include:

1. *Statement of Employment Status.* The usual contract between a nonshareholder employee and the corporation emphasizes that the physician is an employee and may state that the employment is to be a trial arrangement.

2. *Opportunity to Become a Shareholder.* To a limited degree, the employment contract may indicate that if the trial arrangement proves satisfactory, the employee will be awarded the opportunity to purchase shares in the corporation. Many trial employment contracts also will specify the terms for the purchase of shares.

3. *Duties and Responsibilities.* The employment contract usually defines the professional duties expected of the employee by the corporation. Further-

more, the contract may provide a system of professional review and make continued employment conditional depending upon the employee's fulfillment of the terms of the contract.

4. *Determination of Compensation.* Since the incoming physician, in both a legal and a practical sense, will not be able to participate in the major decisions of the corporation, most employment contracts can be quite specific in the rate of compensation due to the physician. The provisions usually allow for increases in the initial employment rate dependent upon the professional development and cooperation of the employee.

5. *Article or Bylaw Provisions.* Any provisions which are stated in the articles or bylaws relating to the trial employment of an incoming physician are either repeated or referred to in the employment agreement.

6. *Restrictive Covenants.* Some professional corporations utilize restrictive covenants in their employment contracts for incoming physicians. The restrictive covenant usually prohibits a departing physician from practicing in competition with the corporation for a certain number of years and within a certain geographic area. The covenant may also contain provisions for payment of liquidated damages, or the waiver of the clause by the corporation if the physician does not wish to remain in the area.

The above suggestions are by no means an exhaustive or mandatory selection of trial arrangements to be provided for in employment contracts. The particular needs and desires of both the group and the incoming physician should be the factors which determine the terms to be included in the employment contract; in some circumstances a professional corporation may not adopt any form of a trial arrangement employment contract.

Employment Contracts for Shareholder Physician. The professional corporation is a separate legal entity that must employ physicians to provide the medical services. With only a few exceptions, the employment relationship between the corporation and the physician is based upon a written employment contract which serves at least two general purposes for the group practice. First, the contract helps to systematize the relationship between the physician and the corporation, which can be extremely complex and can involve salary, medical, and management considerations; and secondly, employment contracts have been regarded as persuasive evidence of the distinct and separate relationship existing between the corporate entity and the professional employee. The terms of the employment contract may be even more important than the articles or bylaws in giving the "look of corporateness" to the medical practice.[101]

The employment contract can be used in addition to the bylaws of the corporation to establish the rights, duties, and obligations of the physician and corporation towards each other. In the professional corporation the traditional forms of employment agreements will vary according to the degree of emphasis placed upon such provisions as, for instance, a reaffirmation of the right of the board of directors to dismiss any employee or officer, or covenants not to compete in order to protect the interests of the professional practice if a physician departs.[102] Employment contracts also may contain any other provisions included in the bylaws that are crucial to the operation of the corporation, such as centralization of management, distribution and control over patients, and possession of patient files. As the collective product of the needs and desires of the corporation and the physicians, further characteristics of the employment contract include possible clauses dealing with procedures for policies governing the allotments and limits of medical practice expenses and obligations; the use and extent of insurance; the regulation of outside professional functions; the basic policies or procedures covering leave, vacation, and other periods of time off; retirement and termination regulations; and the establishment of a professional review structure and stock purchase policies.

One of the most important sections of the employment contract is the provision covering the physician's salary. As with the other provisions of the agreement, any arrangement concerning salary should be the result of the negotiations between the physician and the corporation. Rather than utilizing the general authorization language of salary determination commonly found in a corporation's bylaws, however, the employment agreement usually sets forth specifically all of the policy aspects of compensation for each physician. The following list includes some salary arrangements contained in the *Medical Group Management Association Digest of Medical Group Employment Contracts and Income Distribution Plans:*[1]

1. A varying percentage of cash collected to be paid to the physician along with provisions for determination of employment, permanent disability, military call, and emergency coverage.
2. A stable salary with bonus based on varying percentages of net collections for service seniority and equality.
3. An arrangement for salary equal to a percentage of gross charges for professional services rendered.
4. An equal share plan plus seniority and incentive aspects, with varying mixes of the three for each year of employment.
5. A base salary figured on 40 percent of productivity with a point system to take into account a variety of other factors.
6. A combination salary containing a "base income," "administrative-professional income," and "incentive income."
7. An arrangement including a base salary with longevity increments and trailing increments added to the bonus which is based on bookings.
8. An arrangement using base salary, seniority allowance, special allowances for various qualifications, and a "sliding scale" allowance for monthly clinic billings in addition to a quarterly bonus.
9. A salary using a base plus a bonus for a given level of bookings with further distribution made in relation to bookings below the bonus level.
10. An arrangement allowing for compensation differentiation for various specialties with a point system for longevity and increasing increments of percentage billing for production bonuses.
11. A base salary plus point system with a minimum and maximum level.

The above list refers to various uses of the bonus in salary arrangements. A corporation is taxed on its net profits and any profits distributed in dividends

[1]The digest contains samples of various employment contracts and income distribution agreements for partnerships, corporations, and incorporated associations that the reader may desire to review for his orientation. Sample provisions are not included in this discussion.

will be taxed again to the shareholder. The corporation can, however, adopt a bonus program that is related to the actual employment achievements of the physician. The bonus plan should be well defined and should be presented to the physician prior to his year of practice. If the bonuses are actually "worked for," any objections from the Internal Revenue Service that the bonus plan is a disguised distribution dividend usually can be avoided. The professional corporation's attorney or accountant should be consulted about the use of any bonus system.

Regardless of the method of salary distribution, any compensation made to the physician must be reasonable in order to be allowed as a deductible business expense under Section 61 of the *Internal Revenue Code.* To justify a particular salary as reasonable, the determination of the rate of compensation usually should reflect the employee's special talents and qualifications; the difficulty of the employment and amount of responsibilities assumed; the percentage breakdown of the physician's compensation to the corporation's gross profit and net profit; the prevailing economic conditions; the level of dividend, if any, paid to the shareholders; prevailing rates of compensation in comparable positions for similar professions as well as the salary policy of the corporation to all of its employees; the physician's previous compensation history; and the approval of a board of directors which is independent of any particular shareholder receiving compensation.[103]

A finding by the Internal Revenue Service that a salary payment to the physician shareholder is unreasonable usually will result in a double taxation of the amount considered a dividend distribution. The employment agreement for many professional corporations will contain a provision requiring return to the corporation of the portion of the physician's salary deemed excessive.[104] This reimbursement might avoid double taxation on the returned amount and the repayment might not be considered as income to the particular physician.

The payment of a reasonable salary to a shareholder physician may not in itself allow a full deduction of the salary by the corporation as a business expense. This situation results from the physician's initial contribution of capital, at least in terms of goodwill, to the corporation. Goodwill is commonly referred to as the intangible asset of a medical practice such as a "good name" or "reputation" in the community which can contribute to the success of the corporation. Because goodwill belongs to the corporation and because some of the income generated by the physician is attributable to the corporation's goodwill, any salary payment made to the physician from income received through the corporation's goodwill is actually a return to the physician of his initial goodwill contribution and must be double taxed as a dividend payment.[105]

The forced dividend issue is still under controversy, and until it is resolved, careful planning should include arrangements in the corporation's employment contracts and bylaws to minimize the applicability of a dividend ruling. If the corporation was formed from a partnership, any sale of assets from the partnership would not include goodwill by contract. The physicians or partnership, however, could lease the goodwill to the corporation at a set fee.[106]

The use of employment contracts by the professional corporation serves two purposes. First, the employment relationship between the corporation and the physician is formalized and presented in writing with respective rights, duties, and obligations of employee and employer clarified. Secondly, the employment agreement helps to alleviate doubt concerning the existence of the corporation as the employer and as a bonafide separate legal entity. The employment agreement usually reaffirms the provisions of the articles and bylaws that are relevant to the employment of the physician. Generally, one of the most important provisions of the employment contract for the individual physician employee is the provision establishing his professional obligations and compensation. Although the salary can be determined by a variety of methods, the particular method chosen must reflect a compensation rate that is reasonable. Recently, the Internal Revenue Service has become concerned with salaries for the professional that have, at least in part, contained a possible "disguised" dividend. The employment contract can be used as an instrument to overcome this "disguised" dividend problem.

Dissolution and Liquidation

Either by action of the state or by the resolution of the owners, the existence of the corporation may cease. As with any medical practice, in order to orient and prepare all parties for the possibility of termination, dissolving or liquidating the corporation should be discussed in the early stages of incorporation. Dissolution refers to the termination of the corporate existence, and liquidation refers to the termination by a corporation of its business affairs. If liquidation occurs without dissolution (i.e., the sale of all corporate assets), the corporation usually is terminated as a practical matter, but continues its legal existence.

Voluntary Liquidation. The corporation may be dissolved by the voluntary actions of the board of directors and the shareholders. State law usually provides various simplified procedures which the shareholders and directors may utilize to effect a dissolution. The statutes generally provide that in order for a voluntary dissolution to occur the board of directors must adopt a resolution directing dissolution and submit the resolution to be ratified by a majority of the shareholders. Many states require that the corporation file a certificate of dissolution or other similar document with the appropriate state agency. In addition to the procedure outlined by the state, the articles or bylaws of the corporation may contain provisions directing dissolution to begin if there is an irreconcilable disagreement among the shareholders, upon the death of a sole or leading shareholder, upon an adverse change in the tax or corporate laws, or simply because the reasons which prompted formation of the corporation may no longer exist or seem appealing.[107] Liquidation of the corporation's assets, obligations, and business activities must follow a dissolution. Generally, after a dissolution, the state administration or judicial system may choose to regulate the liquidation procedure.

Involuntary Dissolution. A corporation may be dissolved by state or judicial action, regardless of any desire on the part of the shareholders or directors not to dissolve the corporation. The state may institute proceedings in court to cause a forfeiture of the corporation's charter if the corporation acts outside its expressed or implied powers and purposes, or if the corporation fails to comply with the regulations governing a professional corporation. In most states such a forfeiture due to violation of the regulations will ordinarily occur if the corporation retains a disqualified person as a shareholder or employee; if no qualified person is a shareholder of the corporation; if a withdrawing or disqualified shareholder's interests fail to be transferred to a qualified person or to be redeemed by the corporation; or if a shareholder cannot obtain the consent of the other shareholders for the sale of his interest.[108]

In addition to an involuntary dissolution for failure to follow the state law provisions applicable to professional and general business corporations, statutes in many states provide that a dissolution may occur if an application is made by a shareholder or director. Applications are usually available to general corporations and, by implication, to professional corporations. The use of an application for dissolution is entirely statutory in many states, and the group considering incorporation should consult its attorney for the provisions available in the particular state. The usual circumstances allowing an application for dissolution include a deadlock in the management and operation of the corporation, persistent mismanagement, abuse of authority, fraud in the management, or the expiration of the term of the existence of the corporation.

In most circumstances, an action for involuntary dissolution cannot be brought by the creditors. When the corporation has been dissolved by a court or administrative agency, its affairs usually are placed into the hands of a receiver who is to supervise the liquidation. After the appointment of a receiver, the corporation's creditors may intervene in the liquidation. The receiver has the responsibility of satisfying the creditors and distributing the remaining assets to the shareholders.

Effect of Dissolution. Upon dissolution by either a voluntary or involuntary process under either the directors or a receiver, the corporation can no longer pursue any new business. The corporation continues in existence, however, for the purpose of winding up its affairs, and it must honor its contracts and perform any professional services that were undertaken prior to dissolution. In many instances, the articles of incorporation may outline the procedures for dissolution and liquidation of the corporation, including the distribution of assets. Subject to any provisions of the articles, each shareholder is entitled to a proportionate share of the corporation's remaining assets after payment of the creditors. The distribution is proportionate to the individual holdings of shares, and liquidation of assets may be in cash or by a property distribution. If the corporation has been successful, the distributive share of the assets may exceed the amount of each shareholder's contributions either due to increase in the value of the corporation's property or to accumulated earnings.

A conventional liquidation of a corporation will result in a taxable gain to the shareholders under Section 331 of the *Internal Revenue Code.* The tax ordinarily will be determined by the lower capital gains rates. If the organization has little or no cash items on hand and little or no accumulated earnings and profits, a tax-free liquidation under Section 333 of the *IRC* may be attractive. If the corporation has the opportunity to sell all or most of its assets (as in the case of a younger physician purchasing the corporation practice of another), Section 337 of the *IRC* should be considered. Under this section a sale of the assets of the corporation will be free of tax if a plan of complete liquidation has been adopted prior to such sale, if the liquidation is then completed within twelve months, and if the other requirements of Section 337 are met. There still will be a capital gain on the distribution of the sale proceeds to the shareholders.

The dissolution of a professional corporation can occur by either voluntary or involuntary means. The resolution of the shareholders and directors can cause a voluntary dissolution of the corporation. Upon application to a court or administrative agency, however, a shareholder or the state may cause an involuntary dissolution of the corporation. The shareholders can apply for dissolution when, because of certain events, the corporation can no longer function properly. A state usually requests the forfeiture of the corporation's charter if the professional corporation is found to be in violation of the statutory requirements of the state for an incorporated practice. The liquidation of the corporation's assets may result in taxable gain to the shareholders and prior planning may help to avoid some taxation consequences.

Appendix 5A

Uniform Partnership Act

PART I—PRELIMINARY PROVISIONS

Section 1. [Name of Act]

This act may be cited as Uniform Partnership Act.

Section 2. [Definition of Terms]

In this act,

"Court" includes every court and judge having jurisdiction in the case.

"Business" includes every trade, occupation, or profession.

"Person" includes individuals, partnerships, corporations, and other associations.

"Bankrupt" includes bankrupt under the Federal Bankruptcy Act or insolvent under any state insolvent act.

"Conveyance" includes every assignment, lease, mortgage, or encumbrance.

"Real property" includes land and any interest or estate in land.

Section 3. [Interpretation of Knowledge and Notice]

1. A person has "knowledge" of a fact within the meaning of this act not only when he has actual knowledge thereof, but also when he has knowledge of such other facts as in the circumstances shows bad faith.

2. A person has "notice" of a fact within the meaning of this act when the person who claims the benefit of the notice:

a. States the fact to such person, or

b. Delivers through the mail, or by other means of communication, a written statement of the fact to such person or to a proper person at his place of business or residence.

Section 4. [Rules of Construction]

1. The rule that statutes in derogation of the common law are to be strictly construed shall have no application to this act.

2. The law of estoppel shall apply under this act.

3. The law of agency shall apply under this act.

4. This act shall be so interpreted and construed as to effect its general purpose to make uniform the law of those states which enact it.

5. This act shall not be construed so as to impair the obligations of any contract tract existing when the act goes into effect, nor to affect any action or proceedings begun or right accrued before this act takes effect.

Section 5. [Rules for Cases not Provided for in this Act]

In any case not provided for in this act the rules of law and equity, including the law merchant, shall govern.

PART II—NATURE OF PARTNERSHIP

Section 6. [Partnership Defined]

1. A partnership is an association of two or more persons to carry on as co-owners a business for profit.

2. But any association formed under any other statute of this state, or any statute adopted by authority, other than the authority of this state, is not a partnership under this act, unless such association would have been a partnership in this state prior to the adoption of this act; but this act shall apply to limited partnerships except in so far as the statutes relating to such partnerships are inconsistent herewith.

Section 7. [Rules for Determining the Existence of a Partnership]

In determining whether a partnership exists, these rules shall apply:

1. Except as provided by Section 16 persons who are not partners as to each other are not partners as to third persons.

2. Joint tenancy, tenancy in common, tenancy by the entireties, joint property, common property, or part ownership does not of itself establish a partnership, whether such co-owners do or do not share any profits made by the use of the property.

3. The sharing of gross returns does not of itself establish a partnership, whether or not the persons sharing them have a joint or common right or interest in any property from which the returns are derived.

4. The receipt by a person of a share of the profits of a business is prima facie evidence that he is a partner in the business, but no such inference shall be drawn if such profits were received in payment:

a. As a debt by installments or otherwise,
b. As wages of an employee or rent to a landlord,
c. As an annuity to a widow or representative of a deceased partner,

d. As interest on a loan, though the amount of payment vary with the profits of the business,

e. As the consideration for the sale of a goodwill of a business or other property by installments or otherwise.

Section 8. [Partnership Property]

1. All property originally brought into the partnership stock or subsequently acquired by purchase or otherwise, on account of the partnership, is partnership property.

2. Unless the contrary intention appears, property acquired with partnership funds is partnership property.

3. Any estate in real property may be acquired in the partnership name. Title so acquired can be conveyed only in the partnership name.

4. A conveyance to a partnership in the partnership name, though without words of inheritance, passes the entire estate of the grantor unless a contrary intent appears.

PART III—RELATIONS OF PARTNERS TO PERSONS DEALING WITH THE PARTNERSHIP

Section 9. [Partner Agent of Partnership as to Partnership Business]

1. Every partner is an agent of the partnership for the purpose of its business, and the act of every partner, including the execution in the partnership name of any instrument, for apparently carrying on in the usual way the business of the partnership of which he is a member binds the partnership, unless the partner so acting has in fact no authority to act for the partnership in the particular matter, and the person with whom he is dealing has knowledge of the fact that he has no such authority.

2. An act of a partner which is not apparently for the carrying on of the business of the partnership in the usual way does not bind the partnership unless authorized by the other partners.

3. Unless authorized by the other partners or unless they have abandoned the business, one or more but less than all the partners have no authority to:

a. Assign the partnership property in trust for creditors or on the assignee's promise to pay the debts of the partnership,

b. Dispose of the goodwill of the business,

c. Do any other act which would make it impossible to carry on the ordinary business of a partnership,

d. Confess a judgment,

e. Submit a partnership claim or liability to arbitration or reference,

4. No act of a partner in contravention of a restriction on authority shall bind the partnership to persons having knowledge of the restriction.

Section 10. [Conveyance of Real Property of the Partnership]

1. Where title to real property is in the partnership name, any partner may convey title to such property by a conveyance executed in the partnership

name; but the partnership may recover such property unless the partner's act binds the partnership under the provisions of paragraph (1) of Section 9, or unless such property has been conveyed by the grantee or a person claiming through such grantee to a holder for value without knowledge that the partner, in making the conveyance, has exceeded his authority.

2. Where title to real property is in the name of the partnership, a conveyance executed by a partner, in his own name, passes the equitable interest of the partnership, provided the act is one within the authority of the partner under the provisions of paragraph (1) of Section 9.

3. Where title to real property is in the name of one or more but not all the partners, and the record does not disclose the right of the partnership, the partners in whose name the title stands may convey title to such property, but the partnership may recover such property if the partner's act does not bind the partnership under the provisions of paragraph (1) of Section 9, unless the purchaser or his assignee, is a holder for value, without knowledge.

4. Where the title to real property is in the name of one or more or all the partners, or in a third person in trust for the partnership, a conveyance executed by a partner in the partnership name, or in his own name, passes the equitable interest of the partnership, provided the act is one within the authority of the partner under the provisions of paragraph (1) of Section 9.

5. Where the title to real property is in the names of all the partners a conveyance executed by all the partners passes all their rights in such property.

Section 11. [Partnership Bound by Admission of Partner]

An admission or representation made by any partner concerning partnership affairs within the scope of his authority as conferred by this act is evidence against the partnership.

Section 12. [Partnership Charged with Knowledge of or Notice to Partner]

Notice to any partner of any matter relating to partnership affairs, and the knowledge of the partner acting in the particular matter, acquired while a partner or then present to his mind, and the knowledge of any other partner who reasonably could and should have communicated it to the acting partner, operate as notice to or knowledge of the partnership, except in the case of a fraud on the partnership committed by or with the consent of that partner.

Section 13. [Partnership Bound by Partner's Wrongful Act]

Where, by any wrongful act or omission of any partner acting in the ordinary course of the business of the partnership or with the authority of his co-partners, loss or injury is caused to any person, not being a partner in the partnership, or any penalty is incurred, the partnership is liable therefor to the same extent as the partner so acting or omitting to act.

Section 14. [Partnership Bound by Partner's Breach of Trust]

The partnership is bound to make good the loss:

a. Where one partner acting within the scope of his apparent authority receives money or property of a third person and misapplies it; and

b. Where the partnership in the course of its business receives money or property of a third person and the money or property so received is misapplied by any partner while it is in the custody of the partnership.

Section 15. [Nature of Partner's Liability]

All partners are liable

a. Jointly and severally for everything chargeable to the partnership under Sections 13 and 14.

b. Jointly for all other debts and obligations of the partnership; but any partner may enter into a separate obligation to perform a partnership contract.

Section 16. [Partner by Estoppel]

1. When a person, by words spoken or written or by conduct, represents himself, or consents to another representing him to any one, as a partner in an existing partnership or with one or more persons not actual partners, he is liable to any such person to whom such representation has been made, who has, on the faith of such representation, given credit to the actual or apparent partnership, and if he has made such representation or consented to its being made in a public manner he is liable to such person, whether the representation has or has not been made or communicated to such person so giving credit by or with the knowledge of the apparent partner making the representation or consenting to its being made.

a. When a partnership liability results, he is liable as though he were an actual member of the partnership.

b. When no partnership liability results, he is liable jointly with the other persons, if any, so consenting to the contract or representation as to incur liability, otherwise separately.

2. When a person has been thus represented to be a partner in an existing partnership, or with one or more persons not actual partners, he is an agent of the persons consenting to such representation to bind them to the same extent and in the same manner as though he were a partner in fact, with respect to persons who rely upon the representation. Where all the members of the existing partnership consent to the representation, a partnership act or obligation results; but in all other cases it is the joint act or obligation of the person acting and the persons consenting to the representation.

Section 17. [Liability of Incoming Partner]

A person admitted as a partner into an existing partnership is liable for all the obligations of the partnership arising before his admission as though he had been a partner when such obligations were incurred, except that this liability shall be satisfied only out of partnership property.

PART IV—RELATIONS OF PARTNERS TO ONE ANOTHER

Section 18. [Rules Determining Rights and Duties of Partners]

The rights and duties of the partners in relation to the partnership shall be determined, subject to any agreement between them, by the following rules:

a. Each partner shall be repaid his contributions, whether by way of capital or advances to the partnership property and share equally in the profits and surplus remaining after all liabilities, including those to partners, are satisfied; and must contribute towards the losses, whether of capital or otherwise, sustained by the partnership according to his share in the profits.

b. The partnership must indemnify every partner in respect of payments made and personal liabilities reasonably incurred by him in the ordinary and proper conduct of its business, or for the preservation of its business or property.

c. A partner, who in aid of the partnership makes any payment or advance beyond the amount of capital which he agreed to contribute, shall be paid interest from the date of the payment or advance.

d. A partner shall receive interest on the capital contribution by him only from the date when repayment should be made.

e. All partners have equal rights in the management and conduct of the partnership business.

f. No partner is entitled to remuneration for acting in the partnership business, except that a surviving partner is entitled to reasonable compensation for his services in winding up the partnership affairs.

g. No person can become a member of a partnership without the consent of all the partners.

h. Any difference arising as to ordinary matters connected with the partnership business may be decided by a majority of the partners; but no act in contravention of any agreement between the partners may be done rightfully without the consent of all the partners.

Section 19. [Partnership Books]

The partnership books shall be kept, subject to any agreement between the partners, at the principal place of business of the partnership, and every partner shall at all times have access to and may inspect and copy any of them.

Section 20. [Duty of Partners to Render Information]

Partners shall render on demand true and full information of all things affecting the partnership to any partner or the legal representative of any deceased partner or partner under legal disability.

Section 21. [Partner Accountable as a Fiduciary]

1. Every partner must account to the partnership for any benefit, and hold as trustee for it any profits derived by him without the consent of the other

partners from any transaction connected with the formation, conduct, or liquidation of the partnership or from any use by him of its property.

2. This Section applies also to the representatives of a deceased partner engaged in the liquidation of the affairs of the partnership as the personal representatives of the last surviving partner.

Section 22. [Right to an Account]

Any partner shall have the right to a formal account as to partnership affairs:

a. If he is wrongfully excluded from the partnership business or possessions of its property by his co-partners,

b. If the right exists under the terms of any agreement,

c. As provided by Section 21,

d. Whenever other circumstances render it just and reasonable.

Section 23. [Continuation of Partnership Beyond Fixed Term]

1. When a partnership for a fixed term or particular undertaking is continued after the termination of such term or particular undertaking without any express agreement, the rights and duties of the partners remain the same as they were at such termination, so far as is consistent with a partnership at will.

2. A continuation of the business by the partners or such of them as habitually acted therein during the term, without any settlement or liquidation of the partnership affairs, is prima facie evidence of a continuation of the partnership.

PART V—PROPERTY RIGHTS OF A PARTNER

Section 24. [Extent of Property Rights of a Partner]

The property rights of a partner are (1) his rights in specific partnership property, (2) his interest in the partnership, and (3) his right to participate in the management.

Section 25. [Nature of a Partner's Rights in Specific Partnership Property]

1. A partner is co-owner with his partners of specific partnership property holding as a tenant in partnership.

2. The incidents of this tenancy are such that:

a. A partner, subject to the provisions of this act and to any agreement between the partners, has an equal right with his partners to possess specific partnership property for partnership purposes; but he has no right to possess such property for any other purpose without the consent of his partners.

b. A partner's right in specific partnership property is not assignable except in connection with the assignment of rights of all the partners in the same property.

c. A partner's right in specific partnership property is not subject to attachment or execution, except on a claim against the partnership. When partnership property is attached for a partnership debt the partners, or any of them, or the representatives of a deceased partner, cannot claim any right under the homestead or exemption laws.

d. On the death of a partner his right in specific partnership property vests in the surviving partner or partners, except where the deceased was the last surviving partner, when his right in such property vests in his legal representative. Such surviving partner or partners, or the legal representative of the last surviving partner, has no right to possess the partnership property for any but a partnership purpose.

e. A partner's right in specific partnership property is not subject to dower, curtesy, or allowance to widows, heirs, or next of kin.

Section 26. [Nature of Partner's Interest in the Partnership]

A partner's interest in the partnership is his share of the profits and surplus, and the same as personal property.

Section 27. [Assignment of Partner's Interest]

1. A conveyance by a partner of his interest in the partnership does not of itself dissolve the partnership, nor, as against the other partners in the absence of agreement, entitle the assignee, during the continuance of the partnership to interfere in the management or administration of the partnership business or affairs, or to require any information or account of partnership transactions, or to inspect the partnership books; but it merely entitles the assignee to receive in accordance with his contract the profits to which the assigning partner would otherwise be entitled.

2. In case of a dissolution of the partnership, the assignee is entitled to receive his assignor's interest and may require an account from the date only of the last account agreed to by all the partners.

Section 28. [Partner's Interest Subject to Charging Order]

1. On due application to a competent court by any judgment creditor of a partner, the court which entered the judgment, order, or decree, or any other court, may charge the interest of the debtor partner with payment of the unsatisfied amount of such judgment debt with interest thereon; and may then or later appoint a receiver of his share of the profits, and of any other money due or to fall due to him in respect of the partnership, and make all other orders, directions, accounts and inquiries which the debtor partner might have made, or which the circumstances of the case may require.

2. The interest charged may be redeemed at any time before foreclosure, or in case of a sale being directed by the court may be purchased without thereby causing a dissolution:

a. With separate property, by any one or more of the partners, or

b. With partnership property, by any one or more of the partners with the consent of all the partners whose interests are not so charged or sold.

3. Nothing in this act shall be held to deprive a partner of his right, if any, under the exemption laws, as regards his interest in the partnership.

PART VI—DISSOLUTION AND WINDING UP

Section 29. [Dissolution Defined]

The dissolution of a partnership is the change in the relation of the partners caused by any partner ceasing to be associated in the carrying on as distinguished from the winding up of the business.

Section 30. [Partnership Not Terminated by Dissolution]

On dissolution the partnership is not terminated, but continues until the winding up of partnership affairs is completed.

Section 31. [Causes of Dissolution]

Dissolution is caused:

1. Without violation of the agreement between the partners,

a. By the termination of the definite term or particular undertaking specified in the agreement,

b. By the express will of any partner when no definite term or particular undertaking is specified,

c. By the express will of all the partners who have not assigned their interests or suffered them to be charged for their separate debts, either before or after the termination of any specified term or particular undertaking,

d. By the expulsion of any partner from the business bona fide in accordance with such a power conferred by the agreement between the partners;

2. In contravention of the agreement between the partners, where the circumstances do not permit a dissolution under any other provision of this section, by the express will of any partner at any time;

3. By any event which makes it unlawful for the business of the partnership to be carried on or for the members to carry it on in partnership;

4. By the death of any partner;

5. By the bankruptcy of any partner or the partnership;

6. By decree of court under Section 32.

Section 32. [Dissolution by Decree of Court]

1. On application by or for a partner the court shall decree a dissolution whenever:

a. A partner has been declared a lunatic in any judicial proceeding or is shown to be of unsound mind,

b. A partner becomes in any other way incapable of performing his part of the partnership contract,

c. A partner has been guilty of such conduct as tends to affect prejudicially the carrying on of the business,

d. A partner willfully or persistently commits a breach of the partnership agreement, or otherwise so conducts himself in matters relating to the partnership business that it is not reasonably practicable to carry on the business in partnership with him,

e. The business of the partnership can only be carried on at a loss,

f. Other circumstances render a dissolution equitable.

2. On the application of the purchaser of a partner's interest under Sections 27 or 28:

a. After the termination of the specified term or particular undertaking,

b. At any time if the partnership was a partnership at will when the interest was assigned or when the charging order was issued.

Section 33. [General Effect of Dissolution on Authority of Partner]

Except so far as may be necessary to wind up partnership affairs or to complete transactions begun but not then finished, dissolution terminates all authority of any partner to act for the partnership,

1. With respect to the partners,

a. When the dissolution is not by the act, bankruptcy or death of a partner; or

b. When the dissolution is by such act, bankruptcy or death of a partner, in cases where Section 34 so requires.

2. With respect to persons not partners, as declared in Section 35.

Section 34. [Right of Partner to Contribute From Copartners After Dissolution]

Where the dissolution is caused by the act, death or bankruptcy of a partner, each partner is liable to his copartners for his share of any liability created by any partner acting for the partnership as if the partnership had not been dissolved unless:

a. The dissolution being by act of any partner, the partner acting for the partnership had knowledge of the dissolution, or

b. The dissolution being by the death or bankruptcy of a partner, the partner acting for the partnership had knowledge or notice of the death or bankruptcy.

Section 35. [Power of Partner to Bind Partnership to Third Persons After Dissolution]

1. After dissolution a partner can bind the partnership except as provided in paragraph (3).

a. By any act appropriate for winding up partnership affairs or completing transactions unfinished at dissolution;

b. By any transaction which would bind the partnership if dissolution had not taken place, provided the other party to the transaction:

I. Had extended credit to the partnership prior to dissolution and had no knowledge or notice of the dissolution; or

II. Though he had not so extended creidt, had nevertheless known of the partnership prior to dissolution, and, having no knowledge or notice of dissolution, the fact of dissolution had not been advertised in a newspaper of general circulation in the place (or in each place if more than one) at which the partnership business was regularly carried on.

2. The liability of a partner under paragraph (1b) shall be satisfied out of partnership assets alone when such partner had been prior to dissolution:

a. Unknown as a partner to the person with whom the contract is made; and

b. So far unknown and inactive in partnership affairs that the business reputation of the partnership could not be said to have been in any degree due to his connection with it.

3. The partnership is in no case bound by any act of a partner after dissolution:

a. Where the partnership is dissolved because it is unlawful to carry on the business, unless the act is appropriate for winding up partnership affairs; or

b. Where the partner has become bankrupt; or

c. Where the partner has no authority to wind up partnership affairs; except by a transaction with one who:

I. Had extended credit to the partnership prior to dissolution and had no knowledge or notice of his want or authority; or

II. Had not extended credit to the partnership prior to dissolution, and, having no knowledge or notice of his want of authority, the fact of his want of authority has not been advertised in the manner provided for advertising the fact of dissolution in paragraph (1bII).

4. Nothing in this section shall affect the liability under Section 16 of any person who after dissolution represents himself or consents to another representing him as a partner in a partnership engaged in carrying on business.

Section 36. [Effect of Dissolution on Partner's Existing Liability]

1. The dissolution of the partnership does not of itself discharge the existing liability of any partner.

2. A partner is discharged from any existing liability upon dissolution of the partnership by an agreement to that effect between himself, the partnership creditor and the person or partnership continuing the business; and such agreement may be inferred from the course of dealing between the creditor having knowledge of the dissolution and the person or partnership continuing the business.

3. Where a person agrees to assume the existing obligations of a dissolved partnership, the partners whose obligations have been assumed shall be discharged from any liability to any creditor of the partnership who, knowing of the agreement, consents to a material alteration in the nature or time of payment of such obligations.

4. The individual property of a deceased partner shall be liable for all obligations of the partnership incurred while he was a partner but subject to the prior payment of his separate debts.

Section 37. [Right to Wind Up]

Unless otherwise agreed the partners who have not wrongfully dissolved the partnership or the legal representative or the last surviving partner, not bankrupt, has the right to wind up the partnership affairs; provided, however, that any partner, his legal representative or his assignee, upon cause shown, may obtain winding up by the court.

Section 38. [Rights of Partners to Application of Partnership Property]

1. When dissolution is caused in any way, except in contravention of the partnership agreement, each partner as against his co-partners and all persons claiming through them in respect of their interests in the partnership, unless otherwise agreed, may have the partnership property applied to discharge its liabilities, and the surplus applied to pay in cash the net amount owing to the respective partners. But if the dissolution is caused by expulsion of a partner, bona fide under the partnership agreement and if the expelled partner is discharged from all partnership liabilities, either by payment or agreement under Section 36 (2), he shall receive in cash only the net amount due him from the partnership.

2. When dissolution is caused in contravention of the partnership agreement the rights of the partners shall be as follows:

a. Each partner who has not caused dissolution wrongfully shall have,

I. All the rights specified in paragraph (1) of this Section, and

II. The right, as against each partner who has caused the dissolution wrongfully, to damages for breach of the agreement.

b. The partners who have not caused the dissolution wrongfully, if they all desire to continue the business in the same name, either by themselves or jointly with others, may do so, during the agreed term for the partnership and for that purpose may possess the partnership property, provided they secure the payment by bond approved by the court, or pay to any partner who has caused the dissolution wrongfully, the value of his interest in the partnership at the dissolution, less any damages recoverable under clause (2aII) of the Section, and in like manner indemnify him against all present or future partnership liabilities.

c. A partner who has caused the dissolution wrongfully shall have:

I. If the business is not continued under the provisions of paragraph (2b) all the rights of a partner under paragraph (1), subject to clause (2aII), of this Section,

II. If the business is continued under paragraph (2b) of this section the right as against his co-partners and all claiming through them in respect of their interests in the partnership, to have the value of his interest in the partnership, less any damages caused to his co-partners by the dissolution, ascertained and paid to him in cash, or the payment secured by bond approved by the court, and to be released from all existing liabilities of the partnership; but in ascertaining the value of the partner's interest the value of the goodwill of the business shall not be considered.

Section 39. [Rights Where Partnership is Dissolved for Fraud or Misrepresentation]

Where a partnership contract is rescinded on the ground of the fraud or misrepresentation of one of the parties thereto, the party entitled to rescind is, without prejudice to any other right, entitled,

a. To a lien on, or a right of retention of, the surplus of the partnership property after satisfying the partnership liabilities to third persons for any sum of money paid by him for the purchase of an interest in the partnership and for any capital or advances contributed by him; and

b. To stand, after all liabilities to third persons have been satisfed, in the place of the creditors of the partnership for any payments made by him in respect of the partnership liabilities; and

c. To be indemnified by the person guilty of the fraud or making the representation against all debts and liabilities of the partnership.

Section 40. [Rules for Distribution]

In settling accounts between the partners after dissolution, the following rules shall be observed, subject to any agreement to the contrary:

a. The assets of the partnership are:

I. The partnership property,

II. The contribution of the partners necessary for the payment of all the liabilities specified in clause (b) of this paragraph.

b. The liabilities of the partnership shall rank in order of payment, as follows:

I. Those owing to creditors other than partners,

II. Those owing to partners other than for capital and profits,

III. Those owing to partners in respect of capital,

IV. Those owing to partners in respect of profits.

c. The assets shall be applied in the order of their declaration in clause (a) of this paragraph to the satisfaction of the liabilities.

d. The partners shall contribute, as provided by Section 18 (a) the amount necessary to satisfy the liabilities; but if any, but not all, of the partners are insolvent, or, not being subject to process, refuse to contribute, the other parties shall contribute their share of the liabilities, and, in the relative proportions in which they share the profits, the additional amount necessary to pay the liabilities.

e. An assignee for the benefit of creditors or any person appointed by the court shall have the right to enforce the contributions specified in clause (d) of this paragraph.

f. Any partner or his legal representative shall have the right to enforce the contributions specified in clause (d) of this paragraph, to the extent of the amount which he has paid in excess of his share of the liability.

g. The individual property of a deceased partner shall be liable for the contributions specified in clause (d) of this paragraph.

h. When partnership property and the individual properties of the partners are in possession of a court for distribution, partnership creditors shall have priority on partnership property and separate creditors on individual property, saving the rights of lien or secured creditors as heretofore.

i. Where a partner has become bankrupt or his estate is insolvent the claims against his separate property shall rank in the following order:

I. Those owing to separate creditors,

II. Those owing to partnership creditors,

III. Those owing to partners by way of contribution.

Section 41. [Liability of Persons Continuing the Business in Certain Cases]

1. When any new partner is admitted into an existing partnership, or when any partner retires and assigns (or the representative of the deceased partner assigns) his rights in partnership property to two or more of the partners, or

to one or more of the partners and one or more third persons, if the business is continued without liquidation of the partnership affairs, creditors of the first or dissolved partnership are also creditors of the partnership so continuing the business.

2. When all but one partner retire and assign (or the representative of a deceased partner assigns) their rights in partnership property to the remaining partner, who continues the business without liquidation of partnership affairs, either alone or with others, creditors of the dissolved partnership are also creditors of the person so continuing the business.

3. When any partner retires or dies and the business of the dissolved partnership is continued as set forth in paragraphs (1) and (2) of this Section, with the consent of the retired partners or the representative of the deceased partner, but without any assignment of his right in partnership property, rights of creditors of the dissolved partnership and of the creditors of the person or partnership continuing the business shall be as if such assignment had been made.

4. When all the partners or their representatives assign their rights in partnership property to one or more third persons who promise to pay the debts and who continue the business of the dissolved partnership, creditors of the dissolved partnership are also creditors of the person or partnership continuing the business.

5. When any partner wrongfully causes a dissolution and the remaining partners continue the business under the provisions of section 38 (2b), either alone or with others, and without liquidation of the partnership affairs, creditors of the dissolved partnership are also creditors of the person or partnership continuing the business.

6. When a partner is expelled and the remaining partners continue the business either alone or with others, without liquidation of the partnership affairs, creditors of the dissolved partnership are also creditors of the person or partnership continuing the business.

7. The liability of a third person becoming a partner in the partnership continuing the business, under this Section, to the creditors of the dissolved partnership shall be satisfied out of partnership property only.

8. When the business of a partnership after dissolution is continued under any conditions set forth in this Section the creditors of the dissolved partnership, as against the separate creditors of the retiring or deceased partner or the representative of the deceased partner, have a prior right to any claim of the retired partner or the representative of the deceased partner against the person or partnership continuing the business, on account of the retired or deceased partner's interest in the dissolved partnership or on account of any consideration promised for such interest or for his right in partnership property.

9. Nothing in this Section shall be held to modify any right of creditors to set aside any assignment on the ground of fraud.

10. The use by the person or partnership continuing the business of the partnership name, or the name of a deceased partner as part thereof, shall not of itself make the individual property of the deceased partner liable for any debts contacted by such person or partnership.

Section 42. [Rights of Retiring or Estate of Deceased Partner When the Business is Continued.]

When any partner retires or dies, and the business is continued under any of the conditions set forth in Section 41 (1,2,3,5,6), or Section 38 (2b) without any settlement of accounts as between him or his estate and the person or partnership continuing the business, unless otherwise agreed, he or his legal representative as against such persons or partnership may have the value of his interest at the date of dissolution ascertained, and shall receive as an ordinary creditor an amount equal to the value of his interest in the dissolved partnership with interest, or, at his option or at the option of his legal representative in lieu of interest, the profits attributable to the use of his right in the property of the dissolved partnership; provided that the creditors of the dissolved partnership as against the separate creditors, or the representative of the retired or deceased partner, shall have priority on any claim arising under this Section, as provided by Section 41(8) of this act.

Section 43. [Accrual of Actions]

The right to an account of his interest shall accrue to any partner, or his legal representative, as against the winding up partners or the surviving partners or the person or partnership continuing the business, at the date of dissolution, in the absence of any agreement to the contrary.

PART VII—MISCELLANEOUS PROVISIONS

Section 44. [When Act Takes Effect]

This act shall take effect on the ______________ day of ______________ one thousand nine hundred and ______________.

Section 45. [Legislation Repealed]

All acts or parts of acts inconsistent with this act are hereby repealed.

Appendix 5B

Professional Corporations State Statutes

1. *Alabama*	(Professional Corporations) *Laws 1961*, Act 865 (eff. Sept. 8, 1961); amended by *Laws 1971*, Ch. 184 (effective July 30, 1971); *Ala. Code*, Tit. 46, *Ch. 16*, § 330-345.
2. *Alaska*	(Professional Corporations) *Laws 1968*, Ch. 128 (eff. April 24, 1968); amended by *Laws 1968*, Ch. 75 (eff. Aug. 4, 1969); *Alaska Stat.* Tit. 10, Ch. 45 § 10.45.010-10.45.260.
3. *Arizona*	(Professional Corporations) *Ariz. Rev. Stat.*, Tit. 10, Ch. 3, § 901-909.
4. *Arkansas*	(Medical Corporations) *Ark. Stat. Ann.* § 64-1701 to 64-1717. (Professional Corporations) Ark. Stat. Ann. § 64-2001 to 64-2018.
5. *California*	(Medical Corporations) *Cal. Bus. & Prof. Code*, § 2008.5, 2500-2508, *Cal. Evid. Code* § 994. (Professional Corporations) *Cal. Bus. & Prof. Code*, § 13400-13410, *Cal. Rev. and Tax Code*, § 23038. (Psychological Corporations) *Cal. Evid. Code*, § 1041, *Calif. Bus. & Prof. Code*, § 2907.5, 2995-2996.6.
6. *Colorado*	(Medical Corporations) *Colo. Rev. Stat.*, Ch. 91, § 1-37, Ch. 145, § 1-12.

7. *Connecticut*	(Professional Associations) *Conn. Gen. Stat. Ann.*, § 34-82(1) to 34-82(5). (Professional Corporations) *Conn. Gen. Stat. Ann.*, § 33-182a to 33-182j.
8. *Delaware*	(Professional Corporations) *Del. Code Ann.*, § 8-601 to 8-620.
9. *District of Columbia*	(Professional Corporations) *P.L.* 92-180.
10. *Florida*	(Professional Corporations) *Fla. Stat. Ann.*, § 621.01-621.15.
11. *Georgia*	(Professional Associations) *Ga. Code Ann.*, § 84-4301 to 84-4318. (Professional Corporations) *Ga. Code Ann.*, § 84-5401 to 84-5407.
12. *Hawaii*	(Professional Corporations) *Hawaii Rev. Stat.*, § 416-141 to 416-154.
13. *Idaho*	(Professional Corporations) *Idaho Code*, § 30-102, 30-1301 to 30-3015.
14. *Illinois*	(Medical Corporations) *Ill. Stat. Ann.*, 32 § 631-647. (Professional Association) *Ill. Stat. Ann.*, 106½ § 101-110. (Professional Corporations) *Ill. Stat. Ann.*, 32, § 415-1 to 415-17.
15. *Indiana*	(Medical Corporations) *Ind. Stat. Ann.*, § 25-4901 to 25-4921. (Professional Corporations) *Ind. Stat. Ann.*, § 25-5101 to 25-5111 and *Laws 1973*, H. Act No. 1676.
16. *Iowa*	(Professional Corporations) *Laws 1970*, S.F. 544 (Eff. 7/1/70).
17. *Kansas*	(Professional Corporations) *Kan. Stat. Ann.*, § 17-2706 to 17-2719.
18. *Kentucky*	(Professional Corporations) *Ky. Rev. Stat.*, § 274.005-274.990.
19. *Louisiana*	(Medical Corporations) *La. Rev. Stat.*, § 12-901 to 12-915.
20. *Maine*	(Professional Corporations) *Me. Rev. Stat. Ann.*, 13, § 701-716.
21. *Maryland*	(Professional Corporations) *Md. Code Ann.*, Art. 23, § 430-444.
22. *Massachusetts*	(Professional Corporations) *Mass. Gen. Laws Ann.*, Ch. 156 A, § 1-17. Amendments per *Laws 1972*, Ch. 318 (eff. Aug. 23, 1972) and Ch. 693 (eff. October, 1972).
23. *Michigan*	(Professional Corporations) *Mich. Comp. Laws*, § 450.221-450.235.
24. *Minnesota*	(Professional Corporations) *Minn. Stat. Ann.*, Ch. 319 § 319.01-319.23.

25. *Mississippi*	(Professional Corporations) *Miss. Code Ann.*, § 5390-41 to 5390-53.
26. *Missouri*	(Professional Corporations) *Mo. Stat. Ann.*, § 356.010-356.200.
27. *Montana*	(Professional Corporations) *Mont. Rev. Code*, § 15-2101 to 15-2116.
28. *Nebraska*	(Professional Corporations) *Neb. Rev. Stat.*, Ch. 21 (1943).
29. *Nevada*	(Professional Corporations) *Nev. Rev. Stat.*, § 89.010-89.270.
30. *New Hampshire*	(Professional Associations) *N.H. Rev. Stat. Ann.*, § 294-A: 1 to 294-A: 8.
31. *New Jersey*	(Professional Corporations) *N.J. Stat. Ann.*, § 14A: 17-1 to 14A: 17-18.
32. *New Mexico*	(Professional Corporations) *N.M. Stat. Ann.*, § 51-22-1 to 51-22-14.
33. *North Carolina*	(Professional Corporations) *N.C. Gen. Stat.*, § 55B-1 to 55B-15.
34. *North Dakota*	(Professional Corporations) *N.D. Code*, § 10-31-01 to 10-31-14.
35. *New York*	(Professional Corporations) *N.Y. Bus. Corp. Law*, § 1501-1515 and others.
36. *Ohio*	(Professional Associations) *Ohio Rev. Code Ann.*, § 1785.01-1785.08.
37. *Oklahoma*	(Professional Corporations) *Okla. Stat. Ann.*, § 18-801 to 18-819.
38. *Oregon*	(Professional Corporations) *Ore. Rev. Stat.*, § 58.005 to 58.365.
39. *Pennsylvania*	(Professional Associations) *Pa. Stat. Ann.*, 15, § 12601-12619. (Professional Corporations) *Pa. Stat. Ann.*, 15, § 12901-12914.
40. *Rhode Island*	(Professional Corporations) *R.I. Gen. Laws*, § 7-5.1-1 to 7-5.1-12.
41. *South Carolina*	(Professional Associations) *S.C. Code*, § 56-1601 to 56-1617.
42. *South Dakota*	(Medical Corporations) *S.D. Corp. Laws*, § 47-11-1 to 47-11-21.
43. *Tennessee*	(Professional Associations) *Tenn. Code Ann.*, § 61-105 (*UPA*). (Professional Corporations) *Tenn. Code Ann.*, § 48-2001 to 48-2007.
44. *Texas*	(Professional Associations) *Texas Rev. Stat.*, 32, § 1528f-1 to 1528f-24. (Professional Corporations) *Texas Rev. Stat.*, 32 § 1528e-1 to 1528e-20.
45. *Utah*	(Professional Associations) *Utah Code Ann.*, § 16-11-1 to 16-11-15.
46. *Vermont*	(Professional Corporations) *Vt. Stat. Ann.*, § 11-901 to 11-913.

47. *Virginia*	(Professional Associations) *Va. Code*, § 54–873 to 54–898. (Professional Corporations) *Va. Code*, § 13.1–542 to 13.1–556.
48. *Washington*	(Professional Corporations) *Wash. Rev. Code*, § 18.100.010 to 18.100.140.
49. *West Virginia*	(Medical Corporations) *W. Va. Code*, § 30–2A–2, 30–3–3, 30–3–4b to 30–4–4c.
50. *Wisconsin*	(Professional Corporations) *Wis. Stat. Ann.*, § 180.99(1)–180.99(11).
51. *Wyoming*	(Professional Corporations) *Wyo. Stat.*, § 17–49.1 and 42.2.

Source: The above list was adapted from B.C. Eaton, "Professional Corporations," *Business Organizations*, Vol. 17 (New York: Mathew Bender, 1974).

Chapter 6

Governance

MANAGEMENT STRUCTURE

The management structure of a medical group practice is that network of authority and communication through which the objectives and goals of the organization are transmitted and achieved. It is comprised of owners, policy-making and executive bodies, and administrative and supervisory personnel, aided by advisory committees and staff assistants who also may have incidental management functions. To some extent, this structure is determined by the legal organization of the group from which an individual framework of action is built. Articles of incorporation, the partnership agreement, bylaws, and similar basic documents describe how the organization will be run and by whom it will be run. An organizational chart may be adopted which depicts in graphic form the flow of authority and responsibility within the group. Such documents also describe the parameters of authority and selection processes within the organization. Management policies delineating structure may be promulgated by governing bodies, executive groups, or administrative officials within the organization in the course of discharging their own management responsibilities. These policies can be expressed in the form of memoranda, job description, policy manuals, and other documentation, or simply in orally transmitted instructions or traditionally accepted relationships.

Certain relatively special characteristics of medical group practice affect its management structure. Medical group practice organizations tend to have strong informal as well as formal channels of authority. In common with other scientific or technical organizations, essential group functions can be performed and evaluated only by individuals having technical (medical) training. In some instances, only one individual may possess knowledge essential for the assessment of a given piece of equipment's or quality of an employee's work performance. Conflicts may arise from differing administrative and professional judgments, and it may be that no individual or body within the organization has full competence to arbitrate such differences objectively. The flow of communication and authority within the medical group also can be impeded in many instances as a result of the owner/employee role often occupied by the physician. Even more complex is the common situation in which a physician is elected to or selected for a management role as a board member, department head, or medical director, and yet continues to conduct his medical practice as an employee of the organization.

Figure 6-1 is an organizational chart for medical group practice which can be used as a guide in considering management structure as discussed in this chapter. Additional organizational charts can be found in Chapter 10. Although legal organizational form, facility ownership, and operational mode play significant roles in determining management structure for the group, the personal desires and predispositions of the group's founding members may have an equal, if not a predominant, influence on the management structure. This chapter will point out those considerations necessary in evolving an initial management structure for a forming group practice.

Owners

The owner is that person, group, organization, or agency from which authority to act flows. Legal ownership ordinarily assumes the right to direct and control the organization. This right is sometimes restricted, however, as in the case of the limited partnership, or may be exercised through delegation, as in the case of the corporation. The degree of ownership involvement in management tends to vary with the relationships prescribed by the group's legal form and with the particular circumstances of the medical group. It may range from the selection of a manager or management body to extensive involvement by the entire group in policy-making and administrative action.

Sole Proprietor. At one end of the scale is the sole proprietorship in which a single individual owns and, for all practical purposes, manages the group. The top level of management structure here is greatly simplified, as it rests entirely in the single person of owner. There is no formal decision-making process, such as meetings of the board of directors or other executive bodies appropriate to jointly owned enterprises. Policy is revealed and often created as it is expressed in administrative action. Additional administrative authority found in the organization is derived directly from the owner and exists, barring contractual rights, at the owner's discretion. As the sole proprietorship expands to a large group, professional management may be sought and the management structure may take on the characteristics of other legal forms. The ownership and final authority delegation and control, however, continue to remain with the sole proprietor.

Partnership. The partnership occupies the same management position in the organization as does the sole proprietor. It has complete control and authority over every aspect of operation. The partnership, however, is not a single person, and as an ownership group may be organized in diverse ways to achieve its established mission(s). As discussed in detail in the preceding chapter, medical group partnership interests and authority customarily are shared equally by

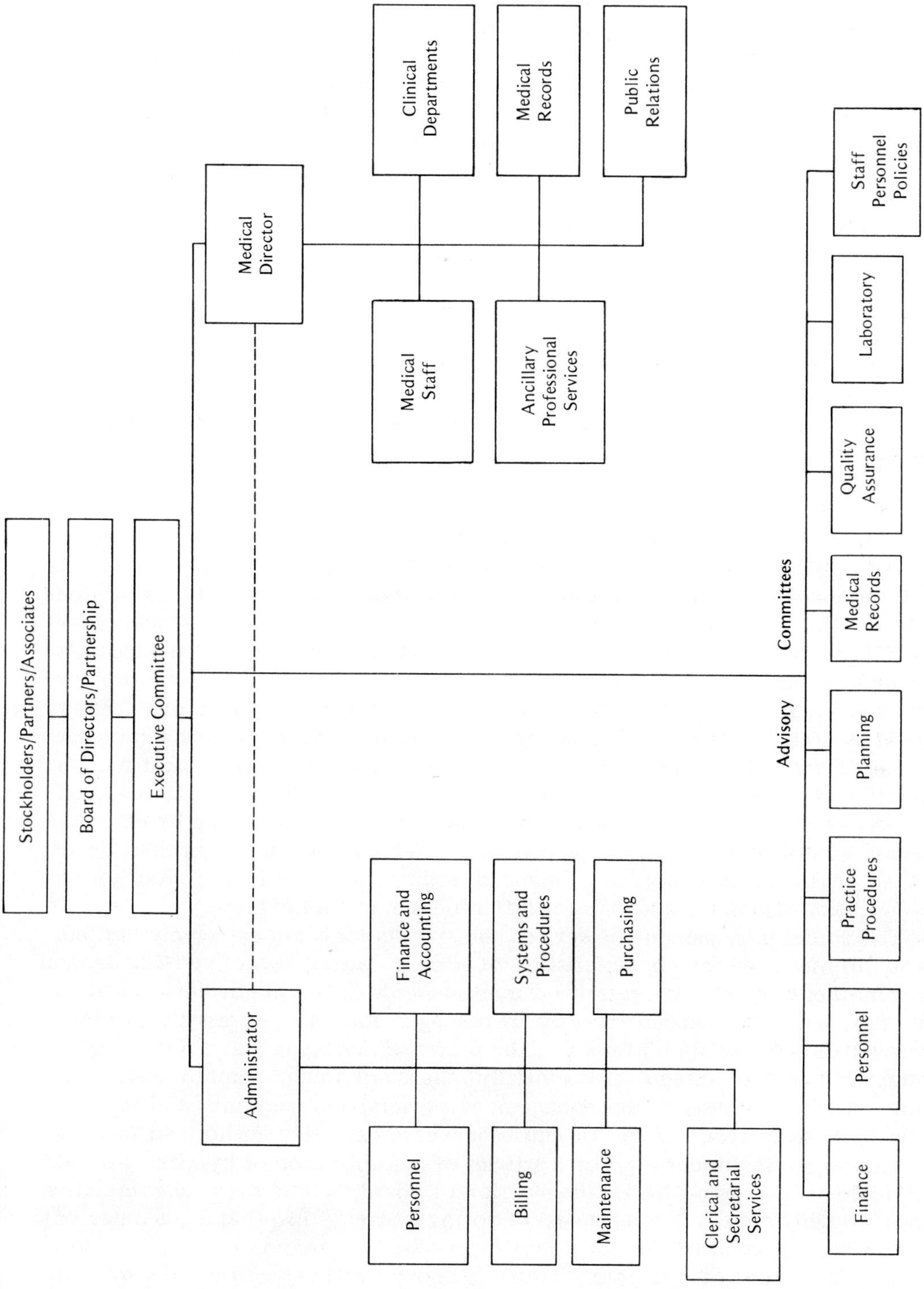

Figure 6–1. Organizational Chart—Medical Group Practice

the physician partners. It is possible, however, for partners to have unequal interests or authority according to the specifics of their agreement. New members usually are brought into the partnership under the terms of the partnership agreement and may or may not be required to purchase a share of the partnership's assets. Acceptance into the partnership usually follows an employment period of a year or two, during which time both the individual physician and the established partners can determine the probable permanence of the association. Depending upon the terms of the original agreement, the addition of a new partner may require the consent of some or all of the existing partners.

The partners, in contrast to the stockholder-owners of a corporation, have direct management authority over the partnership as a business enterprise. They may delegate this authority, but must do so expressly by agreement. In the absence of any agreement, individual partners may be considered legally competent to act for the full partnership in management matters.

Corporate Stockholders. The owners and ultimate management authority of a corporation are, of course, its stockholders. In a medical group practice, they usually achieve this status in a manner similar to the selection process in a medical group partnership; that is, individuals are invited to share in corporate ownership at a time when, usually by custom of the organization, there is reasonable need and mutual anticipation of permanent association. Ownership and the management rights of ownership in a corporation are associated with the purchase of shares of stock of the corporation. Different types of stock may confer different rights, including the right to vote at the stockholders' meetings. The authority of the individual stockholder to affect management is determined by the number of shares of voting stock he owns. Patterns of stock ownership in medical groups vary. For example, in medical partnerships, there is a strong tendency to accord equal representation to each physician owner. Existing variations are sometimes related to seniority; a staff member may be permitted to buy a number of shares of stock according to his length of service with the organization. In some instances, a founding or otherwise senior group of physicians may own a greater number of shares than do the other physician stockholders. Financial ability to invest in the stock of the corporation also may be a basis for differences in stock holdings.

The actual management powers of the stockholders are extremely limited.[1] One of the essential characteristics of a corporation, as defined for federal income tax purposes, is centralized management. Corporate owners, the stockholders, are not involved directly in management, but express their control through election or appointment of the principal managing body of the corporation, its board of directors. Essentially, the stockholders cannot restrict the board in the exercise of its management powers, and they may only remove board members from office for cause or where expressly authorized to do so by the terms of the corporation's articles of incorporation or bylaws. It should be noted that in some states, the election of board members is on a cumulative basis; roughly speaking, the process of voting is arranged so that a given percent of the voting stock of the corporation can elect approximately the same percent of the board of directors.[2] Thus, the power of the stockholders to influence management through election of their representatives to board membership is further emphasized by proportionate holdings of stock.

The stockholders may possess a limited number of other prerogatives in control of their corporation as defined in their articles of incorporation and as permitted by law. For the most part, these pertain to the issuance of stock and other matters which are usually financial in character and directly affect the value of stock. Detailed operating policies concerning internal management are often relegated to the corporate bylaws. Stockholder action customarily is taken at annual stockholders' meetings, although other special meetings may be convened as matters arise within the purview of the stockholders.

Associates. The association form of medical group organization is similar in its management form to the corporation. Its ownership, however, is vested in a group of associates, and in most instances stock is issued to represent ownership interest. Similar to a corporation, the association vests its management authority in an elected or appointed board of directors or executive committee.

Parent Organizations

In some instances, physician groups, although legally autonomous, may be associated with another organization(s) in the delivery of health care. The Kaiser-Permanente system is a well-known example in which health plan, hospital, and physician groups work jointly to provide care to the plan membership. Similar relationships exist in a number of smaller prepaid plans throughout the country. Each element of the joint effort retains its autonomy—there is no umbrella organization to which all segments administratively report. The relationships among elements are closely defined and the ability to act independently is bound by contractual relationships.

Other medical groups operate specifically as departments or functions of a parent organization which retains ownership and ultimate management control. Groups associated with hospitals, for example, may function within the outpatient services section of the hospital under the direction of a physician or lay administrator employed by the hospital. In these instances, the authority of ownership rests in the hospital board of trustees or in the body or agency which selects that board. When medical centers function as a part of or in the form of a nonprofit foundation, representation on the governing body often will include physicians of the group as well as lay representatives of the community or region served. For example, prepaid medical plans which are one form of nonprofit medical service entity, may have on their boards physicians from the group providing service to the plan members. To the extent that such representation is guaranteed by the rules of the organization, the physicians may be said to share in the responsibility of its ownership.

Ambulatory care also may be offered by physician groups who are employed by and serve the personnel of a commercial or industrial enterprise. This organizational model is found most often in locations remote from population centers such as in mining, lumber, and oil exploration and production areas. The Kaiser-Permanente health service complex had its beginnings in the provision of medical service to construction workers on the Boulder Dam. Industrial related group practices also have emerged in well populated areas. The Gates Clinic in Denver, Colorado, is one example. In any case, ownership and ultimate control of the conditions of practice in these industrial situations ordinarily rests with the employer concerned.

Affiliated Organizations. Medical group practices and their owners may be related to and have participatory interest in affiliated organizations which are dependent upon and subordinate to the medical group itself. Perhaps the most common example is the building corporation or building partnership established as a separate entity to own the physicial facilities needed by the group. Not infrequently these independent organizations are established because of the need or desirability for a facility ownership structure different from the medical organization in terms of the individuals represented, the proportions of ownership, and the attendant financing. Pharmacies, optical dispensaries, and other ancillary services, as well as hospitals, may also have ownership representation from the membership of the medical group. Each of these affiliated organizations can be separate administrative units with management control resulting from its own ownership.

Governing Bodies

The authority to direct an enterprise emanates from its owners and in some instances the owners themselves are involved directly in management. When a group is self-governing, in the sense that all or a significant number of its practitioners are its owners, a governing body is recognized or selected to discharge the basic functions of management and policy-making. This governing body may be a board of directors, in the case of a corporation or association, or in the case of a partnership, the partnership itself.

Partnership. The degree to which a partnership chooses to act as a governing body for its own activities is entirely a matter of its own discretion. If the number of partners is small, the partnership most likely will be able to perform in a management role with little or no delegation of authority to subgroups. As the number of partners becomes larger, however, moderately complex matters become increasingly difficult. Larger partnerships, therefore, tend to delegate management authority to other bodies and individuals, to charge advisory groups and administrative staff assistants with the responsibility of investigating and submitting recommendations on matters requiring decisions, and to restrict their own functions to policy-making rather than to specific management action. The management function most commonly retained by the full partnership is that of employment or termination of employment of medical staff members. Since such employment usually is closely related to eventual membership in the partnership itself, its importance to the group is obvious. In many instances the employment or termination of a physician may require more than a majority vote of the partners, even to the point of unanimous agreement. It also is a common practice for the partnership to retain authority to obligate the group for capital expenditures above a given amount, such as for furnishings, equipment, and construction. Policy action usually is taken at partnership meetings which are held periodically in accordance with the terms of the partnership agreement or other adopted procedural rules. A very small partnership may meet only occasionally because its daily association may make it unnecessary to formalize management policy or action. A very large partnership also may meet infrequently because it has delegated all but its broadest functions to others. Partnership organization typically provides for a chairman or president to preside at meetings. Action may be taken by a majority vote or by whatever other manner has been agreed upon. Minutes of all meetings are recorded and filed for reference.

The mechanics of defining which powers the partnership retains and which it relinquishes to others, such as its officers, the executive committee, the administrator, the medical director, special committees, etc., may be contained in the partnership agreement, in other rules of procedure which have been adopted, in individual actions taken at partnership meetings which are recorded in the meeting minutes, in employment contracts, in job descriptions, or simply in the mutual understanding evidenced in the day-to-day administration of the group's affairs.

Board of Directors. The management function of the board of directors of a corporation is essentially the same as that of the partnership in the partnership organization. The greatest difference between the two bodies lies in their composition. The partnership, by definition, is comprised of all of the owners of the medical group; the board of directors, by definition, is required to be a representative body, rather than a committee of the owners as a whole, and, in fact, may not be restricted only to owners. The question of whether all of the stockholders *can* be board members in a corporation recognized as such for federal tax purposes is a practical legal matter about which the group should consult its attorney. Ideally, the principal governing body of any medical group practice includes as many of the practicing physicians of the organization as feasible, relative to the volume and complexity of the matters to be brought to the body for its consideration or action. Often, it is desirable to extend maximum participation to the medical staff in the affairs of the organization. General experience in other organizations suggests that a governing body of fifteen to twenty-five members can function effectively if the matters brought before it are sufficiently broad and adequately researched before presentation.

State law may require a method for electing members of the board which automatically assures a representation of minority stockholders' interest. It may be in the interest of the group to seek further assurance of representation of particular specialties or age groups through use of a nominating committee which, while not restricting nominations for board membership, may present studied recommendations to the stockholders for their consideration. Continuity of membership enhances the capability of a medical group's principal governing body and may be accomplished by the use of staggered multiple-year terms. Arranging for a limitation on the number of terms which one individual may serve on the board also is another possibility.

As in a partnership, the degree of involvement of the board of directors in the active management affairs of the organization is to a significant extent inversely related to the size of the organization and of the board itself; the larger the board, the less the involvement. Involvement also may vary widely in relation to the degree of responsibility accorded to an executive committee, to a medical director or other senior physician, and to the administrator. In any event, major policy decisions usually are made by the board, including decisions regarding employment of medical staff members.

The frequency of board meetings will vary according to the functions of the board. Minutes of corporate board meetings customarily are kept in a somewhat more formal style than those of medical partnerships, although the need for and legal significance of these records is similar in both types of organization. Membership on the board of directors is not necessarily limited to owners of the organization, although board selection is by the stockholders. Physicians working in the group who have not yet attained stockholder status, or for some reason may never do so, may be elected to the main governing body of the organization. Under some circumstances, this arrangement could be regarded as an advantage in structuring the management of the group. In most states, professional corporation laws or medical practice laws restrict board membership to practicing physicians. General business corporations, however, frequently obtain the benefit of effective management counsel by including on their boards members of diverse backgrounds not directly associated with the business of the particular corporation. Some medical centers have reported successful experiences in opening membership on their governing body, in either a voting or advisory capacity, to selected individuals from the community or area which the groups serve.[3] Some medical groups invite their legal counsel to attend meetings of the governing body on a regular basis, and in some instances counsel may be asked to prepare the minutes of the meeting.

Executive Committee. The executive committee of a medical group practice typically is a relatively small group of perhaps three to seven members to which substantial authority for management of the organization has been delegated by the board of directors or the partnership. Ordinarily, the executive committee is comprised of the officers of the corporation or partnership, with any additional members either elected or sitting on the committee by virtue of their appointed position in the organization. Frequently, the medical director and administrator are ex-officio members of the committee but do not necessarily have voting powers. A number of groups ensure continuity of membership on the committee by providing staggered two or three-year terms, which is especially desirable in view of the nature of the committee's responsibilities.[4] Conscious structuring of the committee to represent various medical specialties of the organization also is a familiar feature.

The need for an executive committee often is recognized when it becomes evident that the main governing body, the board of directors, or the partnership, has become too large to deal effectively with the material brought to it for consideration. The degree of authority and responsibility delegated to the committee may vary widely. Even when delegation is substantial, however, matters of broad policy or high sensitivity tend to be referred to the board or partnership for final decision. In such instances, the principal governing body receives the benefit of prior study by the executive committee together with its considered recommendations for action. The executive committee functions both as a management body and, below the level occupied by the board or partnership, as a policy-making body. Management actions might include authorization of additional personnel, approval of specific purchases of a designated character or in a prescribed range, changes in space allocations among departments, the hearing of appeals regarding actions taken by the administrator or medical director, and the approving of recommended changes in departmental fee schedules. At the operating level, policy-making functions tend to involve matters such as setting salary ranges for lay personnel, establishing the purchasing or requisition limits of departments or supervisors, and approving or modifying lay personnel policies.

Meetings of the executive committee generally are held much more frequently than those of the partnership or board of directors, often weekly or biweekly. Minutes of their proceedings usually are recorded and filed. In some organizations, copies of the minutes of executive committee meetings are distributed routinely to the board or partnership, or to the medical staff as a whole, as a means of keeping them informed of actions taken. The administrator and medical director of the group meet with the executive committee to receive guidance and to present matters for consideration and decision. Administrative actions of the committee are transmitted to the organization through these agents, whose related functions are described in subsequent pages. Employment and termination of employment of the administrator and medical director are, however, usually a function of the board of directors or the partnership.

Officers

As discussed previously, the composition of the executive committee typically includes the officers of the group as elected by the principal governing body. Medical practice responsibilities generally restrict these officers from significant involvement in performance of specific duties of office. In most instances, the responsibility for day-to-day operations is delegated to the employed administrative staff.

President. Somewhat contrary to the above generalization, the medical group practice president frequently is an active, part-time administrative officer during his term of office. If the group has no medical director, the president may perform some of the duties of that position. The president performs the usual functions of calling and presiding at meetings of the group's governing bodies, and the administrator and medical director customarily report directly to him as the representatives of these bodies. Inevitably, he is the focal point of problems which occur within the organization and must devote a significant proportion of his time to their resolution or amelioration.

Vice President. The vice president, as in general business organizations, acts for the president in his absence. He also may be designated president-elect, thus assuring that the future president will be experienced in the administrative affairs of the organization.

Secretary and Treasurer. The formal responsibilities of the secretary and treasurer—record-keeping and control of financial affairs—usually are discharged in their names by certain members of the administrative staff. The secretary, however, may exercise some control over these activities through reviewing and signing minutes or other official documents, and the treasurer may control all check signing.

Administrative Staff

Policies adopted and administrative actions taken by the governing bodies are implemented by the administrative staff of the medical group, including the officers to the extent that they function in an administrative capacity. Depending upon the construction of the organization, various administrative positions, titles, and relationships may exist. In the organization chart shown in figure 6–1 the administrator and medical director operate directly under the executive committee and are responsible to that body for certain assigned functions. In many instances, responsibilities will be assigned to department heads or to supervisors who report to the administrator or medical director.

Medical Director. The medical director is the principal channel of communication and authority between the governing body of the organization and the medical staff. He usually is involved in all medical staff personnel decisions and in any administrative acts affecting the practice of medicine. Matters relating to the quality of care, adequacy of staffing, provision of equipment, and personnel and facilities to aid physicians in their practice are within the scope of the medical director's responsibilities. When coordination of effort or resolution of differences is required, he acts as liaison between individual staff members and between professional departments or sections of the group. Ideally, he exercises a leadership role in the definition and achievement of the group's professional goals. The medical director in a given organization, however, may not be designated specifically as such. Some or all of the functions of the position may be assumed by the chairman or president. Even when designated as such, the role of the medical director may vary substantially from group to group. He may be selected on a permanent basis or for a specific period of time, such as one year. In addition to his regular practice, he may assume only a part-time role as medical director, or he may be retained on a full-time basis for that position alone. The degree of his involvement in this essentially administrative role tends to vary with the size and complexity of the group.

Administrator. Responsibility for the direction of nonmedical activities of the medical group usually is placed in the hands of a lay administrator. Personnel, physical facilities, finance, record-keeping, and administrative procedures are within his realm. Customarily, he is responsible for the direction and administrative supervision of all nonphysician personnel. In virtually all instances, the administrator is a full-time, permanent employee of the group. An occasional exception may occur if an individual manages more than one group on a part-time basis or has additional responsibilities such as those of a hospital administrator or health plan director.

The administrator meets frequently with the executive committee or an analogous governing body to render reports, to refer matters requiring consideration, and to receive guidance. He often is directly responsible to the chairman or to the president of the group, and he may share administrative problems and decisions with that office.

Medical Director—Administrator Relationship. As may be imagined, it is difficult to draw a clear distinction between the responsibilities of the medical director and those of the administrator.[5] Virtually all functions of medical group practice have both administrative and medical aspects. For example, compiling, indexing, storing, and moving the medical record may be largely administrative in nature, but the content and format of the record must be considered medical.

Further variations in the division of responsibilities may occur from organization to organization, depending upon the medical director's and the administrator's talents and valuable time.

The functions assigned to the administrator and to the medical director in the organizational chart shown in figure 6–1 are only suggestive of the potential for division of authority. The dotted line drawn between the two positions indicates that each is involved in the administration of functions assigned to the other. In some instances, their administrative responsibility may be virtually equal. Under these circumstances it is essential that the administrator and medical director work together closely and harmoniously. They must be in constant communication, keeping each other fully informed of their respective actions, and consulting prior to taking any action which may affect the other party. Any conflicts arising between them are resolved by the governing body, but the organization cannot function efficiently if chronic conflict exists between these two.

Supervisory and Technical Staff. Depending somewhat upon the size of the group, supervisory positions below the level of the administrator can include credit manager, director of nurses, personnel director, and office manager. These individuals usually report directly to the administrator or, in larger organizations, to the next higher level of administration. They also may meet collectively with the administrator or his immediate staff for joint planning. Other nonsupervisory personnel may offer technical assistance to the administrator or to the medical director at a level of responsibility which characterizes them as members of the administrative staff. The personnel director or comptroller might be considered in this category.

MEDICAL STAFF ORGANIZATION

The organization of the medical staff within a group practice varies widely, particularly in relation to the size of the group. As multispecialty practices grow, department heads may be selected to carry out certain functions such as scheduling time off, coordinating departmental procedures, and representing the department to the group as a whole. Typically, these responsibilities are relatively nominal. As groups grow significantly larger some of the functions once performed by the full group may be dispersed among the departments—for example, planning, involvement in training, continuing education, etc.

Advisory Committees

To assist in its functions of policy and decision-making, the governing body may appoint advisory committees to study or monitor various aspects of the medical group's operations and to make recommendations for action to the governing body. Advisory committee membership is limited in most cases to the medical staff members of the group, with assistance provided by the administrative staff. This limitation, however, is not observed universally.

Advisory committees tend to fall into three broad categories: administrative, professional, and planning. Administrative committees represent the governing body in reviewing administrative activities of the organization, primarily to obtain assurance that these activities are being handled effectively. Their existence and operation not only afford the same extension of the governing body's capacity as may be found in other types of organizations, but also provide an opportunity for involvement of other owners of the group in its management, a characteristic of group practice governance which will be discussed later in this chapter. Professional advisory committees are those formed primarily to provide maximum medical staff input into the administration of areas which directly involve the practice of medicine. Examples as shown in figure 6-1 would be a medical records committee or a laboratory committee. Planning committees are formed to consider broad general directions, both administrative and professional, to be taken by the group. Advisory committees may be of a permanent standing nature such as a general planning committee, or may be appointed for an ad hoc purpose—for example, to consider a single action such as the opening of a branch office. While occasionally advisory committees may be granted or may assume some administrative authority, this role can be dangerous to the smooth operation of the organization.

Informal Organization

Apart from the designated lines and stations of authority, it is well-recognized in management practice that every organization has influential informal structures which do not conform to the nominal organization.[6] Medical group practices are no exception and, in fact, contain some elements of informal structure not commonly found elsewhere.

Medical Leaders. Every enterprise is affected by the quality and strength of its leadership. Frequently, medical groups can be dominated to a marked degree by a single physician of strong talents and personality. Founders of medical groups tend to fall into this leadership role. Observation of existing groups suggests that those having strong, individual leadership grow more rapidly and progress towards well-identified goals more successfully than those in which authority is diverse.

Professional Groups. As with other medical organizations, there are in medical group practices a number of professional groups—physicians, nurses, technologists, therapists. Often, these individuals have external ties which tend to affect their behavior in the group in ways not always consistent with group goals or intentions. Physicians in particular are sensitive to the stated standards of their professional organizations in matters of frequent concern to group practice, such as charging interest on patient accounts, ownership of pharmacies, and, not long ago, association in group practice itself. They also are concerned over, and react to, attitudes of the medical profession in their community, sometimes cherishing peer approval above what appears to be the interest of the medical group practice with which they are associated. In addition, nurses, therapists, and others may conceptualize their roles within the organization on the basis of standards of professional organizations rather than according to their work assignment as defined by the medical group.

Medical Staff. The most notable and unique characteristic of the management structure of the medical group is the ability of its medical staff, as a group and individually, to affect management function. Professionals and technicians (engineers, scientists, etc.) are difficult to mold into administrative conformity in any organization. Physicians in medical group practice tend to be even more independent. Sociologist Eliot Freidson has likened physicians associated together in practice to a "company of equals" in which each member functions in a largely self-regulating manner with minimal acceptance of administrative control by the organization.[7] The business of medical group practice is each physician's service. The physician is in an exceptionally secure financial position in relation to the organization in that he is not financially dependent on it, and frequently sees his affiliation with the group as being financially disadvantageous. More often than not, he is one of the owners of the group and from this vantage point may assume the right to behave administratively in the manner he considers most suitable to his understanding of a given situation.

For these reasons, and perhaps others, physicians of the group can be extraordinarily influential in management affairs. For example, in groups with an institutional ownership base, the wishes of the staff must be carefully regarded in any major administrative action. Such groups frequently make use of advisory committees or committees with some limited administrative authority to assure medical staff involvement in management. In practice, medical directors and administrators will frequently deal individually with each staff member affected by a given administrative action, in advance of the action, to ensure its understanding and acceptance. Whatever the formal intent of the governing body or administration of a medical group, significant sustained action can be taken only with the cooperation and consent of a very substantial majority of its medical staff.

Chapter 7

Facility Ownership

REAL ESTATE AND THE LAW

An informed awareness of the many legal factors involved in real estate and the development of a medical group practice can be helpful to the administration of an emerging group. Activities related to design and construction of the medical facility will be discussed in a later section; in this chapter, several aspects of facility ownership which can govern the medical group's success or failure in acquiring and retaining its place of practice will be explored. No one type of medical group organization is more amenable than another to owning the property on which it practices medicine or to leasing such property. For this reason groups and/or their administrators should be familiar with some of the basic real estate concepts and terms. In each state of the nation, two separate systems of law are enforced, federal law and state law. With few exceptions, federal laws operate uniformly throughout the country. Each state, however, has separate constitutions, laws, and court decisions. While real estate laws may vary somewhat from state to state, the basic legal principles governing real estate transactions are much the same throughout the country. Sources of real estate law include the Constitution of the United States, laws passed by Congress, regulations adopted by various federal boards and commissions, state constitutions, laws passed by state legislatures, regulations adopted by various state and municipal boards, ordinances passed by villages, and court decisions.

The history of modern land law can be divided into two periods. From the time of the Norman Conquest of England in 1066 through the seventeenth century, land law was molded to fit the pattern of a feudal society. The close of the seventeenth century until the present time marks the second period, during which previous feudal social order gradually was replaced by ownership as we know it today. The primary concern of real estate law has been to recognize and protect ownership of land. Because American real estate law stems in large part from the real estate law of England, it is not uncommon for courts today to base their decisions on similar cases that arose in England several hundred years ago. In resolving present-day problems, however, the courts often must evolve new law without the aid of precedence. Because of the complex nature of real estate law, it would be unwise for a group practice to proceed through this legal maze without the counsel and advice of a competent real estate attorney.

Ownership of land may be divided into various types of estates. The word *estate* is used to express the degree, quantity, nature, duration, or extent of interest in land. The highest type of estate is reflected in complete ownership, which is referred to as an estate in *fee simple* or in *fee simple absolute* and means that the owner has title to the property and his ownership is of unlimited duration. As long as he obeys various laws related to such ownership, he may do as he chooses with the property. Upon his death, title will go to his heirs, or, if he leaves a will, to those persons so named in the will. Another form of estate ownership is called *life estate*, which essentially means that the owner can use the land property only during his lifetime; thus, he is a life tenant and is entitled to the reasonable and necessary use of the land during his lifetime, but must not do anything that will in any way injure the permanent value of the property. A life tenant may collect and use the rents of the property, but must keep the property in repair and pay real estate taxes and interest on the mortgage, if applicable. Upon his death, the life tenant's rights in the land cease to exist and revert to the owner or his designee in fee simple.

A third type of estate includes a *lease hold estate*, the specific arrangements of which will be discussed later in the chapter. For purposes of definition, however, assume that the owner in fee simple of a tract of land executes a ten year lease for that property; that is, the owner relinquishes his right to occupy the land for ten years. In return, he receives the lessee's promise to pay a certain amount of rent for the ten year period. The lessee acquires the right to occupy the land in accordance with the provisions of the lease and acquires a lease hold estate in the land.

FORMS OF OWNERSHIP

The responsibilities and liabilities involved in ownership of a group practice facility can vary significantly, depending on the type of organization which has acquired title to property. The organizational form chosen to deliver the group's medical services may differ from the organization which owns property and real estate. Because most states limit interests in medical practice organizations to physicians, most existing group practices select another organization to hold the group's property, thus enabling nonphysicians to participate in the property ownership. Often, groups segregate their medical practice organization from the facility ownership organization in an effort to reduce cross liabilities. Although the corporate form does limit liability in both instances, the forming group's specific circumstances and mission will influence any final ownership decisions.

As discussed in detail in Chapter 5, medical groups are organized legally in one of the following ways: sole proprietorship, partnership, unincorporated association, professional corporation, or foundation. In the sole proprietorship form of medical group organization, the individual owner has the exclusive rights and responsibility of ownership of the medical facility and property. The sole owner makes all of the decisions regarding the facility, its initial acquisition, and subsequent expansion, and he alone is responsible for all capital invested in the property. Because the medical facility is treated as a personal asset of the sole owner, he may sell the property or transfer the assets at his discretion; hence, there is no distinction between the property of the medical group and the property of the owner. It is also the sole owner who assumes unlimited personal liability for the financial aspects of the medical facility.

A medical partnership is an association between two or more persons for the purpose of uniting their property, labor, and skill in the prosecution of specified medical business and the sharing of profits and lossess according to the partnership agreement. It is imperative that the partnership contract or agreement specify the obligations and responsibilities of each partner. In a partnership, every partner is an agent of the partnership for its business purposes. Each partner should remain aware of this contingent liability and each should be sure that the partnership agreement specifically recognizes the conditions and limitations of authorization to commit the partnership to property liabilities. Under a partnership agreement, a tract of land may be owned by two or more persons who are known as cotenants. Persons may own the land as joint tenants, as tenants by the entireties, or as tenants in common.

The association legal form includes some of the desirable features of a corporation and at the same time excludes some of the relatively undesirable features of the partnership form. The articles of association in their original draft form should clearly define the ownership entity through which the property was acquired as well as the limit to which the members of the ownership entity are personally liable.

Essentially, a corporation is a fictitious person vested by law with the capacity of renting property and transacting business as an individual. The stockholders and the board of directors are the constituent or component corporate parts, through whose intelligence, judgment, and discretion the corporation acts. The corporation has a legal life of its own apart from that of its shareholder/member physicians. The shareholders/members may elect a board of directors who in turn may appoint an executive committee vested with management responsibilities (see Chapter 6). With few exceptions, group members in a corporation are not personally liable for corporate debts or for the negligent acts of employees and stockholders. The limitation of individual liability with respect to financial matters, especially pertinent to ownership of the group practice facility, is not available in other organizational forms. Furthermore, neither death nor withdrawal of an individual member dissolves the corporate organization. This continuity of life eliminates the need for reorganization and can greatly simplify property ownership. Nevertheless, a thorough review of state law should be made by any individual or group of physicians prior to incorporation.

A foundation is a nonstock, nonprofit corporation, organized under state law for charitable, scientific, philanthropic, religious, or educational purposes.

The articles of incorporation should provide a means for electing new officers and for replacing those officers who may resign or die. Contracts and other legal documents of the foundation, including the execution of the deeds for the title of property and buildings, must be approved and ordered by the board of directors, signed by the president, and attested by the secretary, as in the case of stock corporations. In recent years, limitations have been placed on the amount of funds that may be accumulated by a foundation. Certain limitations are imposed in order to encourage foundations to engage in the activity for which they are organized. Extreme care must be exercised in using foundation funds to construct or acquire facilities which are to be used by a related group of physicians who pay rent for their use. In addition, tax laws must be examined carefully.

PURCHASING A MEDICAL FACILITY

The purchase of real estate has become a two-step, firmly established procedure: (1) the contract or sale; and (2) the closing—delivery of the deed (instrument), and payment of the agreed price. When the seller plans to build on the land and then convey the land together with a completed structure, all parties concerned will ask that a contract precede the transaction. Even when the sale involves unimproved land or existing structures, the purchaser will need time to investigate the seller's title and to secure financing. Except in cases of fraud, the acceptance of a deed is an irrevocable step. All contracts should contain certain items which are to be considered essential and legally binding, such as:

1. The parties to the agreement must be competent in the eyes of the law.
2. The contract should contain a statement of the consideration—something of value offered by the purchaser. Consideration usually takes the form of money, but personal services, merchandise, other real estate, or any other asset may be equally acceptable.
3. A valid contract must contain an offer and an acceptance. When the price, terms, and conditions are acceptable to all parties, a "meeting of the minds" is said to exist.
4. The purpose for property must be a lawful one. Courts refer to this as "legality of object."
5. Under the statute of frauds, most jurisdictions recognize that a contract has to be made in writing and signed by all principals in order to become enforceable.[1]

The value of the property is obtained by an appraisal, which is an evaluation of property by an impartial, knowledgeable, qualified party who carefully inspects and studies the property and its surroundings. Sound professional appraisals are obtained through the use of certain recognized techniques. The three generally accepted approaches to estimating real estate value are:

1. The *cost* approach—calculated by the replacement value of the property

2. The *market* approach—comparing the property with similar properties and arriving at a conclusion concerning selling price on the open market
3. The *income* approach—concerned with the net return a property will bring

Any combination of these three approaches can be used. In fact, when appraising a given property, all three methods may be utilized and the appraisers may correlate the conclusions to arrive at a comprehensive and knowledgeable single estimate of the property's value. An appraisal report generally follows a basic, recognized form, such as:

1. A letter of opinion, which usually is one or two pages in length and, although informal in nature, contains certain necessary basic facts and conclusions.
2. An appraisal certificate, such as a printed form completed and signed by the appraiser.
3. An affidavit, subscribed and sworn to before a notary public.
4. A combination of an affidavit and certificate.
5. A formal, bound, comprehensive document containing, in addition to complete facts and conclusions about the property, surveys, plot plans, and photographs.

An instrument or note which can be transferred by a sale and endorsement, by assignment, or by delivery is called negotiable. When a negotiable instrument is sold or assigned, the group is transferring the debt or obligation from the original payee to the incoming buyer or assignee. The new, incoming party is referred to as a *holder in due course*, meaning that if the original debtor does not pay as provided for in the agreement, the new holder can sue in his own name. Equally important, the holder is not subject to any defenses available against the original payee. As a result, the note may pass from party to party and may be accepted as a substitute for money. Negotiable instruments are: assignments, bills of sale, bonds, brokerage agreements, construction contracts, deeds, easements, exchange agreements, mortgages, options, promissory notes, and releases. The format of each of these instruments is uniform throughout the states. To identify the instrument which best meets the group's objectives and offers the best ownership protection for its needs, the medical group should work closely with a lawyer who understands both the health field and the legal environment. When making real estate transactions, one's signature, actions, or intentions must be continually verified; consequently, legal instruments such as acknowledgements, affidavits, affirmations, and certificates are in constant use and must be notarized or attested to (witnessed) and sealed.

The practical portion of any real estate acquisition must be defined not only by the services to be offered, but also by the expenses involved. In the outright purchase acquisition of a medical facility, expenses are similar in nature to those connected with the purchase of other properties and buildings to be used for commercial purposes. The basic legal doctrine governing the transfer of land is relatively simple; theoretically, the grantor must execute and deliver a conventional document. In practice, however, land transfers are sufficiently complex to require the services of a number of persons in addition to the immediate parties (seller and buyer). Real estate brokers, attorneys, mortgage lenders, public officials, and others maintain established roles in the process and generally require compensation.

Assuming the facility to be purchased includes both land and an existing structure, the gross purchase price for that package will represent an amount which in the seller's opinion is the fair market value of the package according to current local standards. Because no absolute value can be placed on the reasonableness of the seller's gross purchase price, the acceptability of the price must be judged solely by the purchaser and expressed in terms subject to his need and comparative prices for similar packages in the area. It should be recognized by the purchaser, however, that the gross purchase price must include not only the seller's original acquisition costs and improvement expenses but also the seller's costs and the real estate agent's commission (up to 15 percent), plus a reasonable profit margin for the seller in the transaction.

In addition to the gross purchase price, the purchaser must be aware of additional charges associated with the purchase transaction, generally referred to as ancillary charges. If the purchased facility is to be financed, in addition to the payment of principal plus interest, financial charges will include: mortgage origination fee, appraisal fee, credit report, initial insurance premium such as FHA, etc. Additional costs involved in establishing title and security interests (nonstatutory) will include such items as: bringing the abstract up to date, examining the abstract or original records and certifying or giving opinion of title, title insurance, survey, attorney's fee for drafting the deed, attorney's fee for drafting the mortgage and note or bond, escrow fees, attorney's fee for supervising closing of purchase, etc.

LEASING LAND

Land is a multiservice commodity capable of supplying service after service, *ad infinitum.* If a land owner does not wish to take advantage of the current service potential of his property, that particular service is lost forever. For this reason, it has been a common practice for landlords to sell land services to the highest bidder; the amount paid for such a service is called rent. Until recently, buildings have been leased by their owners for the same reason that landlords lease land—to avoid wasting a service. An individual acquiring fee simple title to a building actually has purchased all the future services of that structure, and having done so, he is under pressure either to use or to sell each service as it is renderable. Within the past decade, however, a new reason for renting buildings has emerged; business managers and health care organization managers alike have found that often it does not pay to own a building when funds could be used more profitably to finance current operations. Recently, many clinics and other health care organizations have begun to transfer title to their land and buildings via a sale to other commercial property purchasers, such as insurance companies, thereby freeing large amounts of funds for use as working capital. Under this type of arrangement, the seller of the building agrees to buy back the use of the building on an annual, rental basis.

The relationship between a landlord and tenant is basically contractual and may span a one to three year period or as long as a ninety-nine-year period. The landlord has the right to receive the rent at the time agreed upon between the parties and can reserve the right to enter the premises to collect rent and to make necessary repairs. The tenant holds possession of the premises in subordination to the rights of his landlord, and the landlord has a reversion in the property so that at the end of the term he receives the property back in good condition, reasonable wear and damage accepted.

The first and most important right of a tenant is the right to "possession and quiet enjoyment," which is comparable to the right of a person who purchases property. Although not mentioned specifically in an oral agreement or in a written lease, this right is implied on the part of a landlord and is inherent in a lease relationship. Just what the possession is that the landlord is required to give can be the subject of much contention in many leasing arrangements involving medical facilities. At the very least, a landlord must give his tenant legal possession; he must have good title and must be in a position to give a free and unencumbered lease for the period agreed upon. If a tenant fails to obtain possession from his landlord he has several remedies available; for example, he may rescind the lease if the premises are not ready for occupancy and recover any rents paid in advance. In the absence of very special circumstances, however, every tenant should insist that there be a clause in the lease that requires the landlord to give actual physical possession. A sample of such a clause is: "The landlord agrees to give tenant actual physical possession of the demised premises at the commencement of the term."[2]

It is customary for a lease to state the purposes for which the premises may be used by the tenant. In the case of a medical facility, a specific description of the use of the facility and nature of the medical practice must be clearly defined. Should the tenant breach the lease by using the premises for other purposes, the landlord may restrain him. On the other hand, if the lease does not specify a particular purpose for which a tenant may use the premises, the tenant may make any reasonable and legal use of them, as long as he does not damage the property or so alter the premises that the landlord's reversion is seriously affected. A tenant may have the right to assign the lease or sublet the premises. In the case of a medical facility, it may be to the medical group lessee's best interest to sublet certain areas of the building, while preserving a reversionary interest in the lease hold estate. In other words, the tenant reserves a portion of the terms for himself.

Important to most medical groups and their patients is the appropriate identification of the group's building or its offices, especially when the prospective space is located in a grouping of buildings and/or when other tenants occupy the same building. Parking rights also must be delineated. The lease arrangement should describe both the internal and the external rights of tenants with regard to directional signs as well as parking space. Often, the group practice can obtain from the landlord physical improvements or renovation of the proposed space. In a new building, for example, the landlord often will shell in space and make funds available to tenants for furnishing internal space to their individual desires. This monetary allowance can take the form of a rent reduction. In existing buildings, a similar allowance can be obtained or the landlord himself might arrange the renovation. The important consideration in either case is that such allowances and terms be contained in the *original* lease agreement. In the case of a building occupied by several tenants and managed by the landlord, the responsibility for cleaning and maintenance services may be assumed by the landlord. First, however, the special requirements of the medical group should be ascertained and assessed in terms of the landlord's ability to furnish such services. The specific rights and obligations of the tenants to the landlord or his agent in providing cleaning and maintenance services also should be enumerated in the lease. Some arrangements involving the lease of medical facilities may include "covenants running with the land," agreements through which one party becomes obligated to another in exchange for benefits. If a covenant or agreement does not touch or concern itself with the land, it merely is a collateral covenant for the benefit of the lessor and personal only to himself. If an estate in land is terminated, the obligations running with the land are terminated unless they occurred during the term of the lease.

Broadly, a lease is any agreement, written or oral, that establishes the relationship of landlord and tenant with respect to well-defined premises. An oral lease is valid in most states if it is made for one year or less. Most states require that a lease for more than one year must be in writing in order to be enforceable or, in some jurisdictions, to be valid. In general, when reference is made to a lease, a written lease is intended. In some respects, a written lease is a conveyance—a transfer of an interest in real property together with certain rights, which usually are some of the incidents of ownership previously discussed. A written lease is comparable to a deed of real property, in that the landlord divests himself or gives up possession to the tenant. A lease also is a contract in that each party to it agrees to do or to refrain from doing certain things. Breaching such covenants may forfeit the lease and subject the offending party to penalties or damages. To be enforceable, a written lease must state certain facts, such as the date of the lease, the names and addresses of the parties, and whether or not one or more persons or corporations are landlord and tenant. Most importantly, it must identify the premises in unmistakable terms, and indicate the amount of rent to be paid, the term of the lease, the rights of renewing the lease, the date rent is due and where and how it is payable, and the obligations of the landlord.

In the absence of specific language to the contrary, rent is not payable until the expiration of the term for which the premises are leased. Most leases, however, require advance periodic payment of rent, generally at the beginning of each month. A lease may require a tenant to pay real estate taxes and water bills in addition to the stated charge for the leasing. Such charges are, by the terms of the lease, considered additional rent, and nonpayment of them subjects a tenant to the same sanctions as does nonpayment of rent. In general, leases prohibit the subletting or assignment of leases without the prior written consent of the landlord, and most leases add that such consent shall not be unreasonably withheld.

A written lease is a complicated legal document. It should be remembered that the landlord or his attorney usually prepares the lease and, in most cases, the form used is one prepared by the local real estate board which generally has the landlord's interest foremost. In most cases, therefore, the tenant or his attorney will want to negotiate with the landlord. A checklist of certain formalities of the lease to be considered includes:

1. If the landlord is a corporate owner or fiduciary landlord, his authority to enter into the lease should be verified.

2. The description of the property should be accurate. Does the lease cover all of the property under discussion, including storage, parking, and miscellaneous space?
3. If the lease is required to be recorded, it must be acknowledged before a notary public. Does it conform to the requirements of the state in which the property is located or the lease made?
4. The duration (or term) of the lease should be well defined. The date of commencement and the expiration date should be clearly stated.
5. The names of the lessor and lessee and other formal details should be checked carefully.

As mentioned above, there are some areas in which the tenant or his attorney may be able to negotiate in order to make certain arrangements in the best interests of the tenant or lessee.[3] Some of the issues to be considered during such bargaining include:

1. The right of the tenant to use auxiliary parts of the building or the premises, such as parking lot, garages, storage areas, and utility rooms should be enumerated.

2. The right of a tenant to assign or sublet should be defined. This is especially important if the term of the lease is long. The right to assign or sublet provides a hedge against financial or other unforeseeable future events.

3. The right of a tenant to install equipment such as air conditioning, laboratory equipment, X-ray equipment, and other electrical appurtenances should be set forth. The landlord's permission in the lease will avoid the need for inquiry about such things at a later date.

4. If property is taken by the city or another governmental unit by condemnation, right of way, etc., the owner of the property is compensated for the loss of his property. Such action could have a detrimental effect on the group practice tenant unless the lease contains a clause which permits the tenant to recover from the landlord compensation for such losses. Some tenants also may be able to negotiate a clause of this nature to protect against loss of fixtures and equipment.

5. In some leases, provision is made for an increase in the rental if the landlord's taxes, water rates, etc., increase. The tenant should attempt to limit the amount of such increases as much as possible by excluding special assessments, salaries of supervisory personnel, and other similar charges. If possible, the tenant should avoid escalator clauses.

6. If repairs or alterations become necessary and are the obligation of the landlord according to the terms of the lease, the tenant may want to have included in the lease a clause permitting the group to make the repairs or changes and to credit these payments with interest against the rents or charges payable.

7. If the tenant makes changes in the premises by installing fixtures or other appurtenances previously mentioned, he usually will not have the right to remove them at the end of the term unless the landlord has agreed to this condition. A tenant should request that he be given this right. Also, if he expects to renew the lease, his right to remove the fixtures should be made to continue at the expiration of the renewal period.

8. The option to renew should be considered. Whether the rent remains

the same, increases a specific amount, or is left open to later negotiation must be determined. Furthermore, for expansion purposes, the group may wish to acquire options or the right of first refusal on additional space within a building occupied by other tenants. Such commitments also could be included in the group's lease agreement.

9. The duty of the landlord to make repairs to the interior of the premises should be well defined. His duty to provide hot water, heat, and air conditioning during certain hours and at certain temperatures should be stated. If alterations are required, a clause in the lease should make completion of such alterations a necessity before the tenants are obligated to take possession and to pay rent. Decisions on fire and liability insurance premiums also must be reached.

10. Arranging an option to purchase should be considered. Giving the tenant the option to purchase the medical facility at a specific dollar amount and applying previous rent to the purchase price are possibilities.

11. It should be ascertained whether the landlord has a valid certificate of occupancy from local authorities and whether the premises are free from violation at the present time. Who is to pay for correction of violations that occur during a tenant's occupancy is another important matter. If it is the tenants' obligation, such payments may be limited to those violations the tenant caused, and if the tenant corrects other violations he may be able to deduct costs from rent due.

12. The issue of zoning of facilities for medical use is of particular importance and will be discussed in detail in Part IV. In the case of leased facilities to be used for the delivery of health care it is important to ascertain if the property is zoned for the use that the tenant intends to make of the premises. If not, the group should explore whether the landlord will agree to obtain a zoning variance and, if unobtainable, whether he will release the tenant from obligation under the lease.

These areas are important to consider before signing a formal lease for a group practice facility. In a city particularly, many rental conditions are prescribed by government statutes which must be carefully scrutinized by competent professionals. Although it might appear that a lease arrangement provides the forming group with additional security in light of start-up uncertainties, it should not be assumed that leasing a facility will relieve the group from liabilities associated with the building. The expenses associated with the leasing of a medical facility have been discussed in some detail in the preceding paragraphs within the context of prevailing terms and conditions surrounding the lease arrangement; however, it may be beneficial for a forming group practice to become aware of expenses it might be expected to incur in addition to the base rent. Additional charges may include escalator provisions to be applied to subsequent term base rents which are predicated on future inflationary factors. Leasehold improvements ordered by the tenant and installed by the landlord might be included as supplementary monthly rental payments or paid in one lump sum by the tenant upon completion of such improvements. The additional expenses related to payment of taxes, utilities, and maintenance services may be included in the base rent or require additional payments by the tenant on a specified basis.

FACILITY OWNERSHIP VERSUS LEASING

Accountants classify land, buildings, and equipment as fixed assets and insist that such assets be recorded in the ledger at cost of acquisition. Land does not depreciate with use, but the usefulness of buildings and machinery does decline with the passage of time. Consequently, at the end of each accounting period a portion of the cost of such properties is transferred to the cost of operation for the current period, and the remainder is carried to the balance sheet to be listed among the assets of the enterprise. Since all fixed assets except land are ultimately charged to the cost of the group's operations, in this context one might conceive of a fixed asset merely as a prepayment of some of the group's future operating expenses. It is generally supposed that when a medical group expends $100,000 for a building with an estimated life of twenty years, the annual straightline depreciation charge of five thousand dollars represents portions of that structure which have evaporated in some mysterious fashion. An alternative way to view this situation is that a building is acquired not because it is a structure, but because it allows the rendering of a series of services deemed essential to the productive operation of the medical organization. Thus, when the organization purchases a building for $100,000, it actually is purchasing the ability to provide a series of essential services. Although a particular group practice building is expected to stand for twenty years, its serviceability to the user may be limited to a shorter period, perhaps only ten years. If one conceives of an expenditure for a building as necessary to acquire delivery potential for a series of services rather than as the simple purchase of a structure, it is not difficult to understand why a building that appears to be in sound condition actually may be almost fully depreciated in a short time. It is necessary to distinguish carefully between "physical" and "use" deterioration. When this definition is applied, the medical group would do well to view its acquisition as an acquisition of ten specific building services useful to the organization, together with certain residual services of no use to the organization but of some possible use to other organizations. This concept of medical facility ownership includes the concept of bundle of services, the basis of which deals with the problem of allocating the original $100,000 purchase price to the various services acquired over a specified time period.

The bundle of services concept of fixed assets necessitates the restructuring of popular concepts of ownership and the value of owning. The services rendered by a fixed asset, rather than the act of holding legal title to the asset, are essential to the productivity of the medical group practice. Sometimes, it is possible to purchase services one by one as they are needed; thus, one service might be purchased at the beginning of one year, the second at the second year, and so on. Because funds expended for each year's services are recovered from patients who purchase the medical group's services during that period, a policy of buying fixed asset services in the period of use greatly reduces the total amount of funds needed at any one time.

It should be clear that owning a fixed asset really means purchasing all the future services which that asset is capable of rendering. In order to enjoy the current service, it sometimes is necessary to buy (or to agree to buy) all the future services. When this is so, an owner-user is forced to run certain risks inherent in legal ownership. For example, since there always is the chance that a change in circumstances may render a specific service obsolete or unnecessary, the group assumes the risk involved in the expectation of a continued need. In addition, a building expected to last twenty years actually may last only eighteen years or less. On the other hand, the group which assumes such risks also has a chance for possible gains inherent in the ownership of the facility itself: the asset may last twenty-five years instead of the originally estimated twenty.

In some types of group practices organized specifically as nonprofit and tax-exempt, the effects of income and property taxes do not apply. For those organizations formed for profit, the implications of purchasing versus leasing medical facilities and equipment can have a serious effect on the organization's financial planning and structure. Outright ownership of a medical facility asset means ownership of all the services that the asset ever will render, but the number of renderable services almost always is uncertain. Hence, a purchaser of a fixed asset, if purchasing an uncertain number of services, is assuming the risk of paying for potentially nonexistent or nonoccurring services. Only the value of a current service can be estimated with any degree of accuracy; consequently, the outright purchaser of a fixed asset is gambling on the value of more remote services. To purchase at once all the services renderable by a fixed asset involves the investment of a sum of capital which is larger than that required for the purchase of each service as it is used, and, of course, the invested capital cannot be used for other purposes. To compensate for this loss, it is customary for lessors to allow interest on prepayments, but the discount allowed in such cases is more apt to coincide with market rates of interest on safe investments than it is apt to coincide with the rates of earnings actually forfeited by the lessee on a prepaid lease. The principal difference between a prepaid lease and outright ownership is that in the former the lessor discounts a specific number of services, whereas in the latter the purchaser discounts all the services. In general, when comparing the advantages of ownership as opposed to leasing, one should consider the loss of earnings in investment and the risks inherent in ownership. In the case of most beginning group practices, the question of ownership versus leasing often is judged exclusively on the availability of large sums of capital required for an initial investment.

A tendency exists for individuals, be they manufacturers, retailers, or health care managers, to prefer ownership of fixed assets even when cost considerations suggest the desirability of leasing. This prejudice lingers because of society's tendency to base social status on the extent of ownership. A clearer understanding of the nature and cost of fixed asset ownership, together with the rise of the large corporate enterprises has had a substantial effect in removing this ownership bias. From the forming medical group's standpoint, the organization's mission should underscore the desirability of critically weighing the choice between a lease agreement and an outright purchase arrangement for property, medical facilities, and equipment.

Chapter 8

Financial Planning

FISCAL CONSIDERATIONS

Financial planning usually begins with the development of fiscal policies and a determination of the accounting period. In addition, the group's legal organizational form, the pooling of group members' assets, and cash management must be considered.

It is essential that a group conduct its practice on a sound business basis if it is to meet the needs of its patients and accomplish its objectives. Facilities and equipment represent necessary expenses of medical practice, but the most significant expenditure is an investment in personnel services. Payments to the physicians, to their paramedical assistants, and to administrative employees constitute a significant amount in any group practice operation. Medical Group Management Association's 1975 Cost Survey reveals that for existing three to ten physician group practices, manpower costs amount to 67 percent of gross annual receipts. Furthermore, an additional 15 percent of gross receipts is related to costs such as payroll taxes, retirement plan costs, and insurance programs. Professional liability insurance is another major expense and one that is extremely volatile (1.7 percent). Taken together with the supplies, fees, and other costs of the practice, it is obvious that there are a number of significant and recurring costs. Generally stated, the overhead or operating expenses in existing three to ten physician groups (excluding physician income) averages 47 percent of gross receipts.[1] Regardless of such costs, however, a group should endeavor to provide services that are reasonably priced. Through efficient and effective financial planning at the outset, benefits will accrue to the group and to its patients and will preclude any need to inflate fees or premiums to cover business inefficiencies.

The first step in financial planning is the formulation of *fiscal system policies* resulting from each of the strategy issues presented in this chapter, and translating the group's financial approach into operating guidelines. Answers to the following questions can provide a basis for fiscal system policies and will help to define the financial system:

1. What business year is to be used?
2. What organizational form is to be used?
3. How will assets now separately owned be merged into the organization?
4. What bank is to be used and how will cash be managed?
5. What method of accounting should be established?

The *accounting period* is the fixed period of time used by the group to compute income. As the group's business year, it should correspond as closely as possible to the usual cycle of business. The accounting period may be a calendar year, a twelve-month period ending December 31; a fiscal year, a twelve-month period ending on the last day of any month except December; or a fifty-two- or fifty-three-week year, which varies according to the day of the week on which the period begins and ends. The selection of an accounting period generally is not as cirtical for medical groups as for other types of business enterprises. General accounting principles suggest that the accounting period coincide with the low point of sales and size of inventory. Although medical groups do encounter seasonal fluctuations, such variations often are not as dramatic as those encountered in other industries. For medical groups who choose a cash basis for recording income, any accounting period would be appropriate; however, for the group choosing an accrual method of accounting, it would be more desirable to close the business year at a time when accounts receivable usually are at their minimum level, because at this time a greater portion of the fees or premiums upon which a tax liability exists has been converted into funds to discharge that liability. The accounting period chosen also may vary according to the legal organizational form of the group and, in order to prevent any substantial deferral of income tax, must be acceptable to the Internal Revenue Service. The professional association, professional corporation, and corporation are tax paying entities, unless tax exemptions have been obtained from the IRS, and usually have no problems concerning IRS approval of a preferred accounting period. The principals and employees of these organizations, however, remain on a calendar year for personal tax purposes.

In recent years, newly formed medical partnerships have not been able to obtain IRS approval for accounting periods which vary more than two months from the calendar year. Because a partnership is not a tax paying entity and files only information tax returns, each partner must report in his personal tax return his portion of partnership income for the calendar year during which the partnership's accounting period closes. Under these conditions it is possible to establish a partnership accounting period which will result in a substantial deferral of taxes. Accordingly, the Internal Revenue Service has not approved accounting periods ending in March, April, May, June, July, August, September, and October. The tax considerations inherent in various legal organizational forms are discussed fully in Chapter 5. When selecting the accounting period, the group also should consider that there are other time periods which are critical to accounting and budgeting, including:

1. Payroll Year
   a. Wages
   b. Withholding Taxes
   c. Social Security Taxes
   d. Federal Unemployment Taxes
   e. State Unemployment Taxes
2. Retirement Plan Year
3. Contract Years
4. Policy Years
   a. Workmen's Compensation
   b. Hospitalization
   c. Life and Disability
   d. Professional Liability.

The Internal Revenue Service requires that the payroll year be a calendar year. Individual payroll records, related reports, and taxes must be reconciled each December 31. Since payroll and payroll related expenses are the most significant portion of overhead costs incurred by medical groups, it is often most convenient to use a calendar year accounting period as well. Accounting and budgeting are simplified to a certain degree when financial activities fall within common time parameters. In fact, time allotments should be staggered only when such variance has a specific advantage, such as:

1. Balancing cash flow by spreading related payments
2. Facilitation of review by group management
3. Availability of records to outside services including legal, audit, and tax services.

A fiscal year accounting period reflects more accurately the group's natural business year and provides an opportunity for an accurate measurement of financial operating results. The usual period of low activity at the close of a fiscal year allows group practice personnel an opportunity to concentrate on the year's closing without the distractions of higher activity periods. In selecting a fifty-two- or fifty-three-week accounting period, the payroll accounting period is the influencing factor. Its advantages are limited to those organizations who pay their employees on a weekly or bimonthly cycle.

For income tax purposes, the accounting period is chosen when the first tax return is filed. If, for example, a calendar year is elected, the books are closed on the December 31 following organization of the group practice, and a tax return is prepared for that period; thereafter, the accounting period will continue to be the calendar year. For accounting periods other than calendar years, the books should be closed and an income tax return should be filed for the period closing the accounting period. This first closing cannot be longer than twelve months from the starting date of group operation; thereafter, the accounting period will continue to close on the selected date.

In any form of group practice, after an accounting period has been established, desired changes usually require approval by the Internal Revenue Service. For example, a partnership must obtain Internal Revenue Service approval to change its accounting period unless the change is to conform with the individual tax years of all its partners who have an interest of 5 percent or more in profits or capital. A partnership's accounting period is not affected by the inclusion of new partners. They continue on their own individual tax year, which usually is calendar; however, they include their share of partnership income in their personal tax returns for the calendar year during which the *partnership year closes.* Professional associations, professional corporations, and corporations also usually must obtain approval to change their accounting periods. If an organization has not changed its accounting period for the past ten years and if certain other conditions are met, an accounting period may be changed without IRS approval, and an accountant should prepare the statements necessary to be filed with the local district director of the Internal Revenue Service.

Organizational structure must be developed to meet the personnel, facility, and equipment needs necessary for quality medical care. Accumulation of capital needs may be filled through the formation of separate clinic related companies. The group's professional activities require operating capital only; however, providing facilities and equipment requires capital accumulation. The use of separate organizations to meet the group's professional needs and its equipment and facility needs offers a significant business advantage. A corporate organizational form may be used to accumulate capital and capital assets, while a professional corporation, professional association, or partnership may be used to provide medical services. In this instance, a corporation can be organized with a relatively low capital outlay, with the physicians of the professional organization investing as stockholders. Capital assets may be purchased with original capital and debt financing and may be leased to the professional organization. All or a major portion of the corporate income after taxes may be retained to meet additional capital asset needs and/or to retire any debts incurred.

As discussed in great detail in Chapters 5 and 7, tax considerations and ownership are key strategic planning issues which strongly influence the group's fiscal rationale. In order to prevent conflicts over rental rates and stock market values, the group should consider maintaining ownership investments in the professional organization and any related organizations as nearly equal as possible. As market values rise over a period of time and the total investment increases, there may be a potential problem in attracting new physicians to the group. Provisions could be developed to allow such investment requirements to be met in annual installments over a relatively long period of time, possibly as long as ten or fifteen years. If the group is organized as a partnership, the joining physician could finance a part of his investment with an interest bearing note payable to the partnership over a prescribed term, thus allowing his ownership to begin at the earliest and presumably lowest market value. Under this arrangement, the cost to a new investor is the interest expense which will be paid on the note, which is deductible when computing personal income tax. Corporations, however, cannot accept note payment because corporate stock cannot be purchased on credit. While third party financing may be used, no financing agreement may be arranged directly with the corporation. The purchase of stock or shares from withdrawing or retiring physicians may be handled through cash repurchase or notes payable over a specified period of time. Gains on sale of stock usually will be taxed at capital gain rates. A senior physician will want to avoid selling his stock in advance of retirement, because the capital gains added to his ordinary income from the professional organization will result in a tax rate which is higher than if the gain is deferred until after retirement.

Whether the group practice is organized as a single or multiple organizational entity, fiscal planning should include provisions for possible excess earnings. Retained earnings of the organization(s) may be used to accomplish one or more of the following:

1. Provide additional assets
2. Provide for updating and replacement of assets as necessary
3. Retire debt financing
4. Retire equity for departing physicians
5. Retire equity of withdrawing physicians
6. Pay dividends or earnings to continuing owners.

The organization may be subjected to substantial punitive taxes for capital accumulations in excess of $150,000 should this excess go beyond the present and planned needs of the corporation. This excess accumulated earnings tax is in addition to regular income taxes. The first $100,000 of excess accumulated earnings is presently taxed at a rate of 27.5 percent and the next $100,000 is taxed at a rate of 38.5 percent.

Physicians forming, or subsequently joining, a new medical group may own personal business assets which can be used beneficially by the group. If these assets are sold to the group, the seller is treated as an outsider in determining whether a taxable gain or loss results from the sale. If the seller has more than an 80 percent interest in the medical group, any resulting gain cannot be treated as a capital gain, and if the seller owns more than a 50 percent interest in the group, no taxable loss is allowed. Another method for transferring assets to the group is the *pooling of assets* in which assets are transferred in exchange for an equity interest in the organization. When assets are exchanged for a partnership interest, no taxable gain or loss in recognized. When assets are transferred for stock ownership, taxable gain or loss is based on the market value of the transferred stock. If the stock has no established market value, however, gain or loss is based on the fair market value of the property transferred.

In the pooling of assets, the collectibility of the accounts receivable of individual practitioners may vary sharply due to the physician's practice, the effectiveness of credit and collection procedures, the efficiency and timeliness of third party billing, or a combination of these factors. When pooling assets, individuals should consider excluding accounts past an agreed upon aging date, disputed accounts, and accounts under litigation or threatened litigation. Furthermore, pooled accounts receivable should be valued after the fact; the equity credit transferred can be based on collections effected within an agreed upon time period, such as 120 days, and reduced by a provision for collection costs.

The pooling plan for fixed assets should be based on organizational need and should include consideration of the specific assets needed, the exclusion of duplications, and the valuation of pooled assets. Equipment planning (see Chapter 27) should identify the fixed asset needs of the group practice, and unnecessary or obsolete assets should be excluded. Where personal assets correspond to organizational needs, criteria for the group selection could be based on highest utility, level of maintenance, and expected useful life. Valuation always should be based on fair market value. An agreed upon value usually is acceptable and provisions for appraisals by third parties can be provided for as necessary. Although organizational objectives are a primary consideration in planning for the pooling of assets, the individual desires and preferences of the principal founders may be difficult to reconcile with group goals, especially when one of the founding physicians brings a large established practice and considerable assets to the new group practice.

Finally, strategies must be developed for actual *cash management.* The group should provide a convenient and well-staffed cashiering service for receiving all payments and should equip its staff with well defined, comprehensive, written policies concerning pricing, credit, collections, check cashing, petty cash disbursements, and cash processing. Each cashier should be assigned funds subject to his individual control and security and should be bonded. Insurance should be carried in an amount sufficient to cover the highest amount of cash anticipated to be in-house at any one time. After cashiering funds are counted and balanced each day, any funds exceeding the imprest balance (an account maintained at a standard balance) should be deposited intact. A deposit copy and receipts totaling the deposit are retained for accounting records.

Because bank services can include account services, financing, retirement plan administration, investment services, data processing services, and even center payroll, the selection of a bank should be based on the ability of the bank to support the total needs of the group. When advantageous, a nearby bank may be used as a temporary depository and transfers may be made to another bank at a later date. Banks can provide specialized expertise and continuity of service, making it often more practical to assign such functions to a bank rather than to center personnel. In arranging financing, the interest and service charges allowable for the group may not provide the bank with an acceptable rate of return. In order to compensate for this deficiency, the bank may require the group to maintain a specified minimum account balance. In determining this balance, the bank usually will compute the additional earnings needed to bring its rate of return to the desired level. Using the current treasury bill rate, the bank then can compute the minimum balance required of the group. Banking services must be tailored to individual group circumstances and local conditions. Delaying consideration of banking requirements too late in the planning stage can result in unwise choices, possibly influenced by physicians who are on boards of certain banks or by friends of group members. If group needs can be met and personal relationships maintained through the selection of one bank, then by all means that bank should be chosen. The group is cautioned, however, not to select a bank solely on personal bias.

Cash management may be expedited by separating certain receipt and disbursement functions. For example, cash receipts may be segregated by using multiple post office box numbers. Clinic letterheads, patient statements, insurance claims, and return envelopes may display different box numbers for various billing classifications. Payments returned to these separate box numbers are functionally sorted as a part of the postal process. Cash disbursements may be segregated by using separate bank accounts, including payroll and refunds, thus allowing separate and special processing, the delegation of responsibilities, and the maximizing of supervision and control. The use of special accounts also facilitates the preparation of bank reconciliations.

The use of a lock box depository system offers yet another means for sorting and delegating responsibilities. When mail payments are made directly to a special post office box, the bank can pick up the post office box and processes all daily deposits at one time. Deposit slips and posting media then can be forwarded by the bank for entry into the group's accounting records. Processing through the bank's proof department and microfilm copying service provides a complete transaction record. An important aspect of internal control is that the bank holds the *only* key to the post office box containing center remittances. Diverting mail payments directly to the bank reduces the clinic's daily processing, balancing, reconciling, and deposit activities. It also can lower average and maximum in-center cash accumulation which, in turn, reduces the required insurance coverage and related premiums.

Another cash management technique utilizes the imprest account, which is an account constantly reimbursed by deposits equal to the checks written against it. It is, therefore, maintained at a standard balance. The following example illustrates a payroll account maintained as an imprest fund:

Beginning Imprest Balance	$ 3,000
Employee payroll checks written for the pay period total $13,185	
A check against the operating account is written and deposited to the payroll account	+13,185
The payroll checks are recorded as disbursements and released to the employees	-13,185
The resulting balance is:	$ 3,000

The balance shown in the general ledger and on the balance sheet will always show the account at its imprest amount. A differing figure indicates that an error has been made or that there has been unauthorized activity in the account.

From the standpoint of managing surplus funds, the forming group practice should consider accumulating cash in a primary account and distributing it as necessary to special purpose accounts. This concentration of funds in one account can be reviewed frequently. Funds temporarily in excess of needs can be invested in short term cash equivalents such as certificates of deposit or treasury bills. Surplus funds should be determined as follows:

Account Balance	$150,000
Less Compensating Balance	-40,000
Less Amount Needed for Operations	-90,000
Available for Investment	$ 20,000

Zero balance accounts are designed to maximize funds available for short term investments. Rather than transferring funds to the special account when checks are written, the transfer is made by the bank as checks against the special account are presented for payment. Some banks are now providing buy back services for treasury bills, certificates of deposit, etc., which further improve investment opportunities by allowing the group to invest for short periods of time. A forming group also must consider the cash management of its retirement plan, which will require strict accounting and reporting and must be managed in careful compliance with regulations. Assignment of the plan's administration, therefore, should be made only to an experienced manager such as a bank's trust department. Finally, the group should investigate methods for recording its business transactions; manual or electronic data processing are two of the alternatives (see Chapter 18).

FINANCIAL ACCOUNTING

After the forming group practice has developed strategies for various aspects of its fiscal program, systems planning and policy issue decisions related to financial accounting must be made, including the accounting system, chart of accounts, books of account, accounts payable, payroll, balance sheet, and income statement. Although all of these interface closely with one another, the following discussion will be segmented to reflect as clearly as possible the decision making process involved in planning.

The Accounting System

The accounting system is comprised of the following processes:

1. *Classifying* financial information involves assigning the data to the correct accounts in an accurate and consistent manner.
2. *Recording* financial information involves compiling a permanent financial record by accumulating data in usable form. Original entries are made in journals and the information then is transferred to the ledger where it is accumulated by account.
3. *Analyzing* financial information involves reviewing the records for correctness and ensuring that the information is understandable.
4. *Reporting* financial information involves transmitting information in an understandable way and in sufficient detail to meet the needs of the user.

An accounting system must provide the information necessary to determine the group's financial position through the compilation of a balance sheet and to compute its income in the form of an income statement. Before establishing an accounting system, however, a method of computing income over a fixed accounting period must be decided upon. The cash method and the accrual method are approaches used most commonly. Modified accounting methods employ some features of both approaches.

When using a cash accounting method, income is recognized when it is received and expenses are recognized when they are paid; therefore, only collected fees are treated as income, regardless of the service date. Patient payments for future services also are treated as income when received and not necessarily when those future services are rendered. Expenses are recorded when paid without regard to the date of order, receipt, or consumption, with the exception of capital asset expenditures or payments which will provide benefits substantially past the end of the accounting period. Payments which are not treated as expenses when paid include the following:

1. *Purchase of Equipment and Buildings.* Expenses are recorded by allocating the costs over a depreciation period, thus spreading the expense over the expected life of the assets. Depreciation does not represent a valuation process; its sole purpose is a means for the allocation of cost.
2. *Purchase of Leasehold Improvements.* Expenses are recorded by amortization of costs over the expected life of the improvements or lives of the leases—whichever is the shorter. Life of the lease may be considered as the original lease term plus any extended option periods when it is anticipated that option extensions will be exercised. In no case, however, should cost be allocated over a period longer than the legal life of the lease.
3. *Insurance Premiums.* Premiums paid for three years of coverage should be spread over the three year period. Premiums for a one year policy usually are recorded in the year paid, although the coverage period may extend far into the next accounting period. Consistently applied, this recognition of expense will not distort income measurement for separate accounting periods.

When using an accrual accounting method, income is recognized when earned and expenses are recognized when incurred. Allocations to future accounting periods are provided for. Operating results can be measured by matching current earnings with their associated costs for the accounting period. Cash receipts and disbursements do not affect the income statement and are accounted for in the balance sheet which describes current financial position. These accounts will fluctuate as collections are received, costs consumed, etc. A combination of cash and accrual accounting may be used if the resulting method is consistently applied and clearly reflects the current financial operation of the group practice. If, for example, a group's bookings are 95 percent individual fee-for-service and 5 percent contract service, 95 percent may be considered income when collected and 5 percent may be considered income when earned. The contract portion of the service is treated on an accrual basis because payment is considered both imminent and assured. Likewise, insurance premiums covering a policy year, which may include three months of the current accounting year and nine months of the next accounting year, may be allocated on an accrual basis, 25 percent to the current year and 75 percent to the following year. Other expenses, however, may be recorded on a cash basis; such expenses as maintenance contracts, renewed for one year periods at various times throughout the accounting year, usually are minimal in amount and may be treated as expenses when paid without material distortion of income in either accounting period.

Once selected, the general accounting plan as well as the accounting treatment of any material item must be used consistently and cannot be changed without Internal Revenue Service approval.

> While the cash basis may be more advantageous from a tax standpoint, the accrual basis lends itself more readily to managerial analysis and control of current operations. There is no prolonged period between production and recognition of earnings and it is far easier to match revenues with the costs applicable to those revenues. Further, the use of the accrual basis greatly reduces the unreasonable periodic results that occur frequently in cash basis data as a consequence of short-term economic conditions. Thus, on the accrual basis, the long-term trends of activity are more readily apparent without being disguised by clinic short-term cyclical fluctuations.[2]

Selection of an accounting method will lead to the establishment of operating policies (see Chapter 10). After such policies have been defined, specific accounting procedures will be required to ensure that organizational objectives are being met. Financial objectives include:

1. Establishment of accountability at the earliest practical point
2. Provision of consistent treatment of accounting detail
3. Provision of adequate documentation of accounting information
4. Provision of accuracy throughout the accounting process.

Established and approved accounting procedures can be included in an accounting manual for reference and for use as an instructional guide to new employees. As new situations develop and accounting decisions are made, the manual can be expanded or adjusted. Most importantly, all procedures should be reviewed periodically for necessary updating; as the practice grows and organizational changes are made, new and better procedures may be possible.

The Chart of Accounts

After having chosen an accounting system, the group must decide upon an appropriate chart of accounts which identifies the official accounting classifications to be used in recording financial transactions of the organization. Account designations provide the terminology to be used in the books of account. The chart of accounts also describes the position and format for each account as it appears concurrently on the balance sheet, income statement, and general ledger. Detailed delineation of account titles makes the resulting chart of accounts a valuable guide to group practice accounting personnel.

In establishing a chart of accounts, the development of a large number of descriptive categories allows the group's accounting personnel to make and apply classifications of accounting entries more easily, accurately, and consistently. Use of a large number of account categories also tends to produce a greater degree of detail, which can lower audit costs and the cost of preparing income tax reports and financial statements. Conveying classification information to others, including group physicians, can be accomplished quickly and easily. Analyzing accounts that are too general, however, most certainly will require clarification, and necessary analysis can be costly in time and effort. Each fiscal year, the chart of accounts can be reviewed for any necessary revisions. When changes are few, comparability of the group's financial position and its operating results remain consistent over time. When changes are necessary, however, they certainly should be integrated immediately.

In the initial as well as subsequent development of a chart of accounts, many variables will influence classification, including the group's organizational type and its choice of accounting method. In Chapter II of the *Clinic Manager's Manual*, Medical Group Management Association suggests a possible uniform chart of accounts; MGMA's accounting committee continues to investigate this area. Appendix 8A of this chapter also contains a sample method for developing a chart of accounts to meet the specific needs of a forming practice. Each account is given an identification number as well as a name. Use of the account number facilitates the allocation of costs to possible cost centers and the processing of accounting data. Furthermore, the use of multiple organizations suggests the segregation of the building and equipment or both into business entities separate from the professional organization. The addition of company codes will segregate effectively such business entities while still maintaining the account number coding. A similar distinction can be initiated by adding department numbers for those organizations electing a method of departmental accounting. Obviously, specific accounts selected to compose the chart of accounts will depend upon the organizational needs of the group.

The Balance Sheet

The balance sheet is a statement of financial position as of a specified date. Its purpose is to present information concerning the assets, liabilities, and net worth of the organization and to present this information in detail sufficient to permit evaluation of financial condition. Balance sheet format always is based on the formula: assets equal liabilities plus net worth. This format is displayed in the following summary balance sheet:

XYZ CLINIC
BALANCE SHEET
December 31, 19___

Assets	$1,000,000
Liabilities	$ 600,000
Net Worth	400,000
Total Liabilities and Net Worth	$1,000,000

Current assets are those assets reasonably expected to be available within twelve months of statement date; current liabilities are defined as liabilities due to be paid within twelve months of statement date, and long term debt represents liabilities due to be paid at some scheduled date past twelve months. Net worth is an expression of owner equity which is called *capital* in partnerships and *stockholder equity* in corporations and in professional associations. For example, in a medical partnership, net worth is presented in capital accounts as shown below:

Capital, Partner V	$80,000
Capital, Partner W	80,000
Capital, Partner X	80,000
Capital, Partner Y	80,000
Capital, Partner Z	80,000
Total Capital	$400,000

Capital is the cumulative total of capital contributed, increased by earnings and decreased by losses and by partner payments. The net worth of professional associations and corporations, however, is established as shown in the following balance sheet example:

	Stockholder Equity		
Stock at Par Value	$ 40,000	(Paid in at Par)	Total from Sale of Shares
Additional Paid in Capital	60,000	(Excess Paid over Par)	
Retained Earnings	305,000	(Earnings less past dividends & restrictions)	
Retained Earnings Restricted	15,000	(Dividend Declared, Not Yet Paid)	
Subtotal	420,000		
Less Cost of Shares in Treasury	20,000	Shares Repurchased	
	$400,000		

Stockholder equity accounts usually contain additional statements which define and disclose information such as the number of shares authorized and the par value per share, the number of shares issued, the number of shares outstanding, and the number of shares in treasury (repurchased—not reissued).

Assets are presented in the order in which they are expected to be available—i.e., in their order of liquidity. Liabilities are listed in the order in which they are expected or required to be paid. An example of this sequence is illustrated in Appendix 8B of this chapter. Because the balance sheet is influenced by the group's legal organization, the accounting method terminology, and the sequence appropriate for financial statement reporting, it is necessary for the forming group practice to relate the chart of accounts and balance sheet to such variables. Referring again to Appendix 8A, the 100, 200, and 300 series accounts are the general balance sheet items; the 400 and 500 series accounts are displayed as they would apply to a partnership's chart of accounts and balance sheet. The 600–900 series accounts are the income statement accounts.

Appendix 8C of this chapter displays a balance sheet which is based on the chart of accounts shown in Appendix 8A. Each balance sheet account is related to the various organizational types and accounting methods. For example, should a group organized as a professional corporation choose an accrual accounting method, the chart of accounts and balance sheet accounts appropriate for that group can be determined by scanning the applicable columns in Appendix 8C. Furthermore, ledger accounts should be included in the general ledger in the same sequence. Maintaining consistency throughout the accounting system assists in providing continuity and expedience in processing recorded, budgeted, and reported financial information.

The Income Statement

The income statement summarizes and thereby measures income and expense transactions for a fixed period of time. Government regulations, taxes, technology, and the state of the economy constantly affect daily business operations. While in the past such factors have introduced many complexities into business systems, basic business objectives of efficiency and solvency have not changed over the years. To achieve these objectives, financial position and operating results must be monitored constantly. The income statement provides a measure of business accomplishment and its purpose is to provide a clear, sufficiently detailed statement concerning earnings for a prescribed period. In terminology, sequencing, and numbering, the accounts used in the general ledger, financial statements, and the chart of accounts should be the same. In Appendix 8A, the 600, 700, and 800 series accounts apply to the income statement and its presentation. Although the sequence of reporting should be based on management need, the examples used here are intended to provide information for analyzing broad categories of income and expenses, including professional and medical personnel, supplies, and general and administrative.

Similar to the balance sheet accounts, income statement accounts vary according to the group's organizational type and its accounting method. For income statement account planning, Appendix 8D of this chapter relates the various chart of accounts/income statement accounts to organizational type and accounting method options. In addition, Appendix 8D contains a sample income statement.

After decisions concerning a chart of accounts/balance sheet/and income statement have been reached, remaining financial planning issues include the books of account, the accounts payable, and the payroll.

The Books of Account

Financial information usually is processed in the following sequence:

1. Source Document
2. Journal ⟩ Books of account
3. Ledger ⟩
4. Report

Information from source documents—charge slips, invoices, receipts, etc.—is entered into accounting journals which provide a sequence listing of financial data to be totaled and balanced for periodic transfer to the general ledger in which the data are assimilated by account. Through this process, information is organized into a usable format for analysis and reporting.

More specifically, journals are books of original entry that provide an assembly point for accumulating detailed financial information. The journal identifies the document source as well as the who, what, where, when, and how of the transaction. Any number of special journals may be used to simplify recording, to allow division of duties, or to provide for better control. Journal entries should be proofed thoroughly to ensure validity of information input into the accounting system. They should be totaled and balanced on a scheduled basis and posted to the general ledger, and the journal format or posting notes should indicate the general ledger account to which information is transferred. A group practice accounting system usually should include the following journals:

1. *Service Journal.* This journal provides a record of services rendered to patients and should include information necessary to support the group's patient and third party billing system.
2. *Cash Receipts Journal.* The cash receipts journal provides a record of cash received, from whatever source or for whatever purpose, and includes information necessary for the proper classification of payment received.
3. *Cash Disbursements.* This journal provides a record of all payments from the group's operating account. These payments should be supported by documents which are properly approved for payment, maintained in vendor files, and usually filed by accounting year.
4. *Payroll Journal.* The payroll journal records employee payments and includes details of pay computation. It must be prepared in comprehensive detail which, when merged with master payroll information, is sufficient to meet the following needs:
   a. Prepare employer wage reports
   b. Prepare unemployment tax reports
   c. Prepare employee W-2 and reconciliation reports
   d. Demonstrate compliance with wage and hour laws
   e. Demonstrate compliance with discrimination laws
   f. Provide information relative to compensation coverage
   g. Provide information relative to group insurance coverage
   h. Report to the Department of Labor on retirement plan coverage.
5. *General Journal.* The general journal receives all entries not recorded in the special journals and typically would include the following types of entries:
   a. Correction of classification errors—moving information between accounts
   b. Recording noncash entries (depreciation, amortization, etc.)
   c. Recording the expiration of prepaid costs—expired insurance
   d. Recognizing changes in condition—writing off bad debts, writing off stale checks outstanding, accruing unbilled expenses such as legal and audit fees
   e. Recording and adjusting entries, and closing entries to close the accounting year.

All journal information is transferred to the general ledger where it is summarized by account classification. The general ledger usually is organized in the following order:

Balance Sheet Accounts
- Assets
- Liabilities
- Proprietorship Accounts

Income Statement Accounts
  Income
  Expenses

Balance sheet accounts are maintained on a continuing basis and adjusted to reflect changing financial position. The income statement accounts are closed at the end of each accounting year and the resultant net gain or loss is transferred to the proprietorship/ownership accounts which reflect owner equity in the organization.

Any number of subsidiary ledgers may be established to furnish necessary detail. For example, accounts receivable may utilize a general ledger control to indicate how much is receivable and a subsidiary ledger to detail from whom it is receivable. Accordingly, the financial information would be processed as follows:

Input Data →	*Journal* →	*Ledger*
Charge Documents Receipts for Payments Adjustments, Refunds, etc.	Input data are sequentially entered. Journal totals are transferred to the general ledger. Journal detail is transferred to the subsidiary ledger.	General ledger carries control total. Subsidiary ledger carries detail which must balance with the general ledger control.

Accounts Payable

Accounts payable represents a strategy or planning issue pertaining to solvency as it relates to accounts receivable and collections. The volume, diversity, and amounts involved in accounts payable make it important to establish a well defined sequence for processing such payments, including these steps:

1. Authorization
2. Documentation
3. Approval
4. Classification
5. Verification
6. Check Writing
7. Review and Payment
8. File and Follow-up

Who among the group has purchasing authority should be decided early in the planning process. Once established, such group prerogatives should be defined clearly. In general, this authority could be delegated as necessary to ensure knowledgeable purchase of goods and service and to provide the necessary follow-up to an order. Certain items are best selected by departmental personnel who have an expert understanding of their special equipment and supply needs. The laboratory and the X-ray and nuclear medicine departments are good examples. In other instances, central purchasing may provide the best expertise. The group must identify those whom it desires to exercise such authority and any necessary limits should be specified. Additionally, those selected should be instructed specifically regarding the accounting classifications pertinent to the goods and services they will be purchasing. Invoices for all payables can be forwarded to the buyer or to the responsible group member and should be marked appropriately to show accounting classification and approval for payment. Such approval would indicate that the items were ordered, that they subsequently were received, and that the quantity, quality, and price are as agreed upon. Approved invoices could then be forwarded to accounting personnel for payment.

All invoices should be reviewed for reasonableness and checked for approval, which usually is indicated on each document. Continuing approval for certain known and recurring payments can be provided in writing and retained in the vendor file. Continuing approvals usually cover routine costs such as rent, utilities, and telephone. Consideration also should be given to verifying invoice calculations. Machine processed invoices usually are correct in terms of extensions and totals; therefore, spot checks may suffice. Regardless of the approach, however, priority should be given to verifying:

1. Vendors who have made errors in the past
2. New vendors
3. Manually prepared invoices
4. Invoices exceeding a specified amount.

The forming group practice also should establish specific payment dates to provide a timely and consistent processing schedule. This schedule would be helpful to the group's authorized purchasers, to those processing payments, and to the person responsible for reviewing and signing checks. Invoices can be batched and totaled periodically. Batch totals then are compared with check totals to ensure accuracy of the total payments. In the process of issuing a check to pay an account as scheduled, a voucher can be prepared to identify clearly the invoices and amounts being paid, assuring that proper credit is given and that detail necessary for account reconciliations is provided. Both the checks and the related documents then can be submitted to the check signer for review. The documents should be returned for filing according to vendor and the checks should be mailed directly. Vendor files should contain source documents supporting all payments. Scheduled reviews of these files help to eliminate duplicate payments and to identify pricing differences. Such differences can be investigated to determine whether they represent pricing errors subject to correction or price changes in need of review. Purchasing policies are discussed in detail in Chapter 16.

The Payroll

Manpower costs will represent the largest single and composite expense item for the group practice. As such, the group's decisions concerning payroll strategy and ensuing policy can have dramatic effects on both the organization and individual involved. Several payroll processing methods are available to the forming medical group. The most common options include:

1. In-house processing by accounting personnel
2. Service bureau preparation under contract
3. Bank processing, as one facet of its service package with the group.

Timeliness and accuracy in paying employees promotes good morale and favorable attitudes toward the organization. Often, the level of efficiency in conducting business with employees sets a standard they will transfer to relationships with patients. When errors occur it is important that the administration's corrections be prompt and consistent. Payroll computations are based upon combined information provided by personnel records, personnel policies, and employee time records. Management of this information is an in-house function which should be assigned to center personnel. The preparation of checks, payroll journals, and wage reports, however, may be handled by center personnel or by an outside agency or service. While the choice between internal or external payroll processing will vary with group circumstances, a traditional argument for internal processing has been control, confidentiality, and assurance of timeliness. On the other hand, service bureaus have developed standard programs and reporting formats which have been tested for accuracy. Because the system meets the needs of many client users it usually can be provided at a very reasonable cost and can provide many of the traditional advantages of internal processing.

An additional payroll consideration involves the wage and hour law which provides for a minimum standard wage to be paid to employees for all the time worked. A time keeping requirement is thereby imposed upon employers to assure compliance with these provisions. While no specific time keeping method is required, time clocks generally are considered an acceptable, accurate and economical approach. Time cards, which are convenient to handle and easily stored, provide a printed record of employee time and can be used conveniently as payroll input. There are many alternative time record systems ranging from simple handwritten entries on a daily/weekly log to direct input of employee time information to a computer via magnetic or optically scanned identification cards.

Although influences within the group will affect the payroll process, the external requirement of the wage and hour law must be adhered to. For example, the law exempts certain classifications of employees from its general provisions requiring that time records be kept. Executive, administrative, and professional provisions in the law establish the criteria necessary for exempt status. Generally, an affirmative answer to each item in the checklist in figure 8-1 would qualify an employee as exempt. Overtime pay is not required for exempt personnel. As a matter of policy, however, some groups may elect to pay overtime to achieve uniformity in pay administration. For example, while registered nurses are exempt as professionals, the group nevertheless may elect to pay them overtime. Nonexempt personnel must be paid for all hours worked based on the following schedule:

	Percent of pay rate
Regular hours to 40	100%
Regular hours exceeding 40	150%
Holiday hours exceeding 40	200%

The law does not require that premium pay be paid for nonworked hours that may be included during the pay period, such as sick leave and nonworked

Executives

yes ( ) no ( ) 1. **Primary duty:** Do you spend 50% or more of your time managing your department?

yes ( ) no ( ) 2. **Supervision:** Do you customarily and regularly direct the work of two or more employees?

yes ( ) no ( ) 3. **Authority:** Can you hire and fire or suggest changes in status of employees under No. 2 above?

yes ( ) no ( ) 4. **Discretion:** Do you customarily and regularly exercise discretionary powers? (This means in excess of those discretionary powers normally required of a routine job.)

yes ( ) no ( ) 5. **Non-exempt work:** Do you spend less than 40% of your time doing routine work?

yes ( ) no ( ) 6. **Salary:** Do you earn more than $155.00 per week?

Administrative

yes ( ) no ( ) 1. **Primary duty:** Do you spend generally 50% or more of your time performing office or non-manual work relating to management policies or general business operations of employer?

yes ( ) no ( ) 2. **Other duties:** Do you regularly and directly assist an executive, or
work under one general supervisor along specialized or technical lines requiring special training, experience, or knowledge, or
execute under only general supervision special assignments and tasks?

yes ( ) no ( ) 3. **Discretion:** Do you customarily and regularly exercise discretion and independent judgment in excess of judgment required for routine completion of job?

yes ( ) no ( ) 4. **Non-exempt work:** Do you spend less than 40% of your time doing routine work?

yes ( ) no ( ) 5. **Salary:** Do you earn $155.00 or more per week?

Figure 8–1. Exempt Employee Checklist

vacations and holidays. Overtime is a financial accounting issue which cannot be budgeted for accurately; therefore, for cost control it must be decided who will determine the need and duration of overtime pay and who will approve it.

PATIENT ACCOUNTING

The next set of strategic planning issues involves accounting of patient services, which encompasses the data required for productivity and/or workload reports, patients' accounts receivable, and credit and collections. The patient accounting process includes the recording, summarizing, analyzing, and reporting of patient information, including the following:

1. *Provider Information*—center and physician providing the service by name, address, and identifying number

Professional

yes ( ) no ( ) 1. **Primary duty:** Do you spend generally 50% or more of your time performing work requiring scientific or specialized study as distinguished from apprentice training and training for routine work (this includes those professions which have a recognized status and which are based on the requirement of professional knowledge through prolonged study)?

yes ( ) no ( ) 2. **Other duties:** Do you perform work predominantly intellectual and varied (not routine) which cannot be standardized in point of time?

yes ( ) no ( ) 3. **Discretion:** Do you consistently exercise discretion and judgment?

yes ( ) no ( ) 4. **Non-exempt work:** Do you spend less than 20% of your time doing routine work?

yes ( ) no ( ) 5. **Salary:** Do you earn in excess of $170.00 per week?

Note:

- New standards regulating the minimum-wage and overtime pay provisions for executive, administrative, and professional employee categories became effective on April 1, 1975.
- Job titles do not have any bearing on exempt classification.

Figure 8-1 (Cont.)

2. *Patient Information*—identification of patient, responsible party, and third party by name, address, and identifying numbers
3. *Service*—description of service, date rendered, place rendered
4. *Transaction*—record of charges, payments, adjustments, and refunds.

Service Reports (S/Rs) are employed to accumulate information necessary for patient accounting and are designed to record information concerning patient services. When services are priced on the S/R it is processed as a charge document and provides the initial input to patient accounting. Service reports may be decentralized (individual charge tickets for each service) or centralized (composite charge ticket for a series of services). When centralized charge tickets are used, they often are prenumbered and issued from a central station in order to account for each document and to fix responsibility for the accuracy of entries. A fixed policy defining the days a service report may be outstanding should be considered. If follow-up visits or extended care is scheduled past the policy period, the original S/R could be released for processing and a new S/R established for future services. Prompt release of S/Rs is necessary to timely accounting and center cash flow. Service report information should be summarized, usually by the physician providing the service, to establish month and year and to date physician booking or workload records, which provide valuable information for budgeting purposes and often can be a significant factor in physician income distribution arrangements (see Chapter 9). After service reports are processed for booking/workload records, they can be entered to individual patient accounts.

Patient accounts are used to accumulate patient transactions necessary to functioning of accounts receivable, third party billing, and credit and collection. A fully paid account does not preclude the necessity of accumulating and maintaining the information. A patient subsequently may request the filing of third party claims or there may be a need to secure credit and collection information during later patient visits. For these reasons, separate transaction documents usually are maintained to provide a clear record of each patient transaction. Example patient transaction documents are shown in figure 8-2. Adopting any of the transaction documents contained in figure 8-2 requires strategic consideration in the planning process. Refunding is one process that often involves considerable time and effort. Credit balances routinely may develop when a patient pays his account and subsequent payments are received from third party payors. The resultant credit balances then require prompt refunding to the patient. Not only the group's approach to refunds (or retention of a credit balance), but also its general credit policy will significantly influence the volume of refund activity.

Productivity and workload, as a function of staff compensation, will be discussed in the following chapter. Although a compensation plan which includes productivity as a component will influence patient accounting, productivity and workload also can be approached strictly from a patient accounting and reporting perspective. The balance sheet reflects a group's financial position at a given date and the income statement measures its financial activity for a specified period of time. Viewed in series, they portray a pattern of financial change and bring into focus developing trends. Financial statements, therefore, can provide indicators of productivity and workload.

	Year 1		*Year 2*		*Year 3*		*Year 4*	
Bookings/ Gross Earnings	$1,500,000		$1,680,000		$1,898,400		$2,164,200	
Less Uncollectible	135,000	9%	117,600	7%	113,900	6%	108,200	5%
Patient Income	1,365,000		1,562,400		1,784,500		2,056,000	
Overhead	737,000	54%	859,400	55%	999,500	56%	1,172,000	57%
Income Available for Distribution/ Surplus	$ 628,000		$ 703,000		$ 785,000		$ 884,000	

One indicator of total workload is expressed by the booking or gross earning amounts for each year. The figures which follow indicate that bookings can show consistent and predictable increases:

	Bookings	*Percent Increase*
Year 1	1,500,000	
Year 2	1,680,000	12%
Year 3	1,898,400	13%
Year 4	2,164,200	14%

	Document	Action
1. Service Report	To record patient charges	Processed as a debit to the patient's account.
2. Receipts	To record all payments	Processed as a credit to the patient's account.
3. Adjustments	To correct charges to wrong account	Processed as a debit to the correct account and as a credit to the account originally charged. Require superb visory approval so that the error level can be monitored and corrected.
4. Discounts	To record policy approved reductions	If discounts are recorded in the organization's books, discounts are processed as a credit to the patient's account. Otherwise, discounts should be deducted fron the S/R and only the net charge entered as a debit to the patient's account.
5. Refund Checks	To refund overpayments	Processed as a debit to the patient's account. Require supervisory approval.

Figure 8-2. Patient Transaction Documents

Workload increases will affect both the medical staff and the employees. Based on the example above, the group would be wise to budget a 15 percent volume increase for the coming year. It must be determined not only what productivity data are deemed meaningful, but also to what extent that data will be used for future planning. In extending the above example, the present center staff probably could absorb a portion of the indicated increases through improved efficiency; however, a measured personnel response to practical growth is necessary. The group should be practical in making personnel increases as indicated by productivity; such increases should be made as necessary both to continue a high level of service and to maximize staff productivity. Furthermore, the example collections show an increasing improvement from year one to year four, reaching a 95 percent collectibility rate, which probably is about as effective a percentage as is attainable on a sustained basis. The figures indicate that credit and collection personnel have been progressively more effective while also dealing with a constantly increasing workload. A higher collectibility percentage may be a signal to review group policies to ensure that they are not overly restrictive.

The productivity example also shows that the overhead rate has continued to climb at the rate of 1 percent per year. To the extent that this increase has contributed to increased bookings, it may be a very acceptable figure. Over the four-year period, bookings have increased 44.28 percent and income has increased 40.76 percent. In terms of results, such increases indicate not only improved efficiency but also effectiveness. In group business affairs, overhead will frequently surface as a topic of discussion. Physicians generally view overhead as the difference in what they earn and what they are paid, especially in a medical partnership. Accountants view overhead as a cost or series of costs not directly identifiable as contributing to the product or service which the organization produces or provides. While overhead may be expressed in different ways, it is important to understand that the term does not imply nonproductive cost. On the contrary, many expenses included in overhead have a very direct impact on workload, productivity, and profitability. Certain items of

Physician Booking Report for the Nine Months Ending September 19___

	This Month	Year to Date	Percentage
Physician A	$ 15,000	$ 130,000	7.80
Physician B	12,000	100,000	6.00
Physician C	14,000	127,000	7.62
Physician D	9,000	95,000	5.70
Physician E	12,000	108,000	6.48
Physician F	15,000	122,000	7.32
Physician G	16,000	115,000	6.90
Physician H	13,000	116,000	6.96
Physician I	11,000	112,000	6.72
Physician J	10,000	99,000	5.94
Physician K	9,000	102,000	6.12
Physician L	14,000	121,000	7.21
Physician M	17,000	118,000	7.08
Physician N	12,000	111,000	6.65
Physician O	9,000	91,000	5.45
Total	$188,000	$1,667,000	100.00
Professional	$151,100	$1,333,600	80.00
Injections, Immunizations	1,800	16,670	1.00
Lab	16,600	150,030	9.00
X-Ray	18,500	166,700	10.00
Total	$188,000	$1,667,000	100.00

Figure 8-3. Physician Booking Report

equipment are associated directly with providing patient care. Purchasing more elaborate equipment may increase the overhead but also may be more than compensated for by increased physician productivity. The same rationale applies to personnel levels or space allocations. Increases may result in increased efficiency and perhaps reduced patient costs.

Obviously, differences exist between groups in organizational structure and staffing, equipment, and facilities policies. Differences also exist in accounting methods and classification of costs. Because of such variances, comparison of overhead rates between groups is not very useful. Even within the same group, comparison of overhead rates for a series of years should be viewed from a cause and effect standpoint. The experience of some existing three to ten physician groups indicates that a 48 percent rate of overhead is not unusual. Overhead ratio comparisons can provide guideline indicators of financial trend and are useful to the extent that they direct the group's attention to the factual components involved. As with overhead rates, it is seldom practical to compare physician compensation and associated benefits with those of other physicians. Many factors affect the professional and personal habits and ultimately the compensation of a professional. Geography, life style, work habits, years of practice, and educational involvement are but a few of the variables. Logical and acceptable progress in group income or individual physician compensation

Procedure Booking Report for the Nine Months Ending September 19___

Procedure Code	Procedure Physician	This Month Count	This Month Amount	Year to Date Count	Year to Date Amount
51962	History and Physical, Comprehensive				
	Physician A				
	Physician B				
	Physician C				
	Physician D				
	Physician E				
	Physician F				
	Physician L				
	Physician O				
	Total				
51963	Physical Exam, Year Check				
	Physician A				
	Physician B				
	Physician C				
	Physician D				
	Physician E				
	Physician F				
	Physician L				
	Physician O				
	Total				
TOTAL BOOKINGS			188,000		1,667,000

Figure 8-4. Procedure Booking Report

can best be evaluated from within—where the facts and figures are available. The following chapter will discuss staff compensation in detail.

One effective measure of physician productivity is bookings or gross earnings for the period. In accumulating patient billing information, the same data can be distributed in a number of different ways to provide productivity and workload data. This information usually is accumulated on a monthly and yearly to date basis as shown in the examples in figure 8-3 and figure 8-4. A history of patient visits also provides a measure of productivity and workload. Acceptable visit increases are indicative of community acceptance and a sound professional reputation. Satisfied patients are the traditional practice builders. More than any other factor, they are responsible for the resultant figures on both new and return patient visits. Visit trends, therefore, could be reviewed continually to determine the direction of movement. Increases may indicate the need for additional budgeting to meet an increasing patient load. A leveling or downward turn should trigger a prompt review to identify possible causes and necessary action. Such evaluations should raise the following questions:

1. Is the medical staff sufficient to meet patient needs?
2. Is the employee staff capable, efficient, and patient oriented?
3. Is the center well equipped? Is equipment well maintained and updated to take advantage of new technology?
4. What is the level and nature of patient complaints? Are they adequately reviewed and satisfactorily responded to?
5. Has the economy or competition created a need for changes in the group's operation?

Departmental reports also could provide a means of measuring volume and ascertaining the primary service rendered in each department. Such reports involve:

1. Statements mailed
2. Claims filed
3. Charts requested
4. Appointments scheduled
5. Maintenance orders answered
6. Employees paid.

Various indicators of productivity can provide objective information which may be sufficient for budgeting activities. Reports on subactivity generally are not used and usually are not worth the cost of file space involved. Such detailed information can be gathered on a test basis as necessary for system reviews, or the group can direct departmental supervisors to explain such activity when necessary.

Accounts receivable information is not only an indicator of productivity, but also is of vital importance in determining financial position, in making management decisions, and in maintaining solvency. The receivable information is accounted for in two ways:

1. *Control.* Accounts receivable in the general ledger is a summary account. Its purpose is to reflect the total amount due from all patients and to serve the function of a controlling account with which individual patient accounts must cumulatively balance. In content, the account consists of journal totals which have been posted routinely to the ledger.

2. *Detail.* The detail consists of the individual accounts established to record the amounts due from each patient. In content, these records consist of entries reflecting specific transactions affecting the individual account balance. Individual patient accounts constitute the subsidiary ledger for accounts receivable and must total the balance in the controlling account. References of general ledger and subsidiary ledger are synonymous with control and detail. The information for both records is based on the accounting journals. Transactions affecting accounts receivable then can be recorded and categorized by transaction type.

a. Transaction types include: charges, payments, adjustments, discounts, and refunds.

b. Totals of each of these categories are transferred to the general ledger (control). Individual entries are posted to each account in the subsidiary ledger (detail).

This segregation can be used to reconcile the control and detail should an imbalance develop. Charges in the detail are totaled for the period and compared with the journal total entered in the control. Payments then are totaled for comparison with the general ledger entry. The process is continued until an error is isolated within a specific type of transaction. The line item entries for those transactions can be checked to locate the specific type of transaction. Accounting entries utilize information detail and cross referencing to provide a clear financial trail. Information should be traceable from any point. The level of detail carried forward must meet financial track needs and ultimate user needs. The record must contain comprehensive information sufficient for patient billing, third party filing, itemized statements, aged trial balances, booking reports, and cashiering reports. Necessary detail for these reports is shown in the schedule in figure 8-5. In this way, subsidiary ledger records serve the accounts receivable record and additionally serve a wide range of patient accounting reports.

Establishing patient accounts is the final strategic consideration affecting accounts receivable. Not only must the account be determined (format, information display, account number), but recognition of responsible party designations is necessary. For example, a patient's account number usually corresponds with his medical record number and may be prefixed or suffixed, to indicate accounting, billing, or collection information. In an effort to account and bill to a family, various individual family account numbers may be linked to a responsible party designation. Furthermore, the requirements of instituting a superbill method of billing may have impact upon patient accounts and accounts receivable. For a detailed discussion of the superbill approach, see Chapter 15. Closely related to patient accounts and accounts receivable is credit and collections. It is perhaps in this area of strategic planning and direction that the group can expect diverse physician predispositions followed by inconsistency in applying any strategy finally decided upon; therefore, a credit and collections strategy is a sensitive issue which must receive honest and careful consideration if meaningful policies are to emanate from the strategy adopted.

Accounting for receivables may indicate that certain portions of those balances are uncollectible. Aging of the accounts organizes the information into a usable form for making overall evaluations on collectibility and for identifying specific accounts for individual review. Separate balances can be distributed into categories of current and various stages of past due. This is illustrated in the example shown in figure 8-6. Because collectibility decreases as age increases, the aged totals and percentages in the example provide very useful valuation information. Accounting entries should record provisions for uncollectible accounts. These entries are reflected in the group's financial statements, which should define as accurately and as fairly as possible the accounts receivable balances considered collectible. Delinquent accounts become the management responsibility of those delegated credit and collection responsibilities. The importance of collection activities in relation to cash flow is obvious; however, the contribution collection personnel can make toward improving patient relations is often underestimated. The collection effort aims not only to collect

Subsidiary Detail	Patient Statement	Itemized Statement	Medical Payment Statement	Third Party Claim	Aged Trial Balance	Booking Reports	Cashiering Report
Center Name	X	X	X	X	X	X	X
Center Address	X	X	X	X			
Center Telephone Number	X	X	X	X			
Center Federal Identification Number				X			
Patient Name	X	X	X	X	X		X
Patient Address	X	X	X	X	X		X
Patient Telephone Number		X			X		
Patient Account Number	X	X	X	X	X	X	X
Patient Credit Code		X			X		X
Responsible Party Name	X	X	X	X	X		X
Responsible Party Address	X	X	X	X	X		X
Responsible Party Telephone Number		X			X		X
Responsible Party Number	X	X	X	X	X		X
Responsible Party Credit Code		X			X		
Physician Name	X	X		X	X	X	
Physician Specialty	X	X		X			
Physician Number	X	X		X		X	
Service Date	X	X		X	X	X	
Service Code	X	X		X		X	
Service Description	X	X		X		X	
Service Price	X	X		X	X	X	
Service Location (clinic, hospital)	X	X		X			
Hospital Admission Date	X	X		X			
Hospital Discharge Date	X	X		X			
Hospital Visit Dates	X	X		X			
Diagnosis				X			
Diagnosis Code		X		X			
Adjustment Date	X	X		X		X	
Adjustment Code	X	X		X		X	
Adjustment Description	X	X		X		X	

Adjustment Price	X	X		X		X	
Discount Date	X	X				X	
Discount Code	X	X				X	
Discount Description	X	X				X	
Discount Price	X	X				X	
Payment Date	X	X	X		X		
Payment Code	X	X	X		X		
Payor	X	X	X		X		
Payment Amount	X	X	X		X		
Refund Date	X	X	X				
Refund Code	X	X	X				
Refund Check Number	X	X					
Refund Price	X	X	X				
Third Party Payor		X		X	X		X
Third Party Address		X		X			X
Beneficiary		X		X			X
Policy or Beneficiary Number		X		X			X
Annual Assignment		X		X	X		X
Benefits Assigned		X		X	X		X
Benefits Not Assigned		X		X	X		X
Date Claim Filed	X	X		X	X		X
Service Period Filed	X	X			X		
Third Party Filee	X	X			X		X
Address to Which Claim Mailed	X	X					
Service Date	X	X		X	X		
Service Code	X	X		X		X	
Service Description	X	X		X		X	
Service Price	X	X		X	X	X	
Physician Code	X	X		X	X	X	
Physician Name	X	X		X		X	

Figure 8–5. Patient Accounting Reports

Aged Accounts Receivable Schedule December 31, 19___

Patient	PAST DUE						
	Total	Current	1-30 Days	31-60 Days	61-90 Days	91-120 Days	Past 120 Days
A	400	400					
B	80			80			
C	1,000	1,000					
D	220						220
E	300				300		
F	150		150				
G	600					600	
H	400		400				
I	90	90					
TOTAL	$650,000	$299,000	$149,500	$123,500	$52,000	$13,000	$13,000
PERCENT	100%	46%	23%	19%	8%	2%	2%

Figure 8-6. Aged Accounts Receivable Schedule December 31, 19___

accounts but also to collect them in a manner that fosters the continuance of good center-patient relationships.

Collection procedures usually are designed to escalate the collection effort as an account cycles through the aging process. This usually begins with reminders and credit messages included on the patient's statement and, if necessary, a follow-up series of collection letters. As the account becomes older, personal telephone calls and conferences may be scheduled as a part of the procedure. This activity is designed to stimulate a patient response which may be payment of the account or the uncovering of information which will lead to subsequent collection. Although some patients will not pay their bills, others have not made remittance because they do not understand the bill, think it is in error, are displeased with some element of the group's service, etc. Certain information provided by the patient delinquent in paying his bill may be valuable to the group for reasons such as:

1. Calling attention to account errors
2. Interpreting information on other action in progress
   a. Insurance being filed
   b. Financial arrangements being made
   c. Plans regarding payment
3. Reporting complaints
   a. Dissatisfaction with service
   b. Unhappiness with charge

Identifying these problems permits necessary corrections and promotes discussion aimed at resolving disputes and misunderstandings. Prompt and fair response can reestablish good patient relations and possibly may even improve them through the demonstration of concern for patient problems. A patient's history of payment provides the primary data base for credit records. General patient evaluation based on address, occupation, employment, etc., may be supplemented as necessary by a credit conference or by ordering credit agency reports. Credit evaluations can be converted to credit codes which define the parameters and procedures to be followed regarding patient financial affairs. Group policies related to the establishment of such codes usually are initiated at patient registration, which will be discussed in Chapter 12. Over time, however, the patient's financial status and attitude toward the group may change. Consequently, credit is not associated only with registration but rather is a potential consideration for the duration of group-patient contact.

Various existing group practices take alternate approaches in their credit and collections strategy. One existing practice provides a new patient with an estimate of charges prior to the completion of the service. This group maintains that providing estimates is not only an obligation, but that it helps patients understand their financial responsibility and assists in collections. Additional information concerning the group's financial policy is provided all new patients upon completion of the registration process (see figure 8-7).

BUDGETING AND AUDITS

A final set of strategic issues involved in financial planning includes group budget and audits. Simply stated, a budget is a financial plan for meeting organiza-

Financial Information

Estimate of Charges:

New patients are invited to request estimates of charges prior to laboratory and x-ray work. This will give you an opportunity to see what tests are scheduled and their estimated cost. You may request an estimate of charges at any time – – now or on future visits. Our cashiers are located on the first floor.

Insurance:

If you have insurance information to submit, our Insurance Department, basement floor, will assist you. We request that you pay us direct and allow the insurance to reimburse you.

Payment:

We ask new patients to start out with an understanding of their payment arrangement. If you are not in a position to pay the charges at the time the work is done, the balance will be payable within 10 days of receipt of your first statement.

Should you wish to discuss finances, please feel free to bring this to the attention of our cashier.

Figure 8-7. Financial Policy

tional goals at acceptable profit, surplus, or loss levels. The group's financial budget is similar to its accounting system in that it allows the structuring of a large amount of financial data and illustrates the interrelationships of these data. Furthermore, the budget provides an orderly format for the presentation of data so that they may be used for management purposes. There is, however, one major difference between the two systems: the accounting system provides data which characterize the *retrospective* operations of the group, while the budget system provides data which illustrate the *prospective* operations of the group. The budget carefully delineates a plan and the accounting system provides information for determining to what extent the plan has been realized. The interdependency between the two systems is apparent, but can pose special problems for the forming medical group which has no accounting data (retrospective) upon which to base a financial budget. As a result, the forming group must base its initial budget on many of the planning assumptions and projected activity described in Chapter 4.

In addition to representing the financial plan, the budget is used for control of that plan. The careful and orderly preparation of a financial budget can delineate goals against which performance can be measured, can set pre-established standards, and can identify and test the planning assumptions against which actual experience is compared in order to modify policies, strategies, and even the group goals and mission. Various financial plans can be represented by a number of different types of budgets. For example, a capital budget provides a plan necessary to predict facility and equipment needs. Capital budgets, however, usually are established to cover a three to five year period. Advanced decisions on major capital needs should be made, providing time for adequate review, orderly accumulation of capital, and arrangement of necessary financing. Associated expenses such as rent, depreciation, interest, taxes, etc. would be included in an operating budget, which perhaps is the most well known plan for financial control. Essentially, an operating budget is an income and expense budget for the accounting period. In other words, it is the financial game plan for meeting operational needs and business responsibilities.

Budgeting usually begins by determining productivity and cash flow in terms of planned demand and capacity. Booking and pay schedules can be developed for each physician resource to project and determine trends in practice growth and compensation progression. With this information, basic projections are made on future bookings and should be adjusted, based on each physician's capacity and availability to accept an increased patient load. Regardless of the method chosen for compensation, such decisions must be made and approved before preliminary budgeting can occur (see Chapter 9). This sequencing permits the definition of necessary levels of effort and the establishment of acceptable short-term financial objectives.

Should the organization include several supervisory levels, supervisors should be informed of the salary schedules and the percentage of pay escalation available for their employees, thus allowing supervisors to develop personnel structures and to define other needs commensurate with the anticipated activity of the group practice. After the initial year of operations, supervisors can submit personnel schedules to administration as part of a budget request. Through a series of conferences and review, budget requests then can be adjusted into an acceptable administrative plan. Personnel schedules for both the medical staff and the employees, and space and equipment schedules also can be prepared. Budget information and formatting concerning medical staff, personnel, space, and equipment then can be submitted to the appropriate insurance agencies or insurance companies for desired coverage and pricing information.

Certain accounts always can be calculated with a high degree of accuracy. These calculations apply known rates to the scheduled staff, personnel, space, and equipment information. Such accounts include social security taxes, unemployment taxes, retirement plan contributions, parking, relocation, personnel agency fees, travel, contract labor, contract services, amortization, depreciation, local taxes, and interest. Other income and expenses may be estimated using current or comparable costs as a guide. One basic approach is to take the last three months of actual expense for a specific account and to annualize it, thus yielding a twelve month cost estimate based on the most current pricing and level of activity. This figure should then be escalated by expected increased volume and estimated price increase. This approach to estimating is shown in the following calculation:

Supply Expense, Actual:			
First Seven Months	$ 6,000		
Last Three Months	4,000	$ 4,000	
Total, Year To Date	$10,000		
To Annualize		X 4	
Base Estimate		16,000	
Estimated Volume to Present Volume		107%	(7% over present 100%)
Base and Volume Estimate		17,120	
Annualized Price Increase per Supplier		110%	(10% over present 100%)
Base, Volume and Price Estimate		18,832	
Budget		$18,800	

The preliminary budget of income and expenses then can be assembled to determine projected net profit, surplus, or loss. The variance of this initial projection indicates the required budget adjustment. Preliminary budget figures should be reviewed completely to determine those expenses which can be cut back with the least impact on efficient operations. To the extent that acceptable profitability cannot be attained through reduced costs, fee increases may be necessary.

Physicians generally recognize their strong obligation to control medical costs through efficient operations and effective services. At the same time, it must be realized that a certain level of fee increase may be necessary in dealing with increased expenses and in maintaining the financial health of the organization. When any necessary adjustment and balancing is complete, the budget should be submitted to members of the group for formal acceptance. The approved budget provides those charged with the group's financial management the authority to manage the organization in accordance with the plan. The budget, however, is a guide and is not necessarily absolute. The group's administration should manage operations to achieve net budget objectives, but variances in one area may be offset in another to meet financial goals. Major variances should be reviewed and approved as budget revisions. In format, the budget should include the same accounts as the income statement, which will facilitate comparison of actual accounts with those budgeted. Meeting budget objectives requires an operating discipline that can be accomplished only with the strong support of the medical staff, the management, and the employees.

After the budget has been established, the need for and frequency of audits must be considered. A financial audit is an assessment of an organization's financial health. Many times such an examination will result in no significant negative findings. During an audit, however, problems or potential problems may be identified. In these instances, the examination is continued to determine the extent and nature of the situation. Over a period of time an audit firm can become more and more familiar with the financial operations of an organization, and previously identified problem areas will be reviewed routinely to determine their current status. Upon completion of the audit, a report is prepared. An opinion on the fairness of the organization's financial statements is issued, based on generally accepted auditing procedures considered necessary under the circumstances. All possible auditing procedures are not employed in any one audit and no guarantee is given that all financial problems will be identified. The audit firm will issue its opinion on whether the financial statements are presented according to generally acceptable accounting principles and whether the presentation is consistent with prior periods. The audit firm also should be required to submit a management letter suggesting any recommended improvements. While the organization's own staff may be efficient in business affairs, there always is room for improvement. It should be recognized that the management letter is intended as constructive criticism and as a recommendation for improving internal operations. These recommendations should be carefully reviewed and only those considered practical should be accepted.

Audits are relatively expensive and do have an impact on overhead. Routine audits are commonly accepted as good business practice and they should be scheduled on an annual basis. Many accountants familiar with group practice operations suggest that the makeup and dynamics of group practice are such that change occurs rapidly. For example, as new physicians are added, others leave, and still others retire. Each arrival and departure carries with it significant implications which are financially important to all group members and to the organization. In addition, the sheer volume of transactions involved in the accounting process makes it difficult to evaluate the correctness of the figures. An audit concerns itself with review, analysis, tests, verifications, and confirmations sufficient for the auditor to express an opinion regarding the fairness of the financial statements. Audit reports provide a convenient and most acceptable form of presenting financial information to banks, mortgage companies, leasing companies, creditors, and others who have a business need for the information. Lastly, the audit provides the sometimes necessary impetus for the group's accounting staff to put matters in order. During the course of the audit, any necessary corrections are made to bring the records to a completely current status. Additionally, a certain amount of instruction occurs during discussions regarding past accounting problems and changes in accounting methods, tax laws, and reporting standards. Working with the auditors involves significant time and workload requirements of the group's accounting staff. These requirements should be understood and accommodated as much as possible.

This chapter has dealt with key strategy issues in financial planning. Most certainly, group practice members should consider employing or contracting with an accountant to provide financial accounting and budgeting services in a manner consistent with established principles, local needs, and group requirements. Before any accountant can provide such technical expertise, however, the forming group practice must have considered its approach or strategies related to fiscal matters, financial accounting, patient accounting, budget, and audits.

Chapter 8 Appendices

Appendix 8A. Chart of Accounts Development Account Number Coding

First Number	Second Number	Third Number
1 Assets	1 Cash	Completes Account Identification
	2 Accounts Receivable	
	3 Notes Receivable	
	4 Inventory	
	5 Prepaid Expenses	
	6 Deposits	
	7 Investments	
	8 Property and Equipment	
2 Liabilities	1 Current Installments of Long Term Debt	Completes Account Identification
	2 Accounts Payable	
	3 Accruals	
	9 Long Term Debt, Deferred Installments	
3 Net Worth	0 Capital	Second and Third Numbers Together are Doctor Numbers
	thru Capital	
	8 Capital	
	9 Stockholder Equity	Completes Account Identification
4 Drawing Accounts	All Drawing Accounts of Doctors	Completes Doctor Number
5 Income Distribution	0 Doctor Income Accounts	Completes Doctor Number
	thru Doctor Income Accounts	
	8 Doctor Income Accounts	
	9 Gain, Year to Date	
6 Income and Income Adjustments	1 Income, Professional Fees	Completes Account Identification
	2 Income, Ancillary Services	

	3 Income, Recoveries	
	4 Income, Contract Services	
	5 Income Adjustments	
	6 Rental Income	
	7 Sales	
	8 Other Income	
	9 Cost of Sales	
7 Expenses	0 Professional and Medical	Functional Classification
	1 Professional and Medical	
	2 Professional and Medical	
8 Expenses	0 Personnel Expenses	Functional Classification
	1 Personnel Expenses	
	2 Personnel Expenses	
	3 Supplies	
	4 Supplies	
	5 General and Administrative	
	6 General and Administrative	
	7 General and Administrative	
9 Expenses	0 Building Expenses	Functional Classification
	1 Building Expenses	
	2 Building Expenses	
	5 Equipment Expense	

Appendix 8B.

Balance Sheet Sequence, December 31, 19___

Assets		Sequence *
Current Assets	$ 400,000	Most Liquid
Deposits	5,000	Next Available
Property and Equipment	595,000	Least Available
Total Assets	$1,000,000	

Liabilities and Net Worth		
Current Liabilities	$ 200,000	Due in 12 Months
Long Term Debt	400,000	Due Past 12 Months
Net Worth	400,000	Capital or Stockholder Equity
Total Liabilities and Net Worth	$1,000,000	

Assets		Sequence *
Current Assets		
Cash	$ 100,000	Liquid
Accounts Receivable	300,000	Liquid Within Short Term
Prepaid Expense	5,000	Consumable, Short Term
Total Current Assets	$ 405,000	All Available Within 12 Months
Property and Equipment		
Land	$ 200,000	Non Liquid, Non Depreciable
Building	600,000	Non Liquid, Depreciable
Equipment	300,000	Non Liquid, Depreciable
Less Depreciation	(505,000)	Depreciation To Date
Book Value, Property and Equipment	$ 595,000	Cost Less Depreciation
Total Assets	$1,000,000	

Liabilities and Net Worth

Current Liabilities		
Mortgage Payable, Current Installments	$ 100,000	Most Enforceable
Notes Payable, Current Installments	50,000	Next Enforceable
Accounts Payable	50,000	Payable but Non Secured
Total Current Liabilities	$ 200,000	All Due in 12 Months
Long Term Debt		
Mortgage Payable, Deferred Installments	$ 350,000	Most Enforceable
Notes Payable, Deferred Installments	50,000	Next Enforceable
Total Long Term Debt	$ 400,000	Due Past 12 Months
Stockholder Equity		
Stock at Par Value	$ 100,000	No Shares x Par Value Per Share
Additional Paid In Capital	100,000	Additional Paid For Shares
Retained Earnings	250,000	Earnings Less Dividends Paid
Less Cost of Treasury Shares	(50,000)	Stock Repurchased, Not Reissued
Total Stockholder Equity	$ 400,000	Net Worth
Total Liabilities and Net Worth	$1,000,000	

* This liquidity sequence is continued in listing the line items within each major section.

Balance Sheet Related to Organizational Type and Accounting Method

Month of ______

Client Number	Company Number	Department Number	Account Number	ASSETS	19__ Prior Year	19__ This Year	*ORGANIZATIONAL TYPE: Sole Proprietorship	Partnership	Professional Association	Professional Corporation	Corporation	*ACCOUNTING METHOD: Cash Basis	Modified Cash	Accrual
xxx	xxx	xxx	100	Current Assets										
			111	Cash, Depository Account	$____	$Debit	X	X	X	X	X	X	X	X
			112	Cash, Operating Account	____	Debit	X	X	X	X	X	X	X	X
			113	Cash, Payroll Account	____	Debit	X	X	X	X	X	X	X	X
			114	Cash, Refund Account	____	Debit	X	X	X	X	X	X	X	X
			115	Cash, Cashiering Account	____	Debit	X	X	X	X	X	X	X	X
			116	Cash, Short Term Equivalents	____	Debit	X	X	X	X	X	X	X	X
				Sub Total Cash	$____	$Debit	X	X	X	X	X	NO	NO	X
			121	Accounts Receivable	____	Debit	X	X	X	X	X	NO	NO	X
			122	Accounts Receivable, Patients	____	Debit	X	X	X	X	X	NO	NO	X
			123	Accounts Receivable, Doctors	____	Debit	X	X	X	X	X	NO	NO	X
			124	Accounts Receivable, Employees	____	Debit	X	X	X	X	X	NO	NO	X
			125	Accounts Receivable, Affiliates	____	Debits	X	X	X	X	X	NO	NO	X
			126	Accounts Receivable, Contract	____	Debit	X	X	X	X	X	NO	NO	X
			127	Accounts Receivable, Trade	____	Debit	X	X	X	X	X	NO	NO	X
			128	Accounts Receivable, Miscellaneous	____	Debit	X	X	X	X	X	NO	NO	X
			131	Notes Receivable	____	Debit	X	X	X	X	X	NO	NO	X
			132	Notes Receivable, Patients	____	Debit	X	X	X	X	X	NO	NO	X
			133	Notes Receivable, Doctors	____	Debit	X	X	X	X	X	NO	NO	X
			134	Notes Receivable, Employees	____	Debit	X	X	X	X	X	NO	NO	X
			135	Notes Receivable, Affiliates	____	Debit	X	X	X	X	X	NO	NO	X
			136	Notes Receivable, Contract	____	Debit	X	X	X	X	X	NO	NO	X
			137	Notes Receivable, Trade	____	Debit	X	X	X	X	X	NO	NO	X
			138	Notes Receivable, Miscellaneous	____	Debit	X	X	X	X	X	NO	NO	X
			141	Inventory	____	Debit	X	X	X	X	X	NO	NO	X
			142	Inventory, Supplies	____	Debit	X	X	X	X	X	NO	NO	X
			143	Inventory, Supplies, Medical-Surgical	____	Debit	X	X	X	X	X	NO	NO	X
			144	Inventory, Supplies, Lab	____	Debit	X	X	X	X	X	NO	NO	X
			145	Inventory, Supplies, X-Ray	____	Debit	X	X	X	X	X	NO	NO	X
			146	Inventory, Supplies, Dental	____	Debit	X	X	X	X	X	NO	NO	X
			147	Inventory, Supplies, Pharmacy	____	Debit	X	X	X	X	X	NO	NO	X
			148	Inventory, Supplies, Other	____	Debit	X	X	X	X	X	NO	NO	X
			149	Inventory, Merchandise	____	Debit	X	X	X	X	X	NO	NO	X
			151	Prepaid Expense, Insurance	____	Debit	X	X	X	X	X	NO	X	X
			152	Prepaid Expense, Maintenance	____	Debit	X	X	X	X	X	NO	X	X
			153	Prepaid Expense, Miscellaneous	____	Debit	X	X	X	X	X	NO	X	X
				Total Current Assets	$____	$Debit								

*Key

X — Applicable
NO — Not Applicable

Client Number	Company Number	Department Number	Account Number	LIABILITIES AND NET WORTH	19__ Prior Year	19__ This Year	*ORGANIZATIONAL TYPE: Sole Proprietorship	Partnership	Professional Association	Professional Corporation	Corporation	*ACCOUNTING METHOD: Cash Basis	Modified Cash	Accrual
xxx	xxx	xxx	200	Current Liabilities										
			211	Mortgage Payable, Current Installments	$____	$Credit	X	X	X	X	X	X	X	X
			212	Notes Payable, Current Installments	____	Credit	X	X	X	X	X	X	X	X
			221	Accounts Payable	____	Credit	X	X	X	X	X	NO	NO	X
			231	Accruals, Payroll	____	Credit	X	X	X	X	X	NO	NO	X
			232	Accruals, Payroll Taxes	____	Credit	X	X	X	X	X	NO	X	X
			233	Accruals, Employee Medical Insurance	____	Credit	X	X	X	X	X	NO	X	X
			234	Accruals, Employee Life and Disability	____	Credit	X	X	X	X	X	NO	X	X
			235	Accruals, Expense, Legal	____	Credit	X	X	X	X	X	NO	X	X
			236	Accruals, Expense, Accounting	____	Credit	X	X	X	X	X	NO	X	X
			237	Accruals, Expense, Local Taxes	____	Credit	X	X	X	X	X	NO	X	X
			238	Accruals, Expense, Income Taxes	____	Credit	NO	NO	X	X	X	NO	NO	X
				Total Current Liabilities	$____	$Credit								
			290	Long Term Debt										
			291	Mortgage Payable, Deffered Installments	$____	$Credit	X	X	X	X	X	X	X	X
			292	Notes Payable, Deferred Installments	____	Credit	X	X	X	X	X	X	X	X
				Total Long Term Debt	$____	$Credit								
			300	Capital										
			301	Capital, Name	$____	$Credit	X	X	NO	NO	NO	X	X	X
			302	Capital, Name	____	Credit	NO	X	NO	NO	NO	X	X	X
			303	Capital, Name	____	Credit	NO	X	NO	NO	NO	X	X	X
			304	Capital, Name	____	Credit	NO	X	NO	NO	NO	X	X	X
			305	Capital, Name	____	Credit	NO	X	NO	NO	NO	X	X	X
			306	Capital, Name	____	Credit	NO	X	NO	NO	NO	X	X	X
			307	Capital, Name	____	Credit	NO	X	NO	NO	NO	X	X	X
			308	Capital, Name	____	Credit	NO	X	NO	NO	NO	X	X	X
			309	Capital, Name	____	Credit	NO	X	NO	NO	NO	X	X	X
			310	Capital, Name	____	Credit	NO	X	NO	NO	NO	X	X	X
			389	Capital, Appropriated	____	Credit	NO	X	NO	NO	NO	X	X	X
				Total Capital	$____	$Credit								

*Key

X — Applicable NO — Not Applicable

Appendix 8C.

Balance Sheet
Month of ______

Client Number	Company Number	Department Number	Account Number	LIABILITIES AND NET WORTH	19__ Prior Year	19__ This Year	*ORGANIZATIONAL TYPE: Sole Proprietorship	Partnership	Professional Association	Professional Corporation	Corporation	*ACCOUNTING METHOD: Cash Basis	Modified Cash	Accrual
xxx	xxx	xxx	200	Current Liabilities										
			211	Mortgage Payable, Current Installments	$____	$Credit	X	X	X	X	X	X	X	X
			212	Notes Payable, Current Installments	____	Credit	X	X	X	X	X	X	X	X
			221	Accounts Payable	____	Credit	X	X	X	X	X	NO	NO	X
			231	Accruals, Payroll	____	Credit	X	X	X	X	X	NO	NO	X
			232	Accruals, Payroll Taxes	____	Credit	X	X	X	X	X	NO	X	X
			233	Accruals, Employee Medical Insurance	____	Credit	X	X	X	X	X	NO	X	X
			234	Accruals, Employee Life and Disability	____	Credit	X	X	X	X	X	NO	X	X
			235	Accruals, Expense, Legal	____	Credit	X	X	X	X	X	NO	X	X
			236	Accruals, Expense, Accounting	____	Credit	X	X	X	X	X	NO	X	X
			237	Accruals, Expense, Local Taxes	____	Credit	X	X	X	X	X	NO	X	X
			238	Accruals, Expense, Income Taxes	____	Credit	NO	NO	X	X	X	NO	NO	X
				Total Current Liabilities	$____	$Credit								
			290	Long Term Debt										
			291	Mortgage Payable, Deffered Installments	$____	$Credit	X	X	X	X	X	X	X	X
			292	Notes Payable, Deferred Installments	____	Credit	X	X	X	X	X	X	X	X
				Total Long Term Debt	$____	$Credit								
			300	Capital										
			301	Capital, Name	$____	$Credit	X	X	NO	NO	NO	X	X	X
			302	Capital, Name	____	Credit	NO	X	NO	NO	NO	X	X	X
			303	Capital, Name	____	Credit	NO	X	NO	NO	NO	X	X	X
			304	Capital, Name	____	Credit	NO	X	NO	NO	NO	X	X	X
			305	Capital, Name	____	Credit	NO	X	NO	NO	NO	X	X	X
			306	Capital, Name	____	Credit	NO	X	NO	NO	NO	X	X	X
			307	Capital, Name	____	Credit	NO	X	NO	NO	NO	X	X	X
			308	Capital, Name	____	Credit	NO	X	NO	NO	NO	X	X	X
			309	Capital, Name	____	Credit	NO	X	NO	NO	NO	X	X	X
			310	Capital, Name	____	Credit	NO	X	NO	NO	NO	X	X	X
			389	Capital, Appropriated	____	Credit	NO	X	NO	NO	NO	X	X	X
				Total Capital	$____	$Credit								

*Key

X – Applicable
NO – Not Applicable

Client Number	Company Number	Department Number	Account Number	LIABILITIES AND NET WORTH (Cont.)	19___ Prior Year	19___ This Year	Sole Proprietorship	Partnership	Professional Association	Professional Corporation	Corporation	Cash Basis	Modified Cash	Accrual
							*ORGANIZATIONAL TYPE					*ACCOUNTING METHOD		
xxx	xxx	xxx	390	Stockholder Equity										
			391	Stock at Par Value	$____	$Credit	NO	NO	X	X	X	X	X	X
			392	Additional Paid In Capital	____	Credit	NO	NO	X	X	X	X	X	X
			393	Retained Earnings	____	Credit	NO	NO	X	X	X	X	X	X
			394	Retained Earnings, Restricted	____	Credit	NO	NO	X	X	X	X	X	X
			395	Cost of Shares in Treasury	____	Debit	NO	NO	X	X	X	X	X	X
			399	Gain Year to Date	____	Credit	NO	NO	X	X	X	X	X	X
				Total Stockholder Equity	$____	$Credit								
			400	Drawing Accounts										
			401	Drawing, Name	$____	$Debit	X	X	NO	NO	NO	X	X	X
			402	Drawing, Name	____	Debit	NO	X	NO	NO	NO	X	X	X
			403	Drawing, Name	____	Debit	NO	X	NO	NO	NO	X	X	X
			404	Drawing, Name	____	Debit	NO	X	NO	NO	NO	X	X	X
			405	Drawing, Name	____	Debit	NO	X	NO	NO	NO	X	X	X
			406	Drawing, Name	____	Debit	NO	X	NO	NO	NO	X	X	X
			407	Drawing, Name	____	Debit	NO	X	NO	NO	NO	X	X	X
			408	Drawing, Name	____	Debit	NO	X	NO	NO	NO	X	X	X
			409	Drawing, Name	____	Debit	NO	X	NO	NO	NO	X	X	X
			410	Drawing, Name	____	Debit	NO	X	NO	NO	NO	X	X	X
				Total Drawing Accounts	$____	$Debit								
			500	Income Distribution										
			501	Income Distribution, Name	$____	$Credit	NO	X	NO	NO	NO	X	X	X
			502	Income Distribution, Name	____	Credit	NO	X	NO	NO	NO	X	X	X
			503	Income Distribution, Name	____	Credit	NO	X	NO	NO	NO	X	X	X
			504	Income Distribution, Name	____	Credit	NO	X	NO	NO	NO	X	X	X
			505	Income Distribution, Name	____	Credit	NO	X	NO	NO	NO	X	X	X
			506	Income Distribution, Name	____	Credit	NO	X	NO	NO	NO	X	X	X
			507	Income Distribution, Name	____	Credit	NO	X	NO	NO	NO	X	X	X
			508	Income Distribution, Name	____	Credit	NO	X	NO	NO	NO	X	X	X
			509	Income Distribution, Name	____	Credit	NO	X	NO	NO	NO	X	X	X
			510	Income Distribution, Name	____	Credit	NO	X	NO	NO	NO	X	X	X
			599	Gain, Year to Date	____	Credit	X	X	NO	NO	NO	X	X	X
				Total Income Distribution	$____	$Credit								
				TOTAL LIABILITIES AND NET WORTH	$____	$____								

*Key

X — Applicable
NO — Not Applicable

Example Balance Sheet Format

__________, 19__ and __

	Last Year	This Year
<u>Current Assets</u>		
Cash, Operating Account	$	$
Cash, Payroll Account		
Accounts Receivable		
Prepaid Expense, Insurance		
Total Current Assets	$	$
<u>Deposits</u>		
Equipment Deposits		
Utility Deposits		
Total Deposits	$	$
<u>Property and Equipment</u>		
Land	$	$
Building		
Equipment		
Provision For Depreciation, Building	( )	( )
Provision For Depreciation, Equipment	( )	( )
Book Value, Property and Equipment	$	$
<u>Total Assets</u>	$	$
<u>Current Liabilities</u>		
Mortgage Payable, Current Installments	$	$
Notes Payable, Current Installments		
Accounts Payable		
Accruals, Local Taxes		
Total Current Liabilities	$	$
<u>Long Term Debt</u>		
Mortgage Payable, Deferred Installments	$	$
Notes Payable, Deferred Installments		
Total Long Term Debt	$	$
Total Liabilities		
<u>Stockholder Equity</u>		
Stock at Par Value	$	$
Additional Paid In Capital		
Retained Earnings		
Less Cost of Treasury Shares	( )	( )
Total Stockholder Equity	$	$
<u>Total Liabilities And Stockholder Equity</u>	$	$

Common stock of $10 par value per share,
100,000 shares authorized.

Number Shares Issued	
Less Number of Shares in Treasury	
Number Shares Outstanding	

Appendix 8C. (Cont.)

Income Statement

For the _____ Months Ending _________

Client Number	Company Number	Department Number	Account Number		19___ Prior Year	19___ This Year	*ORGANIZATIONAL TYPE: Sole Proprietorship	Partnership	Professional Association	Professional Corporation	Corporation	*ACCOUNTING METHOD: Cash Basis	Modified Cash	Accrual
xxx	xxx	xxx	600	Income										
			611	Income, Professional Fee	$_____	$Credit	X	X	X	X	X	X	X	X
			621	Income, Ancillary, Lab	_____	Credit	X	X	X	X	X	X	X	X
			622	Income, Ancillary, X-Ray	_____	Credit	X	X	X	X	X	X	X	X
			623	Income, Ancillary, Optical	_____	Credit	X	X	X	X	X	X	X	X
			624	Income, Ancillary, Physical Therapy	_____	Credit	X	X	X	X	X	X	X	X
			625	Income, Ancillary, Pharmacy	_____	Credit	X	X	X	X	X	X	X	X
			626	Income, Ancillary, Nuclear Medicine	_____	Credit	X	X	X	X	X	X	X	X
			631	Income, Recoveries, Patient Accounts	_____	Credit	X	X	X	X	X	X	X	X
			641	Income, Contract, Services	_____	Credit	X	X	X	X	X	X	X	X
			651	Returns and Allowances	_____	Debit	X	X	X	X	X	X	X	X
			652	Discounts, Charity	_____	Debit	X	X	X	X	X	X	X	X
			653	Discounts, Governmental Programs	_____	Debit	X	X	X	X	X	X	X	X
			654	Discounts, Insurance Only	_____	Debit	X	X	X	X	X	X	X	X
			655	Discounts, Policy	_____	Debit	X	X	X	X	X	X	X	X
				Net Patient Income	$_____	$Credit	X	X	X	X	X	X	X	X
			661	Rental Income	$_____	$Credit	X	X	X	X	X	X	X	X
			671	Sales	_____	Credit	X	X	X	X	X	X	X	X
			681	Other income, Parking	_____	Credit	X	X	X	X	X	X	X	X
			682	Other Income, Telephone	_____	Credit	X	X	X	X	X	X	X	X
			683	Other Income, Vending	_____	Credit	X	X	X	X	X	X	X	X
			684	Other Income, Interest	_____	Credit	X	X	X	X	X	X	X	X
				Total Income	$_____	$Credit	X	X	X	X	X	X	X	X
			690	Cost of Sales										
			691	Inventory, Beginning	$_____	$Debit	X	X	X	X	X	NO	NO	X
			692	Inventory, Purchases	_____	Debit	X	X	X	X	X	X	X	X
			693	Inventory, Ending	_____	Debit	X	X	X	X	X	NO	NO	X
				Total Cost of Sales	$_____	$Debit								
				Total Income before Expenses	$_____	$Credit								

*Key

X – Applicable
NO – Not Applicable

Appendix 8D. Income Statement Related to Organization Type and Accounting Method

Appendix 8D. (Cont.)

Income Statement

For the ____ Months Ending ______

Client Number	Company Number	Department Number	Account Number	EXPENSES	19__ Prior Year	19__ This Year	*ORGANIZATIONAL TYPE					*ACCOUNTING METHOD		
							Sole Proprietorship	Partnership	Professional Association	Professional Corporation	Corporation	Cash Basis	Modified Cash	Accrual
xxx	xxx	xxx	700	Professional and Medical										
			701	Salaries, Doctors	$____	$Debit	X	X	X	X	X	X	X	X
			703	Taxes, Social Security	____	Debit	X	X	X	X	X	X	X	X
			704	Taxes, Unemployment	____	Debit	X	X	X	X	X	X	X	X
			705	Retirement Plan	____	Debit	X	X	X	X	X	X	X	X
			706	Insurance, Hospitalization	____	Debit	X	X	X	X	X	X	X	X
			707	Insurance, Life and Disability	____	Debit	X	X	X	X	X	X	X	X
			708	Insurance, Malpractice	____	Debit	X	X	X	X	X	X	X	X
			709	Insurance, Workmens Compensation	____	Debit	X	X	X	X	X	X	X	X
			710	Parking	____	Debit	X	X	X	X	X	X	X	X
			711	Recruiting	____	Debit	X	X	X	X	X	X	X	X
			712	Relocation	____	Debit	X	X	X	X	X	X	X	X
			713	Personnel Agency Fees	____	Debit	X	X	X	X	X	X	X	X
			714	Travel	____	Debit	X	X	X	X	X	X	X	X
			715	Consultants, Physicians	____	Debit	X	X	X	X	X	X	X	X
			716	Laboratory, Outside Service	____	Debit	X	X	X	X	X	X	X	X
			717	X-Ray, Outside Service	____	Debit	X	X	X	X	X	X	X	X
			718	Film Badge Service	____	Debit	X	X	X	X	X	X	X	X
			722	Dues, Fees, Licenses	____	Debit	X	X	X	X	X	X	X	X
			723	Miscellaneous Professional and Medical	____	Debit	X	X	X	X	X	X	X	X
				Total Professional and Medical	$____	$Debit	X	X	X	X	X	X	X	X

*Key

X — Applicable
NO — Not Applicable

Client Number	Company Number	Department Number	Account Number	EXPENSES	19___ Prior Year	19___ This Year	*ORGANIZATIONAL TYPE: Sole Proprietorship	Partnership	Professional Association	Professional Corporation	Corporation	*ACCOUNTING METHOD: Cash Basis	Modified Cash	Accrual
xxx	xxx	xxx	800	Personnel Expenses										
			802	Salaries, Employees	$_____	$_____	X	X	X	X	X	X	X	X
			803	Taxes, Social Security	_____	_____	X	X	X	X	X	X	X	X
			804	Taxes, Unemployment	_____	_____	X	X	X	X	X	X	X	X
			805	Retirement Plan	_____	_____	X	X	X	X	X	X	X	X
			806	Insurance, Hospitalization	_____	_____	X	X	X	X	X	X	X	X
			807	Insurance, Life and Disability	_____	_____	X	X	X	X	X	X	X	X
			808	Insurance, Malpractice	_____	_____	X	X	X	X	X	X	X	X
			809	Insurance, Workmens Compensation	_____	_____	X	X	X	X	X	X	X	X
			810	Parking	_____	_____	X	X	X	X	X	X	X	X
			811	Recruiting	_____	_____	X	X	X	X	X	X	X	X
			812	Relocation	_____	_____	X	X	X	X	X	X	X	X
			813	Personnel Agency Fees	_____	_____	X	X	X	X	X	X	X	X
			814	Travel	_____	_____	X	X	X	X	X	X	X	X
			819	Contract Labor	_____	_____	X	X	X	X	X	X	X	X
			820	Employee Medical Service	_____	_____	X	X	X	X	X	X	X	X
			821	Employee Meetings and Expense	_____	_____	X	X	X	X	X	X	X	X
			822	Dues, Fees, Licenses	_____	_____	X	X	X	X	X	X	X	X
			823	Miscellaneous Personnel Expenses	_____	_____	X	X	X	X	X	X	X	X
				Total Personnel Expenses	$_____	$_____								

*Key

X – Applicable
NO – Not Applicable

Appendix 8D. (Cont.)

Appendix 8D. (Cont.)

Income Statement
For the ____ Months Ending ______

Client Number	Company Number	Department Number	Account Number	EXPENSES	19__ Prior Year	19__ This Year	*ORGANIZATIONAL TYPE: Sole Proprietorship	Partnership	Professional Association	Professional Corporation	Corporation	*ACCOUNTING METHOD: Cash Basis	Modified Cash	Accrual
xxx	xxx	xxx	830	Supplies										
			831	Data Processing Supplies	$____	$Debit	X	X	X	X	X	X	X	X
			832	Dental Supplies	____	Debit	X	X	X	X	X	X	X	X
			833	Laboratory Supplies	____	Debit	X	X	X	X	X	X	X	X
			834	Laundry, Cleaning, Linen	____	Debit	X	X	X	X	X	X	X	X
			835	Maintenance Supplies	____	Debit	X	X	X	X	X	X	X	X
			836	Medicine and Drug Supplies	____	Debit	X	X	X	X	X	X	X	X
			837	Nuclear Medicine Supplies	____	Debit	X	X	X	X	X	X	X	X
			838	Printing and Office Supplies	____	Debit	X	X	X	X	X	X	X	X
			839	Professional Supplies	____	Debit	X	X	X	X	X	X	X	X
			840	X-Ray Supplies	____	Debit	X	X	X	X	X	X	X	X
			841	Miscellaneous Supplies	____	Debit	X	X	X	X	X	X	X	X
				Total Supplies	$____	$Debit								

*Key

X — Applicable
NO — Not Applicable

Client Number	Company Number	Department Number	Account Number	EXPENSES	19___ Prior Year	19___ This Year	*ORGANIZATIONAL TYPE					*ACCOUNTING METHOD		
							Sole Proprietorship	Partnership	Professional Association	Professional Corporation	Corporation	Cash Basis	Modified Cash	Accrual
	xxx	xxx	850	General and Adminstrative										
			851	Automobile	$_____	$Debit	X	X	X	X	X	X	X	X
			852	Accounting	_____	Debit	X	X	X	X	X	X	X	X
			853	Bad Debts	_____	Debit	X	X	X	X	X	X	X	X
			854	Clinic Meetings	_____	Debit	X	X	X	X	X	X	X	X
			855	Collection Fees	_____	Debit	X	X	X	X	X	X	X	X
			856	Contributions	_____	Debit	X	X	X	X	X	X	X	X
			857	Copy Costs	_____	Debit	X	X	X	X	X	X	X	X
			858	Credit Reports	_____	Debit	X	X	X	X	X	X	X	X
			859	Data Processing	_____	Debit	X	X	X	X	X	X	X	X
			860	Delivery and Messenger	_____	Debit	X	X	X	X	X	X	X	X
			861	Dues, Fees, Licenses	_____	Debit	X	X	X	X	X	X	X	X
			862	Entertainment	_____	Debit	X	X	X	X	X	X	X	X
			863	Insurance	_____	Debit	X	X	X	X	X	X	X	X
			864	Interest	_____	Debit	X	X	X	X	X	X	X	X
			865	Legal	_____	Debit	X	X	X	X	X	X	X	X
			866	Miscellaneous	_____	Debit	X	X	X	X	X	X	X	X
			867	Over and Short	_____	Debit	X	X	X	X	X	X	X	X
			868	Patient Courtesy	_____	Debit	X	X	X	X	X	X	X	X
			869	Patient Parking	_____	Debit	X	X	X	X	X	X	X	X
			870	Postage	_____	Debit	X	X	X	X	X	X	X	X
			871	Publications	_____	Debit	X	X	X	X	X	X	X	X
			872	Storage, Moving	_____	Debit	X	X	X	X	X	X	X	X
			873	Taxes, Franchise	_____	Debit	X	X	X	X	X	X	X	X
			874	Taxes, Income	_____	Debit	X	X	X	X	X	X	X	X
			875	Telephone	_____	Debit	X	X	X	X	X	X	X	X
			876	Telephone Answering Service	_____	Debit	X	X	X	X	X	X	X	X
			877	Travel	_____	Debit	X	X	X	X	X	X	X	X
			878	Recoveries, Expense	_____	Debit	X	X	X	X	X	X	X	X
				Total General and Administrative Expense	$_____	$Debit								

*Key

X – Applicable
NO – Not Applicable

Appendix 8D. (Cont.)

Appendix 8D. (Cont.)

Income Statement
For the ____ Months Ending ______

Client Number	Company Number	Department Number	Account Number	EXPENSES	19__ Prior Year	19__ This Year	*ORGANIZATIONAL TYPE: Sole Proprietorship	Partnership	Professional Association	Professional Corporation	Corporation	*ACCOUNTING METHOD: Cash Basis	Modified Cash	Accrual
xxx	xxx	xxx	900	Building										
			901	Amortization, Leasehold Improvements	$____	$Debit	X	X	X	X	X	X	X	X
			902	Depreciation, Building	____	Debit	X	X	X	X	X	X	X	X
			903	Insurance, Building	____	Debit	X	X	X	X	X	X	X	X
			904	Janitorial Service	____	Debit	X	X	X	X	X	X	X	X
			905	Maintenance Contracts, Building	____	Debit	X	X	X	X	X	X	X	X
			906	Maintenance Contracts, Elevators	____	Debit	X	X	X	X	X	X	X	X
			907	Mortgage Interest	____	Debit	X	X	X	X	X	X	X	X
			908	Pest Control	____	Debit	X	X	X	X	X	X	X	X
			909	Rent, Building	____	Debit	X	X	X	X	X	X	X	X
			910	Repairs	____	Debit	X	X	X	X	X	X	X	X
			912	Repairs, Air Conditiong and Heating	____	Debit	X	X	X	X	X	X	X	X
			913	Repairs, Electrical	____	Debit	X	X	X	X	X	X	X	X
			914	Repairs, Plumbing	____	Debit	X	X	X	X	X	X	X	X
			915	Repairs, Roof	____	Debit	X	X	X	X	X	X	X	X
			916	Repairs, Miscellaneous	____	Debit	X	X	X	X	X	X	X	X
			917	Taxes on Building, Local	____	Debit	X	X	X	X	X	X	X	X
			918	Utilities, Gas	____	Debit	X	X	X	X	X	X	X	X
			919	Utilities, Electricity	____	Debit	X	X	X	X	X	X	X	X
			920	Utilities, Water	____	Debit	X	X	X	X	X	X	X	X
			921	Miscellaneous Building Expenses	____	Debit	X	X	X	X	X	X	X	X
				Total Building Expenses	$____	$Debit								
			950	Equipment										
			951	Depreciation, Equipment	$____	$Debit	X	X	X	X	X	X	X	X
			952	Insurance, Equipment	____	Debit	X	X	X	X	X	X	X	X
			953	Maintenance Contracts, Equipment	____	Debit	X	X	X	X	X	X	X	X
			954	Rent, Equipment	____	Debit	X	X	X	X	X	X	X	X
			955	Repairs, Equipment	____	Debit	X	X	X	X	X	X	X	X
			956	Taxes on Equipment, Local	____	Debit	X	X	X	X	X	X	X	X
			957	Interest on Equipment, Notes Payable	____	Debit	X	X	X	X	X	X	X	X
			958	Miscellaneous Equipment Expense	____	Debit	X	X	X	X	X	X	X	X
				Total Equipment Expense	$____	$Debit								
				TOTAL EXPENSES	$____	$Debit								
				NET INCOME	$____	$Credit								

*Key

X – Applicable
NO – Not Applicable

Income Statement

For the Years Ending December 31, 19__ and 19__

	Prior Year	Current Year
Income		
Income, Professional Fees	$	$
Income, Ancillary, Lab		
Income, Ancillary, X-Ray		
Returns and Allowances		
Net Patient Income	$	$
Expenses		
Professional and Medical	$	$
Salaries, Doctors		
Taxes, Social Security		
Taxes, Unemployment		
Retirement Plan		
Insurance, Hospitalization		
Insurance, Life and Disability		
Insurance, Malpractice		
Insurance, Workmans Compensation		
Travel		
Consultants, Physicians		
Laboratory, Outside Service		
X-Ray, Outside Service		
Total Professional and Medical Expense	$	$
Personnel Expenses		
Salaries, Employees	$	$
Taxes, Social Security		
Taxes, Unemployment		
Retirement Plan		
Insurance, Hospitalization		
Insurance, Life and Disability		
Insurance, Workmans Compensation		
Travel		
Contract Labor		
Total Personnel Expenses	$	$
Supplies		
Laboratory Supplies	$	$
Laundry, Cleaning, Linen		
Maintenance Supplies		
Medicine and Drug Supplies		
Printing and Office Supplies		
Professional Supplies		
Total Supplies	$	$
General and Administrative Expenses		
Automobile	$	$
Accounting		
Clinic Meetings		
Collection Fees		
Credit Reports		
Data Processing		
Delivery and Messenger		
Dues, Fees, Licenses		
Insurance		
Interest		

Appendix 8D. (Cont.)

	Prior Year	Current Year
Expenses (Cont.)		
Legal		
Miscellaneous		
Over and Short		
Postage		
Publications		
Taxes, Franchise		
Telephone		
Telephone Answering Service		
Travel		
Total G and A Expenses	$	$
Total Expenses	$	$
Income Before Federal Income Taxes	$	$
Taxes, Income		
Net Income	$	$

Appendix 8D. (Cont.)

Chapter 9

Staff Compensation

EMPLOYEE COMPENSATION

Unlike many of the subjects discussed in previous chapters, there are numerous alternatives available in the area of employee compensation. These alternatives are well documented in two publications: *MGMA Digest of Medical Group Employment Contracts and Income Distribution Plans*, published by Medical Group Management Association; and *Income Distribution Abstract and Analysis*, published by the American Group Practice Association. Neither manual, however, addresses those compensation alternatives specifically suited to the three to ten physician group. Consequently, to supplement this material and provide a basis for describing considerations appropriate for the small, forming group practice, a number of small group practices with various organizational forms were polled concerning compensation methods, for physician as well as non-physician employees.[a] In this chapter, specific attention will be devoted to the results of that poll which reflect areas important to the decision making process of the forming group and germane to the establishment of staff compensation plans in general. At this point, it is not important to consider the mechanics of establishing wage and salary guidelines, promotion and advancement criteria, and personnel management; these elements are discussed more specifically in Part III. In making initial decisions in the development of a compensation plan, it is necessary to consider the group's established mission,

[a]Of the medical groups listed in Medical Group Management Association's 1974-75 *International Directory* (Denver, Colorado: Medical Group Management Association, 1974), 170 are 3-10 multi-specialty physician groups with in-house laboratory and X-ray facilities. The questionnaire was mailed to 100 of these groups. The response rate to the survey was 42 percent.

planning criteria, organizational form and governance responsibilities, and financial plan. Additionally, during the development of an approach to compensation, it may be discovered that earlier decisions require modification or change consistent with the group formation process.

Physician Employee Compensation

Employee status may represent either a continued or an interim status for the group physician. Usually, interim status is assigned during a trial arrangement period prior to the attainment of full member, shareholder, or partnership status. Physicians joining a partnership may remain in an employed status for varying periods of time, and will be able to become members or partners only after meeting qualifications set by the group.

Salary considerations usually begin with a set of competitive elements, such as salary opportunities and qualification levels. In addition to meeting competitive levels, the amount of compensation paid a new physician, should be based on: training, experience, specialization, board eligibility or board certification, length of practice, group needs, group income projection, and patient and staff acceptance. The desires of group members as well as various external factors also may affect compensation decisions. For example, within a prepayment or fee-for-service setting, employment conditions for the physician, including salary considerations, can vary due to the governance of the organization's structure, the motivation of those individuals who influence administrative decisions, and difficulties encountered in attracting physicians for specific needs. The income level of the employed physician also can be affected by requirements of the group's delivery system mission. Patient satisfaction may rank high in priority on the list of salary considerations. If physician productivity constitutes a high priority, evaluations for salary considerations based on cost effectiveness, as in prepayment, will require an approach different from evaluations based on fee-for-service income.

Salary decisions should be made and the ensuing structure designed with some degree of flexibility so that the group is able to encourage a physician to remain. The evaluation method to be used in assessing the physician employee should be explained to him, preferably when he is interviewed, and certainly when commitments are made to join the staff. Evaluative criteria should be weighed carefully in order to reflect the goals and objectives of the organization and can serve as continuous guidelines during subsequent reviews of the physician's salary status. Included in the criteria for evaluation might be: productivity, group compatibility, patient satisfaction, administrative and organizational interest, educational development, quality of care, cost consciousness, flexibility, potential, and seniority. An employment contract with the physician employee may be desirable to ensure that he understands completely the salary structure of the group. In addition, fringe benefits will continue to play an important role in attracting and retaining the salaried physician and should be considered jointly with salary determinations.

Nonphysician Employee Compensation

Salary guidelines for support personnel are not unlike those which apply in any type of business enterprise where market influences are taken into consideration. Fringe benefits for the nonphysician employee also represent a salary component to be considered carefully. Although group practice salaries and job descriptions may be similar to those found in other medical delivery processess, the need to emphasize the group's goals, objectives, and philosophy to prospective employees is of particular importance. For example, the "team" concept of group practice may preclude the consideration and selection of certain persons who are not oriented toward group goals, regardless of salary levels.

FRINGE BENEFITS

One primary factor to be considered in the setting of salaries is the available benefit package. Benefits represent a significant portion of total compensation, accounting for as much as 5 percent to 25 percent of earnings. In fact, recent Medical Group Management Association unpublished surveys indicate that benefits are in the neighborhood of 10 percent to 17 percent of wages.[1]

Physician Employee Benefits

As in any comparable organization, personnel or fringe benefits for physicians in larger groups are generally more comprehensive than for physicians in smaller groups. Smaller groups tend to channel a greater share of income into their physicians' paychecks.[2] Because of the current lack of any indepth information on fringe benefits in small group practices, the following discussion is based on the authors' recent poll.

Of interest to the forming group will be the advantages which some groups define as fringe benefits. In general, fringe benefits may be classified as any benefit given employees which is above and beyond what is required by law. Nevertheless, because individuals still may disagree on just what constitutes a fringe benefit, the group should consider plans for a variety of benefit options. Physician vacation and sick leave may not be categorized as fringe benefits, particularly in corporate groups. Within the corporate framework, however, overall physician benefits may be greater than in other legal structures. Such benefits may include life, health, disability, and malpractice insurance; and time away for educational purposes and meetings. Pension and retirement plans, reimbursement for job related expenses and medical organization dues, and productivity credit for time spent pursuing post graduate education may or may not be considered fringe benefits. In addition, holidays, staff dues or hospital fees, local privilege tax, no night hours, money purchase plans, the equipping and maintaining of offices, and discounts on dental and optometric services represent potential fringe benefit areas.

The sole proprietorship, professional association, and unincorporated association comprised less than 2 percent of the survey responses. In these categories, benefits were not uniform; they included Keogh, Blue Cross/Blue Shield, vacations, one week leave, life insurance, free lunches, malpractice insurance, disability insurance, pension plans, profit sharing, continuing education, and paid country club dues. Professional associations provided the most generous benefits. Fringe benefits found within the partnership are discussed later in this chapter.

Nonphysician Employee Benefits

Nonphysician employee benefits reflect the economic status of the community and the ability of the forming group to attract employees. Typical nonphysician benefits are vacations (based on length of service), sick leave, holidays, some form of health coverage and/or free medical care provided by the group. Some groups may include pension, retirement, and profit sharing plans.[3] When compared to the benefits offered the small group physician, nonphysician benefits within the small group practice represent a significant component in compensation arrangements, and in intent do not differ greatly from those of medium and large sized group practices.

OVERTIME PAYMENT

In developing a compensation plan, the group also must consider the subject of overtime payment. Paradoxically, the conditions and rates for overtime payment must be communicated to the employees, yet such expenditures constitute a nonbudgetable expense in the financial plan. Generally, for the physician employee in a small group, compensation for extra hours or weekend duty is built into the basic salary, income distribution, or bonus plan. On the other hand, legal statutes require that certain nonphysician and nonprofessional or technical employees be paid overtime for extra hours of work. *Overtime Compensation, Under the Fair Labor Standards Act of 1938, as Amended*, available from the United States Department of Labor, Workplace Standards Administration, Wage and Hour Division, Washington, D.C. 20210, outlines governmental regulations. To avoid complications and confusion, and to provide a basis for adequate compensation planning, it is prudent to indicate clearly which employees according to law must be paid overtime. It also may be wise to have an understanding regarding overtime with other employees whom the law does not require to be so compensated.

Physician Compensation

One need only review documented approaches to physician compensation to discover that the myriad of available methods yield only broad trends rather than explicit configurations. At best, group practice compensation systems are complex and traditionally have been ever-changing. In fact, most existing groups would probably state that they currently are working within a minimum of three distribution plans for physicians—a currently approved plan, the plan most recently used, and a plan considered for adoption. The complexities inherent in alternative compensation methods have been described in various ways:

1. With no concern for internal equity, the organization may find that doctors identify primarily with their specialties and have little concern with overall clinic issues and strategies.[4]
2. Where different specialties are represented, small groups will tend to behave more in the manner of moderate sized clinics insofar as equal distribution of a portion of their income is concerned.[5]
3. As an element of any type of income distribution plan, i.e., equal sharing in-

centive or a mixture including a factor for seniority, recognition and quantifying compensation for non-income producing services such as educational, research, and civic activities is most difficult and often overlooked.[6]

Compensation structures developed in the early stages of a group practice often are dictated by the backgrounds of the physicians involved. Their conclusions will be influenced by a number of factors: medical experience; number of years in practice; habits of practice, including productivity; use of hospitals; specialization; teaching exposure; academic standing of medical schools attended; relationships with other physicians in the community, both personally and professionally; and exposure to and understanding of the community in which they establish a group practice. The physician compensation system should be compatible with the goals and objectives of the medical group, and the degree of flexibility built into the income distribution system will determine how easily modification for maintaining or expanding the group can be incorporated into the plan. Often, the choice of an income distribution system is influenced by the exposure of the principal physicians to others in group practice, either through organizations such as the American Medical Association and the American Group Practice Association, or through local and state medical societies. The knowledge, capabilities, and experience of the individual to whom group physicians entrust the responsibility for managerial aspects of the group practice also may influence the system of physician compensation.

Some basic income distribution methods are outlined briefly below. Most income distribution systems, as they evolve in newly forming groups, will represent some combination of these methods:

1. *Equal distribution.* All of the group's income is distributed on an equal basis among physician partners/shareholders/members after expenses. This system seems to work best for groups that are quite cohesive and cooperative, and produce income sufficient to allow each physician to be adequately compensated. This method, in its pure form, is not widely used today. It is more often combined with other methods of compensation. "Most groups still retain equal distribution in some form and to some degree. There is a definite rationale for some equal distribution on the ground that every group has a degree of economic interdependence."[7] This method or component of income distribution also is referred to as equal shares or share alike distribution.

2. *Productivity.* Income is distributed in a direct ratio to income produced by the physicians in the group. "Observation and direct experience with productivity oriented compensation indicates approximately 40-60% of net earnings for doctor compensation can be effectively distributed on the basis of productivity. Less than 40% tends to be inadequate reward for hard workers and high net earning specialties. More than 60% tends to create strong independent competitive qualities which can limit referral between members of a group and discourage addition of doctors to the group because it represents competition for members which could reduce their contribution to the group's net earnings and consequently their personal compensation."[8] Motivation for high or efficient productivity is the basis of this approach to physician compensation; however, actually employing the productivity parameters can result in the stressing of productivity as the prime ingredient determining compensation.

3. *Percentage.* Income is distributed on a percentage basis taking into consideration a number of factors which may include: equal shares, total bookings, total collections, length of service, and training.

4. *Points.* In this income distribution method, points are assigned for various activities undertaken by the physician and the sum of the points is related to total compensation. Some considerations in the point distribution system are: seniority, group value, training, professional standing, drawing power, patient referral to other physicians in the group, professional charges, publications and research, and administrative ability.

5. *Salary.* This type of compensation requires no explanation except that it usually is combined with other factors such as points, percentage, equal distribution, bonus, etc. A straight salary compensation is employed more frequently when the physician initially joins the group, but is combined with one or more of the above approaches upon his receiving tenure and progressive status.

In the remaining portion of this chapter income distribution plans currently in use in groups of three to ten physicians will be discussed. Although much of the published information on compensation plans is not applicable to the newly forming group practice and represents groups larger than the ten physician size, such reference information can prove valuable in emphasizing to the forming group the need to incorporate flexibility into the compensation plan for the accommodation of future expansion. An analysis of the results of the three to ten physician group poll provides a more appropriate basis for this discussion. The issues to be considered are grouped according to the various organizational forms so that the data is relevant to individual group circumstances. Examples of specific plans as reported by respondents in the poll should be helpful to newly forming groups who face the task of planning and choosing a compensation plan from the many available. The pattern emerging from the poll seems to indicate that physicians in small groups are compensated primarily through salaries; however, benefits, as an element in compensation plans, appear to be more uniform across various group sizes.

Sole Proprietorship

The sole proprietorship is a rare form of organizational structure, yet the income distribution methods utilized within this structure can vary significantly, and can include salary, salary with bonus, points, productivity, or a combination of these systems.[b] Few if any differences in income distribution methods exist between the fee-for-service sole proprietorship and the hospital-based sole proprietorship; the physician in a proprietary prepayment setting, however, usually is a salaried employee. Most proprietorships involved in prepayment are large organizations which employ a physician to provide services on a prepaid-salary basis. An example of sole proprietorship income distribution reported in the authors' survey clearly indicates some of the key considerations:

> After all the expenses are paid and a predetermined amount is placed in reserve for future needs (large fixed expenses such as malpractice insurance, dues, United Fund)

[b]Less than 3 percent of the 170 three to ten physician groups with lab and X-ray that are listed in the 1974-75 MGMA *International Directory* are sole proprietorships. Less than 1 percent of the survey respondents are sole proprietorships.

> the net cash in bank is distributed as follows: all doctors receive a base salary of $350. Then they participate according to the amount of monies collected on an accumulative percentage basis for the year. The more they produce the more they receive. In this method the larger producers also pay a greater percentage of the group's expenses. There is no additional consideration for administrative time, seniority, or board certification.

Medical Partnership

Before professional corporate status was accepted by the Internal Revenue Service, the majority of group practices were organized as partnerships. Adapting the partnership to a corporate form of organizational structure has done little to change the basic motivation and incentive for physicians who work together in a group setting. Consequently, many of the issues discussed below also will apply to other forms of medical group practice organization, particularly the corporate form.[c]

Equal Distribution. Seven of the twenty-one surveyed partnership groups (averaging 6.3 physicians per group) offer equal distribution compensation plans. All the groups distribute laboratory and radiology income equally among the partners. Fringe benefits range from hospital and medical insurance only, to *X* percent of auto expenses; *X* percent of home telephone; physician liability insurance; newspapers, magazines, medical books and medical journals; medical association dues; service club and chamber of commerce dues; payment of expenses for annual physical; payment for income tax service; vacation, based on length of service up to thirty work days; twleve work days per year for medical meetings and postgraduate meetings; ten work days per year for civic meetings as an officer, director, or committee member; and ten work days per year sick leave. In general, in an equal distribution compensation plan, fringe benefits are more liberal than other forms of income distribution found in the partnership framework.

An example of an equal distribution agreement as reported in the authors' poll is as follows:

> A basic drawing account, to be equal among the partners, shall be established at the beginning of this partnership at the term sum of $2,500 per month per partner, payable after closing of business of each calendar month, prorated proportions thereof, and which sum shall continue until change by the vote of the partners, to be done at the annual business meeting of the partnership or such other time as the partners unanimously approve. For convenience, this payment may be referred to as "salary," although it is recognized that it is not a salary by way of compensation of an employee in the conventional sense.
>
> At the end of each calendar quarter, computed from the first of each calendar year (after payments to any terminated partners as provided herein) there shall be distributed to the partners, in equal shares, the net remaining income on hand at the end of such quarter after payment of all the current obligations, debts, and expenses and charges against the partnership or on capital acquisition approved by a majority in interest of the partners. Such distribution shall relieve any partner of his obligation for his prorated share of the losses or obligations of the partnership.

[c]Fifty percent of those groups responding in the survey are medical partnerships. All were fee-for-service and contained an average of 7.4 physicians.

Equal Distribution Based on a Point System. This particular method is used by two of the twenty-one partnerships represented in the poll; one group includes six physicians, and the other seven. An example equal distribution plan based on a point system is as follows:

> Under the point system, a new doctor is on an employed status for a period of two years. His salary and conditions of employment are by unanimous approval of the partners. At the beginning of the third year, the physician may become a junior partner, and his income in proportion to the total earnings of the partnership is as four points are to the total number of points of all the partners. For example, if there were a total of thirty-six points held by all the partners, including the junior partners, and the junior partner in his first year had four points, he would then be entitled to four thirty-sixths or one ninth of the total partnership's profits. Similarly, in his second year as a partner, he would be entitled to five points. In his third year he would be entitled to six points; in his fourth year he would be entitled to seven points, and in his fifth and succeeding years as a senior partner, he would be entitled to eight points.

Laboratory and radiology income also is taken into consideration in the point system. In addition, both of the groups using the point system offer a pension plan. One group offers a month's vacation; both offer study time—one group offers one month's study time, and the other, one week. One group offers paid holidays; the other offers payment of all society and board memberships dues.

Other Distribution Systems Based on Productivity and/or Points. Of the remaining twelve partnership groups (7.1 physicians per group) in the poll, all have income distribution plans which consider productivity as a compensation factor. In these groups, fringe benefits are not as encompassing as in the partnership arrangements cited previously. When asked about fringe benefits two groups stated: "physicians are partners"; another group indicated that "because the clinic is a partnership the amount of fringe benefits is quite restricted in comparison with incorporated practices." Still another group listed "none" under fringe benefits. Typical benefits listed by those groups who do include them are malpractice insurance, and vacation and meeting expenses. Three groups have pension plans, usually Keogh. Laboratory and radiology credit is given to physicians in nine of the groups, and two include lab and X-ray income with other income.

Another example distribution system based on productivity and points is reflected in the following schedule:

Points and Gross Bookings Schedules

Gross Bookings	*Points*
80,000.00	10
83,125.00	10 1/4
86,250.00	10 1/2
89,375.00	10 3/4
92,500.00	11
95,625.00	11 1/4
98,750.00	11 1/2
101,875.00	11 3/4
105,000.00	12

Gross Bookings	*Points*
111,250.00	12 1/4
117,500.00	12 1/2
123,750.00	12 3/4
130,000.00	13
136,250.00	13 1/4
142,750.00	13 1/2
149,000.00	13 3/4
155,250.00	14

This particular schedule has no ceiling, and continues on at 1/4 point increments at $6,250 intervals. During any given calendar month, net profits are computed by deducting the sum of the expenses from the aggregate of all income received by the partnership. The resultant net profit is then distributed among the partners according to the number of points earned by each partner based on his gross production for the twelve months immediately preceding. For example, if the gross bookings of a partner for the preceding twelve months were $80,000, he would have earned ten points, as indicated in the above schedule. He then would be entitled to participate in the net profits of the partnership for any given month in the ratio which his ten points bear to the sum of the total points earned by all the partners. As an example, if the sum of total points earned by all the partners were eighty, and the net profit for the month were $24,000, dividing $24,000 by eighty would yield a value of $300 per point. The partner with ten points, therefore, would receive a total of $3,000 for that particular month. It must be remembered, however, that the amount of net profit to be distributed may vary from month to month. The earned points also will vary in proportion to the amount of a partner's gross bookings for the immediately preceding twelve months.

Percentage Based on Productivity, Length of Service, and Equal Distribution. An example of this type of remuneration for the partners and distribution of the net profits of the partnership is outlined below:

1. Each partner shall be entitled to draw monthly against his profit participation the sum of $1,500.
2. However, if for two consecutive quarterly periods (the dates of which are noted hereafter), the billings of a partner average less than $3,500 per month (computing each quarter separately), said partner's monthly draw for the next quarterly period shall be 60 percent of his average monthly billings for the said two previous quarters. The partners may, by majority vote, allow monthly draws larger than those herein provided for (but in no event more than $1,500).
3. The net income of the partnership shall be accounted for, and distributed as soon as practicable after the quarterly periods ending March 31, June 30, September 30, and December 31 of each year, as set forth hereafter:

   a. After deduction of all monthly draws, 75 percent of the balance of the net income shall be paid in direct proportion to each partner's billings in excess of $1,500 per month. The billings shall be determined by adding the net prorated income from the laboratory and X-ray departments of the clinic to the gross of all other billings. The net prorated income for each partner from the laboratory and X-ray departments shall be the same proportion of the total net income from these departments as each partner's gross billings bear to the total gross billings of all of the partners in these departments.

b. 15 percent of said balance shall be paid in direct proportion to each partner's full years of association with the partnership or its predecessor organizations; except that the maximum proportion shall be limited to twenty years.

c. 10 percent of said balance shall be divided equally among the partners.

Salary and Percentage of Net Profits. In this type of arrangement the physician may be paid a monthly salary of $500 with increases of $150 per month per year until a maximum of $1,250 per month is reached. Within sixty days after the close of each six-month period, the following computations are made:

1. Determine the amount of billings of the partnership during the six-month period.
2. Determine the total amount of billings during the six-month period for services performed by each partner.
3. Compute the respective percentages by dividing the amount resulting from the above computation (2) by the amount resulting from the first computation.

Fifty Percent of Net Profit Distributed Equally, Remaining Fifty Percent Distributed in Proportion to Each Partner's Net Charges. Under this arrangement, net charges are defined as the amount of a partner's total charges to patients, including medical laboratory; X-ray; physiotherapy; electrocardiology; and other medical, diagnostic, and/or treatment, less any fee reductions or adjustment of charges to the patient's accounts. The ratio that a partner's net charges bear to the total net charges of all partners is computed on a calendar year basis. In the event that a partner dies or retires, or if the partnership is liquidated during the year, the net charge ratio of such partner(s) is determined at the end of the month following his death or withdrawal, or at date of liquidation, as set forth in Articles X, Y, and Z of the articles of partnership.

The partners participate in the group's profits as follows: 50 percent of the annual net profit of the partnership is distributed equally to all partners. The remaining 50 percent is distributed in the proportion that each partner's net charges bear to the total net charges of all the partners as set forth in Article Z.

Corporation

Of the forty-two groups responding to the poll, sixteen are corporations, with an average of 8.5 physicians. All the responding corporations are fee-for-service, with two groups offering a prepayment option. One is hospital-based.

The physician can be a salaried employee of a corporation but his relationship to the group is basically the same as it would be in a partnership. For example, only eight of the corporate groups actually use the word *salary* in describing their income distribution system. Nearly every group either considers all physicians to be equal members, or after a specified period of time usually allows a new physician to have an opportunity to achieve an equal basis in the corporation. This latter alternative is implemented in a variety of ways:

1. The physician proceeds through a number of annual longevity steps.
2. The physician pays for shares of stock, thereby eventually giving him equal ownership.
3. After the first year of employment the physician becomes a partner in the corporation.
4. Physicians are hired for one year on a salary basis; after completion of the year they proceed through progress steps to become senior physicians; after four years they are at an equal pay level.
5. A new physician joining the clinic is paid a salary which is considered to have no bonus elements in it; after a year in the group he is eligible for salary bonus elements.

Fifty percent of the corporate groups pay salaries, usually in combination with other distribution factors. Poll results disclose that the income distribution plans for corporations include numerous factors such as points, peer evaluation, bonuses, production, board certification, salary based on previous year's gross production, profit sharing, equal distribution, percentage of productivity, continuing education, maintenance of predetermined quarterly production, longevity, total billings, nonhospital patients (number examined and charged a fee), equal basis, and special consideration for low overhead specialty. Examples of specific income distribution systems for professional corporations responding to the survey are as follows:

Production Basis Distribution. This method of distribution may incorporate the following steps:

1. Gross collections minus adjusted expenses equal gross profit. Adjusted expenses do not include expenses for: physicians drawing accounts, pension expense, profit sharing expense, disability insurance, medical reimbursement expense, or bonuses.
2. An individual physician's gross bookings minus his collection accounts and miscellaneous discounts, divided by the total bookings of all physicians equals his percentage of total bookings. Laboratory and X-ray are included in gross bookings.
3. An individual physician's percentage of gross profits determines his gross income.
4. Individual gross income minus pension and profit sharing contributions, disability insurance premiums, and medical reimbursement expenses determines each physician's adjusted net income for the year.
5. Net income minus drawing account and prior bonuses determines actual income for the year.
6. Bonuses are paid quarterly, and salary checks are issued monthly, using a drawing account.

Straight Salary for Fixed Period Followed by Equal Stockholder Status. The physician is paid a straight salary for two years, and then becomes an equal stockholder, at which time he is no longer paid a cash salary. Upon becoming an equal shareholder, the physician begins to share in the accounts receivable growth of the group. In addition, at the end of two years and upon his obtaining equal corporate status, the physician's compensation is based upon his pro rata share of the group's monthly payroll, the amount of which is set by the board as funds are available and as new members attain equal status. Forty percent is paid at a level (equal) amount, and 50 percent is paid upon percentage of production (bookings) over the past two years, culminating with the most recent quarter's ending. This percentage is based on a comparison among other equal corporate owners. Ten percent of the compensation is based on fifty hours of annual, continuing medical education; if less than fifty hours is used, the value is prorated.

Basic Salary Plus Additional Compensation. Some groups, organized according to the corporate form, pay physicians a fixed monthly salary. Compensation in addition to the salary is determined at the end of each calendar year by first adding up all receipts of the center which have been collected during the year, some of which will be collections on accounts receivable from previous years. From that total are deducted all ordinary expenses, excluding basic salary paid to all stockholders, but including payments made on mortgages and debts; payments made on stock being purchased from department stockholders; severance payments made; disability payments made; any corporate payments on profit sharing or pension plans; and, in addition, $6,000 per year which is deposited in a savings account in the name of the center and intended as a contingency fund. After deductions have been made and distributable earnings have been determined, the distributable earnings are divided among and paid to the stockholders of the corporation as follows:

1. Forty percent is divided equally among the shareholders of the corporation as they exist at the end of each year.
2. Fifty percent is paid to the shareholders in accordance with the production of each during that year. Production includes medical, obstetrical, surgical, consultative services, and injections, but not laboratory, physical therapy, and other similar ancillary services. No credit toward production is given for X-rays, except when the physician ordering the X-rays reads out the film. In that case 40 percent of the total X-ray charge will be credited to that physician.
3. The remaining 10 percent of distributable earnings is paid to the shareholder employee on the basis of longevity. Maximum longevity will be five years. Two percent is allowed for each year up to five years. One year credit is given on longevity for each year of approved residency training, to a maximum of three years; one year credit is given for certification by an AMA approved certifying board. Except as indicated above, credit is given only for medical practice at XYZ Clinic, and for services on a full year's basis. The total longevity of all stockholders is computed first. Longevity of over five years is counted. Each physician then receives his portion of the 10 percent longevity distributable earnings.
4. At the end of each calendar quarter, an estimate of the distributable net earnings for the previous quarter is made and the estimated amount is paid to each professional associate-shareholder at that time by the group practice.

Previous Year's Gross Production. In this plan, physicians are paid a salary based on the previous year's gross production, less overhead. Available cash is distributed at year end to the profit sharing plan for all eligible employees, and cash bonuses are paid to each physician.

Salary Plus Monthly Bonus. Physicians are paid a base salary plus a monthly bonus based on production. The amount of the monthly bonus is determined by the board of directors. In order to qualify for the base salary, the physicians must maintain a quarterly production of a predetermined amount. If any physician fails to achieve this quarterly dollar amount, his base salary for the next quarter is adjusted downward by the percentage amount he failed to achieve during the prior quarter. A maximum of five hundred shares of stock may be purchased by any physician. New physicians who want to become stockholders may purchase one hundred shares per year over a five year period. Adjustment for Medicaid, Medicare, professional discounts, and accounts transferred for collection are subtracted from individual physicians' monthly production.

Total Income Less Expense. One-half of each physician's salary is determined on an equal distribution basis. The other half is derived from each physician's percentage of the total billings he has produced. At the end of the year, if there is a cash surplus it is recalculated into the 50 percent–50 percent formula.

Bonus Salary According to Point System. In corporate groups using this plan, a review of all physician salaries is conducted annually at the completion of the fiscal year, following an audit by an independent accounting firm. After the audit, physician remuneration is calculated and any necessary adjustments in base salaries are made.

The financial productivity (excluding lab tests and X-ray procedures ordered) of each physician is determined, and each department's direct overhead (excluding physician salaries and fringe benefits) is calculated and divided equally among the physicians in that department. Indirect overhead for the department is allocated according to the gross billings. If a physician's financial production exceeds the total expense of his salary, fringe benefits, and his share of the department's direct and indirect expenses, he is then eligible for bonus salary participation and a possible increase in his base salary. That portion of salary and fringe benefits attributable to the time spent on medical practice administrative duties is adjusted from the calculation. Usually, the physician does not receive an increase in base salary if it appears that such an increase will make him ineligible for bonus salary participation a year later. It is through the use of bonus salary participation that physicians are provided with incentive. Bonus salary for those eligible is calculated according to a point system. Factors used to determine points include:

Educational leave (must take eight days minimum for credit)	2 points
Teaching (based on one afternoon a week for six months per year)	2 points
On-call rotation (by department)	2 points
Net production (for each $2,500 production above base expenses)	1 point

Board certification (for duration of certification)	4 points
Subspecialty certification (for duration of certification period)	2 points
Community activities (director—nonprofit corporation)	1 point
Clinic practice administrative duties (officer, committees, etc.)	1 point

Prepayment

Compensation in a prepaid professional corporation is quite similar to that in a prepaid partnership. Variations between the weighing of compensation factors usually are influenced by the degree of fee-for-service income versus prepaid capitation, and by whether prepayment income is in fact received and distributed in a fee-for-service mode. Prepayment philosophy suggests that income will be distributed on some basis other than fee-for-service. The assumption is that payment to the group will be in the form of a capitation payment for provision of medical care and service. Under such circumstances, income distribution is based neither on productivity nor on services rendered, but rather on other criteria more closely related to those used in the evaluation of employed physicians. A group may accept a capitation payment for the care and service of a voluntarily enrolled population, however, and then compensate individual partners or members on a productivity or fee-for-service basis.

The poll results indicate that of all responding three to ten physician groups, less than 1 percent are involved in prepayment. The current Health Maintenance Organization federal law and the concept behind the prepayment mode do not appear conducive to small group involvement. The prepaid medical group usually must assume responsibility for providing a full range of medical and surgical care offered by the prepaid health plan. This extent of care requires a breadth of specialization and primary care which usually is unavailable in the forming group practice.

Hospital-Based Practices

Most of the partnership and corporation compensation elements discussed previously will apply to hospital-based group practices, whether fee-for-service or prepaid. The basic difference usually will be in the manner in which income is distributed from laboratory, X-ray, and other ancillary services. Generally, these services are provided and controlled by the hospital organization; however, if the hospital-based group practice acquires and operates its own ancillaries, the compensation alternatives still differ only slightly, if at all, from those arrangements described previously.

Unincorporated Association and Professional Association

Less than 1 percent of the groups polled were unincorporated or professional associations. Furthermore, responding professional associations distribute income much the same as the partnerships and corporations who responded to the survey. Benefits also are similar to those indicated by the partnerships and corporations. As a further illustration of these similarities, the following example of an income distribution plan for the unincorporated association is presented:

> Physicians receive compensation every two weeks; residual funds are distributed according to the production of each member, with the previous quarter used as a base. Adjustments are made from what is collected and the charges made; Medicare may pay only 90 percent of the billed charges. In addition, individual credit is given for every use of each department, such as:
>
> 50% credit in X-ray; 50% is expense.
> 53% credit in lab; 47% is the cost of operation.
> 80% credit in EKG department; 20% is expense.
> 25% credit in surgery department; 75% is expense.
> 15% of total wages goes into profit sharing.

PROFESSIONAL COURTESY

Those services usually included in the realm of professional courtesy are services provided to group physician staff members and their families. An important issue in this area is whether professional courtesy will be represented by an assignment of insurance benefits, a true courtesy among professionals, or a combination thereof.

Medical and surgical insurance coverage, whether personal or part of a group plan, is becoming more prevalent among physicians and their families. It is assumed, however, that professional courtesy is limited to services provided within the center rather than those that are subject to billing by outside providers. Consequently, while professional courtesy may be rendered and reimbursed through insurance coverage, because the amount received may not equal the usual charges, additional consideration is necessary to determine whether the insurance benefits received by the group will be accepted in full satisfaction of the courtesy service. In addition, for various reasons, not all group physicians and/or their families may be covered by personal or group medical insurance.

The forming group should remember that claims submitted to an insurance company through a group insurance policy, for medical care and service on behalf of the group, could result in policy premium increases. As a result, through premium payments and through the additional costs of preparing and processing claims, the group may be paying premiums for the care they themselves are providing. Although professional courtesy may represent a compensation or benefit to the group physician and his family, it also might constitute a monetary cost as well as a time expense for the group.

Initially, new groups tend to assume attitudes based on the various members' experiences with professional courtesy and payment for such services. Policy decisions are certainly necessary in this area and should be flexible enough to accommodate for the group's growth. The group physician's family may be extended professional courtesy by the group; however, limitations on the amount and degree of services may be required. The following are examples of such limitations in policy:

1. Insurance is filed and payment is retained by the group.
2. Physician's immediate family includes only his wife.
3. All family members receive medical care at no charge and medical drugs and supplies at our cost.
4. Professional courtesy consists only of physician's services not covered by insurance. Ancillary services are billed.
5. Insurance benefits will be accepted as full payment for services; however, special items may be charged at cost (e.g., contact lenses).[9]

In addition to professional courtesy for group physicians and their families, some groups may wish to extend courtesy in varying degrees to group employees and other community physicians and their families. Again, this type of courtesy may represent a form of compensation to the group physician providing the service. For example, in a group setting where productivity is a criterion for the amount of physician compensation and the group elects to provide courtesy service to employees, some method for crediting the providing physician(s) must be devised in order to realize the group objective. The physician contributing courtesy services endorsed by the group may receive credit for those services, as he would for any other patient service. Revenue for the services, however, may or may not be received by the group.

INCOME FROM SOURCES OTHER THAN THE GROUP PRACTICE

The group's organizational agreements, charter, and bylaws usually contain provisions relating to a physician's receiving outside income. In addition, should the group decide to use employment contracts or agreements for group physicians, guidelines relating to outside income probably would be included in the provisions. An example salary agreement is contained in Medical Group Management Association's *Digest of Medical Group Employment Contracts and Income Distribution Plans.* Its treatment of outside income is quite general, but it does contain the implication that such income, if related to medical practice, is considered to be group practice income. In addition to income made available through medical services not rendered within the group practice setting, income received through teaching, research, and honorariums must be accounted for by the group.

In the authors' poll of small group practices, responses regarding outside activities included:

1. Each partner shall perform his duties faithfully and to the best of his ability, and shall devote all of his services in the practice of medicine to the business, and for the account of, the partnership, which shall receive all fees, charges, accounts receivable, payments, salaries and remuneration for said services (partnership).
2. All income which a doctor earns which is connected in any way with his medical expertise is remitted to the clinic and the doctor is given credit for the like amount in his bookings for each month (partnership).

Although the examples cited above indicated that all outside income earned by individual group physicians is considered to be group practice income, the final decision rests with each individual group. The important issue is to ensure that income received from outside sources receives proper and adequate consideration in the group's compensation planning.

This chapter concludes the discussion of criteria for forming and planning the operation of a group practice. The material presented here is designed to assist the planners in making decisions consistent with the group's choice on mission, legal organizational form, management structure, facility ownership, and financial planning. The final chapter in this section is concerned with policy planning and the integration of established goals and objectives into a composite policy plan from which operational decisions can evolve.

❊ *Chapter 10*

Policy Planning

POLICY DEVELOPMENT PROCESS

The process of planning and formulating effective policies is vital to a newly forming medical group practice. Only through group consensus and the careful consideration of policy planning and implementation can a group's founders ensure effective overall operation of the practice in both the present and the future. The previous six chapters have described critical issues involved in the strategic planning activity of a newly formed group practice. While the discussion has focused on the planning process relating to the group's established mission and objectives, it is the result of this process—the strategy or strategies adopted—which provides the basis from which operating policies can be developed. The purpose of this chapter is to provide those individuals contemplating medical group practice with an awareness of the importance of yet another planning process—the development of policies. A discussion of how various policies emanate from the group's mission and a demonstration of how policies provide guidance in the establishment of the group's structure and procedures should serve to emphasize the significance of carefully developing administrative, professional, and patient care policies.

It is important for the forming medical group to be familiar with exactly what policies are and how they differ from other elements to be considered in developing effective policies. The concept of policy is defined as a *statement of operating principles* by which a group intends to realize its objectives and goals. Policies provide a framework whereby the group's definitive objectives and goals can be realized within the constraints of internal and external influences and organizational functions (strategies). The effective use of any policy depends upon its logical and formal process of development. This process is represented conceptually in the following diagram:

1. Group Mission (primary purpose or focus—abstract)
   ↘
2. Group Objectives (more specific—what, how much, and why)
   ↘
3. Group Strategies (how)
   ↘
4. Group Policies (operational guidelines)
   ↘
5. Group Structure (who is responsible)
   ↘
6. Group Procedures (detailed operational instructions)

After establishing a group mission, objectives must be developed which convey to all clinic personnel exactly what and/or how much must be accomplished in both the long- and short-term operation of the group. Members of a medical group appear to feel more satisfied in their interpersonal relationships, and the group itself has a better chance of being successful, if organizational objectives are clearly established and acknowledged by all individuals concerned. Success or viability in this context is defined as the ability to attract and hold physicians over significant periods of time. Donald H. DuBois reports that in order to prevent loss of viability which occurs as a result of role conflict and dissatisfaction, organizational objectives must be congruent with the personal objectives of the group members and must be both known and understood by the members.

> Successful groups were found to have had clearly formulated objectives. These objectives were expressed to recruits willing to serve the stated organizational objectives. In the establishment of group policies and the resolution of management problems, organizational objectives served as a basis for judgement (*sic*). The nature of the objectives served by the highly viable medical groups was distinctly professional. Financial success for physician participants, leisure, professional advancement and relative status all were important aspirations implicit in the group structure, but professional excellence, patient service, and practice of "good" medicine, were the *principal* objectives and the ultimate criteria for decision making.[1]

If policies are to serve as guidelines for the realization of objectives, it is necessary that the group practice be organized to facilitate this process. An employee cannot be expected to abide by or to implement policies for which he is not responsible and of which he is unaware. Policies cannot be effective, therefore, unless the organization is structured to communicate and implement its policies and unless the employees are aware of their responsibilities, authority, and prerogatives. Policies should be formulated by individuals or by a group with the appropriate authority and commensurate responsibility to do so, and should be documented in writing with a provision for periodic evaluation. The effectiveness of clinic policies can be determined only through the measurement of their results; if a policy is not guiding activities in the desired direction, it must be modified, replaced, or perhaps abandoned. Well formulated, well written policies can mean the difference between a smoothly functioning clinic and one in continued crisis or chaos. Flexibility, comprehensiveness, ease of coordination, adherence to professional ethics, and conservation of both physicians' and managers' time constitute the foundations of successful policy formulation.

DETERMINATION OF POLICIES ESSENTIAL TO A MEDICAL GROUP

Although considerable documented information exists regarding organizational policy formulation in general, little of this material applies directly to group practice and its development. As a result, in preparation for this text a list of policy areas relevant to the formation of a medical group practice was compiled through a search of the existing literature and a survey of center administrators. The initial literature search revealed that approximately thirty policy areas are considered important in the area of group practice.

1. Accounting and Billing Procedures
2. Appointment Scheduling
3. Credit and Collection Procedures
4. Third Party Relationships
5. Clinic Organization
6. Clinic Forms
7. Clinic Procedures
8. Communication in Clinics
9. Community Relations in a Clinic
10. Employee Compensation and Benefits
11. Relationships with Consultants
12. Data Processing in Clinics
13. Employees (manuals, job skills, teaching and training)
14. Engineering and Maintenance
15. Equal Employment
16. Medical and Office Equipment
17. Fees and Charges Policies
18. Financial Planning and Management
19. Hospital and Clinic Relations
20. Physician Income Distribution
21. Insurance for the Group
22. Patient Relations
23. Pension Plans
24. Medical Records
25. Personnel Management
26. Physician-Manager Relations
27. Purchasing Policies
28. Physician Recruitment
29. Taxation
30. The group's Long Range Objectives and Growth

Group practice administration activities usually become more uniform when governed by established policies. When activities involving routine decisions by management are regulated by policy, the administrator becomes free to give his attention to more complex activities such as long range planning and market/product research. A subsequent literature review, in the area of group practice administration, resulted in a corollary list of activities more specifically associated with group management activities. These activities closely parallel many of the policy areas listed above:

1. Market Research
2. Product Research
3. Long Range Planning
4. Public Relations
5. Obtaining Working Capital and Collections
6. Recruiting Professionals and Physicians
7. Decisions Regarding Managerial Salaries
8. Devising Work Procedures for Professionals
9. Devising Work Procedures for Non-professionals
10. Promoting/Rewarding Professionals/Managers
11. Employee/Management Development and Training
12. Motivating/Directing Immediate Subordinates
13. Dealing with Personal/Interpersonal Problems
14. Decisions Regarding Charges/Prices for Services, etc.
15. Decisions Regarding New Construction
16. Creating/Changing Professional Jobs/Units
17. Decisions Regarding Changes in Decision/Authority Structures
18. Decisions Regarding Financial/Managerial Information System
19. Influencing Decisions of Board/Owners
20. Arbitration between Internal Units, Departments
21. Influencing Decisions Made by Medical Staff
22. Arbitration between Policy-Making Groups

None of the material reviewed, however, yielded an adequate discussion of policies and/or policy areas critical to group formation, and it became evident that a survey of existing group practices would be necessary. A survey questionnaire was designed utilizing the list of policy areas assembled from the group practice literature, the list of activity areas related to clinic administration, tion, and information derived from interviews with group practice administrators. The resulting questionnaire (see figure 10-1) was sent to a random sample of group practices selected from the Medical Group Management Association's *International Directory* and from the American Medical Association's *Listing of Group Practices.* The respondents were asked to rank in order of importance for a newly forming group the twenty policy areas listed, as well as any policy area considered important but omitted from the survey. The rate of response to the survey was 80 percent. The results of the survey, indicating the numerical ranking of the twenty policy areas by the administrators—with position one as most important to position twenty as least important—are shown in Table 10-1. Approximately one-half of the respondents ranked policy areas associated with

The following is a list of "policy areas." **Please review and add any areas you feel we may not have considered.** Items following each area listed in parentheses are presented as examples of that particular area and are not meant to be all inclusive. **DO NOT PROCEED TO THE NEXT PAGE UNTIL YOU HAVE FINISHED REVIEWING THE POLICY AREAS BELOW.**

1. **ACCOUNTING POLICIES** (Cash or Accrual accounting system, accounting standards and procedures, etc.) __________
2. **POLICIES FOR MEDICAL SERVICE FEES** (Standard fee schedule, deviations from standard charges, discounts and allowances, third party payments, etc.) __________
3. **FINANCIAL POLICIES** (Budgets, long range financing, relationships with banks, group liquidity, capital structure, taxes, outside investments, etc.) __________
4. **INTERNAL CONTROL POLICIES** (Petty cash, cash receipts, cash disbursements, accounts receivable, accounts payable, reports and records, supplies handling, appointments, telephone procedures, etc.) __________
5. **DATA PROCESSING POLICIES** (E.D.P. or machine accounting, evaluating E.D.P. systems, input and output requirements, equipment selection and modification, computer service bureau or in house capability, etc.) __________
6. **CREDIT AND COLLECTION POLICIES** (Open account, installment plans, use of national credit cards, credit restrictions, billing and collection procedures, follow-up routine, aging accounts, etc.) __________
7. **POLICIES TO GOVERN THE ADDITION OR REDUCTION OF PROFESSIONAL STAFF** (Restrictive covenants, buy-in/buy-out policies, etc.) __________
8. **POLICIES TO GOVERN CLINIC GROWTH** (Long-range objectives, periodic review of progress, etc.) __________
9. **POLICIES TO GOVERN ADDITION OF ANCILLARY SERVICES** (Criteria to determine need, schedule for review, patient load required, etc.) __________
10. **POLICIES ON RELATIONSHIPS WITH EXTERNAL CONSULTANTS** (Accountants, attorneys, management consultants, system consultants, etc.) __________
11. **POLICIES ON STAFF CONDUCT BOTH IN AND OUT OF CLINIC** (Referrals to other physicians and sevices both inside and outside the clinic, memberships in civic and charitable organizations, etc.) __________
12. **POLICIES ON FACILITY MAINTENANCE** (Preventive maintenance, operational maintenance, etc.) __________
13. **POLICIES ON ORGANIZATION STRUCTURE AND TYPE** (Developing an organization chart, communicating it to staff, criteria for organization structure, reviewing present organization type, i.e. partnership or corporation, etc.) __________
14. **NON-PHYSICIAN PERSONNEL POLICIES** (Recruiting, selection, orientations, formal and informal lines of communications, training, performance evaluation, promotions, fringe benefits, etc.) __________
15. **POLICIES ON RESOLVING CONFLICTS BETWEEN STAFF MEMBERS AND PATIENTS OR OTHER STAFF MEMBERS** (Grievances, personality conflicts, etc.) __________
16. **POLICIES ON WAGE AND SALARY ADMINISTRATION FOR NON-PHYSICIAN STAFF** (Job descriptions, increases and decreases in compensation, minimum wage, overtime, work week standards, etc.) __________
17. **POLICIES ON PHYSICIANS COMPENSATION** (Income distribution for physicians, bonuses, profit-sharing, etc.) __________
18. **POLICIES TO GOVERN CLINIC PUBLIC RELATIONS** (Who's responsible, relations with patients, relations with community, relations with other health care organizations, staff's relationship with professional organizations, i.e. MGMA, A M A , etc.) __________
19. **PURCHASING POLICIES** (Who's responsible, specifications for equipment and supplies, quantity and quality of purchases, sources of equipment and supplies, relationships with detail persons, inventory control, etc.) __________
20. **POLICIES ON INSURANCE** (Insuring equipment, insuring employees, etc.) __________
21. **OTHER POLICY AREAS:**______________________________

Figure 10–1. Survey Questionnaire Used to Identify Primary Policy Areas in Group Practice Administration

positions eight through twenty at ten or greater; consequently, the following seven policy areas appear to be those most critical to center organization and development:

Position	*Policy Area*
1	Policies on Organization Structure and Type
2	Policies on Physician Compensation

Table 10-1. Final Results and Dispersion of Policy Area Survey

Position	*Policy Areas*	*Median*	*Difference*
1	Policies on Organization Structure and Type	2.64	
2	Policies on Physician Compensation	3.21	0.57
**			
3	Policies to Govern the Addition or Reduction of Professional Staff	5.77	2.56
**			
4	Policies for Medical Service Fees	7.22	1.45
5	Financial Policies	7.45	0.23
6	Accounting Policies	8.33	0.88
7	Policies to Govern Clinic Growth	8.57	0.24
**			
8	Nonphysician Personnel Policies	9.79	1.22
9	Internal Control Policies	10.00	0.21
10	Policies on Wage and Salary Administration for Nonphysician Staff	10.18	0.18
11	Credit and Collection Policies	10.28	0.10
**			
12	Policies on Resolving Conflicts Between Staff Members and Patients or Other Staff	11.75	1.47
**			
13	Policies to Govern Addition of Ancillary Services	12.96	1.21
14	Policies on Staff Conduct Both in and out of Clinic	13.30	0.34
15	Policies to Govern Clinic Public Relations	14.00	0.70
**			
16	Purchasing Policies	15.27	1.27
17	Data Processing Policies	15.86	0.59
18	Policies on Relationships with External Consultants	16.27	0.41
**			
19	Policies on Insurance	17.66	1.39
20	Policies on Facility Maintenance	17.66	-0-

(**Break Point)

Position	*Policy Area*
3	Policies to Govern the Addition or Reduction of Professional Staff
4	Policies for Medical Service Fees
5	Financial Policies
6	Accounting Policies
7	Policies to Govern the Group's Growth

This is not to imply that policy positions eight through twenty are unimportant to group operation; all twenty areas are important for effective planning. The results of the survey, however, strongly suggest that in the initial planning phases some areas are more important than others and should be given commensurate attention. The survey questionnaire (see figure 10-1), also provided an "other policy area" item to allow the respondent either to add policy areas not represented in the survey or to make comments. The responses in this category were evaluated closely and summarized to represent subsets of the twenty policy areas listed on the questionnaire. Table 10-2 lists these subset policy items.

It should be noted that various factors can influence an administrator's perception of the importance attached to any particular policy area. Size of the group practice, its legal organization and operational mode, as well as the age of the group affect policy decisions. Large medical groups may consider policies relating to data processing as highly important because effective operation can be impeded by a lack of well-established guidelines in this area. Smaller groups,

Table 10-2. Subset Policy Items Generated from "Other" Category in Policy Area Survey

Physician Orientation	Bylaws or Articles of Partnership (when group is being organized)
Appointment Scheduling	Relationship of Administrator to Staff and to Ancillary Personnel
In-Service Education	Policies on Clinic Procedures (patient flow, etc.)
Separation or Termination (physicians & non-M.D.)	Examples of various "forms" needed (charge slips, lab slips, registration forms, statements, etc.)
Training (physician and non-M.D.)	Physician Professional Duties (regular duties, weekend, trading duties, attending professional meetings, vacations, extended absences)
Peer Review	Staff Meetings
Financial Reporting	Physician Recruiting (methods of recruiting, i.e., professional search organizations, classified ads, university contacts, etc.; qualification or credential standards)
Governing Board	Policies on Staff Members' Relations (M.D.s)
Vacations for Physicians	Physician Employment Agreements (reciprocal specific obligations of corporation and employees; termination of employment, etc.)
Physicians Personnel Policies (vacation, sick leave, sabbatical leave, meeting time, meeting expense)	Quality of Care
Physicians Benefits (life insurance, disability insurance, medical, and hospital)	Entertainment (who does it, who pays what dollar allowance?)
Recruiting and Indoctrinating New Physicians	Who Authorizes Publications Bearing the Clinic Name?
Administrators Wage, Benefits, Authority, Job Security	Expansion of Facilities (building, departments, staff, equipment)
Management and Supervision of Outside Investments by the Group	Retirement (physician and lay staff)
Establish Policy with Hospitals for Orderly Exchange of Information	Employee Unions: Reaction to Organization Efforts, Negotiating Efforts if Unionized
Establish Liaison with Other Local Clinics	Governmental Relations
Fringe Benefit Plans for Incorporated Groups	Work Day Time Schedules of Clinic and Physicians (hrs. open to public, app't. schedule, absences for vacations, meetings, etc.)
Clinic Building Program (lease, build, size, location)	Teaching and Hospital Affiliation (med. school students in group practice)
Labor Relations	
Limitation to Number of Meetings (local, national, international)	
Medical Records and Review (problem-oriented records)	
Non-Physician Continuing Education (meetings, seminars, courses, etc.)	

however, may find manual systems most adequate and therefore would consider policies relating to data processing relatively unimportant. Requirements associated with legal organizational form can serve as the basis for policies; consequently, policies concerning clinic structure may be more important to a group formed as a professional corporation than to a group formed as a sole proprietorship. In addition, the hospital-based group practice may determine that policies relating to the hospital are of greatest importance; on the other hand, establishing such policies may not be necessary at all if the hospital's existing policies are adopted for use by the group practice. Recently formed groups may be more concerned with immediate operational policy considerations, such as establishing an organizational structure and determining a physician compensation plan, than with long-range policies designed to govern the group's growth.

Geographic location can play a role in policy formation. The size of the community serviced by the group will directly affect the ranking of policies governing clinic growth, addition of ancillary services, and addition to or reduction of professional staff. The size and configuration of the group's physical plant also will influence policy-ranking rationale. If a group practice administrator has been confronted with the transfer of reports and records among satellite clinics, he may be inclined to rank the policies regarding internal control high in importance. An administrator with only one facility and a central record system, however, may not adhere to the same ordering of priorities. The predispositions of the group's policy formulators will greatly influence their assignment of importance to policy areas. Policy formulators with an interest and background in accounting probably will consider that area more important than will those individuals with a primary interest in personnel. A policy making body, such as the executive board or the policy committee, composed of members preoccupied with outside investments, may stress financial policies in their group's development. All of the factors discussed above represent potential influences upon perceived importance, and it should be pointed out that some or all of those mentioned may have affected the administrators' responses in the survey. The results (Table 10-2) can be most helpful if viewed as indicators of potentially important policy areas. The following discussion will consider each of the seven policy areas in the order in which they were ranked in the survey, beginning with the policy area selected by administrators as most important—organizational structure and type.

Organizational Structure and Type

The structuring of authority relationships and formal communication channels in the group practice depend upon the care and planning with which such policies are initiated. A chart of the design and documentation of the group's organizational structure is an important first step. It is imperative that organizational structure be well thought out and thoroughly familiar to all organization members. If properly designed, the organizational chart provides a graphic representation of the lines of authority, responsibility, and formal communication operating within the clinic. In the absence of such a structural design or because of failure to make the design known and understood by all employees, organizational dysfunction can result. An informal communication network or grapevine may develop and may gain credibility, resulting in the transmission

Table 10-3. List of Medical Specialties in Group Practice Used by Medical Group Management Association

Administrative Medicine	Aviation Medicine
Allergy	Cardiovascular Disease
Anesthesiology	Child Psychiatry
Colon and Rectal Surgery	Dermatology
Diagnostic Radiology	Family Practice
Gastroenterology	Forensic Pathology
Internal Medicine	General Practice
Neurology	General Surgery
Obstetrics and Gynecology	Neurological Surgery
Ophthalmology	Nuclear Medicine
Otolaryngology	Occupational Medicine
Pediatrics	Orthopaedic Surgery
Pediatric Cardiology	Pathology
Plastic Surgery	Pediatric Allergy
Preventive Medicine	Physical Medicine and Rehabilitation
Radiology	Psychiatry
Thoracic Surgery	Pulmonary Diseases
	Therapeutic Radiology
	Urology

Other specialties are recognized, but information on them has not been collected by the Medical Group Management Association.

of inaccurate information. If individuals in the group practice develop power inappropriate to their authority, power struggles can ensue, inevitably resulting in conflict.

Organizational charts may be functionally, geographically, or client based. *Functionally* organized group practices usually are established according to departments related to each specialty represented; ancillary services are represented by separate departments or may be grouped under a single department. Although a number of various structural designs is possible, the main criterion for design is the division into departments of those activities having different staff and equipment requirements. Many specialties currently exist and new ones continually come into being. A list currently in use by MGMA is shown in Table 10-3. In addition, Table 10-4 delineates the various services which may be provided in a medical group practice setting. These services usually fall directly under the authority of either the medical director or the group administrator. Specialties and services remain the same regardless of the structural design, but their position in the organization chart and their commensurate authority relationships with other group functions will vary. An example of the functionally designed organization chart is presented in figure 10-2.

To facilitate ease in communication and control, some groups are organized according to *geographical* location. This type of design indicates the physical location of subunits of the organization, often referred to as divisions. The geographic design is used most appropriately when multiple or satellite facilities are involved (see figure 10-3), and usually is combined with other designs. *Client-* or *customer*-based designs are used when one particular client group accounts for a large percentage of the group's activity, as in a prepaid medical plan. If a client group accounts for a large percentage of the clinic's activity, it

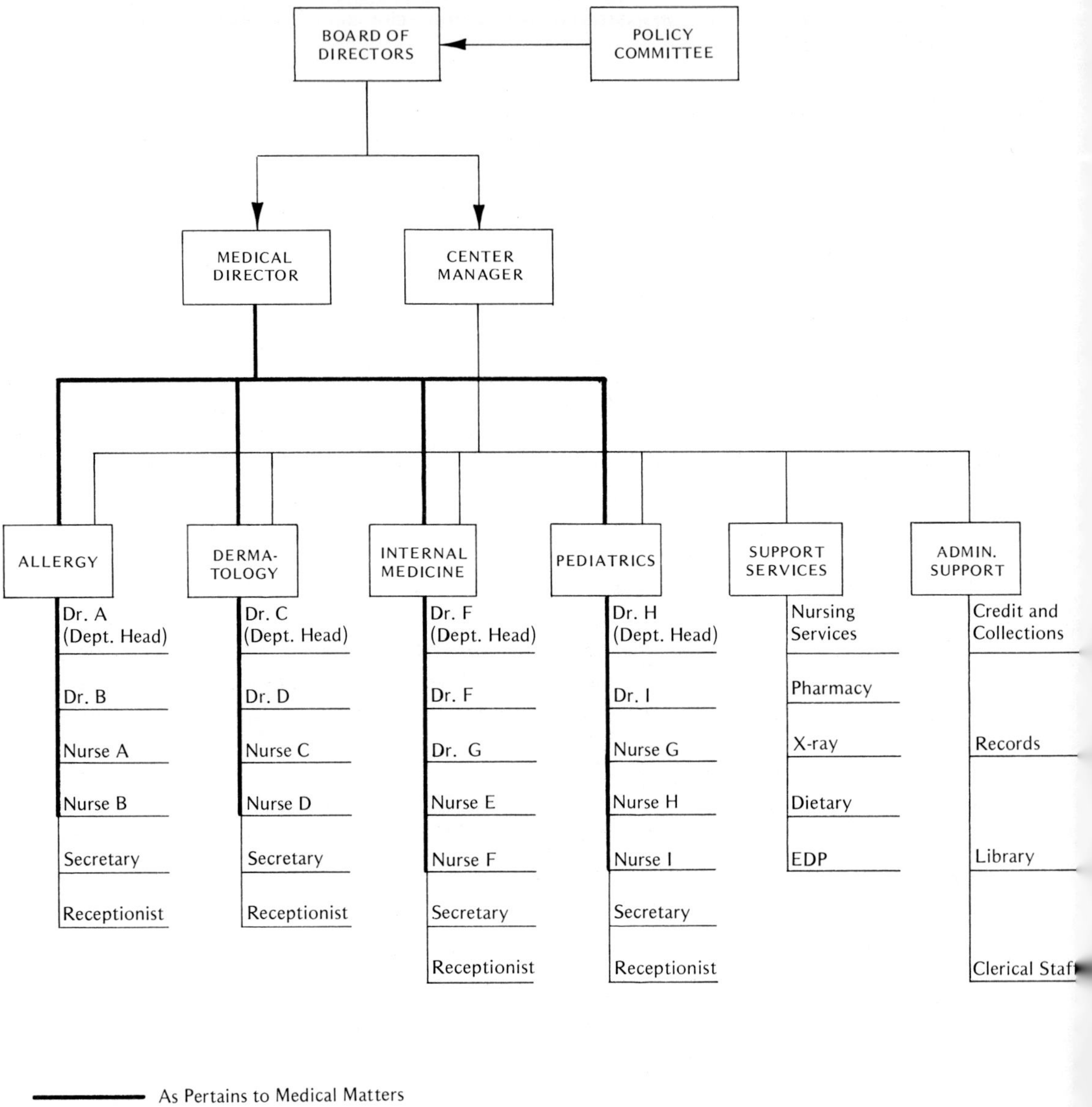

Figure 10-2. Group Practice Organizational Diagram According to Function

may be more efficient and less expensive to establish a facility and department designed exclusively to handle this segment of the group's business.

To better understand the policy development process, consider a hypothetical situation in which a newly formed group proceeds through the process of establishing a mission, determining objectives, creating strategies, and developing policies. The group is composed of four physicians who, with the assistance of an attorney, have adopted the partnership as a legal form. Two specialties are represented in the group, and the needs present in the community (population 40,000) have been determined. The group members have decided to re-

Table 10-4. List of Medical Group Services Compiled by Medical Group Management Association

Diagnostic radiology	After-hours emergency room
Therapeutic radiology	Research and/or education foundation
Laboratory	Center sponsored prepaid medical care program
Pathology laboratory	Dietary services
Isotopes	Home visiting nurse service
Physical therapy	Insurance, credit, and accounting
Pharmacy	
Optical dispensary	
Brace shop	
Dental facilities	
Occupational therapy	
Psychology	
Social work	
Psychiatric social work	

main in the community in which they previously had been in solo practice. Due to the size of the group and a scarcity of capital, a single facility with limited laboratory and X-ray services was designed after consulting with an architect. Two of the physicians have expressed an interest in business matters and have taken related courses at the local university. The remaining two physicians prefer that a professional manager handle the business affairs. It is decided, therefore, to establish an executive board composed of all the partners, with a policy committee comprised of the two business-oriented physicians.

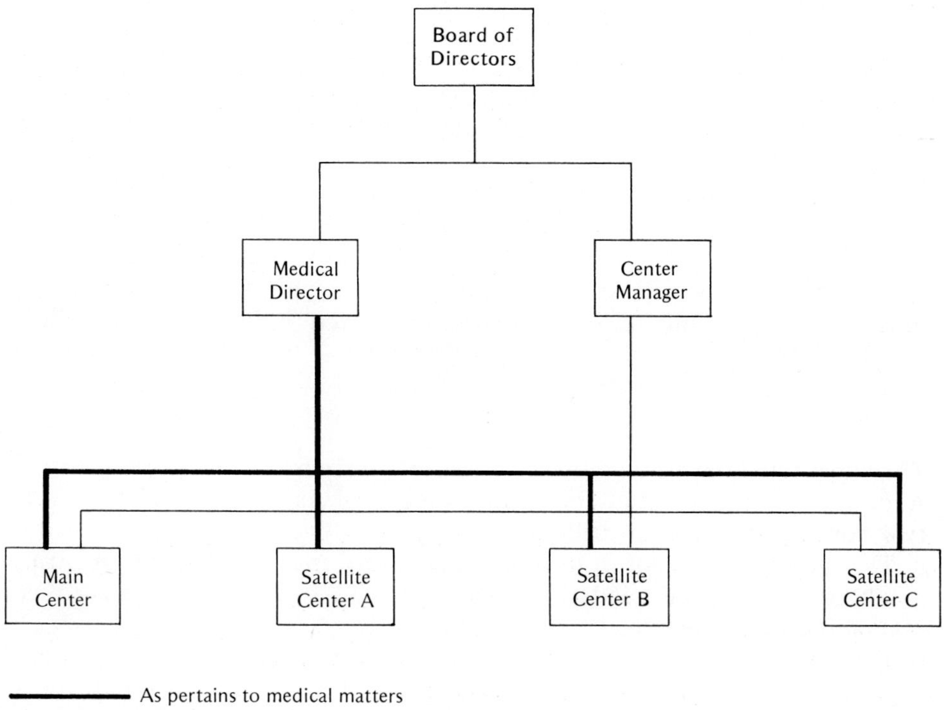

Figure 10-3. Group Practice Organizational Diagram According to Geography

After further discussion the group agrees that a professional administrator is needed. A consensus on the group mission is reached quickly: to provide high quality health care to those members of the community who are capable of providing remuneration under a short-term credit arrangement. *Clinic objectives based on the mission statement* and possible strategies are now developed as outlined in the policy development process (see page 260). In addition to re-evaluating the decision to form a legal partnership in light of the chosen mission and objectives, this newly formed group also is confronted with issues relating to physician recruitment and staff compensation. The final strategies upon which the group has decided, together with the objectives the strategies are designed to fulfill, appear below:

Objective 1: The clinic staff shall provide comprehensive, specialty-oriented medical services of the highest quality, constantly improving in excellence.	*Strategy*: Recruitment to meet patient demand shall focus on board certified candidates. The group shall be organized as a legal partnership.
Objective 2: The clinic shall provide its physicians with an income substantially related to individual productive effort and sufficient to provide an adequate standard of living with relative security in times of disability or retirement.	*Strategy:* All physicians shall receive a monthly salary established by the board and be paid an incentive bonus based on productivity.

The above example is illustrative of the kinds of decisions which initially must be made by forming groups before policy can be established. Continuing the process through the development of policies, consider that the four physicians in this hypothetical situation are practicing in a single facility with limited support personnel; therefore, a functional structural design is most appropriate. A medical director is not recommended for a group that is relatively small and in which medical matters and policies can be discussed with the entire executive board. Although in a group of this size many differing tasks will be performed by each individual, thus eliminating the need for subdepartments and sections with section heads, it will prove beneficial for the administration to delineate tasks assigned to each individual. The resultant organization structure chart is shown in figure 10-4. Policy statements pertaining to this established structure may include:

1. The executive board shall consist of all full partners in the group.
2. A policy committee shall be established and shall consist of no less than two nor more than seven full partners.
   a. This committee shall determine areas, both medical and administrative, where policies are needed, and shall formulate such policies for recommendation to the executive board.
   b. This committee shall be receptive to suggestions concerning areas in which policies are needed, and suggested policies from other partners and group personnel.

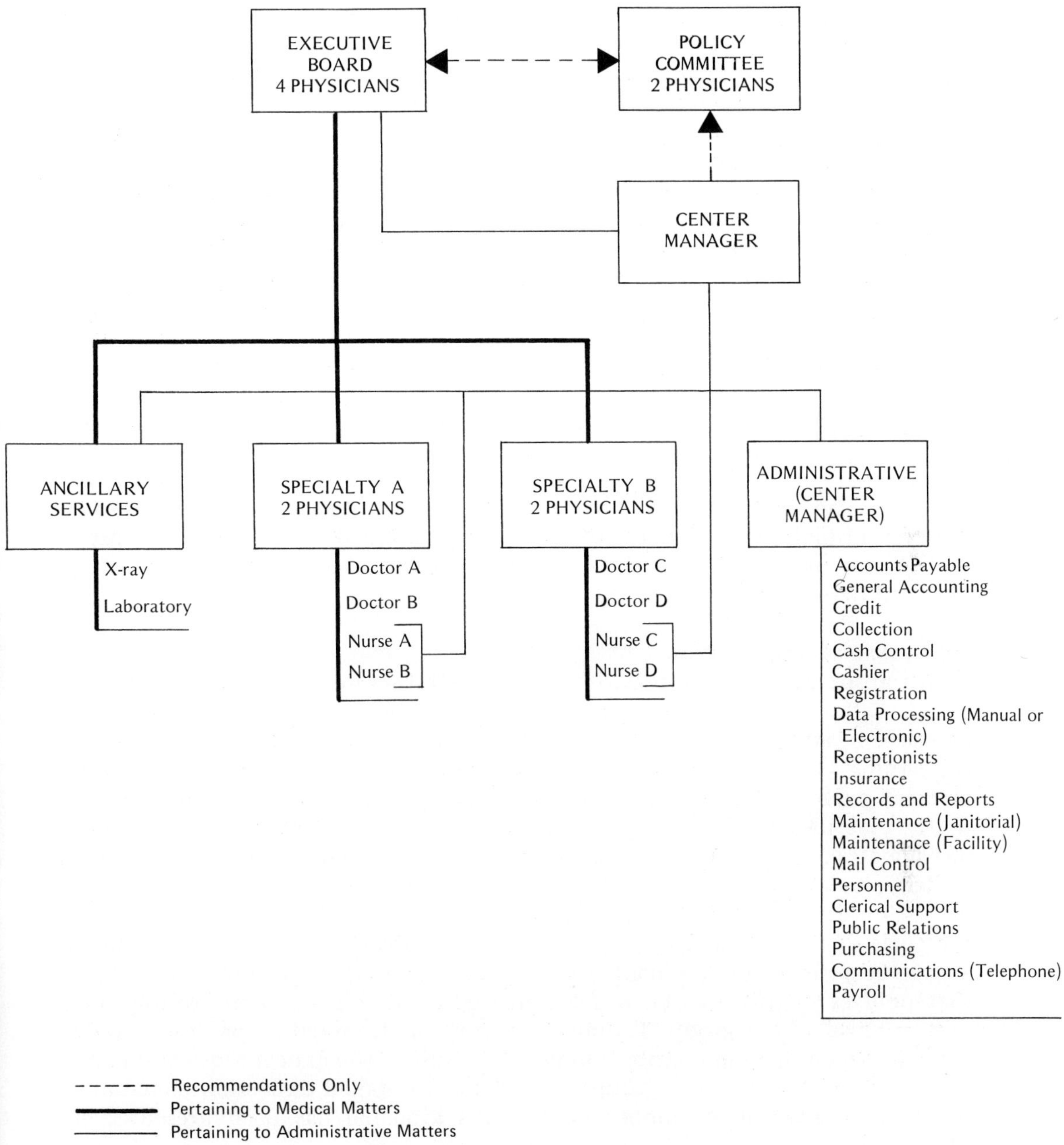

Figure 10-4. Example of Detailed Organizational Chart for Group Practice

3. A group administrator shall be employed and charged with the responsibility for all matters pertaining to the administrative aspects of group operations.
4. The group shall be structured along functional lines with each function being designated a department.
5. Department personnel shall be under the jurisdiction of the group adminis-

trator when administrative functions are concerned and under the executive board when medical matters are concerned.

6. The current organizational structure shall be evaluated annually to determine if it adequately facilitates the achievement of group goals.
7. The existing structure shall be expanded, modified, or completely revamped based upon the results of the above evaluation.
8. The organizational form shall be reviewed at two year intervals with an attorney and an accountant to determine if another organizational form would be more conducive to the achievement of group goals.
9. The organizational chart shall be formally prepared and distributed to all employees.
10. Responsibility and commensurate authority as well as formal lines of business communication shall correspond to those shown in the organization chart.

It would require several volumes to provide a complete set of policy statements for all possible combinations of circumstances in the area of group organization and type. The above example, however, should illustrate the process involved in policy formulation. Evaluation and modification are key concepts in this process; developing effective policies is an evolutionary process, not a revolutionary one, and time and experience are valued allies.

Physician Compensation

In the survey described previously, administrators surveyed ranked physician compensation as the second most important policy area in forming a group practice. In addition, many of the group administrators reported that problems concerning compensation have been responsible for the dissolution of more medical groups than has any other single item. It also was mentioned consistently that in actuality income distribution can be one of the most difficult decisions facing the group. Equal income for all members may be attractive initially, but usually leads to dissension. Careful thought and a great deal of discussion are required prior to reaching consensus on this very crucial matter; the goals of individual group members and the objectives of the group should act as the primary determinants of the plan chosen. It is imperative, therefore, that policies in this area be well-formulated at the outset to ensure the long-term survival of the group. The initial step in the formulation process is to determine which income distribution plan best fulfills the expectations and needs of the physicians and the group's founders. A detailed discussion concerning the various alternative compensation plans available has been presented in Chapter 9.

Primary factors affecting compensation policy are the types of specialties and the predispositions of group members. High producers must be rewarded for their efforts; high revenue generators—specialties involving low patient volume but generating high revenue—also must be recognized. It may be that specialties incurring high relative cost may be required to bear a greater percentage of total group expenses. Finally, compensation for physicians within the group must be reasonably comparable to the compensation received by physicians in solo practice. The approach used in the discussion pertaining to policies on organizational structure and type will be employed again to illustrate the establishment of compensation policies. Additional variables can be added to the hypothetical situation described before; it will be assumed that the four physicians newly organized as partners have agreed to an equal share fund and weighted productivity fund, along with a merit fund and a factor for seniority in the compensation plan.

Policies governing the distribution of partnership income and losses might be established as follows:

Losses. Losses of the partnership shall be shared equally by all partners.

Income. Commencing with fiscal year 19-- the net income of the XYZ Clinic shall be allocated among the partners as determined by the executive committee in accordance with the following guidelines:

1. Each partner shall receive for each fiscal year he has been a partner in the XYZ Clinic the sum of X. This shall be known as the longevity fund.
2. After subtracting this longevity compensation from the total amount to be distributed, the remainder shall be divided among the partners as follows:
   a. Forty-five percent (45 percent) of the remainder, to be known as the equal share fund, shall be distributed to the partners on an equal basis.
   b. Forty-five percent (45 percent), to be known as the weighted productivity fund, shall be distributed to the partners on the basis of the weighted productivity of each partner as it relates to all partners. The weighted productivity figure for each partner is to be computed by the executive committee and made available to the group's accountant(s) for use in this computation.
   c. Weighted productivity is defined as the personal productivity of each partner plus the gross profit resulting from the services of assistants and the ancillary service departments of the clinic.
   d. In computing this gross profit figure the total direct expenses of the X-ray, laboratory, and optical departments shall be subtracted from the gross charges of each of those departments for services rendered to patients. The resulting figures shall be divided by the respective gross charges for such department and the resulting percentages shall be applied as a weighting factor to the charges entered by each partner for the services rendered by the department to his personal production.
   e. For this computation, in no event will the gross profit of X-ray work exceed forty percent (40 percent) of the gross bookings of that department regardless of the actually computed gross profit percentage.
   f. It is further understood that the gross profit percentage computed for the laboratory department also will apply to the charges for services rendered by assistants in providing injections, immunizations, dressings, or other services approved for inclusion in this computation by the executive committee.
   g. The gross profit generated from G. I. fluoroscopy shall be credited to the physician performing the service rather than the partner ordering it.
   h. The remaining 10 percent, to be known as the merit fund, shall be distributed among the partners according to the discretion of the executive

committee. In its deliberations on distribution of this fund, the committee shall recognize seniority, the contributions made by some members of the partnership for their participation in academic spheres of medicine, in scientific publications, and in supervising ancillary services of the group. A partner may request the committee to consider other factors which he feels to be pertinent. The committee shall use the merit fund to correct any inequalities that may become apparent through the operation of the basic formula.

i. Any remaining residue of the merit fund is to be distributed equally among all of the partners.
j. After the committee has computed the individual shares of income due all partners in accordance with the above method, the following shall be deducted from the amount allocated to new partners:
   i. During the first twelve (12) months of partnership status, 15 percent of the average of the earnings of all active partners.
   ii. During the second twelve (12) months of partnership status, 10 percent of the average earnings of all active partners.
   iii. During the third twelve (12) months of partnership status, 7½ percent of the average of the earnings of all active partners.
k. These amounts so deducted from the share of the new partner or partners shall be distributed equally among all other active partners.
l. After the committee has allocated the income of the partnership, each partner shall be informed individually of his earnings for the year. During a period of two (2) weeks any partner who feels that his share of the distribution is inequitable shall have the right to meet with the committee for the purpose of seeking an adjustment in his earnings. If agreement is not reached between the partner and the committee, the partner may appeal the decision of the committee to the partnership.
m. If all partners consent in writing, the two-week period may be waived.
n. The amount of cash to be distributed in any one year shall be determined by the executive committee.
o. The determination of the allocation of net income to the partners shall be completed not later than sixty (60) days following the end of the fiscal year.
p. Each partner shall have a monthly drawing account which must be accommodated to the earnings of the business and to an estimate of his share of those earnings as determined from time to time by the executive committee.

Policies for physician retirement and insurance can be included with the above, although in this example they were omitted for brevity.

Addition or Reduction of Professional Staff

Because the quality of health care provided is only as high as the caliber of physicians practicing in the group, physician recruitment represents yet another critical policy area. Some of the factors universally affecting this area include group type, organizational form, operational mode, physicial facilities, teaching opportunities, and the predispositions of policy formulators. In addition, a group practice must recruit physicians who represent specialties for which the community has an established need and which can be easily integrated into the clinic objectives. If the four physicians in the hypothetical group described earlier have established the providing of the highest quality health care in only two specialty areas as a group objective, recruiting activities naturally would be limited to those two areas. In addition, to accommodate group objectives, the physical plant of the clinic must be capable of housing any equipment required for a specialty or ancillary service before recruitment in the area is undertaken. Finally, the founders must agree as to the need and desirability of acquiring a new physician or professional staff member before active recruitment begins.

Examples of policies in the area of physician and professional staff recruitment are:

1. Requirements for the addition of physician staff shall be reviewed and approved by the executive board prior to active recruiting.
2. Reviewing rosters of available physicians shall be a continual process performed by members of the executive board.
3. Physician recruitment shall be based on documented long range plans, with active recruiting to commence a minimum of one year prior to planned introduction date.
4. Physician employment shall be based on two primary criteria:
   a. High probability of providing quality health care
   b. Compatibility with present staff.
5. Previous academic and professional experience supplemented by personal interview shall be the means used to judge an applicant.
6. Recruiting for the group shall stress the high caliber of health care presently provided and concern for community health care needs.
7. Physician termination shall be discussed and decided upon by the entire executive board. The physician concerned shall have the opportunity to be present and to participate in the discussion of his termination.
8. Termination shall be for either of the following two reasons:
   a. Poor quality health care as determined by peers on the staff
   b. Incompatibility with other staff causing interference with the achievement of stated group objectives.
9. A restrictive covenant shall be agreed to by each physician prior to his acceptance into the group and shall be enforced upon termination, whether voluntary or involuntary.

Policies to govern the admission of new physicians to the status of partner or stockholder also can be included.

Medical Service Fees

In all probability, the patient will remember two things about the group practice: first, the quality of care received, in the patient's opinion; and second, the fee charged for that care. Because some time usually elapses between treatment and the patient's receipt of the bill, the more lasting impression often is made by the billed fee. It is important, therefore, that a fee schedule be developed carefully and consistently. Policies which might be formulated in this area include:

1. Only physicians are permitted to set and enter charges for their services.
2. Any fee, except psychiatric fees, may be adjusted for the patient by the examining physician, whether for a single visit or a series of visits.
3. The available insurance benefits shall not have any influence in the determination of any fees set by a physician.
4. Ancillary departments shall enter all charges for their services according to an established schedule.
5. The group's administrator may adjust fees in accordance with a patient's financial circumstances or any unusual condition.
6. No one other than the physician or the business office is to discuss *any* fee with *any* patient.
7. It is important that, insofar as possible, standard fees for similar services be charged by the group physician.
8. Insurance claim forms should not be completed and delivered to a patient without first being cleared with the business office.
9. When there are third party payor benefits for discounted patients, either the greater of those benefits or the discounted fee will be charged.
10. Fee schedules shall be reviewed and evaluated biannually to determine if adjustments are required to better achieve the group practice objectives.

Medical care discount policies may be desired for the group's physicians and employees, as well as for their dependents. Discounts also may be in order for professional courtesy and other reasons. A discount policy may be represented in the form of a chart for easy reference (see Table 10-5). Policy concerning group physician and employee discounts will be related to the established benefit provisions discussed under personnel systems in Chapter 17.

Policies concerning medical service fees are greatly affected by the predispositions of group founders, which determine the overall philosophy of the fee schedule. If the group members are motivated by humanitarian interests and have little concern for personal gain, they will tend to set fees just high enough to cover cost plus a nominal salary. If they have both humanitarian and financial motives, the fee schedule will reflect this as well. The socioeconomic characteristics of the community also have an impact on medical service fee policy; consequently, a group servicing a ghetto area may not be able to utilize the same fee schedule as does a group in a wealthy suburb.

Regardless of whether physicians record their charges on a centralized or decentralized charge ticket, consistency and compatibility of the entries with other clinic systems may be expedient. It is important to ensure that financial planning and systems development are consistent with the ethical and professional activities of the group's physicians as well as with credit and collection policy, insurance, Medicare, and Medicaid. Such policy statements can be coordinated to be both consistent and compatible with the mission. Regardless of any fee policy or credit and collection policy, steps must be taken to guarantee that emergency treatment is not withheld from any patient, irrespective of his willingness or ability to pay.

If a practice is operating in a prepaid mode, the policies presented above may apply, but would be based on a capitated, longer term basis. Most prepaid practices develop a group based clientele. As a result, policy areas involve the added considerations of utilization, eligibility, terminations, payroll deductions, co-

Table 10-5. Chart of Center Discount Policy Relating to Medical Service Charges

Patient Classification	*Medical Care*	*Injections, Lab & X-ray*	*Psychiatry*	*Psychology, Speech Therapy, Electrolysis*	*Dental, Podiatry,** Refractions*
Clinic physicians and dependents	courtesy care	courtesy care	not provided*	courtesy care	courtesy care** 20% discount
Clinic physicians' parents and parents-in-law	courtesy care	courtesy care	not provided	regular charge	regular charge
Clinic dentist and dependents	20% discount	20% discount	not provided	regular charge	20% discount
Clinic employees, full time	courtesy care	courtesy care	not provided	regular charge	20% discount
Clinic employee dependents (primary wage earner)	courtesy care	courtesy care	not provided	regular charge	20% discount
Clinic employee dependents (secondary wage earner)	20% discount	20% discount	not provided	regular charge	20% discount
Clinic employee, part time (under 20 hrs. per week)	regular charge	regular charge	not provided	regular charge	regular charge
Clinic Drug pharmacist employees	courtesy care	courtesy care	not provided	regular charge	regular charge
Clinic Drug pharmacists' dependents	20% discount	20% discount	not provided	regular charge	regular charge
Clinic Drug non-pharmacist employees	regular charge	regular charge	not provided	regular charge	regular charge
Board members and dependents	courtesy care	courtesy care	regular charge	regular charge	regular charge
Non-clinic physicians and dependents	courtesy care	20% discount	regular charge	regular charge	regular charge
Medical students and dependents	courtesy care	20% discount	regular charge	regular charge	regular charge
Other outside groups: dentists and dental students; nurses, technicians, hospital personnel; clergy and dependents	regular charge	regular charge	regular charge	regular charge	regular charge
Insurance benefits	Will be collected whenever possible. Patients should be asked to assign insurance if they have insurance coverage.				
No discount	Will be available for outside lab, X-ray or other outside procedures, or for ear-piercing.				
*Psychiatry	Initial evaluations or referrals to outside psychiatrists will be provided without charge. No long-term therapy will be accepted.				
**Discretionary discounts	In addition to the above may be given to patients having a direct personal business or medical association with the doctor or the clinic. (Referral doctors, nurses you work with at hospital, etc.)				

payments, group payment, delinquent payments, and risk-sharing. In many existing prepaid groups, actual determination of the premium rates has been established with the assistance of persons or organizations outside of the medical group. Policies are required to govern this initial premium setting process as well as subsequent premium determinations.

Financial Policy

Financial policies are those associated with the acquisition and maintenance of both operating and investment capital. The following list represents those subareas, usually considered in the area of financial policy, for which separate policies should be considered:

1. Preparation, evaluation, and modification of budgets
2. Acquisition of long-term financing—i.e., establishing a credit relationship with a lending organization, initiating an "investment savings account" to which members are obliged to contribute, or devising a system whereby members can buy additional shares of stock
3. Maintenance of relationships with lending organizations
4. Cash flow and working capital
5. Capital structure—i.e., how much equity, long-term debt, and/or short-term debt
6. Equity ownership—separate corporation, limited partnership, foundation
7. Reports to banks, partners, stockholders, etc., on financial status
8. The reporting and payment of taxes
9. The planning for depreciation of the physical plant and equipment
10. Outside investments—i.e., developing an organization to transact such business, center liability, percent time and money devoted to such ventures
11. Audits and reviews of both policies and financial activities.

The financial policy area is too broad and related policies too specific to permit presentation of sample policies in this section. In Chapter 8 a detailed discussion of financial planning has been presented.

General factors affecting policy formulation in the financial area are organizational form, size, and location, as well as the predispositions of the group's founders. The larger the medical group, the greater the capital needs for replacement of equipment, expansion, and investment. The legal, economic, and tax constraints on capital acquisition will be affected by the organizational form; that is, partnership, corporation, association, etc. Different states have different laws designed to regulate financial business transactions. The group practice is subject to these local laws and must budget, invest, and expand in accordance with them. Outside investment is most affected by the predispositions of the group members. If the physicians wish to take all compensation in the form of income and have no desire to join in group investment ventures, the only policy necessary can be expressed by a statement indicating that there will be no joint outside investments. If, however, the physicians are inclined toward outside investment of group funds, a set of policy statements, possibly quite elaborate, must be formulated.

Accounting Policy

Accounting policies are those associated with the recording and reporting of financial information as well as with the maintenance of the balance sheet, the income statement, etc. Accounting information provides feedback on the success or failure of the group practice to meet its economic goals. Policies associated with the recording and reporting of financial information can be separated into four major sub-areas as listed below:

1. Accounting period, whether quarter, annual, etc., and fiscal versus calendar
2. Accounting system used—cash versus accrual
3. Usual accounting routine
4. Standardized accounting and/or specialized accounting.

Each sub-area has an associated set of policy statements. One policy deserving special attention is the establishment of guidelines for the division of accounts used to record the group's expenses. The uniform classification of accounts presented in Chapter 5 offers a workable and well-conceived alternative.

Two documents most often referred to in accounting are the income or profit and loss statement and the balance sheet. The balance sheet provides a financial picture of the organization at any given time while the income statement spans a larger time period. The group's accountant, or bookkeeper with the certification of the accountant, usually is responsible for the preparation of these documents, and policies in this area are dictated by generally accepted accounting principles as outlined by the American Institute of Certified Public Accountants. Policies formulated by personnel in this sub-area are concerned primarily with the timing and packaging of information necessary to compile these reports. The group's accountant can assist in providing most of the necessary information and in many cases both federal and state tax laws will dictate policy.

Group Practice Growth

The haphazard growth of a group practice can be avoided if the founders explicitly state their objectives at the outset. Often it is possible to include a statement on annual growth rate within the broader context of growth objectives. Growth objectives may define the rate and direction of growth, or may simply state that both the rate and direction of growth will be dictated by community health care needs. The latter type of statement then requires a means to determine community needs. Regardless of whether the rate and direction of growth are established *a priori* based on the predispositions of group members, or dictated by some exogenous faction, data must be gathered either to determine the applicability of the stated rate and direction of growth to community health care needs and to evaluate the effects of the growth policy, or, in the latter case, to determine what community needs actually are and to evaluate growth policy. The need for such data results in four sub-areas in which policy considerations are necessary:

1. Data gathering as discussed above
   Policy: Patients will be surveyed annually to determine whether community health care needs are being met.

2. Formulation of policies
   Policy: Growth policies will be developed by the policy committee and will be presented to the executive board for approval.
3. Evaluation of policies and growth objectives; criteria for evaluation—who will establish them and how often
   Policy: Policies will be reviewed semiannually by the executive board in achieving group objectives.
4. Modification—the process by which growth objectives and/or policies are added, modified, or deleted
   Policy: Changes in growth policies will be discussed by the policy committee and will be presented for discussion and approval at the monthly executive board meetings.

Factors affecting growth policies include the socioeconomic characteristics of the community. For example, in an indigent, minority community the probability of obtaining internal or external financing for growth may be low. In addition, such a community may not consider the expansion of a fee-for-service practice appropriate for community needs, nor will the population be able to utilize the additional capacity. As in all policy areas, the formulators' predispositions are extremely important; if group founders do not wish the practice to grow, policies in this area will be minimal. Constraints of time and space do not permit a total delineation of all possible policies for all policy areas. The discussion which has been presented, along with the examples and factors affecting each critical policy area, should provide the policy planner(s) with sufficient information to assist newly forming medical groups.

GUIDELINES FOR POLICY FORMATION: PROFESSIONAL AND PATIENT CARE

The established mission and objectives of the group also will determine and influence policies in the areas of professional staff and patient care. The balance of this chapter will outline additional policy considerations involved in the group's initial formation and development and more directly associated with professional and patient care activities. These remaining policy considerations fall into three general categories: policies associated with providing medical services; policies pertaining to relationships and provisions among the staff and other community physicians; and policies relating directly to patients and their continuous care. Strategic decisions can be made with regard to: the scope of services offered, the cooperation among staff members, the quality of services, the population served, and the announcement of new services, staff, and facilities. If, for example, the established mission is to provide a source for comprehensive medical service, the group's strategies and concomitant policies might include:

Strategy: The medical service shall be as comprehensive as is practical with the intention of eventually including all major specialties and subspecialties.

Policies:

1. The medical staff shall act as a general medical advisor to whom patients may bring all their medical problems.

2. The group practice shall serve as a diagnostic center at which the patient may seek medical evaluation and to which physicians may refer their patients for specialized consultation.
3. The staff shall offer preventive medical care and shall provide facilities for periodic general and special examinations.

Strategy: The medical staff shall be available to those who seek its services, without geographic limitations.

Policies:
1. The staff shall make its services available locally and shall cooperate in the development of the community's medical resources.
2. The staff shall direct its efforts primarily toward that area which supplies a majority of its patients.
3. The staff shall recognize and develop the potential for patients beyond these immediate areas.
4. The staff also shall respond to the needs of the numerous visitors who are attracted to this area.
5. The staff shall display friendly cooperation in solving problems that inevitably arise. While some problems, whether professional or administrative, may be difficult to solve, they may be taken to an individual's advisor, his chief of service, the chairperson of the executive board, or the administrator, all of whom may be expected to offer their cooperation.
6. The staff shall be available to provide services when needed. It is important that the whereabouts of each staff member be known to the telephone operators, nurse, or secretary during the day. The answering service must know where staff members will be when the switchboard is closed; therefore, the staff must keep in touch with the answering service.
7. The staff should respond to all telephone calls, day or night. If the patient who calls has a problem which is outside of a particular specialty, the physician called should assume the responsibility for the patient's care until the appropriate physician has taken over. This responsibility may necessitate a visit to the patient or a telephone call to the proper physician to make the arrangements.
8. The staff should be prompt in keeping appointments. When delays occur, the appropriate nurse or secretary should be notified so that appointments may be adjusted.

Strategy: The announcement of new physicians, new facilities, and new services will be made to the professional and patient community.

Policies:
1. All announcements of staff, facility, and service additions shall be in accordance with the Canons of Medical Ethics and shall be approved by the local medical society.
2. Announcements to professional peers shall be directed to those physicians with whom established relations exist.
3. Announcements to the patient community shall be directed to the group's clientele.

Policies associated with the provision of medical care also include the requesting and movement of medical records within the clinic and possibly to and from the hospital.

Medical Staff Policies

In connection with those policies associated with the provision of medical services, more specific objectives and policies relating to the medical staff include:

Strategy: Medical services shall be provided by a staff working within a cooperative framework of a medical partnership and primarily concerned with patient care.

Policies:

1. A clear, understandable partnership agreement shall be prepared and periodically updated, and shall represent a working agreement between partners, clearly defining their rights and duties, as well as anticipating and providing means to handle future problems.
2. Each partner shall become familiar with the organizational structure and shall conduct all organizational activities accordingly.
3. The partners shall elect an executive board which will meet frequently and will be charged with the responsibility for decision making.
4. Major decisions shall be referred to the partnership for a vote. At any time, the partners may reverse the decision of the executive board by a two-thirds majority vote.
5. Along with the administrator, the chairperson of the executive board is the executive officer responsible for the daily operations of the group practice. The chairperson shall also be an ex-officio member of all committees.
6. Staff members having suggestions or experiencing difficulties shall report first to the chief of their department or section, next to the chairperson of the executive board, then to the executive board, and finally to the partnership.
7. The medical staff shall consist of physicians who are committed to the concept of group practice and agree that group practice offers the following advantages:
   a. The free and easy exchange of medical knowledge
   b. Prompt, formal and informal consultations, so important to the interchange of medical knowledge and patient care
   c. The ability to provide competent and adequate medical coverage
   d. Close fellowship in professional and personal activities.
8. In an effort to constantly enhance and improve the professional scope and quality of departments for overall patient care, new partners shall be carefully selected. Criteria for selection shall be:
   a. Superior training, including the fulfillment of requirements of specialty boards and a desire to pursue as rapidly as possible board certification
   b. Individual personality traits that can be accommodated within the operative framework of the group practice
   c. Primary interest in patient care
   d. Dedication to the basic mission and objectives of the group.

9. Each staff member shall have freedom in the development of his practice as long as it conforms to the general framework of the mission and objectives.
10. It shall be the responsibility of each partner to acquaint patients with his colleagues' qualifications and to protect the good name and reputation of each partner.
11. All members of the medical staff are to assume their fair share of participation in the group's efforts, responsibilities, and objectives, both professionally and in management of the group practice.
12. While the major responsibility is toward the medical care of patients, clinical medical research shall be encouraged whenever practical.
13. The medical staff shall encourage contributions to medical knowledge and teaching through publications in medical journals and through participation in medical meetings, internships, and fellowship programs, as well as regional medical education programs within the clinic.
14. The quality of medical practice shall be maintained at a high level through attendance of postgraduate courses and medical meetings, as well as through planned educational programs within the clinic.
15. The medical staff shall recognize its responsibility to, and shall cooperate with:
    a. Local and regional medical societies
    b. The American Medical Association
    c. Local hospitals
    d. Local welfare agencies
    e. Local pharmacies and representatives of the pharmaceutical industry
    f. Insurance companies and other agencies connected with medical care.

Record-keeping is a costly and time-consuming activity, but is a medical, medicolegal, and often accreditational necessity. Guidelines for the effective recording of patient data and maintenance of such records also should be drafted by the group. Such policy will help to ensure that the records are legible and complete, thereby facilitating better patient care. Other physicians involved can function more efficiently, secretaries can write letters from the record, and future meaningful retrospective studies will be made possible. The physician has the obligation to make sure that the medical records of the group and of the hospitals are current; good records reflect the care rendered and provide a basis for judgment of the physician by his professional peers. In addition, guidelines for the regulation of medical record flow within and among the various medical specialties are necessary to ensure that the objectives of the group are maintained and that the communications in the record not only facilitate professional relationships among the staff but also result in quality patient care.

Policies also may be needed to clarify the relationship resulting from consultations between members of the group. When another physician is called for consultation, confusion sometimes arises concerning exactly who is the consulting physician and who is charging for professional services. The need for policy guidance is amplified when complaints are received from patients who feel they have been charged by more than one physician for the "same" service, or when complaints are received from physicians who wonder why a patient whom they referred never returned. Guidelines to prevent such confusion should prescribe a plan for ensuring that the attending physician indicates clearly to the patient the need for a consultation with another physician. Within the hospital setting, the consulting physician then visits the patient in response to the attending physician's request, and makes his role clear to the patient. The need for additional visits, if any, should be communicated to both the patient and the attending physician. As long as the consultant acts as "second in command," all orders should be written by the attending physician, unless there is a mutual understanding to the contrary.

If it becomes necessary to transfer the care of a patient to the consulting physician, this arrangement should be mutually agreeable to both physicians. The patient should be informed of the reasons for the change, and the attending physician should clarify the reasons for that change to the patient. If proper care of the patient requires continued limited service by the original physician, this should be understood by both the patient and the consultant who has assumed primary responsibility for the case. If the services of the original physician are no longer needed, he should refrain from writing orders and making further charges. It should be clear to the patient, his family, and consulting physician that the original physician is welcome to reenter the case at a later date if needed; however, this reentry should follow the same procedure as that of calling in a consultant.

A problem of patient management within the practice can occur when a patient is referred by the first physician who examines him to another physician, and then perhaps to a third physician. The patient may never find his way back to his original physician, and may be left feeling insecure, not knowing where to turn for help; the original physician may feel ineffectual and frustrated. It should be the responsibility of each consulting physician to direct the patient back to his original physician, who should be informed of the disposition of the patient's problem. Guidance in the form of policy is needed, therefore, to help maintain workable consultation relationships among the staff, and also between the staff and other community physicians who refer their patients to the group practice. Telephone communications can play a role in the consultation process, but not to the exclusion of prompt written reports. Furnishing a pertinent record of the encounter is also one of the obligations of a consultant.

Although not specifically related to the establishment of formal policy, periodic conferences between the group practice physicians can result in better service to patients. Such conferences might entail a telephone call, or a regular weekly or monthly meeting. Specific departments and sections can be urged to initiate such meetings at which the staff can informally discuss its problems and cases; those that occur across departments and sections can be discussed at a more formal conference. It is through such meetings that the physician can broaden his knowledge and can bring into focus a better diagnosis and treatment for a problem case.

Should the group practice become involved in providing medical services to employee groups and/or insurance companies, certain additional referral provisions become necessary. Depending upon the negotiations, the group physician may have complete latitude in the conduct of his examinations and in the extent of the medical report, or procedural latitude may be sharply defined. Although the communication of such guidelines often results in policy determinations, many existing groups who serve such a clientele often assemble what is referred to as "company accounts" or "insurance account" books which convey to the individual physician the extent of the negotiations and scope of pre-arranged medical services.

The group practice physician often will dictate information to be included in the patient's medical record. The dictating and transcribing of this information, both within and outside the practice, may necessitate certain policies to promote cooperation and coordination. Intragroup dictation policy as well as the dictation policies established by community hospitals are important concerns. Hospital policies are influenced heavily by the accreditation requirements of the Joint Commission on the Accreditation of Hospitals; failure by the group physician to comply with hospital dictation policy can result in the loss of his hospital privileges. Many groups incorporate the hospital dictation policy in their policies to ensure productive group practice–hospital relations and to provide guidance and control.

In the course of providing services to the community, many instances can arise in which group physicians are requested or directed to provide written or personal information to the courts. Policy considerations in this area might involve fees charged for testifying in court, for giving depositions, and for providing reports. Attorneys, insurance companies, hospitals, community physicians, and the patient's family also are potential requestors of medical information.

As an efficient and consistent means of providing services, the group may decide to establish distinct departments to offer various special services such as immunizations, vision screening, hearing screening, pulmonary function testing, electrocardiogram, and encephalogram. To guide the staff in ordering these services, policy considerations may be necessary to cover the method of ordering, hours of operation, special instructions, reporting, and charting. Finally, the overall health and periodic physical examinations of the staff as well as the benefits applicable to possible categories of staff employment represent two additional elements in the area of intra-group staff relationships which require attention. Tables 10-6 and 10-7 are examples of policies which outline various staff benefits.

Patient Care Policies

In maintaining a high standard of health care the group will find it advantageous to create an environment which is at once friendly and efficient. The patient should not feel threatened or overwhelmed, but rather should remain secure and confident in the belief that the attention and care he receives in the clinic is of the highest quality. Patient rights, patient consent, and transportation of patients are integral to quality patient care. Policies relating to patient care might be formulated as follows:

1. In all patient contacts the medical staff shall pursue the objectives of the group as well as:
   a. Provide medical coverage for its patients at all times.
   b. Strive to assist other personnel in the efficient handling of patients in all ways, but particularly by keeping the clinic advised of changes in staff-patient scheduling.
   c. Provide patients with coordinated care and reports, particularly when a patient is referred to multiple departments and specialists.

Table 10-6. Example Comparison of Staff Benefits Within a Medical Group

Benefits	*Employed*	*Associates*	*Partner*
Eligibility	Authorized Vacancy	20 months employment Executive committee recommendation 90% vote of partners	1 year as associate Executive committee recommendation 90% vote of partners
Committee Participation	None	May serve as committee member except on executive, income distribution and professional committees Cannot be chairman	Full participation
Travel	2 weeks, $350	3 weeks, $550	3 weeks, $750
Vacations			
After 6 Months	2 weeks		
Under Age 40	2 weeks	3 weeks	3 weeks
Age 40–49 or After 5 Years	3 weeks	4 weeks	4 weeks
Age 50–54	3 weeks	4 weeks	5 weeks
Age 55 and Thereafter	3 weeks	4 weeks	6 weeks
Tenure (with reciprocal notice)	2 weeks	1 year	To retirement
Non-Competition Restrictions	None	6 months, County	6 months, County
Termination	Administrative action	Executive committee recommendation 51% of partners Failure to accept partnership if offered	90% vote of partners
Investment	None	Corporations	Partnership and corporations
Accounts Receivable	None	None	5 year vesting
Retirement Plan	None (1st two years) 5% when eligible	5% clinic contribution	None
One Year Retirement Bonus	None	25% of partner provision	100% of partnership agreement
Wage Restrictions	Percentage wage increase	None on entry, Percentage thereafter	None

   d. Make provisions for a frank discussion of fees, including an estimate of the amount and a mutually agreed upon method of payment.
   e. Maintain a professional attitude and appearance in all patient contacts.
   f. Maintain good ethical relationships with all physicians.

2. The administrative and support staff shall:
   a. Provide courteous, friendly, and prompt attention to patients' needs.
   b. Maintain an efficient appointment system, geared to the patient's needs and best interest.

Table 10-7. Example Comparison of Staff Benefits Within a Medical Group

Staff Benefits	*Salaried*	*Associate*	*Partner*
Sick Leave	One month	One month	Six months
Disability Income	30 day waiting period; 2/3 regular pay	30 day waiting period; 2/3 regular pay	Three months full pay; three months half pay
Medical Insurance	$500 deductible; $300,000 maximum	$500 deductible; $300,000 maximum	$500 deductible; $300,000 maximum
Vacation			
After 6 months	2 weeks	—	—
Under age 40	2 weeks	3 weeks	3 weeks
Age 40–49 or after 5 years	3 weeks	4 weeks	4 weeks
Age 50–54	3 weeks	4 weeks	5 weeks
Age 55 and thereafter	3 weeks	4 weeks	6 weeks
Professional Liability Insurance	$3,000,000	$3,000,000	$3,000,000
Travel	2 weeks—$500	3 weeks—$650	3 weeks—$1,000
Holiday	Six per year	Six per year	Six per year
Retirement	After two years, 5% clinic contribution	1. After 2 years 5% clinic contribution 2. 25% of partner provision	100% of partnership provisions

c. Avoid the inherent tendency of large specialty groups to appear condescending, aloof, and superior, thereby sacrificing individual identification and attention.

3. The business office shall provide an adequate insurance and accounting department.

Because of the increase in malpractice suits, signed patient consent forms as well as the right of patients to be fully informed about possible consequences or hazards involved with certain procedures have become important issues for policy determination. Policy statements in this area might include the following:

1. Each physician shall exercise his own judgment in regard to obtaining a signed consent for any minor surgical procedure to be performed in the clinic. Written consent should be obtained when the patient obviously is hostile or emotionally unstable, or in any other questionable situation.
2. In all cases of elective surgery, the patient shall be fully informed of the chances of success or of possible consequences or hazards.

Figure 10-5 represents an example of a patient consent form.

The transportation of patients includes arrangements for moving them between the clinic and the hospital. The means and methods for such transpor-

XYZ CLINIC

AUTHORIZATION FOR MEDICAL AND/OR SURGICAL TREATMENT

Date ________________, 19___ Time: ______ a.m. p.m.

I, the undersigned, a patient at the XYZ Clinic hereby authorize Dr. ______________________________

(and whomever he may designate as his assistants) to administer such treatment as is necessary, and to perform the following operation ______________________________ (name of operation and/or procedure) and such additional operations or procedures as are considered therapeutically necessary on the basis of findings during the course of said operation. I also consent to the administration of such anesthetics as are necessary, with the exception of ______________________ (none, spinal anesthesia, or other).

Any tissues or parts surgically removed may be disposed of by the clinic in accordance with accustomed practice.

I hereby certify that I have read and fully understand the above AUTHORIZATION FOR MEDICAL AND/OR SURGICAL TREATMENT, the reasons why the above-named surgery is considered necessary, its advantages and possible complications, if any, as well as possible alternative modes of treatment, which were explained to me by Dr. ______________________.

I also certify that no guarantee or assurance has been made as to the results that may be obtained.

Witness ______________________ Signed ______________________ (patient or nearest relative)

Witness ______________________ Signed ______________________ (relationship)

Authorization must be signed by the patient, or by the nearest relative in the case of a minor, or when patient is physically or mentally incompetent.

Figure 10-5. Example Consent Form

tation are important to both the group and the patient. In order to specify the assignment of liability the following policy statements might be proposed:

1. All movement of patients between clinic and hospital must be approved by the attending physician.
2. Patients becoming acutely ill in the clinic should be sent to the hospital via ambulance.
3. Hospital patients cleared by the attending physician to meet an appointment in the clinic should come to the clinic under their own power or assisted by family members.
4. Only in unusual circumstances should clinic personnel be used to transport a patient. The attending physician's approval will be required in such instances.

This chapter has outlined a possible policy formulation process beginning with the establishment of a mission, followed by the determination of suitable objectives and goals, and, finally culminating in productive policy decisions. The success of a medical group practice often is dependent upon its organizational viability. Thoughtful policy planning on the part of a newly forming group can help to ensure long term success both in terms of operation and in the fulfillment of the group members' aspirations and intentions.

Part III

Medical Group Systems Development

Chapter 11

Communications Systems

ESTABLISHING THE COMMUNICATION SYSTEMS

Most individuals underestimate the importance of behavioral processes fundamental to human interaction; it is a universal failing to be unaware of the obvious. Communication represents just such a phenomenon—difficult to define and even more difficult to evaluate. Communication, especially within the framework of a structured organization, appears to be a simple process, but for anyone who has ever been grossly misunderstood, such a simplistic description seems unrealistic. The direction of the communication process also is often misunderstood. When an attempt is made to identify just who has initiated a particular message in a specific situation, it becomes apparent that communication is a two-way dynamic process. A static model or diagram illustrating sender, receiver, and channel bears little resemblance to a heated argument between two persons and even less to a persuasive message televised to millions.

Communication is influenced significantly by both the emotional and the intellectual capacities of the participants, as well as by such cultural attributes as status and power. Within a health care center, communication is probably more complex and has the potential for more dissonance than in any other public service organization. Involved in the communication process are first and foremost the patients, possibly anxious and apprehensive, and secondly, at least two directive groups, the physicians and the administrative staff. Communication events can be initiated by members of each group and dispatched to any person(s) in the other two groups. A free exchange of information between individuals and/or groups should be nurtured by the need for efficient and effective health care delivery and yet, paradoxically, in a setting in which the processing of information has critical implications there may be too little emphasis on effective communication through efficient channels.

Individuals involved in a newly forming group should be particularly aware of the potential for communication breakdown and should take steps to prevent it. Creating an emotional environment which is predictable in terms of group mission, objectives, and policies is one of the first steps. Providing for and eliciting feedback relating to administrative decisions is another, and a third might involve a survey of patient opinion concerning the group's communication effectiveness.

All clinic personnel should be aware of possible problem areas; they need to exert care and patience in dealing with one another and with the group's clientele. Because it may be necessary to document in writing critical information concerning both medical care and costs, many transactions within the clinic may be conducted by using forms specifically designed for a particular purpose. Communication patterns throughout the clinic should be carefully planned and should include a structured method for ongoing evaluation. Individuals responsible for these patterns must remain aware of the need for commonality of understanding among all participants, especially the lay public. For example, medical and accounting terms or symbols should be well-defined and elaborated upon, because differences in the interpretation of meaning and the perception of intent can influence consequential behavior. If an administrator finds that members of one particular department continually fail to implement a particular policy, he should ascertain if the policy is misunderstood or contrary to the perceived objectives of the department. Department heads, through ignorance of the *total* system, may perpetuate procedures which are inhibiting to the long-range goals of the group. Often the clinic management may not have articulated overall group objectives. This information should be readily available with predetermined channels for its dissemination.

The newly forming group will find that first it must give attention to the composition of interclinic and intraclinic communications, and then to the delineation of the routes and channels such information will take. With the organizational channels identified and endorsed, the next step in operational planning is to examine the technological innovations necessary to expedite the flow of information. As a result of electronic advances in the field of communication, the complexity of some of the newer communication channels often can be understood only by specialists. Often, currently available gadgetry is so overwhelming that the necessity of basic systems used daily goes unrecognized. Electronic systems have become an integral part of life, and only when an individual is deprived of their use does their value become apparent. This is especially true in the medical group whose electronic communication system is indispensable to all clinic operations. One of the often cited advantages of group practice is that it facilitates physician interaction and communication. An effective system enables clinic personnel to transmit ideas, results, and requests to one another with speed and accuracy, thus guaranteeing efficient performance of patient services and administrative tasks. The communication system should be designed to enable patients to contact clinic personnel, including physicians, with a minimum of effort and should allow physicians to perform some advisory services without requiring the patient to visit the office.

The Communication Systems Concept

The communications system as a whole, including participants, messages, and channels, is closely intermeshed with clinic operating systems, such as appointments, registration, and medical records. The systems concept as it relates to clinic communications is manifested in various subsystems such as the telephone, a paging system, a dictation system, an intercom system, a clinic newsletter and other instructional sources, routine conversation, etc. Underlying any system of communication are channels for fulfilling the functions of information processing and dissemination. Information in the form of messages must be routed between senders and receivers within the system. Routing, usually prescribed by varying types of physical parameters and defined by policy decisions, should be designed to facilitate both speed and accuracy in communication.

Foremost in the area of clinic communications is the telephone. Communications initiated by patients represent the major portion of messages transmitted by a medical group's telephone system. Studies have shown that 90 percent of all telephone calls to and from a clinic are originated by patients, and only ten percent are originated by physicians and other clinic personnel. Fifty percent of the clinic's telephone call load is in regard to symptoms, with thirty percent of these calls involving acute problems. Forty percent of the clinic's calls concern prescriptions and laboratory results.[1] In terms of convenience alone, the value of an efficient telephone communication system is almost inestimable. In actual dollar cost, communication systems demand a significant amount of clinic expense. In 1973, the Medical Group Management Association *Cost Survey* determined that telephone costs alone are approximately $1,370 per physician per year. In spite of the results of this survey, little comprehensive work has been done in developing guidelines to assist the medical group in evaluating and deciding upon the particular components which will comprise the clinic communication systems.

Word processors comprise a second major communication system within the clinc. Word processing encompasses the recording and transcription of oral communication, whether on paper, on belts, on tapes, or on discs. Dictation equipment can provide both speed and ease in the recording of spoken ideas. The transcription of this recorded material to hard copy involves the typewriter, which, although considered conventional office equipment, actually can vary greatly in its potential for speed and performance capability. Finally, should it be necessary to reproduce a number of copies, a wide array of copying equipment is available currently.

Other subsystems within the communication system include postage handling, data processing, and facsimile equipment. Mailing is an integral part of any group's billing and collections system. Data processing becomes necessary as a wealth of information is assembled for accounting and insurance purposes, as well as for forecasting and research. In some cases, clinic communication systems will be required to interface with other information systems, possibly providing access to a computer data base. Much less common in the typical clinic is use of facsimile equipment which, although not copying equipment per se, is concerned with the transfer of document reproduction from one location to another, typically through electronic means.

The forming group should remember that the human resource represented by the clinic's personnel remains the most important factor in the communication system. Despite the level of present technology, the word processing system, for example, cannot function without the expertise of a human being; thus, the need for those people responsible for operating message transmission and word processing systems in the clinic should not be underestimated. As communications systems become increasingly sophisticated, however, common clerical functions may be assumed by various subsystems. For example, advanced telephone switching features such as automatic call-forwarding, automatic conferencing, and recorded messages can reduce clerical functions while further promoting center goodwill through improved efficiency. The speed and accuracy resulting from a good communications system contributes significantly to community health care. Any increase in ease of access to the clinic and to medical personnel will help to improve community attitudes and will foster goodwill toward the group practice.

Systems Planning

In designing a new facility and in remodeling an existing building(s) it will be necessary to design communication systems which will fulfill the needs of the group and its patients. All components of the system must be compatible with the needs and idiosyncrasies of the group practice members. While no two groups will find their specific needs can be accommodated by identical communication systems, in most cases the analysis of a group's needs and the planning and design of the eventual system can be approached in much the same manner. The traditional problem-solving method works best in a group practice environment. A standardized approach applicable to clinic communication systems design includes eight phases:

1. *Determination of the Basic Parameters of the Needed System.* Minor details surrounding the problem must be evaluated, resulting in identification and definition of the problem or mission.
2. *Statement of Objectives.* The expectations and limitations of the system must be stated clearly.
3. *The Gathering and Analysis of Facts.* From qualified sources, facts relevant to the problem must be assembled. This material, whether verbal or written, then is evaluated and abstracted.
4. *Determination of the Alternatives Available in Developing the Needed System.* The advantages and disadvantages of each aspect of the problem must be reviewed while keeping in mind any potential problems.
5. *Evaluation of Each Alternative.* The assembled facts must be weighed relative to their value to other clinic operations and systems, and then a conclusion must be proposed.
6. *Implementation of the Proposed Communication System.*
7. *Evaluation of the New System Through Observation and User Feedback.*
8. *Continual Modification of the System Based on Repeated Evaluation.* As

feedback on the system is received, it may be necessary to repeat the above steps in order to change the system.

A basic set of criteria is useful in analyzing the qualifications of any given system in relation to the needs of the system's users. Seven basic criteria may be helpful in choosing a particular communication system.

1. The *function* which each system performs must be identified.
2. Some determination of the *distribution* of the actual system, facilities, and benefits must be determined.
3. The *volume* or expected loading of the system must be ascertained.
4. The *form* of the final product must be determined for each end point in the system.
5. Some determination of the *speed* with which the system functions must be calculated.
6. Some judgment also must be made about the *accuracy* with which the system will operate.
7. Most importantly, some determination of the true *cost* of the system must be made.[2]

By Employing the problem-solving approach and by using the criteria set forth above, the group can initiate an analysis of its needs and can begin to plan a communication system for the clinic.

THE TELEPHONE SYSTEM

Often a communications consultant or a representative from a communications firm can be of great assistance in determining the demand requirements for hardware components. Many conveniences included in the proposed telephone system may be personal preference items. While this is to be expected when many different individuals will be using the system, after a determination of the hardware to be used is completed, a cost analysis and comparison analysis should be made.

Present day monitoring devices greatly facilitate the measurement of equipment needs. In order to ascertain the number of trunks necessary to accommodate specific clinic needs, the call rejection rate, the average call holding time, and the amount of peak hour calls must be determined. Usually, telephone company equipment can be used to measure the tolerable number of busy signals. Most often, the call rejection rate is approximately 2 percent for incoming calls and 3 percent or 4 percent for outgoing or intercom type calls. The result of the average call holding time and the number of peak hour calls divided by 100 is referred to as *HCS* or *hundred call seconds*. This figure, along with the call rejection rate, helps determine the number of trunks necessary for a specific traffic load. The telephone company as well as suppliers within the trade have available tables which can aid in the determination of trunk requirements. Blocked call studies also may be implemented to ascertain if each organizational area is receiving adequate station coverage. Stations may be arranged in a rotary fashion so that if a number is dialed and busy, the call will rotate automatically to the next free line. In this way, fewer trunk lines are required, use of all lines is maximized, and service is not diminished. In order to accommodate incoming and outgoing calls at peak times, trunks can be used in aggregate. To project the number of stations and trunks which will be required to fulfill clinic needs, the anticipated traffic load per instrument or employee can be divided by the present and/or expected number of employees or telephone stations.

Ordinarily, voice traffic can be categorized as general incoming and outgoing in-house, outgoing local, and outgoing long distance. When a call comes into the clinic it is important that it reach the correct party quickly and efficiently. Here the switchboard is of prime importance. The impact of frequency and total volume of local outgoing calls will affect the switching unit. If local outgoing traffic is heavy a manual switchboard may not be appropriate. If, however, an operator is handling incoming calls and the outgoing load is light, the system should operate smoothly. Outgoing long distance calls may present a problem. Variables affecting service include the time of day calls are placed; volume at peak periods; and the nature of the calls—that is, person-to-person, station-to-station, or direct dial. Involving the clinic operator and/or long distance operator usually results in a cost of approximately twenty percent more than direct dial calls. The loss of accountability resulting from no assistance from an operator, however, may be compensated for by the lower toll charges. Of course, before any type of switchboard is chosen, the system should be thoroughly evaluated in terms of both utility and economy. Often it proves best to blend several types of service so that outgoing toll calls can be controlled while at the same time the efficiency of the system for incoming calls is maintained.

A telephone company or private supplier representative can be helpful in coordinating installation of the telephone system. Often, it is advisable to deal with only one individual throughout the course of the group's association with the telephone company or with a private supplier. In time, this individual will become intimately aware of the specific needs of the group and often will be more sensitive to various idiosyncracies which must be built into the telephone system. It may require twelve months or more for the installation of cabling and the constructing of a complete telephone system. If a new facility is under construction in a relatively underdeveloped area, the construction time involved in activities such as laying underground cable may be quite extensive. In addition, certain permits may be required from the municipal government. It is best, therefore, to analyze carefully all aspects of the system so that sufficient lead time is allowed.

The telephone communications industry recently has joined other industries in the common practice of offering competitive bids and alternate systems. The Federal Communications Commission rendered a decision in 1968 (The Carterfone Decision) *stipulating that subscribers may lease or purchase their own telephone equipment* while retaining the right to connect this equipment to the national line network for full telephone service. The services available from competitive suppliers include not only intercom and paging systems within the environs of the business, but also in most cases, a complete telephone system.

Competition within the communications industry has stimulated the entry of many new vendors into the field. All manufacturers listed below offer complete lines and wide ranges of telephone equipment and systems, but they by no means constitute a complete list of all producers of telephone equipment.[3]

Ericsson	ITT CESD	No. Telecom	Stromberg
Executone	Lynch	OKI	Teleprompter
GTE	Milgo	Progressive	TeleResources
Hitachi	National Telephone	RCA	TIE
Information Dynamics	NEC Telephone	Reliable	United Busuiness Communications
Interconnect	Norelco	Rollins	Universal

With the growing number of telephone manufacturers has come not only increasing competition among newcomers to the field, but also an increasing challenge to American Telephone and Telegraph Company (AT&T). Since 1969, tariff structures, which are AT&T's price lists, have undergone extensive changes because of this competition.

In general, there are two major categories of telephone suppliers: *telephone utilities* (common carriers) and private *interconnect companies*. Telephone utility company services usually are supplied for an all inclusive monthly charge, while interconnect companies bill on a different basis. Some private suppliers of communication equipment may have offices only in major cities and metropolitan areas; many of the interconnect companies are local, one or two office firms, serving relatively restricted areas. Telephone utility companies, however, are common to all locales. The communications equipment available through both private suppliers and common carriers generally comes from manufacturers in a number of countries including the United States, Japan, and Sweden. Distribution, franchising, financing, and servicing differ according to location and the potential market.

System Considerations. When choosing a particular communications supplier, it is often necessary to differentiate between the types of contract agreements available. Telephone company service contracts generally are considered to be operating leases, cancellable upon relatively short notice. For large systems, however, there are termination contracts covering minimum service periods of two, three, five, or ten years. Interconnect companies sell and lease equipment, as well as offer combinations of these two basic arrangements. The type of contract proposed also is important because the Internal Revenue Service may determine that a "lease" is, in reality, a purchase and sale, and consequently "rental" payments essentially are payments made toward the purchase price which cannot be deducted currently and are recoverable over the life of the property acquired through depreciation deductions. Because any communications contract will spell out warranty terms and usage terms for the equipment involved, and because such terms often are defined strictly and may delineate liability possibilities for the group, it should rely upon a legal advisor and perhaps a communications expert as well. Final resolution for the tax determinations of a communication contract resides with the Internal Revenue Service and the appropriate local tax agencies.

In the remainder of this chapter, certain basic definitions for the acquisition of equipment will be employed. Use of the term *purchase* will imply outright sale and ownership. A *lease* will denote an operating arrangement similar to that offered by the utility telephone company. *Conditional sales* contracts will include installment sales, lease-purchase sales, lease-purchase, or lease-with-buyout options, as well as similar financial lease arrangements.

Contract options generally offered fall into the following categories:

1. *Outright purchase* is characterized by payment upon delivery or upon installation. The purchaser assumes ownership immediately.

2. *Conditional sales and installation purchases* are characterized by payment of principal and interest over a period of years, often stated as a rental or lease amount. In each case, the buyer assumes ownership and considers the equipment as an asset for purposes of depreciation, insurance, etc.

3. *Leases* often are complex. For tax and accounting purposes, however, some leases are designated as financial leases and are treated as conditional sales contracts when certain conditions are satisfied. Otherwise, the lease is an operating or straight lease, because the title to the property is never transferred. Lease payments, rental payments, or monthly service charges are considered operating expenses for income tax purposes. There are many varieties of leases, with many types of provisions for cancellation prerogatives. Common carrier telephone service is most often offered under a straight lease arrangement.

The qualitative aspects of telephone communication equipment also should be explored before a supplier is chosen. Among the major considerations are:

1. *Support Capabilities*. The basic monthly telephone charge will, or should, include a number of component services such as charges for the layout and planning of conduits, poles, and other apparatus. Another such service is user training, which will be on an initial, one time basis, but may become continuous. Several critical questions should be explored: Does the vendor offer these services? Under what circumstances? At what cost?

2. *Maintenance Capabilities*. In the area of maintenance it is especially critical that terms of the contract be well understood. Many questions will arise concerning the maintenance of the communication system. The most basic concern involves repair service, guarantees, parts supply, provisions for catstrophe, and expertise of maintenance technicians.

3. *Financial Stability*. A contract is only as good as the supplier's ability to perform; therefore, the financial stability of a prospective supplier should be investigated thoroughly. It may be wise, however, to make provisions in the contract for the use of the service of another supplier should unforeseen problems arise.

4. *Flexibility*. Because present day technology changes rapidly, the clinic may find it advantageous to investigate provisions for updating the present system. Growth is a realistic probability for any group practice; therefore, it may be necessary to determine and provide for future problems arising from expansion and/or change in location.

As an organization concerned with costs, the clinic should review a number of cost elements associated with owning or leasing telephone communications equipment. Some of these cost considerations are:

Purchasing/Installation. Certain expenses will be incurred prior to, or coincidental with, the installation of the proposed system. A careful study of the contract should clarify exactly what is included in the installation cost. Some commonly used designations are: *installation*, *equipped features*, *optional*, and *capacity*. The precise meaning or meanings of all such terms should be presented in writing and understood before a contract is signed. Typically, the term *installed* refers to that which is included in the quoted price. *Equipped* refers to the number of units of a feature which may be added without a major addition. Features not included, but available at additional expense, are *options*. And *capacity* is the present or ultimate growth capability of the system, usually stated in terms of number of lines or extensions, trunks, and call limitations during the busy hour.

Prices quoted for installation or outright sale may be based on one of several approaches. Total installation cost usually includes labor, materials, profit, cabling, and sometimes a small inventory of spare parts. A contract specifying *materials only* is quoted without labor costs. The materials only approach should be scrutinized carefully because labor expense can amount to 50 percent of the overall system cost, given a margin of error of 10 percent on either side of this figure. The term *cost* as used here refers to the amount billed to the clinic.

Material costs include common equipment, such as the switching cabinet and power plant of a PBX (switchboard), as well as the attendant position(s), station equipment, cabling, and terminals. Another cost factor may be the expense of removing old or existing equipment and wiring. Conduit installation and concealed wiring also may add to the cost of installation. Termination, or disconnection of the system before the contractual time limit expires, is yet another cost which should be provided for in the contract. These costs usually are billed to the customer, but arrangements can be made for this expense to be covered in the original or in the new agreement.

The group's architect will draft telephone and signal drawings. Clinic standards, such as the heights of wall-mounted telephones, will be specified and illustrated on the blueprints. If, after continued consultation with a telephone company or private supplier representative, the group decides to make some changes in the plan, the architect should be notified immediately so that he can incorporate these modifications into the final blueprints. The architect himself may suggest some changes based on his experience. When the installers begin their work, the architect, the telephone company project manager, and the group should be especially careful that no unauthorized changes are conveyed to the installers by the individuals who will be using the equipment in, for example, a specific office area. Usually installers receive orders only from their project manager, so it may be that both the architect and members of the group must channel their requests through him.

The telephone company or the private supplier usually will conduct training sessions for clinic personnel. Depending upon the nature of the system, these sessions may be brief orientations or complex seminars. Continuing education in communication often will result in more effective and efficient use of the system. Many large corporations do not maintain a record of telephone costs.

It will prove beneficial to the clinic, however, if records are kept current, if monthly statements are examined for trends and irregularities, if new developments in the field are heeded, and if traffic studies are initiated on a regular basis. The group should remain aware of actual costs and should analyze these expenses in light of business trends and seasonal influences.

Deposit/Prepayments. Often some downpayment will be required before delivery and installation of the system. Suppliers may call this a *deposit* or *advance payment* which may be included in the first payment, or distributed in equal amounts among the first several payments.

Additions and Rearrangements. Telephone communication systems must change to accommodate new situations and conditions as well as technological advances. Although the basic telephone instrument has remained essentially the same over the years, perhaps with the exception of optional push-button instead of a rotary dial, vast changes have occurred in telephone switching technology and instrumentation.

The consensus of opinion is that costs of updating a communication system can be enormous; such costs typically may be specified in the basic contract and included in lease payments to the telephone company. Provision for updating flexibility in the system may not enable the supplier to keep initial costs to a bare minimum, but such flexibility certainly will contribute to lower future costs for the clinic. A prediction of future financial commitment can be made on the basis of a study of telephone company and interconnect company service charges over the past five or ten years. Realistic cost estimates should be developed for the service provided by the telephone company versus the charges which the interconnect company would bill. Unfortunately, this is not always an easy task.

Maintenance. Depending upon the vendor, differing arrangements may be made for maintenance of the telephone system. Whether the group owns or leases equipment, it may be required to perform certain routine maintenance. The cost of maintaining and repairing communication equipment will be dependent upon a number of factors such as age, environment, and preventive maintenance. Maintenance services supplied by the telephone company are included in the monthly charge. An interconnect company, however, may use one of several approaches. It may train clinic personnel to perform maintenance tasks of varying complexity, or it may include a service contract in the monthly lease payment.

An accurate determination of maintenance probably will be required. The Bell System has developed general maintenance data on some types of equipment, and as experience and competition in the communications systems industry grow, more of this type of information should become available to facilitate planning.

The general maintenance curve in figure 11-1 has resulted from Bell System data.[4] General inferences can be made from this chart; however, as maintenance experience is gathered by the emerging interconnect companies, the Bell System curve may be revalidated or modified to some degree. Assuming com-

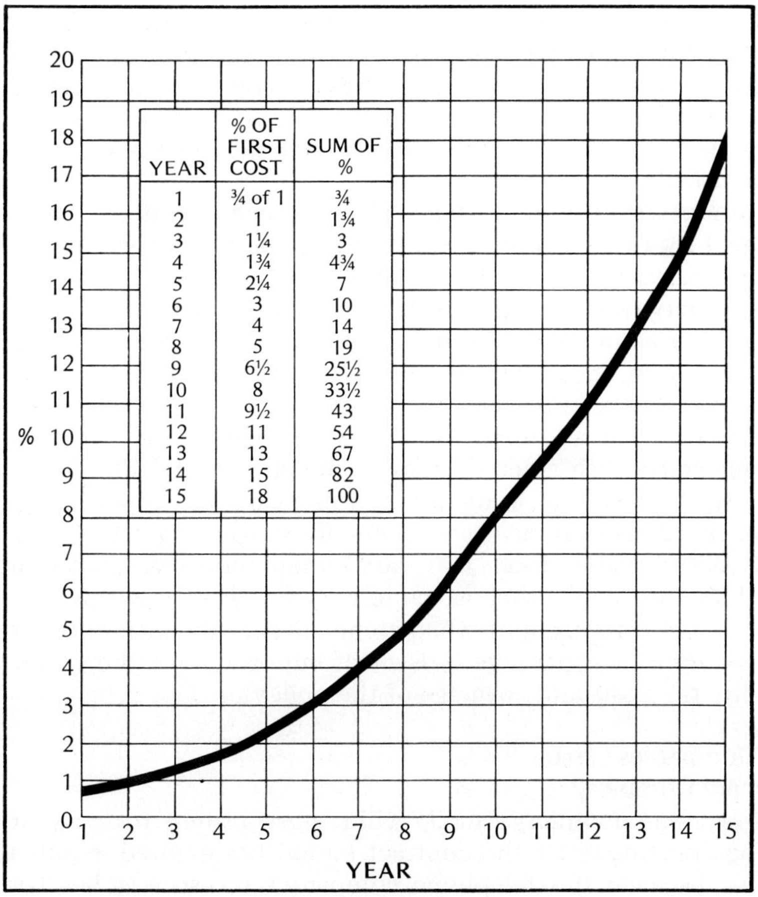

YEAR	% OF FIRST COST	SUM OF %
1	¾ of 1	¾
2	1	1¾
3	1¼	3
4	1¾	4¾
5	2¼	7
6	3	10
7	4	14
8	5	19
9	6½	25½
10	8	33½
11	9½	43
12	11	54
13	13	67
14	15	82
15	18	100

Figure 11-1. The Bell System's General Maintenance Curve

petent installation and servicing of the equipment, maintenance expressed as a percentage of first or total installed costs will represent 100 percent of the investment over a fifteen-year life. Most importantly, from the tenth year on, the range is from 9.5 percent to 18 percent each year. Using this maintenance curve, average costs for maintenance and repair can be estimated for planning purposes. Over a fifteen-year life, the cost of maintaining a communication system will average 8 percent of the original cost each year. On purchased equipment, the first year may be serviced without charge, usually under the manufacturer's warranty. Even with service for routine repair work provided by clinic personnel, rather than telephone company personnel, the savings realized may be relatively insignificant.

Improvements in communication system technology may or may not affect the maintenance characteristics of the telephone systems. Terms such as *solid state*, *space age technology*, and *virtually maintenance-free* can be misleading, and the technology to which such terms refer does not automatically indicate a panacea for maintenance problems. In fact, while technological advances may eliminate some problems, they often generate new and unique ones.

Insurance. Usually, the group must consider equipment insurance when the equipment has been purchased outright. Insurance for telephone communication systems which are leased also is the responsibility of the group, although some vendors do carry blanket policies for their systems. When equipment is leased from the telephone company, however, that company generally assumes all insurance risks.

As with any other type of insurance policy, communications insurance costs are determined by risks, limitations, exclusions, and coverage desired. In addition, policies and coverage vary from state to state. It is best, therefore, to have the group's underwriter carefully review the current insurance situation; even when the supplier assumes the insurance coverage, the group's insurance agent may wish to review the vendor's policy to determine whether the group is sufficiently protected against reasonable hazards. Typically, coverage excludes expendable items such as tubes and similar electronic parts found in power units. In some states, insurance companies apply a fixed deductible amount to actual cost less depreciation, while others will insure only a percentage of some stated value. In 1974 insurance rates generally ranged from $2.00 to $6.00 or more per $1,000 of value. Rates may vary by municipality, neighborhood, city block, and building. Any other extraordinary conditions worthy of examination may be taken into account when companies set the insurance rate. Before purchasing an insurance package it is most important for the group to investigate carefully the costs and coverage of the policy.

Utilities Companies versus Interconnect Company

A local telephone company usually will require a three- to five-year contract for special equipment. After the contract period has expired, equipment rates may decrease because the telephone company's investment has been depreciated. Often special features and new innovations will become standard after the telephone company's initial investment is recovered.

Private telephone equipment manufacturers are relatively new to the market place and have succeeded in creating a competitive atmosphere in telephone service. As a result, Bell System now employs usage sensitive pricing rather than the flat rate of the past. In addition, hardware improvements have been stimulated. The number of equipment manufacturers and the quality of their products have increased steadily. In choosing between a system supplied by the telephone company and one offered by an interconnect company, the decision should be based upon a number of direct comparisons. Inaccurate comparisons often are found in three areas:

1. *Total versus Competitive Charges.* The group should not assume that it can effect a savings in its base telephone bill by purchasing equipment from an interconnect supplier. Charges in the telephone bill for trunk tolls and directory advertising apply to services which the interconnect companies do not offer and which will continue to be billed to the group.

2. *Connecting Arrangements and Certification.* Connecting arrangements currently are required as interface units between most privately obtained equipment and the public message network. Although other alternatives are being discussed, it is only realistic to consider the existing tariff charge for the appropriate number and type of connecting arrangements as part of the interconnect company proposal.

Table 11-1. Comparison of Typical Applicable Costs Between Telephone Company and an Interconnect Company

Telephone Company	*Interconnect Company*
Line Charges	Line Charges Monthly payments on Lease or Loan
Monthly Equipment	Interconnect Devices Installation Charge on Interconnect Devices (One Time Charge)
State and Local Taxes	State and Local Taxes
Federal Excise Tax	Federal Excise Tax Personal Property Tax Business Line Re-termination Charge (One Time Charge)
Telephone Company Equipment Installation Charge (One Time Charge)	Insurance Premium Subtract Depreciation (If Applicable) Subtract Tax Savings Provided by Interest Deduction (If Applicable) Subtract Investment Tax Credit (First Year Only) Maintenance Contract (When Applicable) Other Projected Maintenance Charges (If Any)

3. *Telephone Company Rate Increase Projection.* Any inflationary trend will affect interconnect suppliers as well as the telephone company; consequently, the likelihood of a price increase by all suppliers should be considered.

Telephone company rates, their possible increases, and their effect on the individual clinic situation may be somewhat difficult to predict; a competent representative of the telephone company should be willing to discuss the implications of tariff rates on the individual clinic's situation. For comparison purposes, Table 11-1 displays key cost features for both the telephone company and the interconnect company.

Regardless of the contractual arrangement, a particular area or room must be devoted to actual on-site communications apparatus. Because space represents a definite economic value, the difference between space required by one supplier and that required by another represents a potential cost differential to the group. If privately supplied service is installed, the center must consider the space needed for connecting arrangements. Usually, actual equipment space is planned for, but the group also should allow floor space near the installation for maintenance and repair of the equipment. This space need not be single purpose, but can be a part of a common area. Temperature and noise-control considerations will influence the selection of the space intended for housing the telephone communications equipment.

Utility company tariff schedules determine the optional communication systems available to users; because they have no tariff schedules per se, interconnect companies usually can offer more options and can custom design a system. The actual comparison example, shown in table 11-2, demonstrates

Table 11-2. Feature Comparison Between the Telephone Company and an Interconnect Company

	Bell 608/701	*Bell 300*	*XYZ Corp.*
Direct Station to Station Dialing	x	x	x
Direct Outward Dialing	x	x	x
Attendant Recall and Transfer	x	x	x
Station to Attendant Information Trunks	x	x	x
Call Splitting	x	x	x
Attendant Service Line	x	x	x
Tandem Tie Line	x	x	x
Data Transmission	†	x	x
Attendant Console with Busy Lamp Field		x	x
Direct Station Selection by Operator		x	x
Inquiry During Incoming Calls		x	x
Dial Transfer of Incoming Calls		x	x
Three-way Conference		x	x
Camp-On for Incoming Calls		x	x
Universal Night Answer Any Station		x	x
Ability for Touchtone Instruments		x	x
Visual Indication of Call Processing			x
Attendant Recall on Don't Answer			x
Time Ring-Back on Camp-On Busy			x
Visual Indication of Camp-On			x
Ring-Back on Non-Completed Transfer			x
Reduced Equipment Room Space			x
Individual Station Restriction-Long Distance			x
Trunk Answer Gate			x
Consultation to Outside Trunk			x
Star "Dial 1" Transfer			x
Reset Call			x
Attendant Busy Overide			x
*Inquiry During Outgoing Calls			x
*Dial Transfer of Outgoing Calls			x
*Three Party Conference of Outgoing Calls			x
*MAMS (Message Accounting Management			x
Systems)			x
*WATS Queing (Automated)			x
*Multi Digit Restriction			x
*Ring No Answer Diversion			x
*Key System Trunk			x
*WATS Extender			x
*Code Calling			x
*Meet Me Paging			x
*Dial Dictation—On or Off Premise			x
*Music on Hold			x
Equity			x

*These features not incorporated in system design because not presently required; can be incorporated at a later date as result of future need.

†Significant Limitations.

that in terms of usable features, the interconnect proposal far exceeds the utility system. Although such a display is a good selling point for the interconnect company, it is insufficient for a true comparison of like system alternatives. In making the decision between continuing a utility telephone system and converting to an interconnect system, a group practice of thirty physicians located in Denver, Colorado, compared the two processes and decided in favor of the interconnect system. Cost projections indicate that after eight years with the interconnect system, their telephone costs will drop from $28,000 per year (approximate present cost) to approximately $5,000 per year. Both of these costs are exclusive of trunk lines, directory charges, foreign exchange lines, and hospital tie lines.

THE WORD PROCESSING SYSTEM

As with any other system in the clinic, planning for word processing should include an assessment of needs and a projection of demand. In already existing clinics, a description of the work associated with both medical and administrative communications can be analyzed and is helpful as a basis for planning an efficiently operating system. Newly forming groups may want to consider an analysis of the work load of clinics which are similar to the organization envisioned by the new group. In such an analysis, the tasks described might include typing, transcribing, scanning, shorthand, abstracting medical charts, and supervision. By listing the personnel required, the time spent, and the equipment used, the group can obtain a fairly realistic picture of its word processing activity. Figure 11-2, a form for analyzing work load, was used initially by one group to plan the dictation system and subsequently to evaluate its effectiveness. This type of procedure makes it possible to deploy equipment and personnel in such a manner as to effect the most productive configuration. By ascertaining the kinds, probable numbers, and lengths of reports and communiques produced by each department, a group can determine how many employees are needed and in what locations, as well as what kinds of equipment are needed and in what locations. An estimation of the total cost of the equipment package can be determined and compared to the portion of the budget allocated for that purpose. Then, the best combination of personnel and equipment according to the work load and the situational demands can be designed.

Typewriters

Typewriters are available in models differing greatly in degree of sophistication and effectiveness. The choice of manufacturers and physical features should not be left solely to the discretion of the employee using the machine. When assessing its needs and demands, the group should decide upon a standard for finished copy. The capacity of a machine to meet this standard, together with the considerations of cost, servicing availability, and operator acceptability, should establish criteria for its acquisition.

Major manufacturers of electric typewriters are:

Adler	Olympia
Hermes	Remington Rand
IBM	Royal
Olivetti-Underwood	SCM

Magnetic card and tape equipment is becoming increasingly popular. Compared to the electric typewriter, this equipment has a very high initial cost—

JOB CONTENT ANALYSIS — **SEE INSTRUCTIONS BELOW**

EMPLOYEE'S NAME	POSITION	DEPARTMENT	LOCATION	DATE

TASKS \ TIME	8	9	10	11	12	1	2	3	4	5
	10 20 30 40 50	10 20 30 40 50	10 20 30 40 50	10 20 30 40 50	10 20 30 40 50	10 20 30 40 50	10 20 30 40 50	10 20 30 40 50	10 20 30 40 50	10 20 30 40 50
Transcribing *										
Scanning Recordings										
Logging Recordings										
Playback from Power Typewriters										
Typing (from handwritten notes) *										
Taking Shorthand										
Media Pick-up & Delivery										
Abstracting Charts (includes typing reports)										
MISCELLANEOUS (SPECIFY)										
Supervision										
Breaks & Lunch										

1. Start a new form daily. Change time headings if they do not apply to you.
2. Indicate time spent in the performance of each particular task by drawing a line through consecutive time blocks from its start to its completion.
3. For all "transcribing", indicate the type and quantity of reports being processed (see example):

ⓐ History & physical	ⓙ Pathology reports - Micro
ⓑ Operation report	ⓚ Pathology reports - Gross
ⓒ Discharge summary	ⓛ Medical summaries (to physicians, hospitals)
ⓓ Consultation	ⓜ Medical reports (to attorneys, agencies, etc.)
ⓔ EKG's	ⓝ Insurance reports
ⓕ Radiology reports - Positive	ⓞ EEG's
ⓖ Radiology reports - Negative	ⓟ Nuclear Medicine Scans
ⓗ Progress notes	ⓠ Correspondence
ⓘ Autopsies	ⓡ Other (specify)

*Use red pen or red pencil ıı power typewriter (MT/ST, Itel, etc.) is being used.

EXAMPLE: (Transcribed 2 histories and physicals from 8:30 to 9:00. Then transcribed 2 discharge summaries. Went on break (not shown) at 9:55; returned at 10:05 and began typing a letter handwritten by a doctor. Transcribed 7 progress notes from 11:15 to 12:00).

TASKS \ TIME	8	9	10	11
	10 20 30 40 50	10 20 30 40 50	10 20 30 40 50	10 20 30 40 50
Transcribing *	2ⓐ →	2ⓒ →		7ⓗ →
Scanning Recordings				
Logging Recordings				
Playback from Power Typewriters				
Typing (from handwritten notes) *			→	→
Taking Shorthand				

04210 (REV. 1-75)

Figure 11-2. Form for Analyzing Work Load

$3,000 to $10,000. If both the speed of production and a capacity for storing information are important, the purchase of a power typewriter with an electronic memory might be feasible. If most communications are unique, however, the additional capability of increased speeds of up to 175 words per minute may not be worth expending five to ten times the amount of the cost of a standard electric typewriter. Further advantages of the electronic typewriter include freeing clerical help for other duties through the production of personalized letters with high, error-free speed, as well as automatically produced letters. This also results in less paper and carbon sheet waste. Among current major manufacturers of the electronic typewriter are:

American Automatic Typewriter	IBM
Epsco, Inc.	Lexitron
Friden	Quindata

Dictating Equipment

The recording or dictating system also is a part of the word processing system. Recent technological advances in this field have resulted in increased efficiency due to improvement in transcription speed and accuracy. Nonetheless, certain drawbacks remain, such as the lack of immediate feedback, expensive installation charges for central units, and the tendency for personnel either to underuse or overuse the system extensively.

In choosing the type of dictating equipment to purchase, certain factors demand critical attention. The recording medium—tapes, discs, or belts—can affect efficiency if the system is not standardized throughout the clinic, and to some extent the recording medium will influence the clinic's acquisition of further dictating equipment. Reusability also may be important; if the medium is not reusable, it must be economically feasible for use on a one-time basis. Certain dictating machine features will vary in importance according to the convenience they provide. Some machines are intended only for recording, others for transcription, and still others include both functions. The dictating time capacity of the machine is dependent upon the medium used; and when this capacity is reached, the machine operator will have to interrupt dictation and attend to the machine in order to continue. Other features, such as replay and edit, will vary according to the equipment used. In addition, the potential user will want to determine if backtracking is available, if indexing is manual or automatic, if the erase and re-record can be performed without distortion, and if the equipment can be used on a trial basis before selection.

Some of the same criteria will apply to the choice of dictating systems as will apply to other word processing equipment. In terms of servicing, the group should determine what type of warranty is available, what the service contract entails, the speed and quality of service to be expected, and the financial stability of the dealer. An efficient system will reflect a balance between cost and convenience.

When considering the purchase of dictating equipment, the choice between a central "thought tank" versus individual units can present another dilemma. The central system is costly and must receive the whole-hearted support of the physician group. In addition, the individuals doing the dictating must be

WE FINALLY GOT IT TOGETHER

TRANSCRIPTION THAT IS!

BOTH HOSPITAL AND MEDICAL OFFICE REPORTS WILL NOW BE TRANSCRIBED IN THE NEW TRANSCRIPTION CENTER.

WE'RE PREPARED TO PROVIDE PROFESSIONALLY TYPED MEDICAL REPORTS. HOWEVER, WE DO NEED YOUR HELP.

SEPARATE ALL DICTATION

Please separate your dictation according to the instructions on the labels found on all telephones and dictating handsets.

PROVIDE THE FOLLOWING INFORMATION

1. Your name & the type of report.
2. Patient's name (spell both names).
3. Patient's M.R. number.
4. Dates of admission, operation, etc.
5. State "end of report".

HOW TO OPERATE THE CENTRAL RECORDERS

When you have accessed an open channel, you will hear a faint dial tone.

Telephones in your office or nurses' station

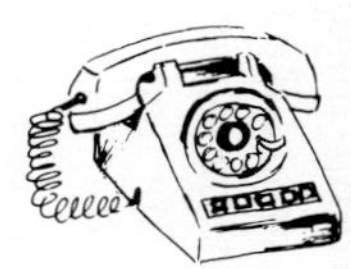

a) Dial the following numbers to access a recorder:
   284 Histories & Physicals
   286 Operation Reports
   288 Discharge Summaries
   290 Outpatient Reports

b) Dial **1** to dictate.
c) Dial **1** to pause.
d) Dial **1** to resume dictation.
e) Dial **3** to reverse & **2** to listen.
f) Correct any errors by:
   - dialing **3** to reverse & **2** to listen.
   - dialing **1** at point of error to dictate correctly.

Dictating handsets

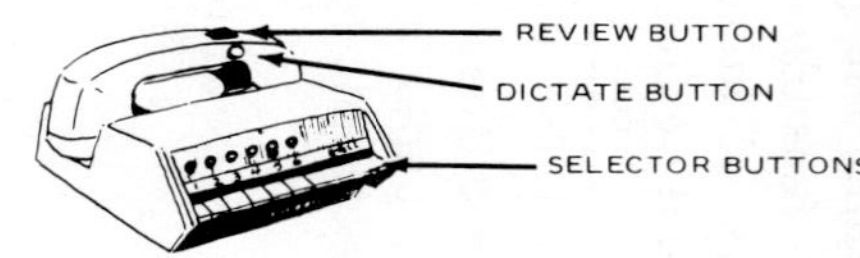

a) Press a "selector button" to access a recorder.
b) Press the "dictate button" to dictate.
c) Push up "review button" to reverse (you will hear double talk).
d) Pull down "review button" to listen.
e) Correct any errors by:
   - following (c) and (d) above.
   - releasing "review button" at point of error.
   - following (b) above to dictate correctly.

Figure 11-3. Pamphlet Designed for Training Center Staff in Centralized Dictation Procedures

trained. A reproduction of a pamphlet used for this type of training appears as figure 11–3. An alternative to centralized dictation is the use of individual desk top recorders, but theft of these items may constitute an unusually high recurring expense. Nevertheless, the assignment of specialties to individual transcribers often produces a more efficient use of time, and personnel can be assigned jobs according to their expertise. Some employees may specialize in transcribing medical histories; others may summarize and abstract data for storage and future retrieval. It may be important to cross-train individuals for different tasks so that morale will not suffer. This arrangement also allows for a concentration of larger groups of workers when a deadline must be met.

Regardless of the system chosen, certain needs must be provided for. The first criterion is that of *availability*; the group must understand what type of access will be provided and what the limitations on this access will be at high-usage times. *Down time* also is an important factor. How many people will be inconvenienced by a breakdown in the equipment? How long might such an inconvenience continue? Centralization will require the general pooling of transcribing personnel, while individual units will allow for decentralization. If a centralized system is adopted the location of the equipment, the amount of surveillance which is needed while the machine is in operation, and the type of notification available in case of malfunction are concerns that must be addressed by clinic planners.

Provisions for interfacing the dictating system with the clinic telephone system will require considering the type of access desired, which in turn may severely limit the choice of equipment. Interfacing an established clinic's present dictating equipment with other makes and models of dictating equipment will become important when expansion is considered. When provided with the proper interface options, often the same type of equipment used for central dictating can be used as answering devices. Both telephone and interconnect companies can provide this type of equipment. The decision often is between an answering service and a recording/answering machine; however, problems with emergency notification, message acceptance, and the capacity to recover messages from a remote location must be ascertained. To make a final choice, it may be necessary to poll each physician within the group. Several system alternatives include portable dictation models ($50 to $400 price range) and desk-type dictation models ($200 to $500 price range). The portable pocket dictation units are especially convenient because they can be carried into the examination room and to the hospital and to the physician's home. Individual units can be taken to meetings and conferences and can be used while traveling. Some dictating machine models do not include a transcribing unit; the cost of transcribing units varies between $200 and $400.

The current major manufacturers of dictation equipment and systems include:

Dictaphone	Sony
IBM	Telefunken
Lanier	Uher
Norelco	

Copying Equipment

The third key element of the word processing system is the copying machine. When purchasing such equipment one should consider:

1. *Cost* per copy (including paper cost)
2. Type of *process* used by the machine (which may be especially important in the copying industry where technological innovation occurs rapidly)
3. General reputation of the particular machine in terms of usage and *servicing*
4. Size of the machine, its *location restrictions* and *electrical requirements*
5. *Quality* and *durability* of copies
6. Variety of *copy sizes* available
7. *Speed* of the machine in producing the first copy and the possibility of *overheating* due to extended production runs
8. Machine *capability* in copying and in reducing photos, colored originals, and material from bound books, and in producing different sized copies
9. Ease of *instructing* new or part-time operators in machine use
10. *Number* of units—one large unit versus several smaller units in various locations
11. *Control* of unauthorized use of machine.

The group can either buy or lease the copying equipment, and differing types of contractual agreements are available. Typically, if a cost evaluation comparison is performed, the time period for comparisons should be fairly brief (three to five years). The purchase price of copying equipment ranges between $500 and $5,000. Major equipment suppliers include:

A.B. Dick	Electrophy	Savin
Addressograph-Multigraph	GAF	3M
Apeco	IBM	Xerox
Dennison	Pitney-Bowes	

Should a lease arrangement be chosen, some of the contractual considerations deserving special scrutiny are the length of the agreement; cancellation privileges; lease/purchase terms; servicing, such as warranty provisions, quality of service, and other contractual arrangements; and updating in the event of technological improvement and change. Here again, the group's attorney or a communications consultant may be of help in providing an understanding of the precise meaning of contractual terms.

PAPER HANDLING SYSTEMS

Certain equipment within the communication system does not lend itself readily to categorization. In some clinics, this type of equipment may be extremely useful, while other clinics may not be able to justify its acquisition.

Facsimile Equipment

Written information can be rapidly and accurately transmitted by facsimile equipment. Although such equipment usually is most useful in a large clinic, it may be valuable for smaller groups to have the ability to transmit handwritten messages, such as prescriptions and laboratory test orders, without the use of a courier. Althought the number of suppliers is limited, several types of facsimile equipment are available. Costs, advantages, and disadvantages should be weighed carefully before any decision is made.

Mail Handling

The mail system is integral to record keeping, correspondence, billing, and collections. As a total system, various types of equipment can be chosen to perform the many functions. Such equipment not only performs the usual stamping and postmarking, but also may display added capabilities such as folding and inserting statements and correspondence, signing checks, and sealing or opening letters.

The typical mail handling system is a series of functions in linear progression, with the complexity of the equipment determined partially by volume considerations. When 3,000–4,000 pieces of mail and multiples thereof must be moved on a per month basis, automated mail handling equipment can save valuable personnel time, expedite mail handling in the post office, and provide a more professional appearance to correspondence. Mail handling equipment may be either leased or bought, and service contracts are available. The arrangements usually stipulate some type of training, and often include application for postage permits and registration of the equipment with the post office. Any contract should be reviewed carefully by competent individuals. As a rule, it is wise to allow for increases in the volume of paperwork which can be handled by the system. Components of the mail handling system may be interfaced quite efficiently with the copying and billing systems. While some of the mail handling equipment may be used only at certain times, its overall value to the group soon becomes apparent.

INDIVIDUAL PAGING AND INTERCOM SYSTEMS

Personnel in the medical field find that the use of paging and intercom devices can be instrumental in providing better service to patients. The paging system may employ a transmitter linked to several pocket receivers. This radio system, which may be acquired through the telephone company or may be established by the clinic and privately licensed, involves wireless transmissions through VHF frequencies with the aid of an antenna. Other pocket paging systems rely on an ultrasonic loop which is installed in areas sensitive to paging. Both systems will require an encoder, transmitter, and individual receivers. With pocket pagers, the size and weight of the unit and the potential distance limitation capabilities must be considered along with features such as one- or two-way voice and multiple address. Radio signal strength, broadcast radius, battery life, reliability, maintenance, telephone system interfacing, and possible interference problems also influence decisions relating to the pocket paging system.

The intercom or speaker type of paging system is limited to an immediate vicinity, and the latter may disturb patients and certain medical specialists. While the location of paging speakers in the cardiology department may be very distracting to the cardiologist, who depends upon being able to discriminate certain sounds for a diagnosis, the radiologist usually would not object to speakers in his department because he depends upon visual rather than audio inspection. If an intercom paging system is part of the clinic's telephone system, one instrument may serve as both intercom unit and telephone. An independent intercom paging system, however, can remove an overburdening amount of traffic from the clinic telephone system, but will necessitate a separate investment and additional maintenance.

Both the speaker system and the pocket paging system can provide for either voice or tone paging. Again, the choice depends upon the personal preference of the clinic physicians as well as a significant cost differential between voice and tone paging. With tone only paging, however, the individual being paged cannot receive voice instructions and must return the call. Often this added step can serve as a double check on activity. When a paging system must be used as part of the telephone communication system, often it is economically sound to have the system serve a dual function. Paging speakers may be used for background music in specified clinic areas and may employ an override feature for the actual paging. The secret of success for a paging/music system is to have an ample number of speakers rather than attempt to cover large areas with only one speaker which may be too loud. In addition, personnel in each area of the clinic should have access to volume controls for their specific area. Similarly, the function of a pocket paging system may be extended to include after-hours coverage. Rather than subscribing to an answering service or sharing a service with another group, the group can employ an operator who will accept after-hours calls and page the proper physician or staff member.

Paging also may be a visual process. Visual paging often is employed for communication between clinic personnel, usually physicians and nurses, and involves the use of colored signal paddles or lights which can be displayed outside the examining room to indicate the status of an examination. These signaling systems have great potential for increasing efficiency when appointment schedules are heavy. Complex systems involving more than three lights/paddles, however, may fall into disuse because personnel do not make the effort to learn and maintain the system.

Various paging systems are available to the group along with various financial arrangements including lease, purchase, and lease-purchase. The price range for intercom units varies between $100 to $500 per unit with a central paging/music system approaching $1,500 to $5,000. Some major manufacturers of paging and intercom systems include:

- Action Systems
- Bell Telephone
- Bogen
- Dictograph
- Executone
- Interconnect
- Medi-Call, Inc.
- Norelco
- Stromberg-Carlson

All communication equipment considered by the group must be seen within the context of other equipment which has been acquired. Overlap and duplication of functions incur costs which usually are nonproductive. Unless overlapping or duplicate equipment is necessary for backup capability, it should not be added to the system. The various elements of the communication system should not be a mere assemblage of dissimilar parts. All devices should be flexible and compatible with other system components, and should offer the user backup capability and convenience.

When investigating communications equipment in general, the group should be aware of economic indicators, such as the rate of inflation and interest rates. Moreover, as discussed in Chapter 27, the basic types of economic analysis—reinvested savings, discounted cash flow, and rate of return—are applicable to all clinic equipment acquisition. Finally, groups involved in medical teaching may qualify for teaching rates or discounts offered by various communication system vendors.

CLINIC PERSONNEL TRAINING AND MAINTENANCE OF THE COMMUNICATION SYSTEM

Modern mechanical and electronic devices will function well only when operated and maintained properly. Individuals operating the clinic equipment constitute an indispensable link between the functioning of the systems and the ultimate effectiveness, reliability, and adaptability of those systems. Thus, it is important that clinic personnel receive thorough and ongoing training in use of the various equipment. Often such education is available on a no-charge basis from the equipment supplier. The group may find it desirable to supplement the vendor-supplied training with certain policies and procedures which are unique to its own situations. If the operator is informed fully as to the advantages and limitations of the system, a positive attitude toward systems operations can be generated. Without proper attitudes and enthusiastic cooperation among personnel, even the best designed systems may fail.

Patient Information Brochure

Patients, as well as clinic personnel, also can profit from a better understanding of the purpose, goals, and available services of the group. Often, this task can best be accomplished through the use of communication brochures or patient information booklets. Appendix 11A suggests some areas which might be covered in a patient information brochure.

Communications Policy

Communication system policy may be recorded formally or simply may be an attitude of the management transmitted orally to employees. Regardless of the method chosen, communication policy should deal with two basic problems which may be encountered in the operation of the systems. The first involves the extent and method of clerical screening; the second involves establishing who will use the system and for what purpose. Actual implementation of these policy decisions probably is most easily accomplished during the personnel training period.

In telephone system development and screening, for example, there are numerous policy considerations pertaining to the disposition of incoming telephone calls to physicians. The disposition of the call may be determined in

			TYPE OF CALL							
			PATIENT							
		DISPOSITION OF CALL	Emergency	Non-emergency	Non-medical	Pharmacists	Hospital	Other Physicians	Business Calls	Personal Calls
1	DOCTOR IS IN THE OFFICE	Immediately, my aide will interrupt me and I will handle the call.	√							
2	DOCTOR IS IN THE OFFICE	Immediately, my aide will interrupt me but she will handle the call.	√							
3	DOCTOR IS IN THE OFFICE	Immediately, my aide will interrupt me but I will instruct her that I will handle the call when I finish what I'm doing.					√	√		
4	DOCTOR IS IN THE OFFICE	I will speak to callers only during certain hours or time periods.			√				√	
5	DOCTOR IS IN THE OFFICE	My aide will keep a list of incoming calls and I will return the calls in clusters whenever I get free time.		√						√
6	DOCTOR IS IN THE OFFICE	My aide keeps a list and I will return calls at a scheduled time. My aide will instruct callers when to expect call.		√						
7	DOCTOR IS IN THE OFFICE	My aide will return the calls after she has spoken with me when I'm not busy.					√		√	
8	DOCTOR IS IN THE OFFICE	My aide will handle the calls without any direction from me.				√				
9	DOCTOR OUT	My aide will contact me immediately and I will determine proper disposition.	√					√		
10	DOCTOR OUT	My aide will accumulate calls and I will dispose of the calls following my "in office" routine.		√	√	√	√		√	√

Figure 11-4. Telephone Call—Physician's Policy Statements

part by its type: patient, pharmacist, hospital, other physicians, business, or personal. While many other factors may influence the disposition of a telephone call, in the policy statements displayed in figure 11-4, *type of call* will be isolated as the only disposition determinant. In the absence of a uniform clinic policy for the screening and disposition of telephone calls, it becomes necessary for personnel to learn the individual policy desires of each physician in the group. A diagram similar to figure 11–4 could be developed as a graphic policy display to those persons handling incoming calls for physicians. This diagram may serve to represent uniform group policy, or each individual physician could have a separate chart to indicate his policy determinations regarding telephone call disposition.

Policy is largely a matter of personal preference and no one correct manner of dealing with the problems encountered can be developed. This may be an area which must be dealt with during the formulation of general clinic policies and upon the actual selection of the specific communication systems to be employed within the clinic.

This chapter has attempted to demonstrate that an effective communication system for providing a crucial link to the patient population is vital to a clinic. Effective integration of the various subsystems involved is critical to efficient clinic operation. For this reason, it is helpful to assume a problem solving approach to planning the group's communication system. The three basic areas which have been dealt with include the telephone system, the word processing system, and the paper handling system. In planning for any and all of these systems, two basic cautions are applicable. First, when legal, tax, and cost questions arise, the group would be well-advised to use the services of a competent professional who specializes in those areas. Second, the group should consider that it is trying to develop a complete and integrated communication system and in doing so should strive to eliminate as many overlaps and conflicts as possible. Communication systems are meant to complement and enhance the functioning of clinic personnel and should facilitate interaction between the group and its patients. To achieve this end, the group always must consider the training, education, and welfare of those people who will operate the systems as well as those who will receive the benefits the systems help to generate. With these ideas in mind, the newly forming group practice should be able to deal effectively with the problems which it encounters in the planning, implementation, and use of its communication system.

Appendix 11A

Topic to be Included in Patient Information Brochure

I. Services Rendered
   1. What is the extent or limitation of professional services rendered?
   2. What about care provided by referring physicians?
   3. What is the policy regarding being seen or cared for by other physicians in the group or physicians who may be covering you?
   4. At what hospitals do you have staff privileges?
   5. Are there nursing home, industrial, school, etc., affiliations that you wish to have the patient know?

II. Hours and Appointments
   1. What are the regular office hours?
   2. What is the patient to do in case of an emergency?
   3. What is the appointment policy for the following:
      a. General episodic care
      b. Physical exams
      c. School physicals
      d. Other
   4. How far in advance should appointments be made?
   5. What if the patient has to be worked in on a given day?
   6. What is the policy on "no-shows"?
   7. What is the policy on "house calls"?

III. The Telephone
   1. List all the necessary phone numbers in a conspicuous manner.
   2. When should the patient call for nonemergency, clinical advice? Define for patient.

3. What kind of screening policies exist?
4. Indicate your procedures on returning patient calls.
5. How should the patient use the telephone in case of a major emergency? During office hours; after office hours?
6. What should the patient know about your answering service or automated answering device?
7. What is your policy about after-hour calls or weekend calls for non-emergencies?
8. What is your policy for giving prescriptions and refills over the phone?
9. What is your policy regarding charging for phone consultations?
10. What is your policy on providing information about patients to relatives, friends, employers, etc.?

IV. Accounting and Credit Service
1. How do you expect payment for services rendered? (If you expect cash or check for first or continued visits, say so clearly.)
2. When are balances due? When will statements be sent?
3. What is your credit privileges policy?
4. How are your fees for services determined?
5. What happens to overdue accounts?
6. What is your policy regarding the preparation of insurance forms? Do you charge for one or more form completions? Do you use a standardized form? Do you employ the "Superbill" concept?
7. What are your assignment policies?
8. What special information do you wish to relate to your Medicare, Medicaid, Welfare, or Workmen's Compensation patients?
9. What is the credit policy for long-term or large bills anticipated?

V. General Center Information
1. Well Baby Care
2. Well Adult Care
3. Periodic Health Exams
4. Maternity Care
5. Medicine Chest Supplies
6. Use of Medications
7. Immunizations—Adult/Children

VI. Some common ailments you may wish to discuss:

General Measures—

Allergies
Antibiotics
Colic
Convulsions
Constipation
Cough
Diaper Rash
Diarrhea
Ear Aches
Fever
Pinworms
Poisoning
Poison Ivy
Rashes
Vitamins
Vomiting

Injuries—

Animal Bites
Bloody Nose
Burns
Cuts
Head Injuries
Sprains, Strains, Muscle Aches, Bruises, Scratches, Abrasions
Broken Bones

Infection—

Chicken Pox
Colds and Flu—General and Babies
Croup
German Measles
Mumps
Red Measles
Strep Throats
Sore Throats
Swollen Glands
Urinary Infections
Vaginal Infections

Chapter 12

Patient Registration Systems

ESTABLISHING THE PATIENT REGISTRATION SYSTEM

Registration, as an early point of communication between clinic and patient, is not only a means of gathering information about the patient but also of transmitting information about the clinic. It is during this early question and answer exchange that the patient receives his first visual impression of the clinic and begins to develop either a positive or negative attitude toward the group, clinic personnel, and available services.

Four basic decisions are integral to the development of a patient registration system—what type and how much data are to be collected, what procedures will be utilized for data collection, what time period will be allotted for each procedure and where registration personnel will be located. When the types and amounts of data have been determined, the group can then estimate the time required to complete each registration event by considering the specific procedures chosen to accomplish registration objectives. In this chapter, the function of the registration process and planning for its efficient interfacing with other clinic systems will be discussed. A number of the various options for collecting, recording, modifying, and retrieving patient information will be presented together with a discussion of the personnel responsibilities inherent in each type of procedure.

During registration, information necessary to begin medical care and service is elicited from the patient and then placed into a permanent record in the clinic. This information provides both a general data base for administrative purposes and a particular reference point for identifying possible patient medical problems. Careful attention should be given to maintaining accuracy in the recording of such information. The patient's *full* name, including his middle name or initial, as well as his address and birth date may provide the means for filing and retrieving medical records. Securing complete information from the patient also contributes to increased accuracy in the transferral of data to data banks for electronic processing. While EDP (electronic data processing) may not be financially feasible for the newly forming group, current trends indicate that alternative EDP systems will become available and will be within the financial capabilities of even the smallest group. In addition, the group should establish a uniform style for the recording of patient name, and all clinic forms should reflect this pattern. The order in which the patient's name will be recorded on the forms must be decided, and should remain consistent across *all* clinic forms. This uniformity also will facilitate future electronic data processing. Throughout this text, various forms have been used as examples. These forms have been assembled from a variety of sources and, therefore, do not reflect the consistency and uniformity which is desirable within a homogeneous setting.

THE REGISTRATION PROCESS

Registration is a requirement for only those patients who are new to the clinic. As subsequent appointments are made with a physician, the patient usually will report directly to the physician's receptionist or nurse. In some instances, however, appointment/reception responsibilities are carried out by the same personnel who are responsible for patient registration. It is necessary, therefore, to determine whether a patient is new or whether he has been seen previously by any one of the group's physicians.

Alternative means available for the acquisition of registration information include a self-explanatory data sheet, a questionnaire, an oral interview, or a combination of these. Regardless of the method chosen, information obtained during the registration process should be in written form before the physician-patient encounter. As an aid to the physician, the registration process also can include questions concerning the patient's previous medical history. A listing of the patient's prior diseases, trauma, and hospitalizations might be supplemented by data on family size and history, patient occupation, and residence information. The patient's medical history can be acquired in various ways, ranging from the completion of a preprinted history questionnaire to the use of an automated history-taking machine. The latter alternative may involve the patient's responding to health history questions as they appear on the screen of a small video display unit (cathode ray tube). Using a simple keyboard the patient can respond positively or negatively to the questions as he reads them on the screen. History information can be stored for future retrieval and usually can be produced in hard copy if necessary. It is anticipated that this procedure will be applicable to the registration process in the near future. When designing a facility, therefore, the group may want to make provision for the later installation of CRT units when this method becomes economically practical. The completion of the health history during registration, most often during the latter stages of the process, should be economical in terms of physician time and should facilitate the physician's reviewing the history with the patient to clarify certain areas, to improve general accuracy, or to seek more complete information.

The registration process also can be helpful to the clinic administrator. Registration information represents one data source for statistics on the usage of facilities, location of the population served, eligibility under third party payor programs, and possibly the credit status of group patients. In addition, the accuracy of registration information enables third party payments to be made more quickly and with less confusion. Insurance companies and government assistance programs often are interested in individual patient and patient population information for identification purposes. The patient population information which is provided to third parties can serve as a part of their data base, thus enabling them to make policy decisions and to render judgments on the extent and effect of the health services provided by the group practice.

If the group chooses to have the patient complete a registration form, as opposed to conducting an oral interview, the decision must be made as to whether the forms will be completed when the patient visits the clinic or mailed to the patient in advance of his arrival, or whether a combination of these alternatives will be used. If preregistration forms are mailed to patients, they either may be returned to the clinic through the mail, if time permits, or delivered by the patient at the time of his appointment. When patients are asked to return completed preregistration material through the mail, a sufficient number of days should be allowed for postal delivery in advance of the patient's appointment. The purpose of preregistration would be thwarted and the goodwill of the group undermined if patients were to arrive at registration only to find that their completed forms had not yet been received by the clinic. If the preregistration form is designed to ascertain the medical complaint or reason for the patient's visit, returning the form through the mail can facilitate the prescheduling of other services deemed necessary before the initial appointment with the physician. For example, new patient visits scheduled with an orthopedist routinely may require that X-rays be taken before the appointment time. With prior information, such X-rays can be prescheduled in advance of the patient's arrival.

Rather than mailing a data or information sheet to the patient for completion, registration personnel can acquire the same information over the telephone, but the health history questionnaire, which is apt to be quite lengthy, might be mailed to the patient and then brought to the clinic at the time of the appointment. Needless to say, when a preregistration or self-explanatory form is used, the patient must be assured of the confidentiality of the information he provides. Issues surrounding the confidentiality of medical records will be discussed in detail in Chapter 14. Examples of preregistration (mail out) and self-explanatory (mail out or in-center completion) registration forms are shown in figures 12-1 and 12-2. A sample history questionnaire for use during the registration process is shown in figure 12-3.

Regardless of whether a self-explanatory form is completed by the patient upon his arrival at the registration area or is completed by clinic personnel through an interview, adequate space within the clinic must be provided for the completion of registration; thus, the system employed to obtain registration data can influence clinic interior design. To many patients registration data is of a personal and confidential nature. If a patient is required to complete the

XYZ CLINIC

We have arranged an appointment for ______________________________ to see Doctor______________ at______ a.m./p.m. ______________. To assist us in making arrangements for the visit, please complete the following information and mail this form to us as soon as possible. This will save you time upon arrival at the Clinic. Please <u>print</u> or <u>type</u> your answers and complete all questions.

1. Name of Patient: ______________________________
   First Middle Last
2. Home address: ______________________________
   Street City State Zip Code

   Phone Number______________
3. Age______ Birthdate______________ Sex ________   ☐ Married ☐ Single ☐ Widowed ☐ Separated ☐ Divorced
4. Name of husband, wife or nearest living relative (if patient is a dependent child, insert father, mother or legal guardian's name)______________________ Relationship to patient:____________
5. Patient's occupation: ______________________________
   Type of work (If retired, please give last occupation)
6. Name, address and telephone number of patient's employer:______________________________
7. Occupation of responsible party: ______________________________
   (If widowed, please give husband's last occupation)
8. Name, address and telephone number of responsible party's employer: ______________________________
9. Referred by:______________________ Have you ever been our patient?__________
10. If referred by a physician, please give his name and address: ______________________________
11. In case of an emergency, whom should we notify (other than immediate family)? Relationship __________
    Name Address Phone Number
12. OUT OF TOWN PATIENTS (Local address, if known)
13. Medicare claim number (if over age 65 and have part "B"): ______________________________
14. Reason for the clinic visit: ______________________________

Merely fold, as indicated, seal and mail <u>as soon as possible</u>. No stamp is necessary unless you wish to air mail this back to us.

We will endeavor to make your visit as pleasant as possible.

Thank you,

XYZ CLINIC

Figure 12-1. Preregistration Form

DATE OF APPOINTMENT	TIME	TYPE OF VISIT	DOCTOR OF PREFERENCE	RESP. PARTY NO.	REGISTERED BY

PATIENT INFORMATION • PRINT FIRMLY & CLEARLY IN COMPLETING ITEMS BELOW •

(circle one) DOCTOR MR MASTER MISS MRS — PATIENT'S FIRST NAME — MIDDLE NAME — LAST NAME — SPOUSE'S GIVEN NAME & INITIAL

PATIENT'S HOME ADDRESS — NUMBER STREET CITY STATE AND ZIP CODE — HOME PHONE NO

PATIENT'S EMPLOYER — PATIENT'S OCCUPATION — BUSINESS PHONE NO

EMPLOYER'S ADDRESS

BIRTH DATE — AGE — RACE — SEX — (circle one) MARR SING DIV WID SEP — SOCIAL SECURITY OR MEDICARE NO IF APPLICABLE — WHO REFERRED YOU TO THE CLINIC OR DOCTOR? — RELATIONSHIP — NAME OF FAMILY MEMBER ALREADY A CLINIC PATIENT — RELATIONSHIP

IN CASE OF EMERGENCY NOTIFY (other than spouse or parent) NAME — ADDRESS — PHONE NO

IF PATIENT IS MARRIED OR IS A DEPENDENT CHILD, COMPLETE ITEMS BELOW:

FULL NAME OF SPOUSE OR PARENT — RELATIONSHIP — SPOUSE OR PARENT'S EMPLOYER

SPOUSE OR PARENTS EMPLOYER'S ADDRESS (number street city state and zip code) — OCCUPATION OF SPOUSE OR PARENT — BUSINESS PHONE NO

WHO WILL BE RESPONSIBLE FOR THE PATIENT'S MEDICAL EXPENSES?

CHECK ONE: ☐PATIENT ☐SPOUSE ☐PARENT ☐OTHER (complete next item below)

IF "OTHER" BLOCK CHECKED ABOVE PLEASE COMPLETE NAME OF PERSON OR COMPANY — STREET ADDRESS CITY STATE & ZIP CODE — PHONE NO

INSURANCE INFORMATION: **TO REQUEST FILING OF CLAIM(S) PLEASE NOTIFY CASHIER.**

NAME OF INSURANCE COMPANY — INSURANCE CO ADDRESS — GROUP NO — POLICY NO

OTHER INSURANCE COVERAGE — GROUP NO — POLICY NO

IF PATIENT RESIDES OUTSIDE OF TOWN, COMPLETE ITEM BELOW:

HOTEL OR LOCAL RESIDENCE — NAME — ADDRESS — LOCAL PHONE NO

REPORT REQUESTED TO DR.

RETURN THIS COMPLETED INFORMATION TO NEW PATIENT REGISTRATION

White Copy - Medical Records
Green Copy - Business Office
Pink Copy - Patient Accounts

Figure 12-2. Registration Form

questionnaire himself, a clipboard and chair may suffice. On the other hand, if the information is to be acquired through an interview, more consideration must be given to privacy. This is not to say that a completely private room or booth is necessary; the partitioning of a registration desk may suffice in creating an atmosphere of privacy or semiprivacy. During the registration process, conditions which contribute to personal embarrassment and lack of privacy should not interfere with the gathering of complete and accurate information.

Interface with Medical Records and Appointments

Although there are various alternatives available in the establishment of the registration system itself, one particular consideration is common to the development of all such systems—the interfacing of the process with other clinic activities and systems.

In addition to acquiring and documenting patient information and medical history, the group may require that registration personnel initiate the medical record for new patients, complete the necessary identification cards, prepare

No. ______

Name ______ Date ______

PATIENT'S HISTORY AND HEALTH QUESTIONNAIRE

FAMILY HISTORY: Have any members of your family ever had the following? If so, please circle below.

Father: Living–Age ______ Condition of Health? ______
Dead–Age ______ Cause of Death? ______
Mother: Living–Age ______ Condition of Health? ______
Dead–Age ______ Cause of Death? ______
Number Brothers: Living: ______ Ages: ______ Dead: ______ Causes ______
Number Sisters: Living: ______ Ages: ______ Dead: ______ Causes ______
Are You Married? ______ Number of Years? ______ Wife's Age: ______ Husband's Age: ______
Health of Husband or Wife? ______
If spouse dead, give age, year, and cause of death: ______
Previous Marriages? ______ Give Dates: ______
Number Children: Boys: ______ Ages: ______ Girls: ______ Ages: ______
All Healthy? ______ Any Dead? ______

Diabetes
Tuberculosis
Headaches
Epilepsy
Cancer
High Blood Pressure
Heart Disease
Stroke
Allergy
Stomach Trouble
Nervous Trouble
Blood Disease
Goiter
Arthritis
Other Diseases

PLEASE LIST HERE PRESENT CONDITIONS OR DISEASES WHICH YOU WISH TO HAVE CHECKED AT THIS EXAMINATION:

______

PERSONAL HISTORY: Please give approximate year of last immunization ("shot") for:

Allergy or severe reaction to medicines, foods, plants, chemicals, etc.: Please list ______

Smallpox ______ Polio ______
Typhoid ______ Influenza ______
Tetanus ______ Other ______

List Average:
Hours worked per day: ______
Hours sleep per night: ______
Days worked per week: ______
Days vacation per year: ______
Number cigarettes per day: ______
Other tobacco per day: ______
Cups coffee per day: ______
Alcoholic drinks per day: ______

Do you take regular exercise? ______
Do you take a rest each day? ______
Approximate date of last vacation: ______
What is you usual weight? ______ lbs.
What is the most you ever weighed? ______ lbs.
At what year or age? ______
Have you lost or gained weight? ______
If so, how much? ______ lbs.

Put a circle around any of the following conditions which you now have or have had in the past:

Skin Trouble	Pneumonia	Worms	Gonorrhea	Measles
Cataracts	Tuberculosis	Dysentery	Hernia (rupture)	Rheumatic Fever
Tonsillitis	Breast Trouble	Colitis	Fainting	Arthritis
Sinusitis	Heart Trouble	Hemorrhoids	Fits or Convulsions	Gout
Goiter	Ulcer	Kidney Trouble	Nervous Breakdown	Anemia
Hay Fever	Jaundice	Kidney Stones	Unconsciousness	Diabetes
Asthma	Gallstones	Bladder Trouble	Paralysis	Cancer or Tumor
Bronchitis	Liver Trouble	Prostate Trouble	Polio	Varicose Veins
Pleurisy	Hepatitis	Syphilis	Mumps	Phlebitis

PAST HISTORY: Please list previous operations, injuries, serious illnesses, etc. and year:

1. ______
2. ______
3. ______

When was your last physical examination? ______ Any abnormality found? ______
Are you under any medical treatment now? ______
List any medications you take now or occasionally: ______

FOR WOMEN ONLY: Menses (Monthly periods): Date last period: ______
Age began: ______
Now occurs about every ______ days
Normal? ______
Discharge? ______
Flooding? ______
Irregular? ______
Painful? ______
Spotting between periods? ______

Age when "change of life" started: ______
Hot flashes? ______
Any history of trouble with female organs? ______
Number of pregnancies? ______
Complications of any pregnancies? (List) ______
Any miscarriages? ______

PLEASE TURN PAGE FOR HEALTH QUESTIONS ON OTHER SIDE

Figure 12-3. Sample History Questionnaire

IF YOU HAVE ANY OF THE FOLLOWING COMPLAINTS, PLEASE CIRCLE (YES.) IF NOT, CIRCLE (NO.) THE DOCTOR WILL ASK ABOUT DETAILS LATER. ANSWER ALL QUESTIONS. IF IN DOUBT, GUESS YES OR NO.

Severe headaches or head pains	Yes	No
Do you need an eye check for:		
Any disturbance in vision	Yes	No
Glasses	Yes	No
Pain or discomfort	Yes	No
Constant noises in ears	Yes	No
Hard of hearing	Yes	No
Ear ache with colds ( ) plane flights ( )	Yes	No
Chronic running ear	Yes	No
Chronic stuffy or runny nose	Yes	No
Chronic dripping from nose to throat	Yes	No
Need to use nose drops frequently	Yes	No
Bad nose bleeds at times	Yes	No
Frequent severe colds or sore throat	Yes	No
Need to clear throat frequently	Yes	No
Any known dental problems	Yes	No
Soreness or bleeding of gums	Yes	No
More than a year since teeth checked	Yes	No
Would you like a dental check during this exam	Yes	No
Sore mouth or tongue	Yes	No
Goiter or thyroid trouble	Yes	No
Metabolism test - too high ( ) too low ( )	Yes	No
Feeling of lump in the throat	Yes	No
Need to take thyroid medicine	Yes	No
Hoarseness at times	Yes	No
Recent or chronic cough	Yes	No
Chronic coughing up of sputum	Yes	No
Ever coughed up blood	Yes	No
Ache all over	Yes	No
Having chills or fever	Yes	No
Severe soaking night sweats	Yes	No
Lived with anyone having T.B.	Yes	No
Worried about your heart	Yes	No
Blood pressure - too high ( ) too low ( )	Yes	No
Pains in heart or chest	Yes	No
Pounding or skipping of heart	Yes	No
Heart starts racing suddenly	Yes	No
Shortness of breath or wheezing	Yes	No
Trouble getting a deep breath	Yes	No
Swelling ankles	Yes	No
Leg cramps in bed or sitting still	Yes	No
Leg cramps while walking	Yes	No
Pain or trouble with swallowing	Yes	No
Gulp your food in a hurry	Yes	No
Poor appetite - recently ( ) always ( )	Yes	No
Nausea or vomiting	Yes	No
Vomiting of blood	Yes	No
Belching, bloating or indigestion	Yes	No
Yellow skin or eyes (jaundice)	Yes	No
Burning or hunger pains in stomach	Yes	No
Use antacids for stomach burning	Yes	No
Soreness or pain in stomach, abdomen	Yes	No
Suspect ulcers or stomach trouble	Yes	No
Cramps in stomach or low down	Yes	No
Loose bowels or diarrhea	Yes	No
Black or tarry stools (bowel movements)	Yes	No
Fresh or bright blood with stools	Yes	No
Mucus (slime or phlegm) in stools	Yes	No
Constipation	Yes	No
Use laxatives ( ) or enemas ( ) frequently	Yes	No
Recent change in bowel habits	Yes	No
Rectal trouble or pain	Yes	No

List any foods which always disagree: ______		
Pain in the kidney region	Yes	No
Get up nights to urinate (No. times ______)	Yes	No
Blood or pus in urine	Yes	No
Albumin in urine	Yes	No
Sugar in urine	Yes	No
Spells of frequent urination	Yes	No
Severe burning or pain on urination	Yes	No
Pains over bladder or low down	Yes	No
Trouble starting urine	Yes	No
Urinary stream has become weak	Yes	No
Hard to empty bladder completely	Yes	No
Lose control of passing urine	Yes	No
Painful or sore genitals (privates)	Yes	No
Swollen or painful joints	Yes	No
Stiffness of muscles or joints	Yes	No
Severe pains in arms or legs	Yes	No
Painful feet	Yes	No
Backache	Yes	No
Pains in neck	Yes	No
Easy to sunburn	Yes	No
Itch or rash (where?) ______	Yes	No
Subject to boils or infections	Yes	No
Subject to athlete's foot, skin fungus	Yes	No
Subject to hives or skin reactions	Yes	No
Easy bleeding or bruising	Yes	No
Mole or sore which is not healing	Yes	No
Swelling, lump, or soreness anywhere on body (where?) ______	Yes	No
Severe dizziness	Yes	No
Numbness or tingling (where?) ______	Yes	No
Twitching muscles (where?) ______	Yes	No
Nail biting	Yes	No
Sleep walking	Yes	No
Bed wetting after age 12	Yes	No
Chronically tired or overworked	Yes	No
Irregular living habits	Yes	No
Can't go to sleep or stay asleep	Yes	No
Nearly always in poor health	Yes	No
From sickly or nervous family	Yes	No
Considered to be a nervous person	Yes	No
Tremble and sweat easily	Yes	No
Have trouble making up your mind	Yes	No
Easily mixed up or confused	Yes	No
Clumsy or have frequent accidents	Yes	No
Feel sad, lonely or depressed	Yes	No
Cry often	Yes	No
Wish you were dead	Yes	No
Worry continually	Yes	No
Upset by little things	Yes	No
A perfectionist	Yes	No
Sensitive or feelings easily hurt	Yes	No
Often misunderstood	Yes	No
Often act on sudden impulse	Yes	No
Easily angered or have violent rages	Yes	No
Frequently keyed up and jittery	Yes	No
Easily scared by sudden noises	Yes	No
Have bad dreams or thoughts	Yes	No
Suspect a serious disease or cancer	Yes	No
Having trouble getting along with someone at home or work	Yes	No

Figure 12-3. (Cont.)

the initial charge ticket(s), and serve as an information resource for new patients. Because medical records personnel must work closely with registration personnel, many groups situate the records and the registration departments in close proximity to one another, or may in fact establish the two activities as one department. If, however, the two activities are spatially separated and registration personnel are given the responsibility of initiating medical records for new patients, carefully designed operating policies and procedures become necessary to ensure coordination and consistency in records preparation. The importance of effective communication between the two departments then increases.

For new patients, the appointment-making system also interfaces closely with the registration process. Whether the appointment system is centralized, decentralized, or some combination of these, the appointments made for new patients must be communicated to the registration personnel so that the patient is expected, the appointment is confirmed, and possible preregistration is facilitated. This aspect of the system is important because lack of information regarding patient arrival necessitates a confirmation of the appointment and displays to the patient uncertainty and a lack of coordination at the time he is forming his initial impressions of the clinic and its operation. Such delays at registration will waste both the patient's and the physician's valuable time. Because appointment personnel will be instructing patients concerning the registration process, coordination between the registration and appointment departments is necessary to ensure that appointment personnel understand the time required for various aspects of the registration process and therefore allow sufficient time for the completion of forms, interviews, etc., before the appointment time.

The determination of the order in which patients are to be registered is a very important procedure which can cause difficulty when queues occur and policy is not well defined for the registration personnel. Basically, there are two possible alternatives: first-come-first-served or by appointment time. One major drawback of the first-come-first-served approach is that it is possible for patients farther back in the queue to have appointment times which are in fact earlier than those of patients who are at the front of the line. On the other hand, difficulty also can be encountered when using the appointment time approach as new patients waiting to be registered observe later-arriving patients with earlier appointment times being registered ahead of them. "Walk-in" or "drop-in" patients further compound delay for patients who hold confirmed appointments. For a new patient arriving at the registration desk without an appointment, registration personnel usually must obtain an appointment and then verify that no previous medical record exists for that patient. After these tasks have been completed the routine registration process can begin.

In order to maintain accuracy, patient identification cards should be prepared by personnel who are responsible for the initial preparation of the medical record for new patients; these individuals may be involved in the registration process as well. The card itself may be made of either paper or embossed plastic/metal. Should the embossed card alternative be chosen, many options in card size and thickness are available from card manufacturers. In addition, embossing equipment manufacturers offer a variety of card design alternatives, and imprinting equipment is available in varying degrees of sophistication and capability. It will be necessary to maintain certain standards among all elements of this system; for example, the embossing and imprinting equipment must be compatible with the size and thickness of the identification card. The minimum amount of information on a patient identification card usually includes the patient's name and his chart or account number for continued reference and use. The card may be held by the patient, may be affixed to his medical record, or may be placed in an alphabetical file. Often, when one of the latter two approaches is used, a duplicate card is issued to the patient. If patients are consistent in the use of their identification cards, clinic personnel can save considerable time in locating a patient's chart or account number, and the accuracy of patient information accumulated by the clinic can be improved. The embossed cards present the added benefit of reducing transposition errors. If the identification card or a duplicate is held by the patient, the clinic must explain to him carefully the purpose of the card and its usefulness when making clinic appointments and when dealing with the clinic business office. Often it is helpful to treat the card as if it were a credit card by indicating to the patient that just as use of a credit card will result in more efficient service when charging merchandise, likewise use of a patient identification card will result in prompt and efficient attention when he seeks service at the clinic. It should be remembered, however, that the patient card is designed to be used primarily for identification rather than for credit. In fact, the charging of some services may be in conflict with the group's collection policy. Unless patients are instructed in the use of their cards, the group cannot expect the identification card system to result in economic or time saving benefits.

Alternative Approaches to Registration Systems Design

Registration activity usually involves only new patient appointments, but because return patient as well as new patient appointments must be coordinated with the medical records department, a medical record requisition form should be designed which, through routing procedures or duplicate copies, can serve a dual or even triple purpose. For example, the medical records requisition form shown in figure 12-4 is printed in triplicate and serves three functions:

1. Requisition of the chart for return patients
2. Notification of registration of a new patient appointment
3. Medical record department verification to registration personnel that new patient's status has been validated against the master file to ensure that a duplicate chart is not prepared.

When time constraints make a written procedure impractical or impossible, requisition and verification of information can be conveyed orally between departments.

As new patient information is received by registration personnel, that information must be organized and retained for retrieval at the time of the patient's arrival. A daily log is one procedure used to fulfill this need. When registration personnel receive information in written form, such as through a medical records requisition form, the data must be transferred to the log; if the information is received orally, it can be entered in the log directly. Such logs can be established inexpensively and can be designed to include the infor-

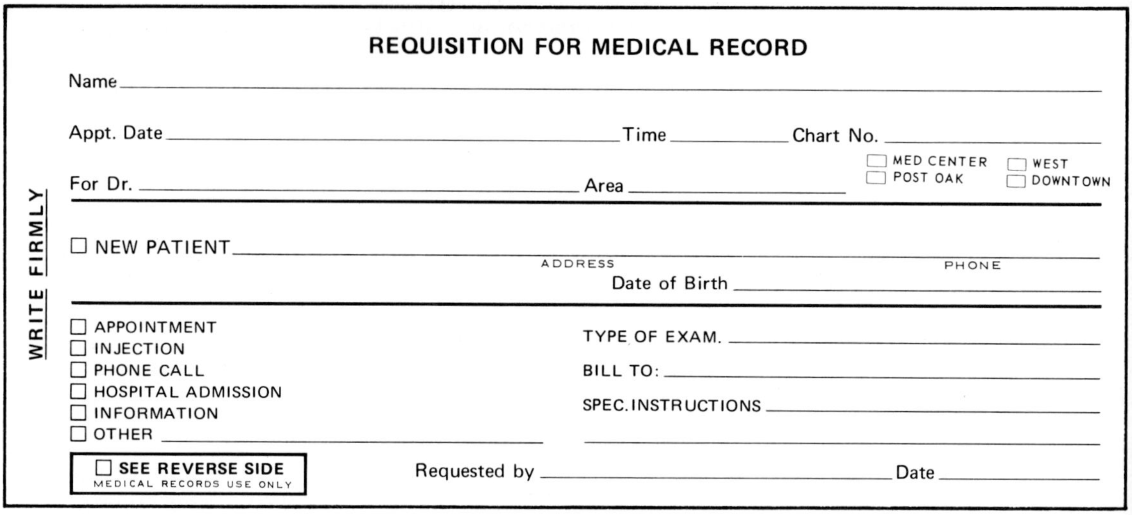

REQUISITION FOR MEDICAL RECORD

WRITE FIRMLY

Name ______________________________

Appt. Date ______________ Time ________ Chart No. ________

For Dr. ______________ Area ________ ☐ MED CENTER ☐ POST OAK ☐ WEST ☐ DOWNTOWN

☐ NEW PATIENT ______________ ADDRESS ______________ PHONE

Date of Birth ______________

☐ APPOINTMENT
☐ INJECTION
☐ PHONE CALL
☐ HOSPITAL ADMISSION
☐ INFORMATION
☐ OTHER ______________

TYPE OF EXAM. ______________

BILL TO: ______________

SPEC. INSTRUCTIONS ______________

☐ **SEE REVERSE SIDE** MEDICAL RECORDS USE ONLY

Requested by ______________ Date ________

Figure 12-4. Form for Requisitioning Medical Records

mation necessary to acknowledge the appointment, to determine if a medical record exists for the patient, and to begin the patient preregistration process if necessary. Usually, these logs are prepared for each day and can be organized internally according to time, physician, etc. The primary disadvantage to the log approach results from patient cancellations, changed appointments, and broken initial appointments. As appointments are canceled the patient's name usually is blanked out; changed appointments must be reentered in another time slot and often in another daily schedule; and broken appointments must be indicated on the log, especially when the center wants to ascertain why new patients may fail to keep initial appointments. The log also must be annotated for those patients who keep their appointments. Poor design and organization can easily result in a log that is difficult to read due to changes and cancellations, difficult to maintain alphabetically for ease in retrieval, and cluttered with verification, check, double check, and other markings. The readability of the registration log at the end of a day's activity becomes even more important if the group decides to rely on the log for the retrieval of certain information for statistical or other purposes.

An alternative to the use of a daily log relies heavily upon the use of the written requisition/notification form (see figure 12-4). The organization of these forms alphabetically or by day, time, or physician is similar in purpose to the handwritten log. Rather than a list, however, registration personnel utilize a "deck" of forms. In addition, to expand this second alternative into a third consideration, upon receipt of the appointment notification, a registration card can be prepared for each new patient (see figure 12-5). The information contained on the record requisition/appointment notification form (see figure 12-4) is repeated on the registration card and occupies a greater percentage of the area, the intent being that information recorded on the registration card be consistent, whether received orally or through a written procedure. If the information is received orally it is recorded directly on the card; if received in writing, the written notification is simply attached to the card by a pressure

CARD FRONT

REGISTRATION

TAB

PLACE REQUISITION CONFIRMATION HERE

Doctor ______________ Type of Exam ______________ Chart No. ______________

New Patient ______________ ______________
ADDRESS PHONE NO

____
DATE OF BIRTH

Remarks: ______________

____

☐ Pre-registered | ☐ By Phone | ☐ By Mail ______________ DATE MAILED ______________ DATE RETURNED

☐ Cancellation | ☐ Change ______________ DATE ______________ TIME ______________ DOCTOR

MR/MRS	LAST NAME	FIRST NAME	MIDDLE INIT	APPOINTMENT DATE	TIME

REVERSE SIDE

REGISTRATION CHECKLIST

Check

☐ 1. Determine if pre-registered. If yes, chart is in pre-registration bin. If no, proceed:

☐ 2. Complete Patient Information Sheet from next successive chart and attach original copy to the front of KS Form 3-B. Place the copies in file, unless credit is questionable. If questionable, then stat the credit copy (pink) to the Credit Department.

☐ 3. If visit is NPC, an Internal Medicine consult, or a new patient of Dr. Eichhorn, initiate a History and Health Questionnaire. All Pediatric NPC's and Neurology consults for children receive a Pediatric History and Physical Questionnaire.

☐ 4. Complete two ID cards and insert one card in the pouch on the inside back of the chart.

☐ 5. Initiate an SR. Imprint the SR with the other card and enter the date, doctor, type of visit, and OT/OTM/ Station 3 if appropriate on the SR. (If the appointment is for Dermatology, Ophthalmology, or Electrolysis, check with Registration personnel before initiating the SR.)

☐ 6. Paper clip the SR to the front of the chart and determine that the record contains the following items: ID card in pouch, Information Sheet attached to KS Form 3-B, Miscellaneous envelope, and an Instruction Sheet for the use of the ID card.

☐ 7. Give the patient one of the ID cards and briefly explain its use. Also hand the patient the instruction slip on the use of the ID card, a Patient Information Booklet, and a Financial Information Booklet.

☐ 8. Give directions to the appropriate floor, hand the chart to the patient, and ask the patient to check-in at the reception desk.

THE ABOVE CHECKLIST PROCEDURE FOLLOWS CONFIRMATION OF APPOINTMENT AND RECORDS CHECK.

Figure 12-5. Registration Card

sensitive tab or by some other type of adhesive. Preregistration, cancellation, and appointment change information also is contained on the card. An information checklist can be printed on the reverse side of the registration card (see figure 12-5) to serve as a guide for new, substitute, or partially trained personnel.

As a further refinement of this system, on the front of the card at the lower edge, space can be designated for the patient's name, and the date and time of his appointment. This design facilitates the arrangement of registration cards in a file similar to the one shown in figure 12-6. The cards may be filed either alphabetically by day, by time, or by some combination thereof. In the file shown in figure 12-6 the cards for one day are organized within the tray. Each day of the week can be represented by a separate tray. As a new patient arrives to be registered, his card can be located easily and it contains all of the necessary registration information, including appointment notification and medical records check. As patients preregister, cancel, or change appointments, their cards can be annotated and either removed from the file due to cancellation or transferred to another tray due to appointment change. The registration cards, whether organized as a deck or in a file, can save personnel time and can reduce transposition inaccuracies because as appointment changes or cancellations

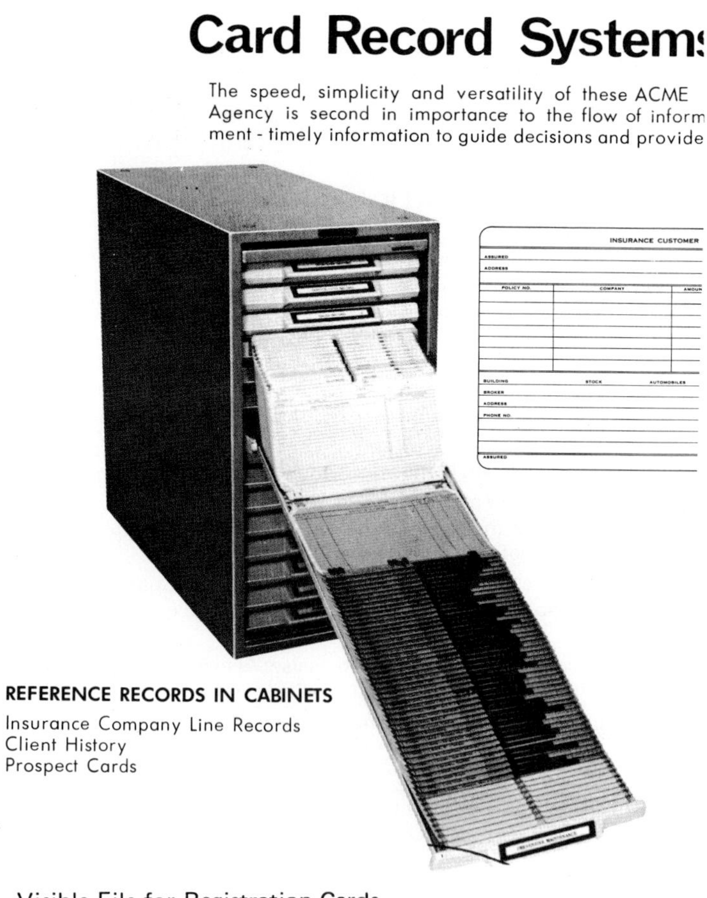

Figure 12-6. Visible File for Registration Cards

ALLERGIES

RECORD OF PATIENT VISITS & DIAGNOSES

DATE SEEN	PHYSICIAN OR DEPARTMENT	DIAGNOSIS	CROSS INDEX	CODE NO.

Figure 12-7. Patient Information Sheet

occur, the individual cards can be moved about within the system. While there are many advantages to the visible file system, its primary disadvantages are that it is significantly more expensive than the log system and it requires continued organizing on the part of the registration personnel.

Maintaining and Updating Patient Registration Information

Registration information usually becomes part of the new patient's medical record. There are various methods available for accomplishing this; for example, the registration form shown in figure 12-2 can be attached to a patient information sheet within the medical record (see figure 12-7). To be used effectively, patient data must be kept current. Inaccuracies, changes, and omissions occurring over a period of time can result in faulty judgments, distorted communications, and even total communication breakdown. For example, a change in patient address and telephone number left uncorrected on the registration form can result in a loss of contact between the clinic and the patient. During subsequent visits by the patient to the clinic, inaccuracies and omissions can be identified in several ways. Clinic personnel, perhaps the receptionist, can contribute to the maintenance of accurate data by confirming with the patient information previously supplied by him. Signs and supplemental forms provided in the patient reception and registration area will alert patients to the need for accurate data and will facilitate their voluntarily providing updated information.

Inaccuracies in registration data also may be discovered when billing or informational material mailed by the clinic to the patient is returned as undeliverable for a reason such as an improper or incomplete address. This situation can be remedied immediately by an outreach follow-up phone call to the patient. If the patient cannot be reached to substantiate information, clinic personnel may want to mark that patient's records in some manner in order to call attention to the fact that certain information in the record is not current. The situation then can be rectified when the patient again visits the clinic.

PATIENT RIGHTS AND RESPONSIBILITIES

Positive patient attitude toward the clinic and the foundation for a long-term patient-clinic relationship can be established by ensuring that each patient is aware of his rights and responsibilities. The group may find it advantageous to develop a brochure or pamphlet which briefly but clearly outlines these rights and responsibilities. Such a brochure might be designed specifically for distribution to new patients during the registration process. As discussed in Chapter 10, the patient may have certain justified expectations in the following areas:

1. Respect for the patient and the patient's dignity
2. Confidentiality of the information given to the center by the patient
3. Reasonable fulfillment of appointment requests
4. Expectations concerning type of treatment and facility usage
5. Patient's privilege to request consultation and/or transfer to another physician within the clinic.

On the other hand, the patient also has certain responsibilities and duties in his relationship with the group, such as:

1. The providing of accurate personal information and subsequent changes in that information when necessary
2. Agreement to pay for services rendered when requested to do so or notification to the clinic of mitigating circumstances which may necessitate some type of negotiation in regard to a payment schedule
3. Willingness to abide by the corrective actions taken by the clinic in case of a default in the above responsibilities
4. Punctuality in keeping appointments or, if an appointment is to be cancelled, prompt notification of the clinic of the cancellation so that the time may be released for another patient's use.

Providing the patient with a basic outline of his rights and responsibilities may save both the clinic and the patient from future unpleasant experiences. The patient aware of his rights and responsibilities is better able to evaluate his relationship with the group. Through well-planned policies and through the use of signs or notices designed to remind employees of patient expectations, the group can help to maintain its obligations to patients.

REGISTRATION POLICY

Establishing procedural guidelines is helpful to registration personnel and will contribute greatly to an orderly registration process. Depending upon the clinic's patient population, it may be difficult to validate registration information. Nonetheless, in all cases every effort should be made to maintain the accuracy of patient information. Personal identification should be required and patient addresses should be verified and updated continually. In addition, information on third party coverage and patient credit status is important to the proper management of the clinic.

Policy and procedures can be especially important in the movement of patients throughout the facility. Within the clinic, registration personnel are usually the first individuals the patient contacts and through whom he forms a first impression of the clinic as a whole. Clinic personnel should be aware that they are performing a service to the patients, and in performing this service they should remember the patient's right to courtesy, confidentiality, and privacy.

The close interdependence between registration, appointments, medical records, and patient accounts will require carefully developed policy procedures to produce the coordination, communication, and consistency necessary for efficient operation. If both the group and the patient begin their association with mutual understanding, a long and satisfactory relationship undoubtedly will follow and can be maintained as long as both parties cooperate in providing the information which is a requisite to quality health care.

Chapter 13

Patient Appointments, Scheduling, and Referral Systems

ESTABLISHING THE PATIENT APPOINTMENT, SCHEDULING, AND REFERRAL SYSTEM

The appointment-making process has the potential for fulfilling a vital public relations function for the clinic because it is during this process that the first transfer of information between the group and the patient usually occurs. The health service rendered to the patient is set in motion with a preliminary analysis of his problem and the scheduling of an appointment with the appropriate physician. Effective appointment scheduling enables the physician to operate at an efficient medical service level; it should greatly reduce both slack times and overloads, and should contribute significantly to the quality of patient care. Similarly, the scheduling of ancillary services (laboratory, radiology, EKG, etc.) ordered by group physicians, and the referral of patients by, to, and between group physicians can be administrated in a smooth and orderly fashion, thereby achieving efficiency in operation and patient service.

APPOINTMENTS

The patient, the physician, and, indirectly, the clinic administrator benefit from an established appointment system. For the physician, a well-designed appointment system provides information necessary to organize more efficiently the health care services in the clinic. For example, using a group time block to appoint patients requiring similar services to a schedule can organize the rendering of such services more efficiently and can reduce the amount of unproductive time between the rendering of dissimilar services. Accurate appointment information regarding the time as well as the type of patient visit can reduce the physician's free time and can increase productivity. An appointment system also can enhance the effectiveness of health care by documenting prior notice of patient visits, thus providing time for the physician to prepare himself for dealing with new or continuing health problems. Consequently, with the clinic's overhead rate fixed, greater physician productivity results in greater cost effectiveness.

Patients consider their time as valuable as the physician's. By enabling the patient to know exactly when he can expect to receive health service, the well-planned appointment system offers the additional advantage of minimizing waiting time, thereby allowing the patient to utilize the balance of his day more effectively. A patient can appoint himself to the physician of his choice, can expect the undivided attention of that physician for the period of his appointment, and should be encouraged to see the same physician on subsequent visits.

In a newly formed medical group, information provided by the appointment process can be especially useful in assessing various aspects of group operation. By surveying weekly or monthly schedules of departments and physicians, management can gain an overview of efficiency in the functioning of departments, and physicians and can plan for better use of clinic resources and facilities. Clinic management also may gain insight into areas that require expansion, modification, or reduction. In addition, clinic ancillary staff personnel may benefit from an efficient appointment system. An appointment schedule alerts certer ancillary staff personnel to prepare in advance for required services by retrieving medical records, preparing an encounter form, and requisitioning necessary equipment.

The Appointment System

In making an appointment the responsible staff person performs four basic steps:

1. *Determines* the patient's condition, medical complaint, and/or requests
2. *Assigns* the patient to departments and physicians based on the information received in the first step
3. *Schedules* the patient to an appointment time
4. *Completes* the necessary clerical functions associated with making the appointment.

Additional steps may be required of these personnel depending on varying circumstances. For example, added apointment activity could be the provision of fee information, explanation of credit policy, and the request of third party payor information.

The clerk or receptionist must elicit from the patient or the referring physician the patient's "symptoms" as well as other information that applies to the particular case. Specifically, this information should serve to elucidate the complaint, disease, or condition to be treated, and which physician(s) the patient specifically desires to see. When this information has been obtained, appointment personnel can assign the patient to the proper department and, if appropriate, to a specific physician. Using general appointment policy and procedures, appointment personnel then schedule the patient into an array of available time slots. Necessary clerical procedures must be carried out and appropriate requests must be completed as determined by the department involved, and possibly by the specific physicians within that department. For example, in the case of a new patient appointment, registration personnel should be made aware of the patient's anticipated arrival time so that patient preregistration can proceed efficiently. In the case of a return patient, the medical records department must be notified of the appointment time so that the medical record may be sent to the appropriate place in time for the appointment.

Appointment rules and procedures employed by appointment personnel generally fall into several categories. These rules should be in writing and should be an understood policy of the group. Various appointment procedure categories include:

1. *Type of appointment*—when assigning appointments of a particular type, the service to be performed constitutes the criterion for the actual determination of the time needed. For example, a complete physical examination generally will require a greater amount of time than will a routine office visit for medications follow-up.

2. *Geographic location of patient's residence*—the scheduling of appointments can be influenced by the patient's geographic proximity and accessibility to the clinic. The distance a patient must travel to come to the clinic should be considered when the appointment is made. If it appears necessary that the patient see *two* different physicians and appointments are not open for both consultations on the same or successive days, every effort can be made to fit the patient into schedules which are already filled.

3. *New patient or return patient*—the appointment process may be influenced by a determination of what information is required; certain procedures are then included or omitted. For example, new patients require the initiation of a medical record, whereas return patients already have a record established.

4. *Age and condition of patient*—after the urgency of the patient need is determined the scheduling of an appointment is performed accordingly. For example, emergency appointments usually are worked into a schedule that is considered to be filled.

5. *Group patient*—the appointment process may be influenced by the type of service stipulated by a group contract. In time, the group usually will be performing medical care and services (preemployment examinations, executive physicals, etc.) for companies or other organizations on a contract basis which necessitates the performance of preestablished services.

In general, the functions and procedures outlined above include most appointing situations and serve to delineate the appointment process. Not every appointment making encounter, however, will involve all of these functions or procedures. For example, when appointment personnel receive a request for further appointments from an internal source, such as a physician, the *determine* and *assign* steps already have been performed. In addition, when an appointment request is received by mail, often it is impossible for the clerk to determine anything further about the patient's condition or to request information other than that already provided in the letter.

Ideally, the clinic appointment system should be able to handle all potential appointment requests. If the appointment process is heavily dependent upon more than one person and consequently upon the communication between those persons, errors in the transfer of information may occur. In establishing the appointment process, it is important, therefore, that efficient communication and information transfer take place. The transfer of appointment information flows through several channels, i.e., from patient to appointment personnel, from appointment personnel to departments, from departments to specific physicians. Several other channels may be included if ancillary services are involved. At each one of these channels information may be stopped or distorted. In addition, the greater the number of channels, the greater the probability that such a problem will occur. Because no single method for determining the relative importance of the various communications channels is valid for all clinics, the appointment process itself and the space utilized by appointment equipment and personnel vary among clinics.

In order to facilitate information acquisition and distribution, a method for appointment system organization must first be chosen. The alternatives available to a medical group include a centralized appointment system, a decentralized (departmental) appointment system, or a combination thereof. Each alternative system represents an attempt to direct both the patient and information pertinent to the medical treatment of the patient to the proper destination within the clinic.

Centralized Appointment Systems. This method involves the centralization of the clinic appointment system in one location and the performance of the appointment making process by personnel assigned only to that function. Centralization offers a number of advantages in the scheduling of appointments. With the appointment process and authority located in one place, multiple appointments can be made by a single appointment person without checking available openings by telephone or routing the patient to multiple locations. Internally, the system proves to be more efficient, especially when a physician or a nurse wants to make more than one appointment for a patient who is in the clinic. A centralized system appears to be efficient in the eyes of the patient because all arrangements can be made at one location and the "run-around" syndrome can be avoided; however, when the centralized appointment-making facility is located in an area away from public view and the main patient flow, patients already in the clinic may find it inconvenient to schedule return appointments. Some existing groups handle this situation by having internal appointment telephones available for use by patients. An additional consideration involves the logistics of providing patients with appointment reminder cards containing information such as physician, date and time of appointment, and instructions for cancellation or change of the appointment.

With a centralized appointment system all scheduling records are located in one place. Appointment personnel, therefore, have access to the schedules of *all* clinic physicians. Because visibility of times available for appointments is greater, personnel have less difficulty in finding an opening to meet a demand. Centralized appointment systems result in less confusion for other center departments interfacing operationally with the appointment system because all actions or questions related to appointments can be directed to personnel in one location as opposed to various personnel in several locations. With scheduling personnel centrally located, departmental variations in scheduling preferences are somewhat reduced, allowing more effective implementation of appointment policy, procedures, and control. Centralization of personnel into an appointment-making pool creates a more manageable and more flexible workload and provides more opportunity for section coverage when needed because of personnel absence due to illness, vacations, etc. Finally, centralization allows for personnel specialization in the appointment-making procedures and is separate from the reception function usually associated with decentralized appointments.

Decentralized Appointment System. Some distinctive advantages also can be realized with a decentralized or departmental appointment system. Appointment personnel specialize by scheduling only a few types of appointments and consequently may have fewer policies and procedures to deal with than do centralized appointment personnel. Decentralized appointment personnel not only can become expert in making the type of appointment for which they are responsible but also are more knowledgeable about the activities of their department and its physicians. As a result, they often are more flexible in the appointment-making process and know better when they can and cannot "work in" another patient. Departmental appointment personnel may be better able to schedule the amount of time needed for patient follow-up visits because they are more familar with both the patient's needs and departmental procedures. Eliminating the need for the patient to contact a central appointment office may facilitate patient relations and eliminate some intraclinic communication. Finally, a better understanding of departmental physicians and their time allocations for follow-up, return, and new visits, can result in more efficient time utilization.

Hybrid Appointment System. Hybrid systems represent a combination of centralized and decentralized appointments tailored to specific areas of the clinic. Although a variety of combinations may exist, groups often choose to decentralize appointments for dermatology and ENT because of their high volume of work in appointments, while centralizing appointments for the remainder of medicine and surgery. The majority of existing appointment systems could be categorized as hybrid systems depending upon the specialty mix and needs of the group. In the small, newly formed group practice the trend has been first toward centralization of the appointment process with eventual branching or total commitment to decentralization as patient volume increases and specialty mix broadens. Some large clinics, however, do continue to maintain a centralized process.

The Appointment-Making Process

In addition to the selection of a workable appointment system, there are various other considerations essential to the appointment process. Routing of patients within the clinic can present certain difficulties. In order to schedule an appointment time, the appointment clerk must acquire from the patient certain pertinent information such as the medical problem involved and the particular physician the patient would like to see. Most appointment personnel employed by existing medical groups are less conversant and knowledgeable in medical procedures than is the nurse or aide. For example, a request for a GU consult appointment may be routed by appointment personnel to the OB/GYN department instead of the urologist. Often, the patient himself does not know or fully understand the specific problem and, consequently, cannot communicate the information needed for the appointment person to make the proper determination of the necessary service. Also it is possible that the symptoms which the patient does relate are so vague that appointment personnel can determine neither the department nor the physician to which the patient should be directed. It is possible that the prospective patient consciously may withhold information about his problem from appointment personnel because he either is uneasy with the appointment person or is unwilling to discuss his problem with anyone but the physician. On the other hand, the patient may be willing to discuss his problem and may have an actual insight into it, but may be unable to communicate adequately with the appointment personnel on the telephone, by mail, or in person. Finally, the patient may demand to be appointed to a specific physician's schedule, even though this physician is in a specialty field completely unrelated to the patient's problem or complaint. These potential difficulties suggest areas in which appointment personnel must be trained, in which systems must be effectively designed, and in which procedures must be outlined for the acquisition of assistance when problems arise. Because appointment personnel sometimes have difficulty obtaining the information necessary for appropriate appointment-making, information acquisition systems and procedures may require refinement. For example, procedures may differ when the appointment maker is not the patient, but rather the patient's relative or a friend.

In the area of appointment scheduling, *static problems* (problems which are continuously present) as well as *dynamic problems* (those problems which are independent of existing conditions and policies) may emerge. Static problems can include:

1. Incorrect routing of the patient
2. Incorrect amount of time scheduled per appointment
3. Problems arising from centralization, decentralization, or a combination thereof
4. Difficulty in schedule rearrangement as new appointments alter the existing situation
5. Inaccessibility of the data base (patient information)
6. Clerical error (due to transposition and other causes)
7. Policies which are inappropriate or insufficiently extensive
8. Incomplete scheduling of patients
9. Lack of feedback from departmental personnel on the success or failure of current appointment scheduling.

While such static problems indicate areas requiring policy determination, dynamic problems in the appointment-making process are independent of existing conditions and usually cannot be regulated directly by clinic policy. Dynamic problems may be:

1. Patient fails to keep appointment
2. Physician late
3. Patient late
4. Actual time patient spends with doctor is unpredictable
5. Late cancellations by patients
6. Other departmental failures, such as availability of medical records, return of test results, etc.
7. Failure to fully integrate into the system the time it takes to perform and report tests
8. Lack of scheduling information visibility (such as not being able to tell at a glance which physicians are occupied at which times)
9. Physician called away to hospital due to emergency and/or delivery
10. Telephone calls to physicians, corridor consultations, and unavoidable interruptions.

Although both static and dynamic problems do arise, some naturally are more serious than others. A determination of the extent and seriousness of each problem can be made by recording the amount of patient and physician waiting time each problem causes. Rockart's study indicates that the most time consuming problems are:[1]

Static:	*Time Average:*
Incorrect routing	17 min.
Incorrect time assignments	28 min.
Clerical error	14 min.
Dynamic:	
Other department failure	12 min.
Test time not understood in system	12 min.

A cursory examination of these problems reveals that each can be attributed to a communication breakdown either between the patient and the clinic or within the clinic itself. When the group is evaluating alternative appointment processes, the implications of each approach in terms of solving problems such as those noted above should receive careful consideration.

Unscheduled appointments represent another potential problem area. A recent study by the Oregon Region of the Kaiser-Permanente Medical Care Program demonstrated that in their major departments of medicine, surgery, and pediatrics unscheduled appointments increased 33 percent between 1964 and 1971.[2] Specifically, the Kaiser study revealed that relative to scheduled visits, unscheduled visits decreased with the age of the patient, both for males and for females. For males, however, 50 percent of the total visits from birth to age 44 were unscheduled. The only female age category comparable to these male statistics was that of from birth to age 19. In general, it was found that females use services on a scheduled basis more often than do males, particularly after age 19.

Injuries and diseases of an acute nature usually were handled on an unscheduled basis and no evidence of abuse of the appointment system was determined; that is, individuals using unscheduled services were not found to be using the medical care system inappropriately. The proportion of unscheduled visits was highest on Mondays (44 percent) and Saturdays (41 percent). Patients with few scheduled visits tended to have few unscheduled visits, and those with several unscheduled visits were likely to have many scheduled visits. The researchers therefore concluded that unscheduled use does not seem to be a substitute for scheduled use, but rather an additional means of taking advantage of available medical care services.

Although the Kaiser study conclusions represent results from a system unique to the nature of the Kaiser-Permanente practice, the study does indicate that unscheduled use can pose a major problem in undermining the appointment process itself. Likewise, problems generated by unscheduled visits soon have profound effects on those departments which interface with the appointment process, such as registration and medical records. In certain instances, physician assistants, nurse practitioners, and nurses may be able to assist effectively in handling an overload "add on" schedule either by telephone or by office visits. In other instances, when the schedule has become overloaded, the group may decide to have appointment personnel direct unscheduled patients to other group physicians.

Planning the appointment process involves decisions which not only shape the process itself but also influence the functioning of other systems within the clinic, particularly when difficulty occurs. Because the problem most often encountered is one of information transfer, either between patient and clinic or between departments and/or staff members within the clinic, the group will want to establish an appointment system which facilitates this process and which can reduce if not eliminate potential problems.

Preregistration. Preregistration of patients involves certain administrative activities prior to the patient's arrival which are based on information collected through the appointment process. The actual process of preregistration may be performed either by appointment or by registration personnel. In smaller group practices, however, these two administrative functions may be handled by the same department.

If a large percentage of the patient appointments is made two to four weeks in advance, the clinic may be able to send out a preregistration form by mail to the patient before his clinic visit. Thus, clinic personnel tentatively schedule the patient on the basis of the information obtained over the telephone or through the mail, and then mail out the preregistration material for return, either by mail or in person at the time of the appointment. If the material mailed is returned to the clinic before the patient's appointment, many administrative activities, such as the establishment of an account and the preparation of the medical record, can be completed in advance of the patient's arrival.

The material to be mailed should be simple and self-explanatory, yet detailed enough to gain accurate administrative and possibly medical information about the patient. If preregistration is used, the patient must have confidence that an accurately completed form will reduce his waiting time at the clinic. Effective preregistration also can eliminate the communication problems encountered during verbal exchange between patient and clinic personnel. An example of a preregistration form is shown in figure 13-1. Should it be decided to acquire the patient's medical history through the preregistration process as well, a health questionnaire can be included with the preregistration form. An example of an abbreviated questionnaire is shown in figure 13-2. In addition to

We have arranged an appointment for ________________ to see

Doctor ________________ at ______ am/pm ________________. To assist us in making arrangements for this visit, please complete the following information and mail this form to us as soon as possible. This will save you time upon arrival at the Clinic. Please **print or type** your answers and complete all questions.

1. Name of Patient: ________________
   First   Middle   Last
2. Home address: ________________
   Street   City   State   Zip Code
3. Age ____ Birthdate ________ Sex ______ ☐ Married ☐ Single ☐ Widowed ☐ Separated ☐ Divorced
4. Name of husband, wife or nearest living relative (if patient is a dependent child, insert father, mother or legal guardian's name) ________________ Relationship to patient: ________
5. Patient's occupation: ________________
   Type of work (If retired, please give last occupation)
6. Name, address and telephone number of patient's employer: ________________
7. Occupation of responsible party- ________________
   (If widowed, please give husband's last occupation)
8. Name, address and telephone number of responsible party's employer: ________________
9. Referred by: ________________ Have you ever been our patient? ________
10. If referred by a physician, please give his name and address: ________________
11. In case of an emergency, who should we notify (other than immediate family)?
    ____
    Name   Address   Phone Number
12. OUT OF TOWN PATIENTS (Local address, if known)
    ____
13. Medicare claim number (if over age 65 and have part "B"): ________________

Please see the reverse side of this form. Merely fold, as indicated, seal and mail **as soon as possible**. No stamp is necessary unless you wish to air mail this back to us.

We will endeavor to make your visit as pleasant as possible.

Thank you,
X Y Z Clinic

PLEASE FOLD AND MAIL

Figure 13–1. Preregistration Form

No. ______________________________

Name ______________________________ Date ______________________

PATIENT'S HISTORY AND HEALTH QUESTIONNAIRE

FAMILY HISTORY: Have any members of your family ever had the following? If so, please circle below.

Father: Living–Age ________ Condition of Health? ________________

Dead–Age ________ Cause of Death? ________________

Mother: Living–Age ________ Condition of Health? ________________

Dead–Age ________ Cause of Death? ________________

Number Brothers: Living: ______ Ages: __________ Dead: ______ Causes ______________

Number Sisters: Living: ______ Ages: __________ Dead: ______ Causes ______________

Are You Married? ______ Number of Years? ______ Wife's Age: ________ Husband's Age: ______

Health of Husband or Wife? ________________

If spouse dead, give age, year, and cause of death: ________________

Previous Marriages? __________ Give Dates: ________________

Number Children: Boys: ______ Ages: __________ Girls: ________ Ages: ________

All Healthy? ________________ Any Dead? ________

Diabetes
Tuberculosis
Headaches
Epilepsy
Cancer
High Blood Pressure
Heart Disease
Stroke
Allergy
Stomach Trouble
Nervous Trouble
Blood Disease
Goiter
Arthritis
Other Diseases

PLEASE LIST HERE PRESENT CONDITIONS OR DISEASES WHICH YOU WISH TO HAVE CHECKED AT THIS EXAMINATION:

____

____

PERSONAL HISTORY: Please give approximate year of last immunization ("shot") for:

Allergy or severe reaction to medicines, foods, plants, chemicals, etc.: Please list

____

____

Smallpox ______		Polio ______	
Typhoid ______		Influenza ______	
Tetanus ______		Other ______	

List Average:

Hours worked per day: ________	Do you take regular exercise? ________
Hours sleep per night: ________	Do you take a rest each day? ________
Days worked per week: ________	Approximate date of last vacation: ________
Days vacation per year: ________	What is you usual weight? ________ lbs.
Number cigarettes per day: ________	What is the most you ever weighed? ________ lbs.
Other tobacco per day: ________	At what year or age? ________
Cups coffee per day: ________	Have you lost or gained weight? ________
Alcoholic drinks per day: ________	If so, how much? ________ lbs.

Put a circle around any of the following conditions which you now have or have had in the past:

Skin Trouble	Pneumonia	Worms	Gonorrhea	Measles
Cataracts	Tuberculosis	Dysentery	Hernia (rupture)	Rheumatic Fever
Tonsillitis	Breast Trouble	Colitis	Fainting	Arthritis
Sinusitis	Heart Trouble	Hemorrhoids	Fits or Convulsions	Gout
Goiter	Ulcer	Kidney Trouble	Nervous Breakdown	Anemia
Hay Fever	Jaundice	Kidney Stones	Unconsciousness	Diabetes
Asthma	Gallstones	Bladder Trouble	Paralysis	Cancer or Tumor
Bronchitis	Liver Trouble	Prostate Trouble	Polio	Varicose Veins
Pleurisy	Hepatitis	Syphilis	Mumps	Phlebitis

PAST HISTORY: Please list previous operations, injuries, serious illnesses, etc. and year:

1. ____
2. ____
3. ____

When was your last physical examination? ________ Any abnormality found? ________

Are you under any medical treatment now? ________________

List any medications you take now or occasionally: ________________

FOR WOMEN ONLY: Menses (Monthly periods): Date last period: ________________

Age began: ________	Age when "change of life" started: ________
Now occurs about every ________ days	Hot flashes? ________
Normal? ________	Any history of trouble with female organs? ________
Discharge? ________	Number of pregnancies? ________
Flooding? ________	Complications of any pregnancies? (List) ________
Irregular? ________	
Painful? ________	Any miscarriages? ________
Spotting between periods? ________	

PLEASE TURN PAGE FOR HEALTH QUESTIONS ON OTHER SIDE

Figure 13–2. Patient's History and Health Questionnaire

IF YOU HAVE ANY OF THE FOLLOWING COMPLAINTS, PLEASE CIRCLE (YES). IF NOT, CIRCLE (NO).
THE DOCTOR WILL ASK ABOUT DETAILS LATER. ANSWER ALL QUESTIONS. IF IN DOUBT, GUESS YES OR NO.

Severe headaches or head pains . . . . . Yes No
Do you need an eye check for:
  Any disturbance in vision . . . . . Yes No
  Glasses. . . . . Yes No
  Pain or discomfort . . . . . Yes No
Constant noises in ears . . . . . Yes No
Hard of hearing . . . . . Yes No
Ear ache with colds ( ) plane flights ( ) . . . . . Yes No
Chronic running ear . . . . . Yes No
Chronic stuffy or runny nose . . . . . Yes No
Chronic dripping from nose to throat . . . . . Yes No
Need to use nose drops frequently . . . . . Yes No
Bad nose bleeds at times . . . . . Yes No
Frequent severe colds or sore throat . . . . . Yes No
Need to clear throat frequently . . . . . Yes No
Any known dental problems . . . . . Yes No
Soreness or bleeding of gums . . . . . Yes No
More than a year since teeth checked . . . . . Yes No
Would you like a dental check during this exam . . . . . Yes No
Sore mouth or tongue . . . . . Yes No
Goiter or thyroid trouble . . . . . Yes No
Metabolism test - too high ( ) too low ( ) . . . . . Yes No
Feeling of lump in the throat . . . . . Yes No
Need to take thyroid medicine . . . . . Yes No
Hoarseness at times . . . . . Yes No
Recent or chronic cough . . . . . Yes No
Chronic coughing up of sputum . . . . . Yes No
Ever coughed up blood . . . . . Yes No
Ache all over . . . . . Yes No
Having chills or fever . . . . . Yes No
Severe soaking night sweats . . . . . Yes No
Lived with anyone having T.B. . . . . . Yes No
Worried about your heart . . . . . Yes No
Blood pressure - too high ( ) too low ( ) . . . . . Yes No
Pains in heart or chest . . . . . Yes No
Pounding or skipping of heart . . . . . Yes No
Heart starts racing suddenly. . . . . . Yes No
Shortness of breath or wheezing . . . . . Yes No
Trouble getting a deep breath . . . . . Yes No
Swelling ankles . . . . . Yes No
Leg cramps in bed or sitting still . . . . . Yes No
Leg cramps while walking . . . . . Yes No
Pain or trouble with swallowing . . . . . Yes No
Gulp your food in a hurry . . . . . Yes No
Poor appetite - recently ( ) always ( ) . . . . . Yes No
Nausea or vomiting . . . . . Yes No
Vomiting of blood . . . . . Yes No
Belching, bloating or indigestion . . . . . Yes No
Yellow skin or eyes (jaundice) . . . . . Yes No
Burning or hunger pains in stomach . . . . . Yes No
Use antacids for stomach burning . . . . . Yes No
Soreness or pain in stomach, abdomen . . . . . Yes No
Suspect ulcers or stomach trouble . . . . . Yes No
Cramps in stomach or low down . . . . . Yes No
Loose bowels or diarrhea . . . . . Yes No
Black or tarry stools (bowel movements) . . . . . Yes No
Fresh or bright blood with stools . . . . . Yes No
Mucus (slime or phlegm) in stools . . . . . Yes No
Constipation . . . . . Yes No
Use laxatives ( ) or enemas ( ) frequently . . . . . Yes No
Recent change in bowel habits . . . . . Yes No
Rectal trouble or pain . . . . . Yes No

List any foods which always disagree: ________________
____
Pain in the kidney region . . . . . Yes No
Get up nights to urinate (No. times ________) . . . . . Yes No
Blood or pus in urine . . . . . Yes No
Albumin in urine . . . . . Yes No
Sugar in urine . . . . . Yes No
Spells of frequent urination . . . . . Yes No
Severe burning or pain on urination . . . . . Yes No
Pains over bladder or low down . . . . . Yes No
Trouble starting urine . . . . . Yes No
Urinary stream has become weak . . . . . Yes No
Hard to empty bladder completely . . . . . Yes No
Lose control of passing urine . . . . . Yes No
Painful or sore genitals (privates) . . . . . Yes No
Swollen or painful joints . . . . . Yes No
Stiffness of muscles or joints . . . . . Yes No
Severe pains in arms or legs . . . . . Yes No
Painful feet . . . . . Yes No
Backache . . . . . Yes No
Pains in neck . . . . . Yes No
Easy to sunburn . . . . . Yes No
Itch or rash (where?) ________________ Yes No
Subject to boils or infections . . . . . Yes No
Subject to athlete's foot, skin fungus . . . . . Yes No
Subject to hives or skin reactions . . . . . Yes No
Easy bleeding or bruising . . . . . Yes No
Mole or sore which is not healing . . . . . Yes No
Swelling, lump, or soreness anywhere on body (where?)
________________________________ Yes No
Severe dizziness . . . . . Yes No
Numbness or tingling (where?) ________________ Yes No
Twitching muscles (where?) ________________ Yes No
Nail biting . . . . . Yes No
Sleep walking . . . . . Yes No
Bed wetting after age 12 . . . . . Yes No
Chronically tired or overworked . . . . . Yes No
Irregular living habits . . . . . Yes No
Can't go to sleep or stay asleep . . . . . Yes No
Nearly always in poor health . . . . . Yes No
From sickly or nervous family . . . . . Yes No
Considered to be a nervous person . . . . . Yes No
Tremble and sweat easily . . . . . Yes No
Have trouble making up your mind . . . . . Yes No
Easily mixed up or confused . . . . . Yes No
Clumsy or have frequent accidents . . . . . Yes No
Feel sad, lonely or depressed . . . . . Yes No
Cry often . . . . . Yes No
Wish you were dead . . . . . Yes No
Worry continually . . . . . Yes No
Upset by little things . . . . . Yes No
A perfectionist . . . . . Yes No
Sensitive or feelings easily hurt . . . . . Yes No
Often misunderstood . . . . . Yes No
Often act on sudden impulse . . . . . Yes No
Easily angered or have violent rages . . . . . Yes No
Frequently keyed up and jittery . . . . . Yes No
Easily scared by sudden noises . . . . . Yes No
Have bad dreams or thoughts . . . . . Yes No
Suspect a serious disease or cancer . . . . . Yes No
Having trouble getting along with someone at home or work . . . . . Yes No

Figure 13–2. (Cont.)

using the postal system, the telephone may be employed in the preregistration process, especially when time does not permit the mailing and returning of materials. Although telephone preregistration does not readily permit the acquisition of medical history, the information requested on the preregistration form can be elicited from the patient and recorded on the form. Because of patient availability, however, it may be necessary to conduct a portion of the telephone preregistration process in the early evening hours.

Service Time Interval. The service time required for each patient often is estimated inaccurately. When physician appointment time is scheduled by using only two time categories, such as fifteen minutes and thirty minutes, the patient will receive an appointment for one of these two time intervals. This dual category method presents the appointment secretary with the choice between only two time periods for the patient, both of which may be unsuitable to the actual patient need. The practice of using dual categories stems from the belief that each patient's ailment is unique and under most circumstances will not lend itself to preliminary categorization and service time estimates. To reduce the ambiguities and inaccuracies present in the dual category scheduling process, however, some medical groups have attempted to further categorize patient ailments and assign to each ailment a specific service time interval. With the help of the group's physicians, a basic set of five, ten, twelve, etc., ailment categories can be identified. Among these categories might be complete history and physical, new patient office visit, or return patient office visit. Physician estimates of actual service time needed for such ailment categories have proven to be accurate. After the major categories have been established, a set of modifying factors may be developed to help the appointment personnel better estimate the actual service time required by each patient based on his ailment category. The modifying factors may add to or subtract from the initial time estimation for the category to which the ailment was assigned.

When simple category assignment rules and service time modifier rules are available in a clear and concise form, appointment personnel are able to make patient appointments for a time period which in most cases will meet the patient's needs. The resultant increase in accuracy will eliminate both patient and physician waiting time. In establishing time intervals, consistency should be maintained for all center physicians. The establishment of unique time interval criteria for each group physician, even when the clinic is utilizing a decentralized appointment system, often produces confusion and consumes greater amounts of clinic personnel time.

Organization and Visibility. A third consideration in establishing appointment process involves the organization of each physician's appointment schedule. Many existing clinics have experienced problems because their appointment schedules do not lend themselves readily to a quick and accurate visual inspection to determine which physician time slots already are assigned and which remain available. Often, appointment personnel are required to page through a book or clipboard while the patient waits on the telephone, thus engaging a telephone line which might be used to schedule other appointments or to deal with an emergency. In other instances, the patient may be standing impatiently at the appointment desk during this process.

With regard to appointment forms and their organization and display, several alternatives exist. The simplest form used to record appointments usually contains the date and the physician's name followed by a series of horizontal lines corresponding to the established time intervals. These forms can be placed into books or attached to clipboards which are organized according to physician. As appointments are demanded, the appropriate book or clipboard is identified and the patient information entered. The primary advantage of this form of appointment organization is that the schedules can be arranged on a countertop so that appointments for various physicians can be made simultaneously by various appointment personnel; but this system does result in the production of a number of charts for the same period of time, which may not be simultaneously visible to the appointment clerk.

One means of solving both the visibility and the organization problem is through the use of an open card file system arranged by physician on overlaid sections. Appointment times for each physician are shown by month, week, and day, with the edge of each day card showing those appointment times available (see figure 13-3). With this type of visible system, when an appointment is made the appointment person completes the patient information in the proper time slot on the body of the card and then blocks out the corresponding time period on the edge of the card with a pen or felt tip marker (see figure 13-4). Such a system enables appointment personnel to see at a glance which physician times are open for the day, week, and month. Other than the expense involved in purchasing the cards and the equipment, the primary disadvantage to the visible system is that it can be readily accessed by only one person at a time. Consequently, the possibility for more than one person to simultaneously assign multiple appointments is nonexistent.

Regardless of the process chosen, the appointment information must be communicated accurately to the patient to ensure that there are no misunderstandings about the appointment time. Appointment reminder cards usually are prepared and given to patients who are in the clinic and are scheduling future appointments. Since this process is not possible for telephone appointments, it is necessary to make certain that the information is communicated clearly and accurately, and is repeated if necessary. The process of canceling or rescheduling appointments when the physician is occupied with an emergency also must be established. The process by which appointment personnel are to schedule patients who do not have a physician preference must be clarified as well. These patients may be assigned to one particular physician, such as the physician whose schedule is least full on the requested date, or they may be equally distributed by using a "round robin" approach.

The importance of the appointment-making system cannot be underestimated because this is the process by which the physician's time is allocated. On the surface, appointment-making may seem to involve no more than the assigning of specific time frames to individual patients, but in reality the appointment system is deceivingly complex and must be well coordinated with other operating systems within the clinic. Because appointment personnel are scheduling the primary commodity of the group practice, the physicians' time and service to the patients, policy considerations concern the maintenance of an efficient appointment-making system and the management of appointment personnel. Depending upon the needs of the group, various appointment processes

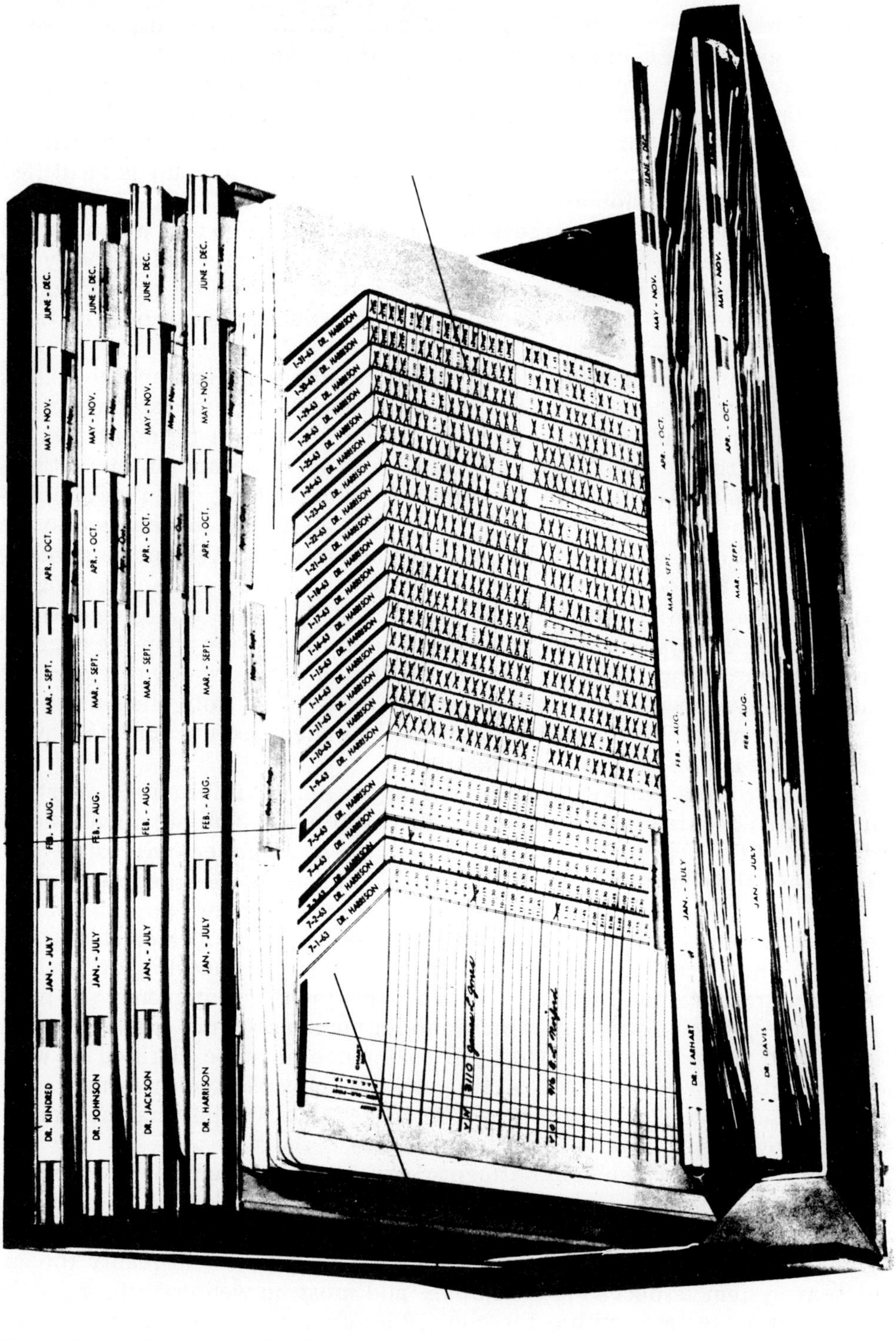

Figure 13–3. Open Card File System

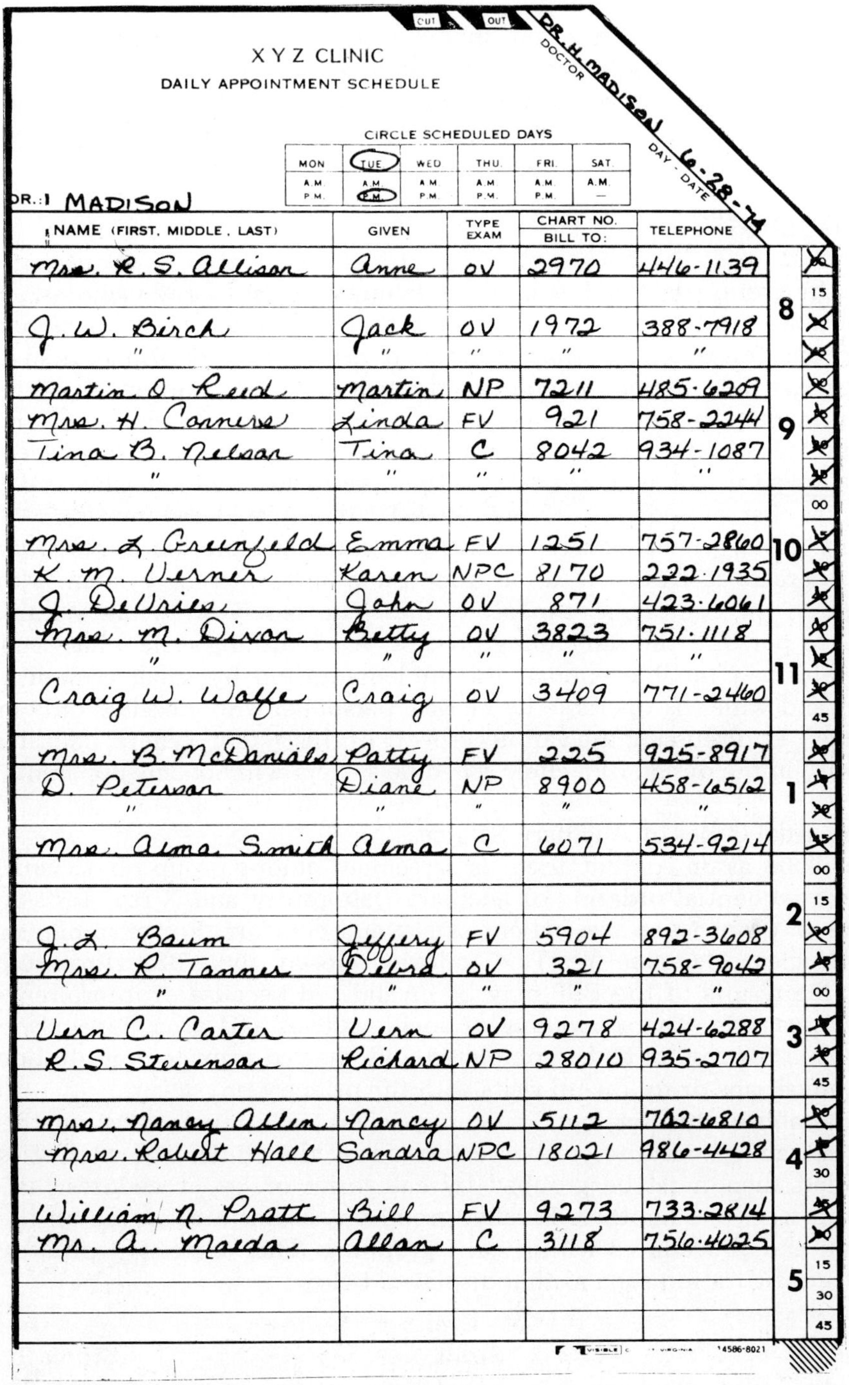

XYZ CLINIC
DAILY APPOINTMENT SCHEDULE

DR. H. MADISON — DOCTOR
DAY - DATE 6-28-74

CIRCLE SCHEDULED DAYS: MON, **TUE** (circled), WED, THU., FRI., SAT. — A.M. / **P.M.** (circled)

DR.: MADISON

NAME (FIRST, MIDDLE, LAST)	GIVEN	TYPE EXAM	CHART NO. / BILL TO:	TELEPHONE	HOUR	
Mrs. R. S. Allison	Anne	OV	2970	446-1139		
						15
J. W. Birch	Jack	OV	1972	388-7918	8	
"	"	"	"	"		
Martin O. Reed	Martin	NP	7211	485-6209		
Mrs. H. Conners	Linda	FV	921	758-2244	9	
Tina B. Nelson	Tina	C	8042	934-1087		
"	"	"	"	"		
						00
Mrs. L. Greenfield	Emma	FV	1251	757-2860	10	
K. M. Verner	Karen	NPC	8170	222-1935		
J. DeVries	John	OV	871	423-6061		
Mrs. M. Dixon	Betty	OV	3823	751-1118		
"	"	"	"	"	11	
Craig W. Wolfe	Craig	OV	3409	771-2460		
						45
Mrs. B. McDaniels	Patty	FV	225	925-8917		
D. Peterson	Diane	NP	8900	458-6512	1	
"	"	"	"	"		
Mrs. Alma Smith	Alma	C	6071	534-9214		
						00
					2	15
J. L. Baum	Jeffery	FV	5904	892-3608		
Mrs. R. Tanner	Debra	OV	321	758-9042		
"	"	"	"	"		00
Vern C. Carter	Vern	OV	9278	424-6288	3	
R. S. Stevenson	Richard	NP	28010	935-2707		
						45
Mrs. Nancy Allen	Nancy	OV	5112	762-6810		
Mrs. Robert Hall	Sandra	NPC	18021	986-4428	4	
						30
William N. Pratt	Bill	FV	9273	733-2814		
Mr. A. Maeda	Allan	C	3118	756-4025		
						15
					5	30
						45

Figure 13–4. Daily Appointment Schedule

can be implemented. There are many well-conceived computer appointment processes which not only serve to schedule appointments, but also perform information transfer and access functions. Regardless of the method employed in the appointment process, however, the foregoing should help to delineate considerations relevant to the designing of an appointment system.

SCHEDULING

When the group practice has in-house laboratory and X-ray facilities, a patient may require multiple appointments, either for laboratory tests, X-ray examinations, consultations, or perhaps follow-up visits. Clinic personnel then must be able to schedule patient appointments in a medically correct sequence. Most appointment personnel, having had little or no medical training, often find it difficult to schedule tests, examinations, and consultations in proper order, with allowances for required service time, reporting time, and interval time to guarantee that subsequent or previous tests are not rendered invalid.

Many group practices refer to this appointment function as *scheduling* and often segreate it from the usual doctor-appointment-time system. Moreover, because of the complexities involved, these clinics rely on specially trained personnel to perform the scheduling process. A scheduling system has been developed which is flexible enough for implementation by small as well as large groups and which is operable by clerical personnel who have had only minimal training.[3] In discussing the various aspects of this sytem, general considerations necessary in the design of a clinic schedule system will become apparent.

Sequential Order of Ancillary Services

It will be assumed that there is agreement among group physicians on the need for sequential ordering of ancillary (laboratory and X-ray) tests and procedures in order to ensure patient safety and comfort. For example, should a 131_I (Nuclear Medicine Test) be followed closely by a BSP (Bromsulphalein Test), the results of the BSP may be invalidated because of interference from the 131_I capsule. The scheduling of ancillary tests and procedures also should allow time for results to be completed and charted prior to consultations with other physicians or follow-up visits with the primary physician.

To establish this system, clinic physicians first must agree on the ancillary tests and procedures to be performed by the clinic. The ancillaries to be scheduled then must be grouped by categories or by procedures that could interfere with one another. Finally, group physicians must agree on the order of tests and procedures within each grouping. This three-step process might yield a configuration such as that displayed below:

	Group 1	
BSP	Stool	Stomach
Procto	Chest X-ray	Small Bowel
131_I Capsule	KUB	Cardiac Series
131_I Count	Sinus	Esophagus
IVP	Spine	GI Consult
Urology Consult	Gall Bladder	
IVC	Colon	

Group 2
Podiatry
Mammogram 2-Hour
Pap Smear
Tissue Study
Nuclear Med. Scan
24-Hour Urine

Group 3
Skull X-ray
EEG
ENG
EMG
Neurology Consult

Group 4
Diag. Tubeless Gastric
2-Hour Sugar

Group 5
EKG
Audio Testing
Pulmonary Function
Physical Therapy
Bone Marrow
Electrolysis
Dental
Psych./Psychol.

Group 6
Fasting Tests Lab

Group 7
Routine Lab Tests
Injections
Dietitian

In taking these preliminary steps in establishing a scheduling system it is important that flexibility be built into the grouping of ancillary tests and procedures. Figure 13-5 is a flow chart which graphically represents test and procedure groupings. The established order in each grouping flows from left to right. An example sequence might be a BSP, followed by a Procto, followed by a 131_I. As the clinic grows, new tests and procedures may be added to those already available; conversely, discontinued tests must be deleted with minimal impact on the overall operation of the system. This addition and/or deletion of tests also is facilitated through use of a flow diagram such as displayed in figure 13-5.

Assignment of Numbers to Each Ancillary Service Procedure

Although the flow diagram alone can serve as an excellent guide for the scheduling personnel in appointing ancillary services, the system can be further refined by superimposing a matrix over the flow diagram (figure 13-5), thereby assigning a number to each test or procedure; for example, BSP=110, Procto=111, and 131_I=120 (see figure 13-6). Because the number assignment corresponds to sequence in the flow diagram, the scheduling technique is further simplified. In each case, a lower-numbered ancillary is scheduled before the higher-numbered ancillary. For example, a 110(BSP) is scheduled before a 111(Procto), and a 111(Procto) is scheduled before 120 (I 131 uptake). Provision is made for expanding the chart by using three-digit numbers which allow for an increase of nine test designations per item. Flexibility in number assignment also is maintained; for instance, if a new procedure is needed which should be scheduled after an Urology Consult (131) but before an IVC (140), the new procedure could be numbered 132 or 140 with the IVC redesignated as 141. Because this numbering corresponds to the scheduling order of ancillaries, it is adaptable to a computerized scheduling system, if and when the scheduling volume so dictates.

After a logical order and corresponding number have been assigned to each test and procedure, scheduling personnel must be made aware of any special

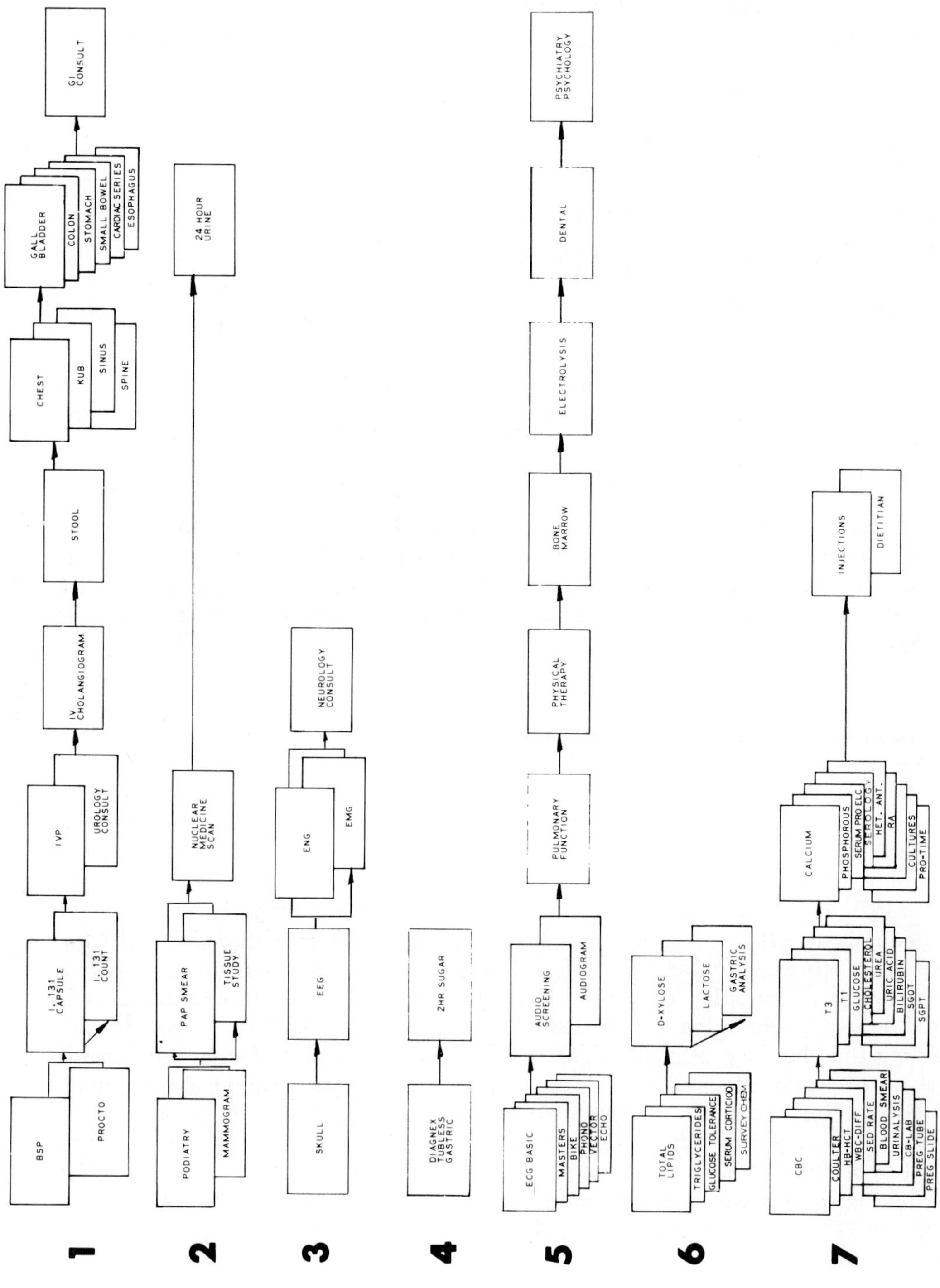

Figure 13-5. Ancillary Tests and Procedures

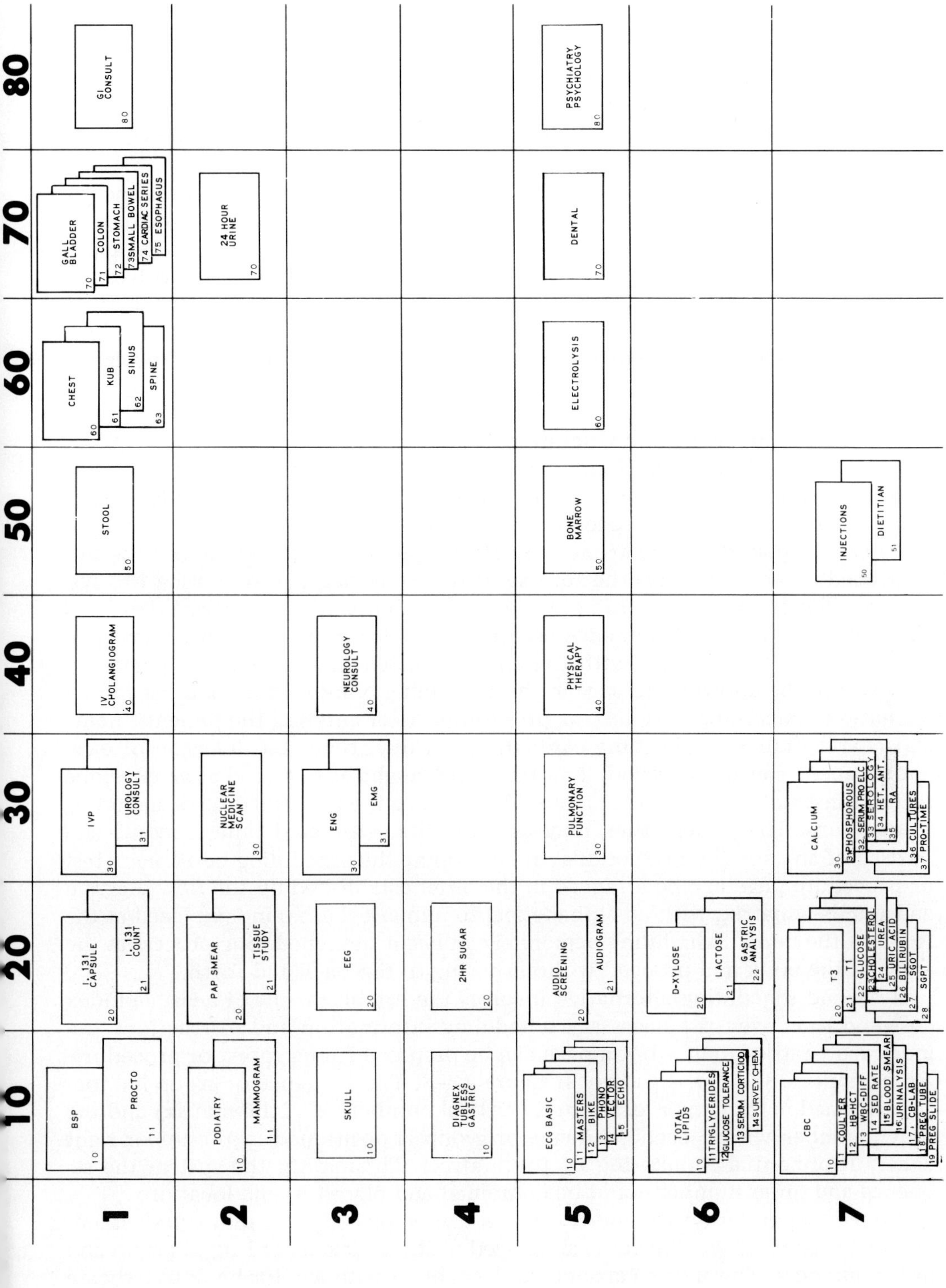

Figure 13-6. Number Matrix Superimposed on Ancillary Test and Procedures Flow Chart

instructions concerning the proper appointing of each ancillary. For example, the instructions for a BSP may be as follows:

1. Time required is one hour
2. Do not schedule before 9:00 A.M. or after 4:00 P.M.
3. Patient must fast from 10:00 P.M. the night before
4. The appointment for the BSP is made with the ordering doctor's nurse.

Because scheduling personnel often receive questions from patients concerning ordered tests and procedures, it is advisable to provide personnel with some information about each test and procedure. For example, a BSP is a Bromsulphalein Test; that is, a procedure to determine liver function. It involves the injecting of a dye substance and the drawing of a blood specimen after 45 minutes have elapsed. With this information available, scheduling personnel are better able to answer patient questions and can better understand the various tests and procedures they are scheduling.

The Scheduling System in Operation

A scheduling instruction book can be utilized to convey the proper information to a patient concerning the nature and requirements of his ancillary tests. Each test or procedure can occupy a different page in the manual, and instructions can be placed on the front of each page, with information about the test or procedure contained on the reverse of the same page. In operating the system, ancillaries ordered by the physician can be entered on a patient time card (see figure 13-7) in the sequence established by the flow diagram (refer again to figure 13-5). Beginning with the ancillary listed first, scheduling personnel can refer to the appropriate page in the scheduling book for instructions and information concerning that test or procedure. After entering the patient's name and chart number on the time card, the date, day, time, and location of each appointment can be recorded. The time card might be designed as an envelope to hold instructions and other material related to the scheduled tests, including medications. The patient then may be given the completed time schedule and advised of any special instructions. In developing the scheduling book, each test or procedure page can be arranged in the order established by the flow diagram and number matrix, with an alphabetical to numerical cross index placed at the front of the book. Scheduling personnel can begin the scheduling process at the front of the book and proceed without having to flip back and forth.

A second scheduling alternative involves the establishment of a visible index designed to convey the necessary scheduling information and instructions. An index card rather than a book page can be prepared for each test or procedure. An example BSP card is shown in figure 13-8. The sequence or group number is positioned in the upper left corner (vertical numbering of the matrix) and the order number within each sequence or group is positioned in the upper right corner (horizontial numbering of the matrix). To simplify the system the sequence and order number could be combined and placed in one location.

After its completion the index card set can be placed in an index desk stand, shown in figure 13-9. The cards are placed in this index according to group and order numbers. The index carriers can be tabbed with a color bank to indicate

XYZ CLINIC

APPOINTMENT SCHEDULE AND INSTRUCTIONS

CHART NO.____________________

NAME____

DATE	DAY	TIME	FLOOR	APPOINTMENTS

PLEASE GIVE US TWENTY-FOUR HOURS NOTICE IF YOU ARE UNABLE TO KEEP THESE APPOINTMENTS.

CLINIC HOURS:

MONDAY - FRIDAY — 8:00 - 5:00
DAY OR NIGHT: CALL 526-2671

Figure 13–7. Patient Time Card

the absence of a particular card in the order set and an alphabetical to numerical cross index can be developed and attached to the base of the desk stand.

When scheduling personnel make use of the book-page scheduling system, the requested ancillaries must be arranged in sequential order before the book is used to retrieve the instructions. Using the visible desk stand method, however, scheduling personnel take the requested ancillaries information, which is not in sequential order, and simply offset the corresponding index cards in the desk stand. The alphabetical to numerical cross-index is helpful here because the cards must be maintained in the stand in numerical order sequence. When all cards for ancillaries requested have been offset, the scheduling person can refer to the beginning of the set of index cards, take each offset card in succession, acquire the scheduling information and schedule the tests and/or proce-

Sequence	**Examination/Procedure**	**Order**
1	BSP	10

Time Required	**Misc.**
1 hour	Do **not** schedule before 9:00 a.m. or after 4:00 p.m.

Decision Rules:

Schedule before I131 Uptake
IVP
IV Cholangiogram
Gallbladder

Instructions:

Must **fast** from 10:00 p.m. the night before (no food, nonalcoholic liquids only) Maximum BSP's daily = 20

Department: Ordering Dr's. nurse **Floor:** (Variable)

Telephone: (Variable)

REVERSE SIDE OF CARD

BSP BROMSULPHALEIN 1-10

This is a procedure to determine the functioning of the liver. It involves the injection of a dye and the subsequent taking of a blood specimen 45 minutes later.

The patient must **fast** from 10:00 p.m. the night before.

Figure 13–8. Sample Scheduling Card Designed for Visible File System

dures on a scheduling time card. The visible scheduling system has the same disadvantages as the visible appointment system, i.e., the system's establishment requires a moderate initial expense and the stand can be accessed by only one scheduling person at any one given time.

Although two alternative approaches to the implementation of a scheduling

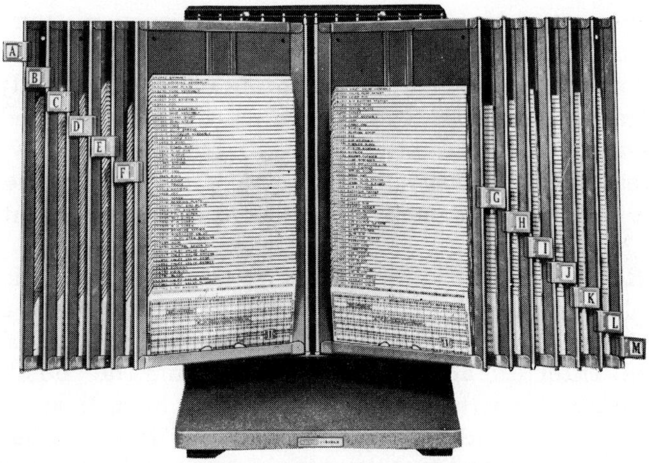

Figure 13-9. Index Desk Stand

system have been introduced, certainly there are many other variations. Before any system can be put into practice, group members must agree upon a logical sequence of ancillary scheduling. The flow chart and matrix design introduced here can be helpful in this process. Pertinent information concerning the nature and requirements of ancillary tests and procedures then must be conveyed to the appropriate personnel to ensure that scheduling policy is maintained.

REFERRAL

Referrals and intragroup consultations represent one of the key advantages to medical practice in a group setting. Because neither an individual physician nor the average group can provide the full spectrum of medical services to patients, referral relationships must be established between physicians and between organizations. Often, during the development as well as during the actual operation of a medical group, little consideration is given to the referral activity, but attention to this area is necessary if patients are to receive quality medical care and if the group is to continue receiving referrals from outside sources. Variables affecting the physician's decision to refer his patient to another physician include not only the nature of the patient's illness and its relationship to the scope of the physician's practice, but also the patient's socioeconomic characteristics and his psychological needs. A physician treating two patients who suffer from the same illness may decide, after weighing all social and psychological factors, that only one of the patients should be referred to a consulting physician. On the other hand, the primary physician also may decide to refer both patients, but because of individual characteristics he may send each patient to a different specialist. Community attitudes as well as type of community also will influence the referral process. A high level of referral activity may or may not be valued within a community as an indicator of the availability of quality health care. In addition, factors such as community size, rural versus urban characteristics, and availability of transportation will contribute to the amount of referral activity.

Professional courtesy and conduct regarding referrals generally fall into three categories: intraclinic referrals, those from external sources, and hospital referrals or consultations. Although Chapter 10 treats the policy considerations affecting professional courtesy and referrals, it is necessary here to approach these activities from the perspective of the initial establishment of the system.

Intraclinic Referrals. Consultations may occur among physicians within the group. Referral patients will require appointments and perhaps scheduling. The group must decide if these patients will be treated with a priority different from those who enter the appointment system from the "outside." The physician or his nurse usually is the person initiating the intraclinic referral; consideration must be given to the appointment-making process, especially when the appointments are centralized and the requester uses the telephone. Are internal referrals going to be made on a designated line in central appointments or will the calls be received in the same manner as those directly from patients?

Responsibility for the direction of patients is yet another important consideration of internal referrals. Determinations must be made concerning the physician in charge and the communications involved. For example, the means through which the referring physician transmits results of the work performed or information concerning work ordered must be developed. Communication failure between group physicians can result in the duplication of services and costs and can waste both physician and patient time. Existing groups employ various methods to convey information concerning services already performed. Among these are special referral forms, centralized order sheets with a referral tear-out copy, and the patient's medical record. Of prime importance in this communication process is an explanation or reason for the referral—a guideline for the consulting physicians.

Structuring the internal referral process also involves the manner in which the consulting physician returns primary responsibility for the patient to the referring or primary physician. It can happen that a patient will prefer the services of the consulting physician to those of the referring physician and therefore will choose to remain in the care of the consultant. An orderly and well-understood process to deal with such circumstances should be developed.

While the newly forming group may consider the development of procedures and systems for the handling of intraclinic referrals to be of secondary or minimal importance, the experience of both existing and dissolved group practices indicates that internal operations and procedures can cause far more conflict than can activities associated with external individuals and organizations. Physicians often take one another for granted and as a result fail to communicate effectively.

Refferals to and from External Sources. In most cases, referrals to specialties within the newly formed group are essential if the practice is going to continue. A system of handling referrals from external physicians becomes necessary if efficiency and consistency in clinic operations are to be maintained. The group should consider not only the method of appointments and scheduling for patients referred by external physicians, but also whether or not these patients will be registered, if and how a medical record will be established for them, how possible X-ray films, reports, and laboratory files will be maintained, how billing and credit will be effected, and finally, how follow-up visits will be handled. Each of these systems difficulties should not jeopardize the referral relationship which is developing or existing between the center and external physicians.

Group practice is often criticized by solo practitioners for pirating private patients upon referral. While medical ethics certainly provide guidance for these circumstances, various clinic systems should not present the overt appearance of seeking to assume responsibility for the continued care of other physicians' patients. For example, groups often develop mailing lists for new service announcements as well as other follow-up visits for certain medical procedures such as immunizations. The group should develop effective procedures to ensure that referred patients do not receive such service announcements and are not advised to come to the clinic to be given, for example, a flu shot. On the other hand, ethics also dictate that the patient should maintain freedom of choice regarding his private physician. Should the referred patient prefer the services of the group, he certainly is free to make that choice and should be welcomed. Regardless of center procedures, the patient's own choice often may be perceived as pirating by the referring physician. Consequently, the group should remain aware of the possible effect of procedures and established systems upon the referral relationship.

The procedure for referral of clinic patients to external physicians also requires attention. For example, how are appointments made with external physicians? Who makes them? Will a consultation report be prepared by the consulting physician? To whom will this report be sent? How will the report be filed in the medical records? Of special concern are referrals to external physicians whose specialty and/or subspecialty is represented within the group. Although this situation is related more directly to professional policy, procedures will be necessary to maintain these relationships on a consistent and equitable level. When patients are referred to physicians outside the group, possible conflicts or complaints about the referral may occur. How these complaints will be recieved and whether or not they will be reported to the consulting physician must be decided. Although such complaints may follow the channel established for group physicians, the outside individual or organization must be dealt with in some manner by the clinic. Will the clinic representative be the referring physician, the senior physician, the medical director, the administrator, etc.?

Referrals to and from external sources are certain to become daily occurrences in clinic operations. Effective patient care upon referral, favorable public relations, and ethical relationships among group members and their professional peers may be dependent upon clinic referral systems and procedures. The group should remain aware of possible areas of referral conflict and should evaluate other areas requiring specific referral procedures and systems for efficiency and consistency in the referral process.

Hospital Referrals. While hospital referrals and consultations involve both intragroup and external referral considerations, the primary concern is the manner of rendering reports and recording appropriate charges for billing purposes. For example, should a group physician perform a hospital referral for another group physician, how will the service be recorded and the charge applied? In this instance, it is likely that the referral will be recorded and billed on the primary physician's charge ticket because it represents a group bill. If the referral were accomplished for an external physician, the group physician would bill the patient for the referral. Any action to the contrary may constitute fee-splitting.

Referral Reports and Consultations

As with all clinic services, referrals should be documented and become a part of the patient's medical record. It is essential that a report also be made to the referring physician. For intraclinic referrals, the report prepared for the medical record could well serve as the report to the referring physician. For external physicians, referral reports customarily are more formalized than internal progress notes. Usually, reports to external physicians are dictated and typed on formal stationery. In many instances, however, a photocopy of the progress notes will suffice. While in some cases it may be appropriate for the consulting physician to telephone the referring physician and render a verbal report, documentation of the referral remains necessary and such telephone consultations should be followed up with a written report. In addition, prompt attention in this area can stimulate even more referral activity in the future.

Referral information among clinic physicians can be hindered by the "taking for granted" syndrome. Physicians who daily work closely with one another may delay the preparation of referral reports to one another because they expect to transfer the information verbally in the hallway, over lunch, or at a social gathering in the very near future. In this situation, procedures may be in order to ensure that clinic physicians provide the same degree of promptness in written reports to one another as they would for reports to external physicians. Of course, clinic physicians should not refrain from consulting with one another informally, but such practices may delay formal documented consultation reports by days or possibly weeks and can be as harmful to the patient as actual technical incompetence on the part of the physician.

APPOINTMENTS, SCHEDULING, AND REFERRAL POLICY

Essential to effective operation of the appointment, scheduling, and referral processes is the development of procedure and policy guidelines. Such policy guidelines usually center around the actual mechanical operation of the appointment, scheduling, and referral processes and patient flow techniques. Although covered in detail in Chapter 10, several procedural and policy considerations can be reiterated here.

First, the clinic management must abide by the ethics and traditions governing the operation of a medical practice, even if these ethics and traditions are incompatible with the principles of business efficiency. Second, facility design and capacity will have a definite influence on determinations of patient routing and patient flow policy. Problems of poor design or inadequate space cannot be solved simply through policy determination; rather, a thorough understanding of the facility as it relates to clinic operating systems points the way to alternate solutions for design and space problems. Within the context of goals and objectives, appropriate policy and procedures can be generated.

A third consideration involves clinic size and specialty mix. Specialties of the group's physicians will dictate the types of procedures used in patient appointments, scheduling, and internal referrals. Variations in group size, and the communication problems which usually occur as group size increases, will have significant bearing on the type and number of policies necessary. Consideration of clinic size and specialties may be particularly critical when a decision must be made as to whether the group will use a centralized or decentralized appointment and scheduling system.

A fourth consideration concerns the nature of patient ailments. Usage patterns and expectations are affected by age, sex, and socioeconomic background. If certain diseases and ailments are found more frequently in the area served by a particular group, the group may have to adjust its procedures and policies to accommodate such an imbalance. Treatment of the patient remains the primary consideration; but should an imbalance necessitate a high level of referrals due to nonrepresentation of certain specialties or services, the group may alter its established mission, objectives, and policies to meet the demand. Such an alteration in policy would be certain to change both the systems and procedures.

During the actual process of developing appointment, scheduling, and referral procedures, management should allow for variations in physician preferences and physician compensation. For example, the clinic fee schedule, whether a flat-rate or graduated-complexity system, can have significant effect upon the number of patients which each physician may be expected to see in one day and also may determine the actual appointment time intervals which the physicians use. If patients are charged a flat-fee per visit, the physicians may be required to see a minimum number of patients per day to cover their overhead costs. If a scale of graduated-complexity is used, an average fee may be calculated which would indicate the number of patients a physician must see to cover his overhead. Alternatively, appointments of different types may be credited with an agreed-upon number of treatment units and the specified number of treatment units per day to cover overhead. The appointment, the scheduling, and even the referral processes which the group develops may have a direct effect upon physician reimbursement; the group may find it advantageous, therefore, to determine the physician reimbursement plan before finalizing an appointment, scheduling, and referral system.

The appointment and scheduling process and patient flow within the clinic may influence one another greatly in terms of policy determination and procedure. Clinic personnel who operate the systems must remain continually aware that the patient's attitude toward the center may be heavily influenced by his experience in making appointments, in being scheduled, and in being referred. In a business sense, the patient is a customer without whom the clinic would cease to function; therefore, it must develop and maintain a professional manner in patient-clinic communications, courtesy, and knowledge of job tasks and responsibilities.

In summary, as with the development of policy and procedure which guides and controls any other clinic operations, appointment, scheduling, and referral processes must be developed with an awareness of the needs and desires of the patient, the physician, and the clinic management. Generally, the administrator wishes to establish systems which will provide for the greatest possible efficiency at the lowest possible cost. The physician wishes to have available systems which enable him to provide quality health care, while allowing for flexibility in dealing with unexpected problems. The patient expects the clinic's systems to provide him with quality health care, while permiting him to use his time effectively. In formulating and establishing actual appointments, scheduling, and referral policies and procedures and in attempting to consider all points of view, the policy and systems planner(s) may find, upon occasion, that the perspectives of physician, patient, and clinic administrator are not always compatible, and compromise is sometimes necessary.

Chapter 14

Medical Records System

DEVELOPING A MEDICAL RECORDS SYSTEM

In establishing a system for medical records, group physicians face a number of important decisions concerning the types and amounts of data to be collected, the format for recording data, the method of record storage, and the system for record retrieval. All of these decisions will be influenced by the scope of the group's purpose in data collection, the various inputs to the system, and the facilities and equipment available for record storage and retention. This chapter will outline specific aspects of the system which must be considered by group members. Throughout the development process, as decisions are made, two important factors must be borne in mind. First, medical records must be *usable*. The most sophisticated system available will prove worthless if records are not easily accessible, organized, and meaningful. Secondly, the medical records system should be established with an eye toward the future. *Flexibility for growth* not only will prove economically beneficial for the group, but also will result in a constant level of system efficiency.

The Importance of Medical Records

The main objective in establishing and maintaining medical records is to facilitate the continued care of the group's patients. Physicians cannot be expected to remember in detail the ailments, diagnoses, and treatment of each patient they see. The record, therefore, as a history of a patient's medical treatment, serves as a reference source for the physician and helps to ensure continuity of care for the patient. Often, within one clinic a diversity of medical specialties may be represented. As the patient moves among the various clinic specialties and departments, a continuous chronicle of his medical problems is compiled in his record. Thus, the patient may be assured of comprehensive health care for his present problems, as well as preventive health care to forestall possible future health problems. If the clinic is family oriented, a medical record may include not only individual patient data but also data on the various members of that patient's family. From these data can be abstracted a family health profile which may be useful in retrospective studies of social problems as well as in continued general health maintenance.

Medical records also are important in protecting the physician and patient against various medicolegal entanglements. A medical record may be a physician's as well as the patient's only evidence concerning a diagnosis, a prescribed medication, or a particular treatment rendered; therefore, it may be crucial in a court decision. Needless to say, this possibility underscores the need for accurate, legible, well-organized medical records. The effective control and retrieval of medical records also is necessary because the record department often is interfaced with other clinic systems, such as insurance and billing registration, appointments and scheduling, and referral; consequently, the recording of data concerning diagnosis and treatment as well as the maintenance of current patient information (address, credit status, employment) are important activities, and the necessity for standardized forms and procedures cannot be overestimated.

In addition to serving as a tool with which the physician can render quality medical care to the patient, and to providing medicolegal protection for both physician and patient, the medical records department may offer the research-oriented physician a wealth of data. While not all groups will be engaged in this type of activity, it nevertheless remains possible for the physician to consult the records of patients whose previous diagnoses and treatment may bear direct relevance to a case with which he is presently concerned. Medical records also are influential in accreditation processes and are integral to the external as well as internal assessment of the quality of medical care offered by group physicians and the clinic as a whole. External reporting requirements, such as those generated by Professional Standards Review Organizations (PSROs), have necessitated the refining and updating of medical data collection in order that an accurate measurement of health care may be made. In addition, review requirements of Medicare, Medicaid, and other third party payors have added impetus toward the standardization of medical records. Internal peer review conducted by auditing committees also relies upon complete, meaningful, and standardized records of medical care.

Basic Components of the Traditional Medical Record

Data contained in a medical record generally falls into four categories: patient information; notes; drugs, tests, and procedures; correspondence and administrative data. While these categories do not necessarily reflect the sequencing of information within the record, they do represent basic information areas which provide the framework for a usable medical record.

Patient Information. In Chapter 12, the patient registration system is discussed in detail. The patient's initial contact with the clinic will generate at least two forms for inclusion in his medical record: the registration form and the patient history form. The registration form may be quite brief and simple (see figure 14-1), or it may be more complex and designed to serve a dual or even triple function. Figure 14-2 is a registration form completed in triplicate, with copies intended not only for the patient's medical record, but also for the business office and the office of patient accounts. A third possibility for the recording of patient registration information is to have the registration form imprinted directly onto the inside cover of the medical record jacket. While this latter approach may be convenient for registration personnel, as time passes the record jacket will become worn and the information illegible. In addition, corrections usually must be made as patient address, place of employment, etc., change. A form which can be detached from the record and replaced with a new, clean copy may prove more practical than replacing the chart jacket, thereby disturbing the contents of the entire record and risking loss of other forms. Regardless of the alternative chosen, in designing the registration form the group will want to include space not only for the patient's *full* name (including his middle initial), his address and telephone number, and, possibly, his social security number, but also for insurance information, responsible party designation, and, if a family record is being maintained, for the names of family members who already are patients of the group. The registration form also should have space designated for the patient's chart number, which may be assigned at the time of registration or later by the medical records department. Maintaining accurate and complete patient information is important for billing purposes as well as for quick and efficient medical record retrieval.

The second form usually initiated at the time of registration is the patient history, which is used to gather data concerning the past and present medical condition of the patient and his family through questions concerning past illnesses and surgery, X-ray, allergies, immunizations, and the present condition of physiological systems—i.e., cardiac, respiratory, etc. Figure 14-3 is an example of an adult health history questionnaire. Pediatric health histories usually vary somewhat from this model. It is also possible to use a history questionnaire designed for computer use. A third possibility involves the use of a small video (CRT) unit and keyboard. As questions are displayed on the screen to the patient, he depresses the key which corresponds to his intended response. The history information is then stored in the computer and can be retrieved by the physician either on a video screen or in hard copy. If the group does adopt this type of electronic data processing, or considers it for the future, it also might want to extend the system to include patient registration as well. Newly forming groups of three to ten physicians probably will not be considering such a sophisticated approach for immediate implementation, but should be aware of such technology in planning for the future.

Although questions concerning allergies and drug sensitivities do appear on the health history questionnaire, when the record is initiated it often is wise to underscore any condition of this type either by applying to the front of the chart cover a pressure sensitive tab indicating the allergy or sensitivity, or by stamping the chart cover with conspicuous lettering. The dates and results of certain tests and procedures and Medicare or Medicaid applicability, as well as the existence of medical problems which require constant follow-up or are being monitored in a research project, also can be indicated by applying a label to or by stamping the chart cover.

Finally, the patient registration form and the patient health history may be

CHART # ____________ DATE ____________

MISS
MRS.
MR. ____
Last Name First Middle Maiden

ADDRESS ____
Street, Rt., or Box City State Zip

AGE ______ BIRTH DATE ____________ SEX ______ RACE ______ RELIGION ____________ NO. OF CHILDREN ______ PHONE ____________

EMPLOYER ____________________

YOUR OCCUPATION ____________________ ADDRESS ____________________

HUSBAND, WIFE, FATHER, OR MOTHER (RESPONSIBLE PERSON):

____ RELATIONSHIP ____________
Last Name First Middle

ADDRESS ____
Street, Rt., or Box City State Zip

OCCUPATION OF RESPONSIBLE PERSON ____

EMPLOYER ____________________ ADDRESS ____________________

NAME OF HOSPITAL INSURANCE ____

MEMBER OF FAMILY *NOT* RESIDING AT YOUR ADDRESS:

____ RELATIONSHIP ____________
Last Name First Middle

ADDRESS ____

HAS ANY MEMBER OF YOUR IMMEDIATE FAMILY BEEN A PATIENT HERE? ____________
Yes or No

NAME OF THAT PATIENT ____

SIGNED ____________________

Figure 14–1. Registration Form

DATE OF APPOINTMENT	TIME	TYPE OF VISIT	DOCTOR OF PREFERENCE	RESP. PARTY NO.	REGISTERED BY

PATIENT INFORMATION • PRINT FIRMLY & CLEARLY IN COMPLETING ITEMS BELOW •

(circle one) DOCTOR MASTER MISS MR. MRS. | PATIENT'S FIRST NAME | MIDDLE NAME | LAST NAME | SPOUSE'S GIVEN NAME & INITIAL

PATIENT'S HOME ADDRESS NUMBER, STREET, CITY, STATE, AND ZIP CODE | HOME PHONE NO.

PATIENT'S EMPLOYER & ADDRESS | PATIENT'S OCCUPATION | BUSINESS PHONE NO.

BIRTH DATE | SEX | AGE | RACE | (circle one) MARR SING DIV WID SEP | SOCIAL SECURITY OR MEDICARE NO. IF APPLICABLE | WHO REFERRED YOU TO THE CLINIC OR DOCTOR? | RELATIONSHIP | NAME OF FAMILY MEMBER ALREADY A CLINIC PATIENT | RELATIONSHIP

IN CASE OF EMERGENCY NOTIFY (other than spouse or parent) NAME | ADDRESS | PHONE NO.

IF PATIENT RESIDES OUTSIDE OF HOUSTON, COMPLETE ITEM BELOW:

HOTEL OR LOCAL RESIDENCE | LOCAL PHONE NO.

IF PATIENT IS MARRIED OR IS A DEPENDENT CHILD, COMPLETE ITEMS BELOW:

FULL NAME OF SPOUSE OR PARENT | RELATIONSHIP | SPOUSE OR PARENT'S EMPLOYER

SPOUSE OR PARENTS EMPLOYER'S ADDRESS (number, street, city, state and zip code) | OCCUPATION OF SPOUSE OR PARENT | BUSINESS PHONE NO.

WHO WILL BE RESPONSIBLE FOR THE PATIENT'S MEDICAL EXPENSES?

CHECK ONE: ☐PATIENT ☐SPOUSE ☐PARENT ☐OTHER (complete next item below)

IF "OTHER" BLOCK CHECKED ABOVE, PLEASE COMPLETE: NAME OF PERSON OR COMPANY | STREET ADDRESS, CITY, STATE, & ZIP CODE | PHONE NO.

INSURANCE INFORMATION: TO REQUEST FILING OF CLAIM(S) PLEASE NOTIFY CASHIER.

NAME OF INSURANCE COMPANY | INSURANCE CO. ADDRESS | GROUP NO. | POLICY NO.

OTHER INSURANCE COVERAGE | GROUP NO. | POLICY NO.

REPORT REQUESTED TO DR. NAME | ADDRESS

RETURN THIS COMPLETED INFORMATION TO NEW PATIENT REGISTRATION MEDICAL RECORDS

RETURN THIS COMPLETED INFORMATION TO NEW PATIENT REGISTRATION BUSINESS OFFICE

RETURN THIS COMPLETED INFORMATION TO NEW PATIENT REGISTRATION PATIENT ACCOUNTS

Figure 14–2. Multi-Copy Registration Form

PATIENT'S NAME ______ BIRTH DATE ______ SEX ______ S. M. W. D.

ADDRESS ______ TEL. NO. ______

INSURANCE ______ REFERRED BY ______ OCCUPATION ______

INSTRUCTIONS: PUT ☑ IN THOSE BOXES APPLICABLE TO YOU AND IN THE "YES" OR "NO" SPACE. IF LINES ARE PROVIDED WRITE IN YOUR ANSWER.

FAMILY HISTORY

	FATHER	MOTHER	BROTHER				SISTER				SPOUSE	CHILDREN					
			1	2	3	4	1	2	3	4		1	2	3	4	5	6
AGE (IF LIVING)																	
HEALTH (G) GOOD (B) BAD																	
CANCER																	
TUBERCULOSIS																	
DIABETES																	
HEART TROUBLE																	
HIGH BLOOD PRESSURE																	
STROKE																	
EPILEPSY																	
NERVOUS BREAKDOWN																	
ASTHMA, HIVES, HAYFEVER																	
BLOOD DISEASE																	
AGE (AT DEATH)																	
CAUSE OF DEATH																	

PERSONAL HISTORY

HAVE YOU EVER HAD . . .	NO	YES	HAVE YOU EVER HAD . . .	NO	YES	HAVE YOU EVER HAD . . .	NO	YES
☐ SCARLET FEVER ☐ SCARLATINA			☐ GONORRHEA ☐ SYPHILIS			ANY ☐ BROKEN ☐ CRACKED BONES		
DIPHTHERIA			ANEMIA			RECURRENT DISLOCATIONS		
SMALLPOX			JAUNDICE			☐ CONCUSSION ☐ HEAD INJURY		
PNEUMONIA			EPILEPSY			EVER BEEN KNOCKED UNCONSCIOUS		
PLEURISY			MIGRAINE HEADACHES			☐ FOOD ☐ CHEMICAL ☐ DRUG POISONING		
UNDULANT FEVER			TUBERCULOSIS			EXPLAIN		
☐ RHEUMATIC FEVER ☐ HEART DISEASE			DIABETES					
ST. VITUS DANCE			CANCER					
☐ ARTHRITIS ☐ RHEUMATISM			☐ HIGH ☐ LOW BLOOD PRESSURE			ANY OTHER DISEASE		
ANY ☐ BONE ☐ JOINT DISEASE			NERVOUS BREAKDOWN			EXPLAIN		
☐ NEURITIS ☐ NEURALGIA			☐ HAY FEVER ☐ ASTHMA					
☐ BURSITIS ☐ SCIATICA ☐ LUMBAGO			☐ HIVES ☐ ECZEMA					
☐ POLIO ☐ MENINGITIS			FREQUENT ☐ COLDS ☐ SORE THROAT			WEIGHT: NOW ONE YR. AGO		
BRIGHT'S DISEASE			FREQUENT ☐ INFECTIONS ☐ BOILS			MAXIMUM WHEN		

ALLERGIES

ARE YOU ALLERGIC TO . . .	NO	YES	ARE YOU ALLERGIC TO . . .	NO	YES	ARE YOU ALLERGIC TO . . .	NO	YES
☐ PENICILLIN ☐ SULFA DRUGS			ANY OTHER DRUGS			ANY FOODS		
☐ ASPIRIN ☐ CODEINE ☐ MORPHINE			EXPLAIN			EXPLAIN		
☐ MYCINS ☐ OTHER ANTIBIOTICS								
☐ TETANUS ☐ ANTITOXIN ☐ SERUMS			ADHESIVE TAPE			☐ NAIL POLISH ☐ OTHER COSMETICS		

SURGERY

HAVE YOU HAD REMOVED . . .	NO	YES	HAVE YOU HAD REMOVED . . .	NO	YES	HAVE YOU . . .	NO	YES
TONSILS			☐ OVARY ☐ OVARIES			HAD HERNIA REPAIRED		
APPENDIX			HEMORRHOIDS			HAD ANY OTHER OPERATIONS		
GALL BLADDER			EVER HAVE A TRANSFUSION . . .			BEEN HOSPITALIZED FOR ANY ILLNESS		
UTERUS			☐ BLOOD ☐ PLASMA			EXPLAIN		

X-RAYS

EVER HAVE X-RAYS OF . . .	NO	YES	DATE	DISEASE PRESENT
CHEST				
☐ STOMACH ☐ COLON				
GALL BLADDER				
EXTREMITIES				
BACK				
OTHER				

Figure 14–3. Patient Health History Questionnaire

SYSTEMS

DO YOU NOW OR HAVE YOU EVER HAD	NO	YES	DO YOU NOW OR HAVE YOU EVER HAD	NO	YES
ANY ☐ EYE DISEASE ☐ EYE INJURY ☐ IMPAIRED SIGHT			KIDNEY ☐ DISEASE ☐ STONES		
ANY ☐ EAR DISEASE ☐ EAR INJURY ☐ IMPAIRED HEARING			BLADDER DISEASE		
ANY TROUBLE WITH ☐ NOSE ☐ SINUSES ☐ MOUTH ☐ THROAT			BLOOD IN URINE		
FAINTING SPELLS			☐ ALBUMIN ☐ SUGAR ☐ PUS ☐ ETC. IN URINE		
CONVULSIONS			DIFFICULTY IN URINATION		
PARALYSIS			NARROWED URINARY STREAM		
DIZZINESS			ABNORMAL THIRST		
HEADACHES: ☐ FREQUENT ☐ SEVERE			PROSTATE TROUBLE		
ENLARGED GLANDS			☐ STOMACH TROUBLE ☐ ULCER		
THYROID: ☐ OVERACTIVE ☐ UNDERACTIVE ☐ ENLARGED			INDIGESTION		
ENLARGED GOITER			☐ GAS ☐ BELCHING		
SKIN DISEASE			APPENDICITIS		
COUGH: ☐ FREQUENT ☐ CHRONIC			☐ LIVER DISEASE ☐ GALL BLADDER DISEASE		
☐ CHEST PAIN ☐ ANGINA PECTORIS			☐ COLITIS ☐ OTHER BOWEL DISEASE		
SPITTING UP BLOOD			☐ HEMORRHOIDS ☐ RECTAL BLEEDING		
NIGHT SWEATS			BLACK TARRY STOOLS		
SHORTNESS OF BREATH ☐ EXERTION ☐ AT NIGHT			☐ CONSTIPATION ☐ DIARRHEA		
☐ PALPITATION ☐ FLUTTERING HEART			☐ PARASITES ☐ WORMS		
SWELLING OF ☐ HANDS ☐ FEET ☐ ANKLES			☐ ANY CHANGE IN APPETITE ☐ EATING HABITS		
VARICOSE VEINS			☐ ANY CHANGE IN BOWEL ACTION ☐ STOOLS		
EXTREME ☐ TIREDNESS ☐ WEAKNESS			EXPLAIN		

IMMUNIZATION - EKG

HAVE YOU HAD . . .	NO	YES	HAVE YOU HAD . . .	NO	YES
SMALLPOX VACCINATION (WITHIN LAST 7 YEARS)			POLIO SHOTS (WITHIN LAST 2 YEARS)		
TETANUS SHOT (NOT ANTITOXIN)			AN ELECTROCARDIOGRAM WHEN		

HABITS

DO YOU . . .	NO	YES	DO YOU USE . . .	NEVER	OCC.	FREQ.	DAILY
EXERCISE ADEQUATELY			LAXATIVES				
HOW ?			VITAMINS				
AWAKEN RESTED			SEDATIVES				
SLEEP WELL			TRANQUILIZERS				
AVERAGE 8 HOURS SLEEP (PER NIGHT)			SLEEPING PILLS, ETC.				
HAVE REGULAR BOWEL MOVEMENTS			ASPIRINS, ETC.				
SEX - ENTIRELY SATISFACTORY			CORTISONE				
LIKE YOUR WORK (HOURS PER DAY) ☐ INDOORS ☐ OUTDOORS			ALCOHOLIC BEVERAGE				
WATCH TELEVISION (HOURS PER DAY)			COFFEE (CUPS PER DAY)				
READ (HOURS PER DAY)			TOBACCO: ☐ CIGARETTES (PKS PER DAY)				
HAVE A VACATION (WEEKS PER YEAR)			☐ CIGARS ☐ PIPE ☐ CHEWING TOBACCO				
HAVE YOU EVER BEEN TREATED FOR ALCOHOLISM			☐ SNUFF				
HAVE YOU EVER BEEN TREATED FOR DRUG ABUSE			APPETITE DEPRESSANTS				
RECREATION: DO YOU PARTICIPATE IN SPORTS OR HAVE HOBBIES WHICH GIVE YOU RELAXATION AT LEAST 3 HOURS A WEEK.			THYROID MEDICATION: ☐ NO ☐ YES, IN PAST ☐ NONE NOW NOW ON GR. DAILY				
			HAVE YOU EVER TAKEN . . .				
			☐ INSULIN ☐ TABLETS FOR DIABETES ☐ HORMONE SHOTS ☐ TABLETS ☐ NO				

WOMEN ONLY

MENSTRUAL HISTORY . . .				NO	YES
AGE AT ONSET			ARE YOU REGULAR: ☐ HEAVY ☐ MEDIUM ☐ LIGHT		
USUAL DURATION OF PERIOD DAYS			DO YOU HAVE ☐ TENSON ☐ DEPRESSION BEFORE PERIOD		
CYCLE (START TO START) DAYS			DO YOU HAVE ☐ CRAMPS ☐ PAIN WITH PERIOD		
DATE OF LAST PERIOD			DO YOU HAVE HOT FLASHES		
PREGNANCIES . . .	NO	YES		NO	YES
CHILDREN BORN ALIVE (HOW MANY)			STILL BORN (HOW MANY)		
CESARIAN SECTIONS (HOW MANY)			MISCARRIAGES (HOW MANY)		
PREMATURES (HOW MANY)			ANY COMPLICATIONS		

EMOTIONS

ARE YOU OFTEN . . .	NO	YES	ARE YOU OFTEN . . .	NO	YES
DEPRESSED			JUMPY		
ANXIOUS			JITTERY		
IRRITABLE			IS CONCENTRATION DIFFICULT		

Figure 14-3. (Cont.)

completed by registration personnel or the nursing staff. In the case of the health history, the physician may complete the form at the time of the patient's initial physical examination. Unlike other forms in the record, however, it is possible that the patient himself may have sole responsibility for the completion of these forms. Group physicians should remain aware of the patient population whom they expect to serve. Often, bilingual forms will be necessary so that patients do not find it difficult or impossible to communicate with clinic personnel. Accommodating these special patient needs undoubtedly will result in a favorable image for the group in the community.

Progress Notes. Among the various notes contained in the patient's medical record are progress notes, which are intended to be a prose record of the physician's assessment and treatment of the patient's various health problems. As such, progress notes represent an integral part of a patient's medical record. In order for the patient to receive consistent care over an extended period, progress notes must contain pertinent, complete information which has been compiled systematically and is legible. In addition, to be most effective, progress notes must be uniform in nature of content. Ideally, any group physician should be able to read a patient's progress notes and thereby ascertain exactly the course of that patient's treatment throughout the various specialties represented within the medical group. Typically, progress notes include information concerning the patient's complaint or reason for his visit to the group; the results of any physical examination; any tests, procedures, or medications ordered by the physician; any diagnoses made by the physician; and any other information—subjective or objective—considered relevant by the physician. Within the medical record, the progress notes may be organized chronologically or by specialty. When the latter alternative is chosen, the record often becomes fragmented and, consequently, the continuum of the patient's medical history is interrupted. While chronologically organized notes do reflect the patient's course of treatment, some specialists maintain that they find the notes of other specialties superfluous in their treatment of the patient. Often, a combination can be the best alternative. Specialties, such as dermatology and allergy, as well as hearing, ophthalmology, and dental, can be kept as separate records or as discrete units within one record, perhaps color coded for ease in identification. Notes for the remaining specialties may be kept chronologically, with each physician rubber stamping and/or initialing his notes.

All notes, whether by specialty or chronology, should be conspicuously dated and the progress note sheets should be arranged with the most recent sheet forward. The notes may be handwritten by the physician on specifically designed forms or on plain, unruled paper. As records leave the medical records department, personnel can place a blank progress note sheet in each record, if necessary; or, as records arrive at their destination, the physician's nurse can check the record to ascertain if a new note page is needed. Regardless of who has this responsibility, the patient's full name and chart number should be recorded at the top of each new sheet.

As the clinic grows and patient load increases, the group may want to consider the benefits of dictating progress notes. Dictation is discussed in detail in Chapter 11. To reiterate only briefly, the group physicians can consider a variety of options in this area, ranging from individual desk top units to a central dictating system interfaced with the clinic's telephone system. Transcribing may be assigned to *trained* clinic personnel, or may be done on a contract basis through an agency. The group may subscribe to a dictating service which provides the dictating units or telephone interface as well as the transcribing service. As the transcriptions are completed by clinic personnel or received from the transcribing service they must be inserted into the patient's record. The group must decide who will have this responsibility—the physician's nurse or medical records personnel.

Diagnostic Summary Sheet. The medical record also may contain a diagnostic summary sheet which serves as an abbreviated guide to the patient's medical history since his first visit to the group for care. Figure 14-4 is a sample diagnostic summary sheet which is designed to include a record of all the patient's immunizations. Trained medical records personnel or the physician's nurse usually are responsible for recording the pertinent information on this type of form, including the applicable diagnostic code number. Group physicians will have to decide upon a uniform diagnostic code. Available systems include: *Eight Revisions of the International Classification of Diseases, adopted for use in the United States (ICDA-8)*; the *Hospital Adaptation of ICDA, H-ICDA*; or the *Current Procedural Terminology for Naming, Coding and Reporting Medical Services (CPT).* As an alternative, some groups may establish their own codes or may use a code preferred or required by a third party payor(s). The physician can indicate in the progress notes whether or not he wishes a diagnosis to be coded and recorded. Often, the patient's record will leave the medical records department with an encounter form or record of charges attached (see figure 14-5), a copy of which will eventually reach the accounting department for the compilation of charges, preparation of the patient's bill, and/or insurance processing. The physician can indicate the appropriate diagnostic and/or procedural code on this form; however, after only one patient visit it is possible that nothing more than a tentative diagnosis can be made, which may or may not be confirmed upon subsequent appointments.

Group physicians may decide that maintaining a diagnostic summary sheet in every medical record is not worth the additional time and expense involved. Within the larger, research oriented group, however, the data recorded on this type of form can be helpful in tracing the course of various diseases. The diagnostic summary sheet also may aid in fulfilling such reporting requirements as internal medical audit or external accreditation and PSRO reporting. Finally, availability of diagnostic information can prove beneficial in obtaining third party payor reimbursement. The ability or willingness of clinic personnel to execute this type of coding activity might determine eligibility for participation in programs such as the National Ambulatory Medical Care Survey (NAMCS), a symptom classification system designed to identify and order the reasons patients visit ambulatory care centers.[1]

Consultation and Referral Notes. When an attending physician requests another physician to examine and render an opinion concerning his patient, referral and consultation notes are generated. In referring his patient to another physician, the primary physician must indicate to the consulting physician the areas in which he desires an opinion. He may indicate in the progress notes that

Name ____________________ No. __________

DATE SEEN	PHYSICIAN OR DEPARTMENT	DIAGNOSIS	CROSS INDEX	CODE NO.

Figure 14–4. Record of Patient Visits and Diagnoses

YR. CK. (Yes) (No) (Active) (Inactive) M.D.							
YR. CK. CARD							
HAD YR. CK.							
D. P. T.							
D–T (Adult)							
DIPHTHERIA-TETANUS							
MUMPS							
RUBELLA							
POLIO SABIN							
MEASLES							
SMALLPOX							
TYPHOID							
INFLUENZA/COLD							
TUBERCULIN TEST							
TYPHUS							
CHOLERA							
YELLOW FEVER							
OTHERS:							

RECORD OF PATIENT VISITS & DIAGNOSES

DATE SEEN	PHYSICIAN OR DEPARTMENT	DIAGNOSIS	CROSS INDEX	CODE NO.

Figure 14-4. (Cont.)

PATIENT'S NAME	CHART NO.	DATE	BILL TO:	
	CHANGE OF NAME		COMPANY NO.	CODE 1 2 3 4 N/R
	CHANGE OF ADDRESS		PHONE	SPECIAL INSTRUCTIONS
	XYZ CLINIC	Post Oak ☐ West ☐	Downtown ☐	INTERPRETER: ☐
	• BEFORE RELEASING SR •			GIVE ESTIMATE ONLY: ☐
	RETURN TO ORIGINAL DOCTOR FOR REPORTS TO BE CHARTED			CALL ☐ WRITE ☐ REPORTS

CODE	LABORATORY(1)	FEE	CODE	LABORATORY(1)	FEE	CODE	X-RAY (2)	FEE	CODE	NUCLEAR MEDICINE (6)	FEE	CODE	PROFESSIONAL (4)	DATE	M.D.	FEE	PHONE NO:
15	CBC	8					CHEST (PA) (LAT)		190	T_3	10		NEW( ) RETURN( ) PATIENT				YEAR CHECK: YES ☐ NO ☐
107	SED RATE	8				31	KUB	18	213	T_4	15		COMPLETE EXAM S( ) L( )				
410	COULTER	5				54	SKULL	30		THYROID UPTAKE			FOLLOW-UP				
12	BLOOD SMEAR	10				53	SINUS	23					NEW PATIENT-OFFICE VISIT				
139	URINALYSIS	5				60	SPINE CERVICAL	30					PRE-EMPLOYMENT				
80	OB LAB	20				62	SPINE-LUMBAR	35		SCANS: LIST			FAA				
53	PREG. TEST	8				29	IVP	40					CONSULTATION - OFFICE				
59	GLUCOSE TOL	23				25	GALL BLADDER	30					CONSULTATION - OFFICE				
222	SURVEY-CHEM.	21				67	STOMACH		CODE	TREATMENT(3)	FEE						
13	GLUCOSE	5				20	ESOPHAGUS		76	DIETARY			OFFICE VISIT S( ) L( )				
137	UREA	7				69	SMALL BOWEL	45					OFFICE VISIT S( ) L( )				
138	URIC ACID	7					(AIR COLON CONT)		75	PHYSICAL THERAPY							
44	ELECTROLYTES	32															
39	CREATININE	8															
104	SGOT	10							67	DRUGS:							
105	SGPT	10															
31	CHOLESTEROL	7											HOSPITAL SERVICE				
131	TRIGLYCERIDES	13	CODE	INJECTIONS(3)	FEE	CODE	PROFESSIONAL (4)		DATE	M.D.	FEE		@ $ /DAY (REG. CARE)				
77	LIPOPROT. ELECT.	17	45	TETANUS (S) (B)	5		PROCTO( )						TO				
146	CALCIUM	7	157	D-T ADULT (S) (B)	5		ECG( ) MASTERS( )						@ $ /DAY (ICU CARE)				
89	PHOSPHOROUS	7	14	DPT	5		ERGOMETER( ) WITH CONSULT( )						TO				
47	PROTEIN ELECT.	17	37	POLIO ORAL (S) (B)	4		PULMONARY FUNCTION( ) WITH CONSULT( )										
276	SEROLOGY	8	49	TYPHOID (S) (B)	5	115	EEG				35		HOSPITAL (HISTORY & PHYSICAL)				DIAGNOSIS CODE(S):
63	HET. ANT.	8	42	SMALL POX	5		AUDIOGRAM - ENT						HOSPITAL CONSULTS				
98	R.A.	6	30	MEASLES	10								NO. OF VISITS				
215	ANA	20	105	MUMPS	10	168	TISSUE STUDY				17.50						
96	PRO-TIME	5	139	RUBELLA	10								SURGERY:				
84	PAP SMEAR	8	152	RUBELLA MUMPS	10	184	PREG. SLIDE				5						DOCTOR(S) INITIAL HERE →
121	STOOL	10	161	RUBELLA MUMPS & MEASLES	15												INSURANCE ONLY ☐
			9	CHOLERA	5		OCC. HEALTH SCREENING:						SPECIAL PROCEDURES:				MEDICARE ASSIGNMENT ☐
	CULTURE		59	YELLOW FEVER	10		AUDIO. SPIROMETRY										
			56	TINE TEST	4		VISUAL. TONOMETRY										DISCOUNT:
			22	GOLD	4		URINE								GRAND TOTAL		REASON:

Figure 14-5. Encounter Form

he is requesting a consultation, record all the pertinent information on a consultation request form (see figure 14-6), and then forward it along with the patient's record, or a copy of the record if the referral is outside the clinic, to the consulting physician. Ideally, the consultant, after examining the patient and reviewing his record, renders an opinion which he records on a consultation report. The report, along with the patient's record, is then returned to the primary physician, perhaps via the clinic's medical record department. Often, the consultation request and report are recorded on one form. The request and the report usually are filed chronologically in the progress notes. Within the clinic, it also is possible for the attending and consulting physicians to communicate with one another via only the progress notes, thus eliminating the need for additional forms. The professional courtesy involved in consultation reports is considered in Chapter 10, but often the referral process does not operate according to the established ideal. Usually, as each record is returned to the medical records department for filing, medical records personnel check it for completeness and proper order. Because physician colleagues can exchange information over the telephone or at social gatherings, consulting physicians may be slow in compiling formal reports and medical records personnel may be assigned the task of acquiring formal, written reports for inclusion in the patient's record.

Hospital Discharge Summaries. A patient's medical record also may contain reports concerning hospital admissions, including any surgery performed on the patient. Figures 14-7 and 14-8 are examples of this type of report. The hospital regularly compiles discharge summaries and surgical records for its own files, and the group physician, as attending physician, can request copies. Often the group can establish a formal relationship with a hospital, whereby copies of such reports are automatically forwarded to the group's records department or to the attending physician.

Previous Record Summaries. Due to the mobility of present day society, not every patient will maintain a lifelong association with one medical group. One individual may have several medical records established, not only in different states or perhaps countries, but also within the very same city. While the medical record does contain a patient history questionnaire, more specific information on past illnesses might prove most enlightening and helpful to the physician. The patient, therefore, should be encouraged to allow his present physician to contact his previous physician(s) and request that any other medical records the patient has established be forwarded to the present physician or to the medical records department of the clinic. These notes, usually in abstract and/or photocopy form, are then incorporated into the patient's present record and serve as a reference source for the physician in his attempt to formulate a total clinical picture of a patient.

As new physicians enter the group, arrangements must be made for incorporating patient records which the physicians may bring with them into the clinic's present system. As patients of these physicians come to the clinic, a new record may be established for them, with the older record being abstracted or photocopied and included as a previous record summary. Similar circumstances may exist as the initial group is forming. For example, some physicians

REQUEST FOR RADIOLOGICAL CONSULTATION

PATIENT'S LAST NAME–FIRST NAME–MIDDLE NAME

DATE OF REQUEST | STATION NO. | X-RAY NO.

DATE OF BIRTH | SEX M F | HT. ____ WT. ____

EXAMINATION REQUESTED:
GB, UGI, BE, IVP, SINUS, L.SPINE, C. SPINE, CHEST-PA/LAT

OTHER:

PERTINENT CLINICAL HISTORY, OPERATIONS, PHYSICAL FINDINGS, AND PROVISIONAL DIAGNOSIS

REQUESTED BY

CONSULTATION REPORT:

RADIOLOGIST ____

XYZ Clinic

8X10 ____ 14X17 ____ 7X17 ____ TOTAL ____
10X12 ____ 11X14 ____ 14X36 ____ TECHNICIAN ____

Figure 14–6. Radiological Consultation Request Form

Date Admitted: Date Discharged:

Provisional Diagnosis:

Final Diagnosis:

Operation:

Brief History And Essential Physical Findings:

Significant Laboratory, X-ray And Consultation Findings:

Course In Hospital With Complications, If Any:

Condition, Treatment, Final Disposition On Discharge And Prognosis:

Family name:	Room No.:	Hosp. No.:

Attending physician:

, M.D.

Figure 14-7. Discharge Summary

ROOM ________ CHART NO. ________

PT. ________________________ SEX ________ AGE ________ DATE ________

SURGEON ________________ ASSISTANT ________________ ANES. ________________

Op. Began ________ .m. Op. Ended ________ .m. Anes. Began ________ .m. Anes. Ended ________ .m.

Anesthesia: General ________ Spinal ________ Local ________ Agent ________ Amt. ________

Scrub Nurse ________________ Circulating Nurse ________________ Sponge Count ________

Catheters ________________ Packs ________________ Needle Count ________

Drains ________________________________ Tissue: Yes ______ No ________

Medications and Fluids ____

____

PRE-OP DIAGNOSIS ____

____

POST-OP DIAGNOSIS ____

____

OPERATION ____

____

OPERATIVE PROCEDURE:

____
SURGEON

Figure 14–8. Surgical Record

previously in solo practice may bring patient records with them to the group. The medical record system chosen by the group must be developed to accommodate what may be widely divergent record formats of the member physicians. Such records may be "redone" on demand, as indicated above, or the group may decide to reformat all extant records at the outset.

Ancillary Service Reports. In his treatment of a patient, the physician may order a variety of laboratory tests, procedures, and medications. The progress note usually will indicate the physician's plan for treatment and, therefore, will include information concerning the various tests, medications, etc. ordered. The record also may contain one or more master lists specifically designed for the recording of physician's orders. To avoid unnecessary duplications, all tests, procedures, and medications ordered by the physician can be noted briefly on this form, along with the date of the patient's visit. The encounter form or record of charges also may serve as an order sheet and record of work in progress.

Often, a multicopy form is used to order various laboratory tests and procedures. One copy of this form is the actual order form indicating to ancillary personnel what tests or procedures should be carried out. Another copy may be used by the billing department, and a third copy, after serving as a report to the physician, may be included in the patient's medical record. In order that any physician treating a patient can ascertain the results of laboratory work completed for the patient, all laboratory reports can be accumulated in a specific place within the medical record. They may be attached in shingle fashion to a backing sheet (see figure 14–9) or, if the clinic is anticipating the future microfilming of records, they may be attached to a backing sheet so that each individual report is visible. Combination requisition-report forms also may be used for procedures involving physical therapy, pathology, cytology, radiology, EKG, and nuclear medicine (see figure 14–10). Often, the medical record will contain a form specifically designed for the recording of immunizations. This type of information is especially important in pediatric records.

As the group develops the medical records system, it must consider the effective interfacing of medical records with ancillary services. Not only must procedures be established for ordering tests and procedures and avoiding duplication, but responsibility must be assigned for filing test and procedure reports in the record and for calling attention to abnormal results. The patient's record may be returned to the records department before ordered tests are completed. In this case, records personnel may be responsible for filing reports in the record. As results reach the record room, the master list indicating work in progress will be helpful in determining if ordered tests and procedures are in fact being completed. If test reports have not been sent to the ordering physician, records personnel may be responsible for informing the physician of abnormal results. It also is possible for the physician's nurse not to return the patient's record to the records department until all reports have been received. The nurse may screen results, file the reports in the record, and send the record back to the records room. While bulky EKG and EEG tapes and X-rays may be kept on file in their respective departments, the reading reports of these procedures will be included in the patient's record. Again, the group must develop clearly defined operating procedures for the filing of such reports.

Family Name	First Name	Attending Physician	Room No.	Hosp. No.

NAME Room No. Hosp. No.

Physician

Test Required

Technician Director of Laboratories

Date

MISCELLANEOUS

CHEMISTRY

URINALYSIS

BACTERIOLOGY

SEROLOGY

GLUCOSE TOLERANCE

HEMATOLOGY

Figure 14–9. Laboratory Reports

No. ______________________

Date ______________________

NAME ____ Age ______________________

ADDRESS ____

Referring Physician ____

Examination of ____

____

History ____

____

____

Report of Examination Date ______________________

______________________ Roentgenologist

Figure 14–10. X-Ray Requisition

Date ______________________

To ____

____

I hereby authorize you to release to ______________________

____

____

any information including the diagnosis and records of any treatment or examination

rendered to me during the period from ____________ to ____________

____________ Signature ____________

____________ Witness ____________ ______________________

Figure 14–11. Record Release Form

Correspondence and Administrative Information. A patient's medical record may contain various items of correspondence which are related only peripherally to the actual record. This material may be kept together at the back of the record or may be placed in a separate envelope within the record. Other administrative items often found within the medical record include a chart status form which indicates what physicians and departments have been in possession of the record in the past and, therefore, who might be held accountable for any missing information. In addition, a record release form (see figure 14–11) is placed in the record to facilitate release procedures when necessary. The record also may contain a plastic patient identification card which usually is embossed at the time of patient registration (see Chapter 12). The patient card may be kept in a specially designed pocket on the inside of the back of the chart and is usually used to imprint clinic forms with the patient's full name and chart number. Patient date of birth and address are sometimes included on the card.

The Medical Record Jacket. The chart jacket itself should be durable and designed as a functional aspect of the total system. Specifications to consider include:

Size: The most versatile folder size measures nine to nine and one-half inches by eleven and one-quarter to eleven and three-quarters inches, excluding tabs.

Tabs: The type of records storage and the filing system employed by the group will dictate the design of folder tabs. If filing cabinets are used, tabs can be straight across the top of the folder in full, one-half, or one-fifth cut. If folders are being filed in open shelves, tabs usually are cut vertically along the side, but the folder may have a horizontal, straight-across tab as well. Tabs are used most often for the recording of patient filing number and other patient identification data, and generally it is practical to have tabs double strength reinforced.

Style of Folders and Fasteners: Chart covers may be designed as large envelopes, but most are of the open-book variety and include some type of fastener at one or more positions within the folder. Fastener clasps of various sizes can be attached at the inside top of the front and back covers. If the folder is scored or bellowed along the crease line, a fastener can be attached to or embedded in the folder parallel to the crease and on the inside back cover. Folders may be designed with pockets attached on the inside covers. Such pockets usually are intended to hold plastic or metal identification cards. It also is possible to place items loosely into the folder. Papers may be stapled or clipped together but not actually attached to the folder. For maintaining organization within the folder, however, the use of one or more fasteners is most practical.

Folder Weight and Durability: The weight of a folder is measured in point stock. One point equals 1/1000 of an inch. Folders are available from eight to fourteen points; ten to eleven point thickness is usual for medical record use. Folders may be made of bleached or unbleached material. Initially, bleached folders may be more attractive; however, unbleached folders will not show finger prints and are stronger because chemicals have not weakened the paper. Another alternative involves the use of plastic vinyl folders which, while expensive to acquire, will not become worn over time and will not require frequent replacement.

Printing on the Folder: Some chart folders may be purchased with filing system numbers preprinted (and color coded) onto the folder's tabs. Space also may be designated on the outside of the folder for patient identification data such as patient name, address, responsible party designation, electronic data processing number, and allergy and drug sensitivity warnings. Some folders have the complete patient registration form printed on the inside front cover. The folder also can display a simple activity gauge consisting of a printed column of years. At the time of the patient's first visit of the year, the appropriate year is checked. This system facilitates pulling inactive records and segregating them from active charts. In addition, chart status forms and master lists for immunizations and prescriptions may be printed directly on the chart. The record cover also may display a brief explanation of the filing or color coding system in use so that medical record personnel have a convenient reference source.[2]

Medical Record Order or Sequence

Components of the traditional medical record may be integrated or may be arranged sectionally. Components of the integrated record such as progress notes, laboratory reports, etc., are arranged chronologically, thus allowing the record to reflect the medical history of the patient. Often, however, this method of sequencing the information can be overly time-consuming for the physician who simply wants to know what laboratory tests have been performed recently for a particular patient. Scattering information throughout the record also can result in communication breakdown. For this reason, a sectional arrangement of the various record components may be preferable. Depending upon the type of chart cover used, record components may be arranged in a variety of ways. If the patient registration form is not actually imprinted upon the chart itself, it should be contained at the very front within the chart and should be followed by the patient health history. If a standard file folder is being used, the registration and history may be attached to the inside front cover. The next component of the record usually is the progress notes, which are kept as a unit in reverse chronological order. They may be attached to the folder with a metal fastener or may be held together as a unit but not actually attached to the file. Laboratory reports and radiology, pathology, etc. reports usually follow the progress notes, with hospital discharge summaries toward the back of the record. Correspondence can be kept at the very back of the record along with various administrative items such as release forms and chart status forms. To further differentiate the various components of the medical record, each type of form may be printed on a different color of paper or, if all material is attached to the folder, tabbed chart dividers may be used.

The Problem-Oriented Medical Record

The problem-oriented medical record (POMR) was developed in response to a need for increased usability of the medical record for the patient, and clinic, in terms of internal auditing, PSRO, and accreditation. The problem-oriented medical record differs in format and in sequencing of components from the traditional or source-oriented medical record (SOMR). Proponents of the POMR contend that it reflects more of the physician's decision-making process and that it more readily facilitates the *systematic* displaying and retrieval of medical data. Information within a source-oriented record usually is filed according to the source from which it came—i.e., laboratory, hospital, attending physician, consulting physician, etc. In a POMR, patient *problems* are the basis for the organization of information. This basic conceptual difference is reflected in the fact that a part of POMR is a table of contents referred to as a problem list (see figure 14-12). Abnormal data are recorded on the POMR problem list and become an organizing principle of the record.[3] Similar to the page numbers in a table of contents, the dates of problem onset and resolution act as reference points. Components of the POMR include the *data base*, the *master problem list*, the *initial plans*, and the *progress notes.* The data base is similar to SOMR health history and also may include the results of a complete multiphasic screening of the patient. Ideally, the patient's numbered problem list should include *all* problems—active as well as inactive or resolved.

Patient problems usually fall into one of four categories: a diagnosis, a physiological finding, a symptom related by the patient, or an abnormal laboratory finding. As problems become clarified, their status on the problem list can be modified. Each problem on the list should have a correspondingly numbered initial plan for the collection of further data and/or for treatment of the problem. Progress notes for each problem also should be correspondingly numbered. Each progress note usually contains subjective data provided by the patient, objective data and interpretation made by the physician, and an indication of immediate follow-up plans. Various tests and procedural reports can be filed within the record and the results can be indicated on flow charts. Recording physiologic variables and drug dosages on a single sheet may help the physician recognize important trends in the patient's health. The various components of the POMR usually are arranged in the order in which they are discussed here. Similar to the traditional SOMR, various colors of forms or chart dividers may be used to distinguish the different sections of the record, and considerations for basic file folder specifications remain the same as for the more traditional record.

Although the POMR offers many advantages in terms of structuring the medical record and facilitating audit procedures, it is possible that the POMR format may encourage a fragmented response to *individual problems* rather than an integrated approach to the patient's *total* health situation. It also is possible that confusion may arise when various users of the chart renumber problems and cross reference data applicable to more than one problem.[4] As group

Problem	Onset	Active Problem	Inactive Problem	Resolved Problem	Date

Figure 14–12. Master Problem List

planners approach the development of a medical records system it is important for them to remember that variables such as format of the record, sequencing of record components, style of forms, and the type of record jacket cannot be considered in isolation. A decision concerning one aspect of the record has direct impact on subsequent decisions. It is equally important that all group members accept and are willing to work with the record format chosen. The group, therefore, should investigate thoroughly all available options before reaching any final decisions.

Centralized versus Decentralized Filing

As indicated previously, information contained in the medical record may be integrated or may be arranged sectionally. Progress notes for all specialties may be kept chronologically as a unit, or for certain specialties, such as dermatology, notes may be kept as a separate unit in the patient's file. In a multispecialty group, it also is possible to maintain completely separate medical records for each patient within each specialty. Such decentralization and compartmentalization of information, however, does not facilitate continuity in the care of the patient and is really contrary to some of the motivation behind *group* practice. Interrelationships between medical problems and symptoms may go unrecognized, various tests and procedures may be unnecessarily duplicated, and prescribed medications may conflict dangerously. Some multispecialty groups decentralize only a portion of their medical records, such as dermatology, radiology, and orthopedics. Centralized storage of medical records seems to be a logical extension of the POMR concept. Filing records in one location aids in quality control, in standardization of procedures, and in auditing. In addition, if a group is considering a central dictating unit, centralized medical record storage can facilitate the process of transcription.

If the group is considering interfacing its medical record activity with that of the hospital, forms and procedures control will be difficult unless a centralized medical record system is employed. A combined hospital/medical group record represents a great step toward the ultimate goals of record standardization, completeness, and continuity. The Uniform Medical Record System of Boone County Hospital in Iowa is an excellent example of the *unit record* rationale. The philosophy of this program is recounted here in part.

> We believe each patient should have a single medical document that accompanies him through life. It should deal precisely with all his medical problems and care rendered, be it via hospital or outpatient care, and should be the major vehicle of communication among all members of the health care team.
>
> The main purpose of the Uniform Medical Record System is to facilitate communication, understanding, and interpretability between physicians, nurses, and other allied medical personnel in terms of what the patient's problems have been and are through greater precision in medical record documentation.
>
> It is our belief that "the medical record determines the nature of medicine itself" and should make explicit the reasoning behind diagnostic and therapeutic activities undertaken on behalf of the patient. The medical record should be the central vehicle for a rigorous systemization of medical care planning and delivery. We believe good records = good communication = continuity of care.[5]

When attempting to establish a unit record relationship between group and hospital, crucial decisions concerning the system include:

1. *Format of the Record.* The Boone County program uses a problem-oriented framework. The group and the hospital may prefer a more traditional or source-oriented format. The important point is consistency; if all organizations involved do not use the same record format, the unit record system will not be operable.

2. *Forms.* After the group and the hospital have decided upon a mutually agreeable record format, it should not be difficult to select or to design the various forms necessary for recording medical data. If the institutions involved do not use the same forms in similar ways, communication will become ineffective and the purpose of the unit record will be undermined.

3. *Transportation.* It must be decided if both the hospital and the group will maintain a copy of each record, or if only one institution will maintain the record. If the latter alternative is chosen, it must be decided which organization will keep the record and how it will be transported to the other organization. If the former alternative is chosen, differences between hospital and group filing methods must be accommodated. For example, if both hospital and group are using a form of terminal digit filing, but the hospital is assigning patient numbers serially and the group is using social security numbers, the patient will have a dual identity in terms of his assigned numbers. When hospital and group communicate concerning a patient's file, the patient's number will not necessarily be enough to identify him. It may be that both hospital and group will have to maintain a cross-file geared toward each other's numbering systems.

Procedures for the exchange of information between group and hospital also must be coordinated. Often, groups that do not use a unit record system will receive very fragmented information from the hospital. Consequently, laboratory tests and physical exams may be repeated unnecessarily. Formal procedures for the exchanging of medical data between hospital and group must be established. Photocopies, carbon copies, and multicopy forms are possibilities. Long-distance telecopiers are yet another alternative. It may be wise for the group and the hospital to develop a check list of potential missing material which can be used by both institutions to assess their own records as well as to inform the other institution that it has been late in forwarding data. In addition, a combined, hospital/group dictating system can facilitate the inclusion of all progress notes, emergency care notes, post-operative reports, and discharge summaries in the patient's record.

Filing Systems

Medical records, whether centralized or decentralized, may be filed in alphabetical sequence according to patient name, or in numerical sequence according to the patient identification number usually assigned at the time of registration. A third filing system, soundex, is phonetically based and includes numerals as well as color coding. *Alphabetical filing* simply involves filing records according to the spelling of the patient's last name, first name, and middle initial. The basic advantages of filing alphabetically are that the system is simple and easily understood and that a cross index is not required to locate a record. The misfiling of records, however, is a continual problem, and it is crucial for locating a record that records personnel have the patient's full name correctly spelled. As the group practice grows, there may be, for example, more than one John R. Jones represented in the file. In such instances, additional information is necessary to locate the specific record requested. In resolving this type of difficulty, many existing groups include other short indicators on the medical record folder such as date of birth or father's first name. When using alpha filing, a projection of record growth is necessary to determine how much space to allocate for medical record storage. Such growth will occur somewhat randomly within the boundaries of the alphabet.

Numeric filing includes straight numerical, middle digit, and terminal digit alternatives. *Straight numerical* filing is a method by which consecutively-numbered medical records are placed in the file in exact sequential order. Straight numerical filing is relatively simple—any individual who can count can easily learn and operate the system. Disadvantages of the system include the following:

1. If only the patient's name has been given to record room personnel, when retrieving records, a cross-index is needed to ascertain the record number. In the case of more than one John R. Jones, the charts will not be next to one another in the file, and the cross-index must include differentiating information, such as date of birth.

2. Straight numeric filing represents a time chronology; the most recent records are at the end of the file and, because these records usually are the most active, the work of records personnel will be more concentrated in this newer section of the file.

3. Errors due to the transposition of digits is a common occurrence. When retrieving files, this difficulty can be alleviated by verifying patient name according to the record requisition slip before forwarding the record to the requestor.

In *middle digit* filing, consecutively assigned six-digit record numbers are divided into three groups of two digits each, with the middle group of digits representing the primary filing digits. For example, in the record number 123456, the middle digits 34 are the primary filing digits, 12 are the secondary digits, and 56 are the tertiary digits. The record bearing number 12–34–56 would be filed as number 56 behind file guide 12–34 (in section 12 of section 34 of the file). Middle digit filing has not been widely used by traditional group practices, yet compared to straight numerical filing, middle digit filing does offer more practical distribution of active and inactive records throughout the file. It allows for the placement of no more than 100 consecutively numbered records together in any one section (12–34–00 through 12–34–99). Thus, personnel can be assigned to specific file sections and if misfiling does occur, the record remains in a 100-block section, in this case section 12–34. Middle digit filing works most effectively with numbers not exceeding six digits. For example, when seven digits are used (1234567), the secondary group of digits expands from two to three (123–45–67) and a sequence of 1,000 file guides (000–45 to 999–45) becomes necessary. From six to eight times more space is required for a 1,000-division section than for a 100-division section. This problem may be overcome by performing an additional sorting operation or by employing terminal digit filing.

In *terminal digit* filing, consecutively issued six digit record numbers are

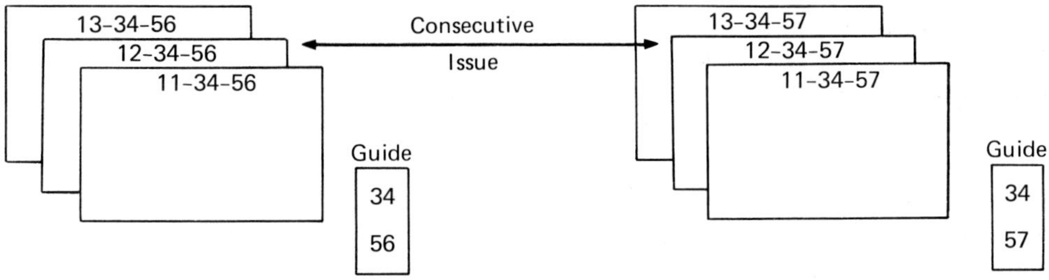

Figure 14-13. Example of Terminal Digit Filing

divided into three groups of two digits each and filed first by the last two (terminal) digits. Essentially, the terminal digit filing method effects a near perfect distribution of the most recent records among other records in the file. For example, record 12-34-56 would be filed first by the terminal digits (56), next by the secondary or middle digits (34) and finally by the first two digits (12). Under a terminal digit filing arrangement, two consecutively issued medical records numbered 12-34-56 and 12-34-57 would be filed as shown in figure 14-13.

Although the record numbers were issued consecutively, there would be 100 file guides (34-56 to 34-57) and 10,000 records or spaces between the records numbered 12-34-56 and 12-34-57. Obviously, since all groups will not be able to accommodate such extensive filing space, it is possible to use file guides which have the secondary digits broken down into multiples of ten (00-56, 10-56, 20-56, etc.). The advantages of terminal digit filing are that the distribution of records in the file eliminates personnel concentration in an area of most active (recent) files, and that personnel responsibility can be assigned to specific file sections. In addition, the number of digits in the record number is of little or no consequence. For example, the seven-digit number 1234567 would be broken down as 123-45-67. The primary and secondary groups of digits remain at two. Thus, guide indexing is unchanged and a 100-division sorter may still be used (00-67 to 99-67). Terminal digit filing is, therefore, amenable to a nonclinic generated number such as social security number, telephone number, etc. One of the disadvantages of terminal digit filing is the difficulty in converting existing records to a terminal digit system. Also, misfiling within a range of 100 to 10,000 records is possible.

Soundex filing combines alpha and numeric filing through the use of color coding. By applying a number and color to phonetically based alphabetical groupings, a patient name can be assigned a serial filing number and corresponding color pattern. The phonetic basis of the number/color pattern is illustrated in the following example:

Color	*Number*	*Alpha Groupings*[a]
Red	1	BFPV
Orange	2	C, G, J, K, Q, S, X, Z
Yellow	3	DT
Green	4	L
Blue	5	MN
White	6	R

[a]Note that vowels (A,E,I,O,U) and W,H,Y are omitted and represented by an O.

For the name John R. Jones the numerical designation would be 252 (JNS in Jones)-2 (1st initial, 1st name)-6 (middle initial). The color coding would be orange, blue, orange, orange, white. Ideally, a record can be retrieved via name or patient number. Essentially, the soundex method allows for the alphabetical retrieval and numerical/color refiling of medical charts. The main advantage of the soundex method is its flexibility of design, but its major disadvantage is complexity.

Some groups oriented toward family medical practice find it beneficial to have a complete *family* record available as a unit. When an alphabetical or phonetically based filing method is used, it is possible either to accumulate the medical records of all family members into *one folder* filed according to the responsible party designation or to file a *series of separate folders* for family members under the rubric of the responsible party. When using straight numerical, terminal digit, or middle digit filing, the family may be issued one number and all records may be kept in one folder. Alternatively, if the records are kept as a series of folders on the shelf, each family member may be issued a different numerical suffix for filing purposes. Existing groups have found that one folder for an entire family can become unwieldy and can prove dysfunctional when two members of the same family must be seen at the same time or within a short span of time. Maintaining a series of family folders differentiated only by a suffix to the family record number also poses difficulties as children are married or establish separate households. When using a straight numerical system, however, it is sometimes possible to issue consecutive numbers to family members, and when using an alpha system it is feasible to subalphabetize family members according to first and/or middle name.

Color Coding

As indicated above, filing may be further systematized by the addition of color coding, which increases speed and filing accuracy and also reduces time required to locate misfiles. File folders may be color coded in various ways. The complete folder may be of a certain color; the folder tabs may be printed in various colors; or colored tape may be applied to the folder tabs. Color coding an alphabetical filing system may simply involve establishing, at the most, twenty-six (less for groupings of letters) color combinations which can be imprinted on file tabs or taped onto tabs. A straight numerical system may be color coded in various ways. For example, in a 10,000 folder file, folders may be divided into ten distinct groups of 1,000 by coding each folder with a solid bar of one of ten colors across the top (drawer file) or down the side (shelf file). A simple system such as this reduces possible misfile to 10 percent of the total file. A middle digit or terminal digit system may be coded by relating color to the primary group of filing digits, either to the left-hand digit or to both digits of the primary group. Folders already imprinted with color and numerals may be purchased as a complete system along with corresponding file guides. It also is possible to apply colored tape to the folder. Often, this alternative is chosen to code the right-hand digit of the primary group of filing digits, whether middle or terminal. The potential of color coding for a medical records filing system is vast. It is possible for a forming group to design a filing system complete with color coding tailor-made to the group's specific needs. Companies specializing in filing systems can be helpful to medical groups in determining system parameters. Of course, group members should remain aware that commercial consultants naturally will attempt to sell their own products. It may be wise, therefore, to arrange presentations from several such companies before reaching any decisions.

Records Storage

Systems decisions related to the design of the record jacket, the degree of centralization/decentralization, the filing method, and the degree of color coding used heavily influence methods of records storage. There are two basic types of records storage—standard file cabinets or open shelves. Variations of these two methods include rotary mechanical or electrically operated tub files (capable of holding approximately 15,000 files each) and circular, Lazy Susan type open shelf files.

For forming groups, the storing of records in file cabinets has been the most common approach because of readily accessible equipment and the limited amount of patient records. As a practice grows, however, the number and thickness of the medical records also increase, and efficient storage becomes a primary consideration. The planning of storage space can influence to a great degree the design of the facility. For example, the potential weight of thousands of medical records will influence the location of the records department within the facility as well as affect the construction of the file room floor, especially if the department is located above ground level. In addition, two file cabinets totaling four linear feet in width accommodate the same number of charts as an open shelf file which requires only three linear feet of space, and, if the group decides to color code charts for ease in retrieval and filing, open shelves will prove more amenable to the coding system.

Accessibility and working space are additional planning considerations for the medical records department. For example, a file cabinet with the top drawer opened and filled with records can become unsteady and will be awkward for some personnel to handle. The continuous noise of opening and closing file drawers and the difficulty of more than one person at a time using the same cabinet are design problems that may interfere with the operation of an efficient system. The open shelf file system, however, eliminates many of these disadvantages and does not create additional cost burden. This method also is more flexible in its arrangement potential, and can help in maximizing the available space. Aisle space or work area between the files should generally measure between thirty and thirty-six inches in width. Using valuable space for aisles, however, lessens the amount of footage available for filing area. Some existing clinics place files, whether open shelves or cabinets, on tracks or rollers so that the files are arranged back to back with no intervening aisle space. As files are needed, the appropriate shelves or cabinets can be moved so that an aisle is created. This type of system is rather costly and does not readily lend itself to rearrangement and the accessing of several files at the same time. Record growth projections and determining space required per file are discussed more fully in Chapter 26.

Chart Requisition Process

The requisition process associated with the retrieval of the patient's medical record is vital to the effective delivery of health care services in any setting.

There are two overriding concerns in the implementation of such a process—the logistics of locating and moving the records and the assignment of recipient priority. Chart requests generally are initiated at the appointment desk as a result of information recorded in the daily logs. Most groups have established a protocol for alerting the medical records department a day or so in advance of the patient's arrival. Additional guidelines must be determined for securing the records of "add-on" patients who arrive unannounced and sometimes require emergency treatment, or those who call on a given day requesting an appointment for that day. Under these circumstances, and depending upon the means for transporting the records, it may be necessary to hand-carry the record or to deviate in some way from the usual procedure. It is especially important that priorities concerning the individuals requesting the record, the time the record is needed, and the reason it is needed are clearly stated and understood by all personnel in the practice. Obviously, top priority is given to the attending physician at the time of the patient's visit. "Add-on" chart requisitions should indicate the purpose for which the chart is needed, the name and position of the person requesting it—physician, nurse, secretary, etc.—and the time at which the chart must be available (see figures 14-14 and 14-15). Special care should be taken to make sure that the patient's *full* name, including first name and middle initial, is properly spelled and recorded. For daily, routine chart requests, this responsibility generally is assumed by the appointment personnel; for "add-ons," the responsibility is assumed by the individual making the special request.

Cross-Index. If the medical records are filed alphabetically, the record can be pulled from the file as soon as the patient's full name is known. As medical record holdings increase in size and complexity, other methods of filing, such as phonetic and numerical indexing, may be used. The use of other types of filing systems necessitates creating a cross-index which references the numbers and possibly sounds assigned to each name. There are various ways to establish such indexes, depending upon the amount of information recorded and the efficiency requirements of the system. Some indexes are made up of ordinary filing cards which can be any of a number of sizes depending upon how information is stored on each card. When demographic and billing information is recorded on the card, constant updating is necessary to maintain accuracy. Some clinics deliberately use small plastic cards or visual strip indexes to restrict the amount of data contained on each element and to decrease the amount of time necessary to retrieve essential patient information. Plastic identification cards embossed with the patient's name and record number can effectively eliminate errors in transposition. They can be used to imprint patient information on all documents and forms required during each patient visit, such as encounter forms, lab reports, and charge slips. If the record itself does not already contain a card, the file card may be attached to the chart and can be routed along with the record to each department serving the patient. If the clinic uses a computer and has established an accounting file of keypunched cards, a duplicate of each punched card, interpreted with printing, can be used for cross-indexing by the medical records department. Any type of card can be stored in an automated card index. Such systems do

WRITE FIRMLY

Name ______________________________

Appt. Date ______________ Time ________ Chart No. ____________

For Dr. ______________ Area ______________ ☐ MED CENTER ☐ WEST ☐ POST OAK ☐ DOWNTOWN

☐ NEW PATIENT ______________________________
ADDRESS PHONE

Date of Birth ______________

☐ APPOINTMENT
☐ INJECTION
☐ PHONE CALL
☐ HOSPITAL ADMISSION
☐ OTHER ______________

TYPE OF EXAM. ______________
BILL TO: ______________
SPEC. INSTRUCTIONS ______________

☐ SEE REVERSE SIDE
MEDICAL RECORDS USE ONLY

Requested by ______________ Date ______________

REVERSE SIDE

TO ______________ AREA ______________

WE ARE UNABLE TO SEND THE REQUESTED RECORD

☐ OUT TO ______________ DATE ______________

☐ AT POST OAK AND WILL BE REQUESTED ON NEXT TRIP.

☐ IN REMOTE STORAGE. WILL BE SENT TO YOU ON

____

☐ NO RECORD. SUPPLY ADDITIONAL INFORMATION.

THANK YOU.
MEDICAL RECORD DEPARTMENT

BY ______________ DATE ______________

Figure 14–14. Requisition for Medical Record

have the disadvantage, however, of permitting only one person to retrieve cards at one time. Patient information for cross-indexing also can be stored on microfilm or microfiche with readers not only in the medical records department but also at various stations throughout the clinic. This type of file is often generated by computers and can be easily updated on a routine schedule.

If a change in the system of filing the medical records is being implemented, records should be converted to the new system before they are sent to the various clinic departments. Thus, although two systems are extant in the med-

CLINIC NO. ______ BIRTH DATE ______

NAME ______
(PRINT) LAST FIRST MID. INITIAL

FLOOR [2] [3] [4] [5] [6] [7] [8]

REQUESTED BY ______

DATE OF APPOINTMENT ______

TIME OF APPOINTMENT ______

CHECKED OUT TO ______ DATE ______

MEMO ______

RECEPTION DESK COPY

RECORD ROOM COPY

RETURN RECORD WITH THIS SLIP ATTACHED TO INSURE THAT THE RECORD GETS TO ITS DESTINATION.

Figure 14–15. Multi-Copy Appointment Record Request

ical records department itself, only records filed according to the newer system are routed throughout the clinic. Clinic personnel, therefore, are not exposed to the confusion of two different filing systems.

Chart Routing. Any medical record routing system can be only as efficient as the physicians in the group allow it to be. The records department cannot prevent physicians from putting records in their desks or from carrying them home in a brief case. Records personnel can, however, keep accurate records of the routing of all records and the group can establish policy which allows medical records personnel to search offices and departments for needed and missing records. Many medical record departments have found that maintaining accountability can be significantly improved by using multi-copy requisition/routing slips (see figure 14–15). One slip is attached to the record and indicates the departments requesting the record, the date of the order and the time for receiving it. Another copy is filed in the record room. Routing information also may be recorded on cardboard out guides which can be inserted in place of the

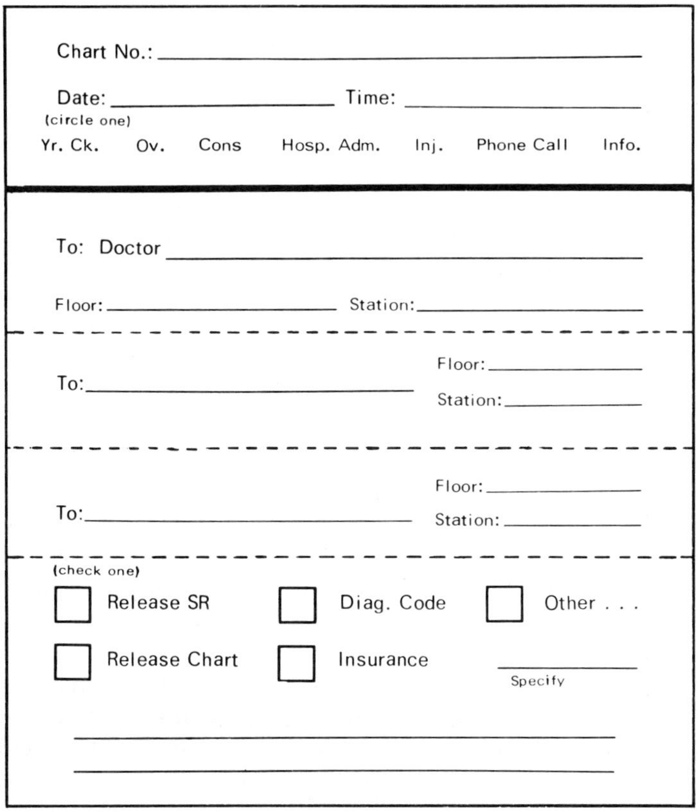

Chart No.: ______

Date: ______ Time: ______

(circle one)

Yr. Ck. Ov. Cons Hosp. Adm. Inj. Phone Call Info.

To: Doctor ______

Floor: ______ Station: ______

To: ______ Floor: ______ Station: ______

To: ______ Floor: ______ Station: ______

(check one)

☐ Release SR ☐ Diag. Code ☐ Other . . .

☐ Release Chart ☐ Insurance ______ Specify

Figure 14-16. Chart Routing Form

records as they are removed. Often, out guides are made of plastic and have a pocket for a copy of the requisition/routing slip. When a single copy routing slip is used (see figure 14-16), a record of the routing can be maintained in a log in the medical records room. To further maintain accountability, each nursing station can keep a log noting the date and time each record is received and when it is either sent to the department indicated next on the routing slip or returned to the medical records department.

Chart Transportation. Once the medical record has been located, pulled, and processed for routing, how it is to be transported to its various destinations within the clinic must be decided. Some groups have the patient carry his own record as he visits each department with which he has an appointment. This method supposedly guarantees that the record will be at the right place at the right time. Other groups may rely on personnel to hand-carry the record. Especially in larger facilities, this latter method represents an inefficient use of personnel time and, on a cost basis, it may be more feasible for the group to invest in an automated transport system. Vertical transport systems generally are cheaper than those used for horizontal transport of materials. Vertical gravity chutes and simple box lift conveyors can be used to transport records to and from upper floors. This arrangement facilitates the more effective space allocation of record storage areas in subground levels, thus freeing ground and upper level floor space for offices and laboratories. The cost of lateral movement of materials is based upon the length of the routes, the size requirements of material to be transported, and the number of turns or bends in the channels. Pneumatic tube installations for both vertical and horizontal transport can be very expensive, particularly if the system is installed after the facility has been built. Other types of motorized conveyors may be less costly and more practical, depending upon the configuration of the facility and the requirements for the system. Protection against loss because of jam-ups as well as protection against violation of confidentiality are additional considerations associated with mechanized transport.

Refiling Records. Medical record departments should establish policies which govern the return of the record and its prompt refiling. Some departments require that at the close of the day *all* records be returned to the record department where each is checked for proper order and missing material. Records personnel also may forward billing information to the business office at this time. In addition, information received from hospitals must be included in the patient's medical record. Medical records personnel should examine carefully each piece of information and, operating under very specific guidelines, can be authorized to dispose of duplicate copies which only serve to clutter the record folder.

If there is an indication that laboratory or X-ray work may be in progress, the record is held in a specific area of the department until the information resulting from that work is received. This material should be checked to determine if there are any abnormal test results which must be immediately reported to the attending physician. Specific individuals should be responsible for carrying out each function—checking the sequencing of content, ascertaining if work in progress is completed, flagging abnormal test results, and refiling the record. Some groups will have established procedures whereby all records are held at the various nursing stations until work in progress reports are received and the physician has seen the results. The record is then sent back to the medical records department where personnel check for missing material and put the record in order before refiling. When using this system, records personnel are not responsible for flagging abnormals because test reports are sent directly to the physicians. One disadvantage of this arrangement is that conflicts and confusion may arise when records are not centrally available to be routed to other clinic areas and are delayed at one point or another because test results have not been returned. Using the medical record department as a "clearing house" does result in more efficient movement of the medical record throughout the clinic. Records personnel, however, have the additional responsibility of flagging abnormals, and the importance of this task necessitates their adhering to specific operating policies and procedures.

RECORD MAINTENANCE AND RELEASE POLICIES

When developing a medical records system, it should be remembered that there exist various legal statutes concerning the maintenance and release of medical information. Every state requires that hospitals and other health care institutions initiate and maintain medical records; however, the language and scope of such statutes may vary from state to state. Although the value of medical records is such that they no doubt would be kept regardless of any legislation, maintenance laws help to safeguard the legitimate interests of everyone involved with a record—patient, physician, nurse, hospital, insurance company, etc. The advent of government sponsored Professional Standards Review Organizations (PSROs) further underscores the importance of maintaining the security and reliability of medical records. In addition, the United States Department of Health, Education and Welfare will be playing an ever-increasing role in establishing standards for the maintenance of standardized medical records.

In addition to governmental statutes and influences in the maintenance of medical records, various professional organizations associated with the practice of medicine have developed guidelines for medical records. The clinic accreditation program of the American Group Practice Association (AGPA) considers the medical record to be the single most important measure of the quality of care provided by a clinic, and has explicit requirements in the area of medical records maintenance which encompass the areas of patient identification, clinical notes, diagnostic coding, health history, and clinic/hospital record interface. Information in the record must be sufficient to support the diagnosis and to justify any treatment rendered. In addition, the attending physicians must be readily identifiable. The AGPA also strongly encourages clinics to establish a medical record committee or to use their peer review committee to monitor records standards. If a group is considering a unit record arrangement with a hospital, hospital record requirements, as outlined by the Joint Commission on the Accreditation of Hospitals, will be of major importance.

The Retention of Medical Records

One of the greatest concerns of any group practice in relation to patient records is the appropriate length of time to retain a medical record. While the most important reason for *maintaining* a medical record is to ensure continuity and quality in medical care, the most important reasons for *retaining* a medical record are to provide an accurate basis for testimony in a malpractice suit and accurate data for retrospective studies of specific diseases or procedures. In some states, retention of the record is governed by law which may encompass any or all of the following: civil law, state statutes, public health agencies, state boards of medical examiners, or a professional practice insurance carrier. A group practice must decide upon active versus inactive criteria and storage methods commensurate with the goals of the practice.

Record Activity and Storage. Some groups, such as university-based practices, may be willing to invest in easily accessible long-term storage in order to provide data for graduate studies. Most groups, however, probably will decide upon a period of active retention which spans at least the seven years from the date of last treatment for adult records, and for the records of minors, one year after the eighteenth birthday. In a number of states, courts have ruled that the one-year statute of limitations on a malpractice action does not begin until the patient discovers the injury resulting from the physician's alleged wrongful act. In addition, the death of a patient does not signal the end of the active status of his medical record. On the contrary, the time involved in estate settlement may result in the record's remaining active for as long as five years and sometimes even longer. In view of all of these circumstances, records really should never be totally destroyed, but rather placed indefinitely in some type of inactive storage.

The nature of record inactivity will be influenced by whether the group operates primarily under a prepaid or under a fee-for-service mode and also will be dependent upon the characteristics of the patient population—numbers of indigent, children, elderly, etc. Many providers have a rule of thumb for determining the active status of a particular record. This rule generally is based upon the length of time since the patient's last visit. The group could decide that the records department would purge the active file of the records of all patients who have not returned to the clinic in the past five years. These so-called inactive records then could be either microfilmed or stored in economical warehouse storage. Records felt to be least inactive might be stored on-site, while records determined to be most inactive may be stored at a remote site. The criteria for deciding the method of storage could be cost based on the average number of records pulled. When records are microfilmed, the material usually is reduced to its essential elements and photographed. All duplication, insurance forms, and old normal X-rays are culled. Lab slips are summarized and hospital records may be destroyed on the theory that they are available from the hospital. While microfilming is a fairly expensive process, it does facilitate ready access to the information. Before investing large amounts of time and money on microfilming, however, the group would be wise to ascertain state statutes regarding the admissibility of microfilmed records as evidence in legal actions. If microfilm does not constitute legal evidence, records must be maintained in their original form. Computer storage of inactive records is also a possibility; however, decisions must be made concerning the amount, type, and form of the information to be stored.

Purging the Files. When the basis for retiring and retaining the records has been decided upon, the actual logistics of purging the file may be planned. If the records have been assigned numbers, and filed serially, the date a particular number was assigned can be determined and all the records prior to that number/date can be examined for level of activity. If alphabetical, phonetic, or middle/terminal digit filing has been used, however, inactive records will be scattered throughout the files. As the files are purged, out guides indicating the status and location of the record can be placed in the vacant slots.

Confidentiality of Medical Records

Because the relationship and communication between physician and patient is privileged, the record of that relationship is confidential. The physicians' code of ethics, licensing laws, and various confidential communication statutes protect against the disclosure of the contents of medical records to persons or agencies who are not properly authorized to receive such information. Only when a patient consents to the release of medical information concerning him does he waive the protection afforded him by law. It is important to note that the scope and uniformity of confidential communication statutes vary from state to state. For example, protection may be limited to only that information acquired professionally. In some states, the confidential privilege applies in civil law actions only; in other states, criminal action is included. Some statutes protect only that information recorded by a licensed physician. Other statutes extend the protection to information acquired by other health professionals, including the physician's assistant, the nurse, X-ray and laboratory technicians, and sometimes even the pharmacist. In establishing medical record policy, therefore, it is important that the group thoroughly understand the laws of its state in regard to record privilege.

In order to release the contents of a patient's medical record to a third party, the patient must first authorize the disclosure via a signed, dated release form (see figure 14-11). In the case of minors, a parent, guardian, or legal representative must authorize the release. If the record is of a deceased individual, the executor of the estate usually must authorize the release. Individuals and organizations requesting medical record information include patients' attorneys, various governmental agencies, health departments, law enforcement agencies, and insurers. Unless otherwise indicated by law, a patient's medical record cannot be given to these individuals without prior consent of the patient.

Medical Records in Court. A medical record may be required as evidence in a civil or criminal action. In such cases, the record department will be served a *subpoena duces tecum* which requires the presence of a specific record and a witness in court on a certain date. In some states, it is possible for the medical records custodian simply to certify the record and not actually be present in court with the record. In preparing the record for court, all extraneous information or information not specified in the subpoena should be removed. In some states, a certified copy of the record can be submitted to the court. Photocopies, microfiche, microfilm, and/or photographic copies of microfilmed records may be admissible as evidence. The group should be aware of state laws concerning microfilmed records before making any decisions concerning inactive records storage. If the record must be submitted to the court in its original form, each page should be clearly numbered, and a notation of the total number of pages submitted, along with an itemized list of the record's contents, should be filed in the records room. It also is helpful to make a duplicate of the record to leave on file in the clinic. A more detailed discussion of the logistics involved in preparing a record for court can be found in *Handbook on Release of Information and Reporting from Medical Records* (1970) which is published by the Illinois Medical Record Association.

Patient's Right to His Medical Record. With malpractice litigation on the increase, the patient's right to see or be in possession of his medical record is of growing concern to health care providers and to patients. Legally, the medical record is the property of the physician or physician group. The patient neither owns his record nor has any legal right to see it. He does, however, have a humanistic right to the information contained in it. In the past, it has been felt that access to his own medical record may mislead the patient and in some instances actually threaten his health. While it is generally agreed that the patient is entitled to information about his health and medical treatment, he needs guidance in understanding and using his record. Some individuals maintain, therefore, that such information should be given to the patient only by the physician and only at his discretion. In some states, with no expressed reason, a patient may authorize his legal representative to see and even copy the patient's medical record. In most states, however, the patient first must file suit indicating a basis for his attorney to examine the record. In many states, there must be just cause for the release of a medical record. For example, in an attempt to see his own record, a patient cannot merely authorize its release to his neighbor who has absolutely no valid or legal reason to be in possession of the record.

The legal situation surrounding the issue of the patient's right to his record remains in a state of flux. As of March 1975, in forty-one states patients can obtain their records through litigation. In three states, records can be obtained through an attorney. In one state, the patient must show good cause and in one state the record is not available until after the patient has been discharged from care. In three states, the patient is either implicitly or explicitly allowed direct access.[6] There appears to be a growing trend toward allowing the patient unrestricted access to his own record. In an attempt to stem the wave of malpractice suits, some professionals have suggested that the patient initial his record at each physician-patient encounter, thus indicating his knowledge and approval of treatment. Other individuals concerned with the maintenance of records in a mobile society have suggested that the patient be in possession of his record and totally responsible for it.

As patients are allowed ever-increasing access to their records, the pressure for recording information accurately, completely, and clearly will grow. The right to see his record, however, may only confuse the patient unless diagnoses and health evaluations are expressed in language which is understandable to the lay public, while at the same time explicit and meaningful to the group physicians.

The medical records department has the potential to interact daily with almost every other clinic department. A well-conceived records system can expedite this interaction, while a hastily and poorly designed system can create disorder in any one or all of a number of clinic areas. Well-maintained, precise, and complete records have ramifications for effective, productive clinic operation. Ultimately, good records mean quality patient care.

Chapter 15

Charge Systems

PATIENT ACCOUNTING SYSTEMS

It would be unwise for any group practice to underestimate the importance of charge systems, billing and collection procedures, and insurance processing methods. The impact of these systems on the financial stability of the group is easily recognized; not as readily apparent, however, is the impact that these systems can and do have on the physician-patient relationship. No matter how the patient is billed, the amount of the fee charged and the manner in which he is asked for payment often represent in a very real and personal way the medical care he has received. The design of any patient accounting system should be characterized both by its *effectiveness* in guaranteeing the financial stability of the practice and by its *sensitivity* to the psychological needs and socioeconomic limitations of the patient.

Fee Schedules and Charge Systems

It is readily apparent that the fees to be charged by the medical group for its services are not nationally or even locally standardized. Establishing fees in the forming group is dependent upon conditions within that group. There are, however, certain direct costs that can be identified, especially those resulting from laboratory and X-ray services and from other resources such as personnel (see Chapter 4). Unlike most commodities and even some service-oriented businesses, more than the cost of providing the service or the commodities must be considered. The determination of fees should be influenced by the patient's reaction to the charge and his ability to pay promptly without undue hardship, as well as whether he returns to the group for further care and refers his family and friends to the group. Generally, there are three basic methods of establishing fees for the group's services: according to the patient's ability to pay, through use of a fee schedule with a charge range for each service, or through use of a schedule of fixed fees for each service. These methods may be combined in various configurations to yield yet a fourth alternative in fee setting.

One basis for establishing the amount of a fee which remains in use after many years is the patient's ability to pay. The fee charged for a service can vary widely, not necessarily because of a variance in physician time and effort but rather because of a divergency in the ability to pay among patients in the group practice's population. To use this method effectively, and to keep overdue accounts at a minimum, the group must formulate a fee range for each service offered. To develop an accurate and sensitive system for ascertaining a patient's actual ability to pay, the clinic may have to rely on outside sources such as credit agencies. On the other hand, the group may be able to develop an effective self-administered questionnaire which elicits from the patient a statement concerning his salary as well as various other determinants of his ability to pay.

Recently, several factors have stimulated a trend away from determining fees based on the patient's ability to pay. Insurance programs such as Blue Shield and union welfare plans have published fee schedules which keep the public well informed of average fees charged anywhere in the nation. Second, group practices throughout the country have discovered that an increasing percentage of their patients come from the same geographic area and occupy the same economic level; thus, the range of fees charged for a particular medical service has narrowed. A third influence has been that more and more patients are covered by some form of medical insurance, including the Medicare, Medicaid, and Maternal and Child Health Programs, which not only increases the buying power of the patient's medical care dollar, but also forces standardization of fees through the publication and application of a standard schedule of benefits to be paid for specific medical services. In addition, fees charged by other physicians in the area also can influence the forming group's fee schedule. In many instances, the amount charged for comparable services by other providers (physicians, hospitals, etc.) in the community represents the most significant influence. Fees charged must be competitive in order for the group to maintain its viability.

Cost of Service

The service provided by medical laboratories and X-ray departments lends itself to a fairly straightforward method of fee determination. Because so much of the service provided consists of physically identifiable components such as equipment and supplies, the actual cost of providing laboratory and X-ray services can be established, resulting in a fairly standard schedule of fees roughly reflecting the group's cost in providing such services. Those responsible for setting fees should bear in mind, however, that some services cannot be charged for on the basis of cost alone; a patient volume less than projected, inflation in the cost of supplies, and the replacement of equipment necessary to perform the service are intervening variables which may be cyclical, thereby not justifying long-term cost/fee adjustments. In these cases, the patient's ability to pay perhaps should take priority in establishing or modifying the fee. Losses incurred as a result of performing these services can be compensated for by other service fees which equal cost plus a profit margin. The group's administrator can alert physicians to remain aware of the cost basis of fees, of fees that are inconsistent with those charged by other physicians in the area, and of fees which may cause poor public relations. In some groups, if the administrator has the authority to review any fee charged a patient, he also may have the authority to adjust the fee within the patient's ability to pay. A standing committee comprised of physicians and the group administrator may be formed to review fees periodically and to monitor patient reaction to them.

When fees for the group's services are based on the cost to provide those services, the group is always aware of its deficit, break-even, or surplus situation. Furthermore, as the cost of operating varies, the group has an identifiable basis for adjusting and justifying its fees. Thus, depending upon its financial objectives (see Chapter 3), the group retains control of the implementation and adjustment of its fees.

Physician services tend to vary greatly in time and expenditure of effort; a standard schedule, therefore, should provide for a minimum (perhaps just covering costs) and maximum in the range of fees to be charged for each type of service—e.g., office visit, comprehensive physical examination, etc. On the other hand, rigid fee schedules often are felt to be impersonal and inflexible. Furthermore, such schedules preclude the physicians' setting fees, even though they are in the best position to determine the value of services. If a standard schedule is used, each physician in the group should be kept well informed of the range of fees to be charged. Services can be assigned a code designation to be used by the physician in relaying to the billing personnel the type of service performed. If the physician wishes to adjust his fee he can do so by adding a modifier of a specified type to the basic code. Such a coding scheme should be used with caution in that it does require some monitoring to ensure uniformity, but it does offer the advantage of allowing each physician to participate in determining the fee for his service.

Some groups may find one or a combination of the many relative value studies now available useful in establishing a standard fee schedule. The *California Relative Value Study* (1964, 1969, and 1974 editions) is a result of a survey of physicians to ascertain the relative value of specified services on a predetermined scale. Such studies can provide an indication of the uniformity needed within the group's pricing structure. It must be remembered, however, that a relative value schedule does not in itself determine the actual charge. By assigning the service's relative value a monetary value determined on the basis of cost, plus perhaps profit or reserve, a standard fee schedule can be determined.

Prepaid Plans

There are a number of manuals and publications available that describe in detail the parameters to be considered in developing a prepaid plan. Some of these are listed in the bibliography for this chapter. Prepaid plans can assume many different configurations and organizational characteristics and usually are based on the principle of providing medical care to all enrollees for a predetermined and prepaid fee or premium.

In general, there are two basic methods for determining a group's prepaid premiums (on either a community or group rating basis). One method is by acquiring the services of an actuary who will use the plan's benefits and corresponding manual rates to compile a premium. By using data accumulated by many recent prepaid plans, actuaries are now in a better position to make use of general insurance experience in compiling premiums which usually take into consideration the services to be provided, marketing efforts, administrative services, and a contingency reserve.

A second method for determining premiums involves tailoring the premium rate to the group's cost of providing the medical service. For a newly forming group this cost will be based upon a number of assumptions—the type of population to be served, the average number of times each person will visit the group practice facility, and the cost associated with each visit. A method for projecting the cost of each visit based upon the resources required for particular types of individuals (for example, adults or children) was discussed in Chapter 4. A rate to cover services provided by the group can be computed in the following manner: multiply the estimated cost for each visit by the projected number of visits per year and divide by twelve, yielding the monthly premium rate for a particular population.

$$\frac{\text{Cost/visit} \times \text{Estimated number of visits/year}}{\text{12 months/year}} = \text{Rate/month}$$

Example:

Adult Premium

$$\frac{\$24.89\text{/visit} \times 4.4 \text{ visits/year}}{\text{12 months/year}} = \$9.13 \text{ premium rate per month.}$$

If the enrollment in the plan is projected to be 1,650 adults, the group should expect to receive in prepayments each month:

$$\$9.13 \text{ per adult} \times 1{,}650 \text{ adults} = \$15{,}064.50 \text{ each month.}$$

Example:

Child Premium

$$\frac{\$24.89\text{/visit} \times 3.2 \text{ visits/year}}{\text{12 months/year}} = \$6.64 \text{ premium rate per month.}$$

If the number of children enrolled in the plan is projected to be 880 children the group should expect to receive in prepayments each month:

$$\$6.64 \text{ per child} \times 880 \text{ children} = \$5{,}843.20 \text{ each month.}$$

Certainly there are many other methods as well as variations of the ones discussed here for computing premium rates. It is important to remember, however, that if the group's marketing of the plan is to be successful, the rate must be competitive with the charges levied by other providers in the community—other prepaid groups, fee-for-service groups, and hospitals. On a premium basis, the plan also will compete with those offered by insurance companies. Negotiations for a prepaid plan should not be completed by the group with an employer (group rating) or a community until the group has some idea of the cost of providing its services to the enrollees. In addition, the premium rate also must be adjusted to accommodate the cost for contracted services as well as any other costs such as administration, hospitalization, other specialty care, drugs, etc. This contractual agreement between the plan and the consumer lists the services to be provided by the organizing physician group in a benefit package. There may be a number of services that the organizing medical group is unable to provide. If the group can contract for these services with other providers, the services can be included in the benefit package. Determining the appropriate premium charge is very important in maintaining the stability of the group, for premiums generate the revenue to cover the cost of providing all of the medical services in the benefit package. Groups organized to offer a prepaid plan should be aware that such plans are subject to many regulations. Some states require that a plan fall under the jurisdiction of the insurance commissioner and adhere to the financial regulations imposed on health insurance companies. For example, the establishment of appropriate reserve ratios, rates, and solicitation or marketing methods may be regulated by civil statutes, insurance law, and medical practice statutes. Because regulations on prepaid plans vary from state to state, the organizing group should seek appropriate legal and financial counseling before attempting to price and market a prepaid plan.

The Health Maintenance Organization Act of 1973 (Public Law 93-222) commits the federal government to provide for the development of health maintenance organizations (HMOs) for a trial period. The act provides for financial assistance through grants or contracts for planning and development projects as well as for feasibility studies. The act also includes a statement which stipulates that an employer with twenty-five or more employees must offer his employees the option of joining an HMO if one is available. There are a number of qualifications an HMO must meet before assistance can be provided by the 1973 act, including the offer of a comprehensive range of basic health care services, and encompassing eye examinations and preventive dental health care for children. Supplemental health care services, such as coverage for care in extended care facilities and routine dental care, can be provided for with an additional premium. The fees charged must be affixed uniformly under a community rating system which, stated in an oversimplified manner, requires a similar rate for all individuals and families in the community who are applying for the plan. The community rating system does not allow for the actuarial differences that comprise most insurance premiums, such as risk of employment, age, sex, etc. It should be understood, however, that a prepaid plan need not meet the requirements of the HMO act unless the plan is seeking federal assistance under the HMO act. Regulations adding to and modifying the law are presently being written and also should be reviewed. A group offering prepayment has a written contract with its patients or employer to provide certain services. In a fee-for-service setting, usually no written contract exists. Prepaid contracts can be written and premium levels can be determined which cover varying time periods—five months, six months, one year, etc. Contract law and its interpretation are important in prepayment and require expertise usually not available within the group itself. Actuarial assistance is abundant from outside experts such as insurance companies but it is unusual to find an actuary who understands group practice and how it differs from hospitalization underwriting. Additionally, insurance companies (other than Blue Shield) have not provided coverage for outpatient services; therefore, experience is lacking in such pricing on a premium or prepaid basis.

Charge Methods

In a fee-for-service group there are three basic methods for compiling and recording charges for patient services: the centralized charge method, the decentralized method, and a combination or hybrid charge method. The type of charging method used by the group depends largely upon its objectives and its general accounting system and financial reporting system. (see Chapter 8). The efficient and comprehensive reporting of charges is invaluable for the productive analysis of periodic financial statements. The method used to determine the fees to be charged can be employed in combination with differing methods of recording charges—whether centralized, decentralized, or hybrid. Thus, the physician may have a varying degree of responsibility in assigning charges no matter what the fee schedule or charge method may be.

When charges are centralized, they are entered on one form which may specify scheduled fees and their range, or the provider may be allowed to enter the fee. This method requires a timely reporting system throughout by various center departments using the form and an efficient transmission of that service information to the billing point. Recording on a single form all the services performed for the patient not only simplifies the billing procedure and charge ticket control through prenumbering, but also reduces the chance of repeating tests and procedures (duplicate charges) by different departments providing treatment to the patient. If the centralized form remains a part of the record, it is transported "round robin" to the various departments providing treatment to the patient for illness, injury, routine medical, and/or surgical episode. In some groups, such information is conveyed via a combination routing and charge slip which is generated when the patient registers and is sent to all departments where he may require services. To avoid duplication of effort in transporting this form and the medical record, the form usually is attached to the record and is not removed until the termination of the patient's care or until the end of a billing period. Upon the patient's dismissal, the charge slip can be sent to the billing point, usually the business office, for computation of the patient's statement of charges (see figure 15-1). If the group maintains central medical records in which all records of physician visits and all laboratory and X-ray reports are included, the medical record of each patient can stand alone as the possible source document for compiling charges. A physician can indicate the fee to be charged for his service in coded form by an appropriate marginal note in the medical record. In this way, personnel in the business office are not responsible for determining from the physicians' progress notes the amount of time and effort the particular medical visit required. More importantly, the system allows for fees to be set by the

PATIENT'S NAME	CHART NO.	DATE	BILL TO:	
	CHANGE OF NAME		COMPANY NO.	CODE 1 2 3 4. N/R
	CHANGE OF ADDRESS		PHONE	SPECIAL INSTRUCTIONS
	XYZ Clinic	Post Oak ☐ West ☐	Downtown ☐	INTERPRETER: ☐
	• BEFORE RELEASING SR •			GIVE ESTIMATE ONLY: ☐
	RETURN TO ORIGINAL DOCTOR FOR REPORTS TO BE CHARTED			CALL ☐ WRITE ☐ REPORTS

CODE	LABORATORY(1)	FEE	CODE	LABORATORY(1)	FEE	CODE	X-RAY (2)	FEE	CODE	NUCLEAR MEDICINE (6)	FEE	CODE	PROFESSIONAL (4)	DATE	M.D.	FEE	PHONE NO:
15	CBC	8					CHEST (PA) (LAT)		190	T_3	10		NEW ( ) RETURN ( ) PATIENT				YEAR CHECK: YES ☐ NO ☐
107	SED RATE	8				31	KUB		213	T_4	18		COMPLETE EXAM S ( ) L ( )				
410	COULTER	5				54	SKULL			THYROID UPTAKE			FOLLOW-UP				
12	BLOOD SMEAR	10				53	SINUS						NEW PATIENT-OFFICE VISIT				
139	URINALYSIS	5				60	SPINE CERVICAL						PRE-EMPLOYMENT				
80	OB LAB	20				62	SPINE-LUMBAR			SCANS: LIST			FAA				
53	PREG. TEST	8				29	IVP						CONSULTATION-OFFICE				
222	SURVEY-CHEM.	21				25	GALL BLADDER						CONSULTATION-OFFICE				
13	GLUCOSE	5				67	UGI		CODE	TREATMENT(3)							
137	UREA	7				20	ESOPHAGUS		76	DIETARY			OFFICE VISIT S( ) L( )				
59	GLUCOSE TOL.	23				69	SMALL BOWEL						OFFICE VISIT S( ) L( )				
138	URIC ACID	7					BE (AIR CONT)		75	PHYSICAL THERAPY							
44	ELECTROLYTES	·32															
39	CREATININE	8															
104	SGOT	10							67	DRUGS:							
105	SGPT	10															
31	CHOLESTEROL	7											HOSPITAL SERVICE				
131	TRIGLYCERIDES	13	CODE	INJECTIONS(3)	FEE	CODE	PROFESSIONAL (4)		DATE	M.D.	FEE		@ $ /DAY (REG. CARE)				
77	LIPOPROT. ELECT.	17	45	TETANUS (S) (B)	7		PROCTO ( )						TO				
146	CALCIUM	7	157	D-T ADULT (S) (B)	7		ECG ( ) MASTERS ( )						@ $ /DAY (ICU CARE)				
89	PHOSPHOROUS	7	14	DPT	7		ERGOMETER ( ) WITH CONSULT ( )						TO				
47	PROTEIN ELECT.	17	37	POLIO ORAL (S) (B)	5		PULMONARY FUNCTION ( ) WITH CONSULT ( )										
276	SEROLOGY	8	49	TYPHOID (S) (B)	7	115	EEG				35		(HISTORY & HOSPITAL PHYSICAL)				DIAGNOSIS CODE(S):
63	HET. ANT.	8	42	SMALL POX	7		AUDIOGRAM - ENT						HOSPITAL CONSULTS				
98	R.A.	6	161	RUBELLA MUMPS & MEASLES	17								NO. OF VISITS				
215	ANA	20	9	CHOLERA	7	168	TISSUE STUDY				17.50						
96	PRO-TIME	5	59	YELLOW FEVER	12								SURGERY:				
84	PAP SMEAR	8	111	PPD	7	184	PREG. SLIDE				5						DOCTOR(S) INITIAL HERE →
121	STOOL	10	22	GOLD	4												INSURANCE ONLY ☐
			56	TINE TEST	5		OCC. HEALTH SCREENING:						SPECIAL PROCEDURES:				MEDICARE ASSIGNMENT ☐
	CULTURE						AUDIO. SPIROMETRY										
							VISUAL. TONOMETRY										DISCOUNT:
							URINE								GRAND TOTAL		REASON:

Figure 15-1. Patient Charge Slip

person in the best position to make the judgment—the physician. Thus, a centralized charge method can be used in combination with a standardized fee schedule which can be modified to some degree by each individual physician. If fees are based on the patient's ability to pay, however, that ability must in some way be ascertained.

A decentralized charge method is characterized by separate procedures whereby each department and/or physician charge for the individual services they perform on departmental charge forms. Charging procedures which are not uniform across departments can create problems of control. The preparation of insurance claim forms and, in the final analysis, the efficient gathering of data to provide an accurate financial picture of the group also become complicated. The decentralized method of charging, however, can be functional and fairly efficient if every department is brought under a uniform billing procedure and fee schedule which is modified and appropriate for each specialty. Individual department charges also can be more closely associated with the cost of operating each particular department. An efficient bookings reporting system, such as centralized charging for services with assignment of charges made by department or even by individual physicians, can accomplish the same task with far less medical department effort and as much if not more accuracy.

When a decentralized method for recording charges is used, the assignment of charges by departments may become complex if patients' ability to pay is used as a criterion. In such cases it may be expedient to have registration personnel assess a patient's ability to pay, record the information on the medical record, and forward it to individual departments. To maintain consistency in fees charged, each department then can use a standard fee schedule or a range of charges for specific services, with options for modification by the provider. The patient should be made aware of the potential fee so that he knows what is expected of him and, as a consequence, is prompt in paying his bills.

A hybrid charge method may offer the best potential for meeting the objectives of any group. Individual departments can be given specific procedures to follow in reporting their service charges to a central billing point. Such procedures may include the use of a standard form throughout the center and may or may not require individual departments to determine their fees. If a standard fee schedule is used, the laboratory and the X-ray department usually have very little need to report the fee to be charged, but only what services have been performed. Physician fees, which may vary as a result of time and effort expended, can be reported on a centralized reporting form or coded within the medical record as was discussed previously. Again, there is no real need for the physician to set the fee; he need only indicate a variance from the standard allotment for the type of service. If fees are based on the patient's ability to pay, services could be reported to a centralized point; credit counselors, the business office manager, or an individual delegated the proper authority can set the fee. The standard service reporting form usually can be sent directly to the central billing point as soon as services are performed or can be held with the patient's medical record until the end of his period of care. This charging method promotes accuracy in the reporting of services performed by forcing each service department to report its services in a standard way. It also creates more time for the department to provide medical care by allowing the central billing point to determine fees and to bill the patient efficiently and fairly. The method of accumulating charges is especially important in a prepaid group, as well as in groups which are fee-for-service and prepaid, or in a prepaid plan which has several exclusions or co-payment charges. Charges may be processed and accounted for as in the fee-for-service mode but are not billed for prepaid patients. For example, prepaid plans may use a centralized charge ticket for services covered under the prepaid plan and may initiate a decentralized ticket for excluded or co-payment services.

CREDIT, BILLING, AND COLLECTIONS

After the group has established the method of charges, it must establish a credit policy and a billing system, which constitute significant cost items especially when computer billing is used. No organized group will dispute the fact that a considerable dollar volume can be locked up in unpaid patient accounts and that this problem can be compounded by an inefficient billing and collection system.

Credit Policy

Medical Group Management Association's *Medical Credit and Collections Manual* (1974) is an up-to-date, comprehensive collection of credit and collection methods and ideas. Its introduction includes several reasons that detail the importance of a group credit policy:

1. The group's credit policy must include the means for extending sufficient credit so the patient without insurance coverage or savings will be able to obtain treatment when he needs it.
2. The group's credit policy must be understandable to the patient so that he will feel responsible to pay within the time agreed upon.
3. The group's credit policy must include a mechanism for grouping payees according to credit status in order to assist the business office in determining with reasonable accuracy the difference between those who can and will pay, those who will pay when they are able, those who cannot pay, and those who can but will not pay.
4. The group's collection policy must provide for the collection of sufficient money to maintain the center and satisfy the physicians in the group.
5. The group's collection policy must be firm enough to be effective.
6. The group's collection policy must be temperate enough to not irritate those who intend to pay, thus jeopardizing further visits or the positive public relations effect of satisfied patients.

Within the framework of credit policy, as outlined above, several variables are important:

1. Is the policy written or unwritten?
2. Is the policy consistent yet flexible?
3. Is there a finance charge? If so, what are the terms?

4. Is bank financing used?
5. Are time payments used?
6. Are patients encouraged to use a monthly budget plan if payment in full is not possible?
7. Is adequate credit information obtained at registration?
8. Are all patients given a financial interview?
9. Is this policy described in a brochure, etc.?
10. Is there a staff member available to serve as a credit counselor?

By presenting the patient with a credit policy written in easily understood terms, many future collection problems can be prevented. If the patient understands the policy as it is intended, he also will understand what is expected of him. If collecting an account becomes a problem, the group has a firm basis to press for payment. Every collection department should be aware of the law of contracts which outlines specific duties concerning contracting parties, and of the federal Truth in Lending Act, effective July 1, 1969, which requires disclosure by creditors of their dollar finance charges and the annual percentage rates on the credit transactions. Even when no interest charges are made on patient accounts, if a patient agrees to pay for medical services in more than four installments, the arrangement is within the scope of the Truth in Lending Act. The group's credit policy may be posted in the business office, made available in brochures or pamphlets given to the patient at registration (see figure 15-2), and restated on the billing statement sent to the patient. It is important that group employees also understand the credit policy, and professional and paramedical personnel should be aware of possible changes in patient credit status.

If a group charges on the basis of the patients' ability to pay, it is advisable to conduct a financial interview which should be completed before service is given so that sufficient time is allowed for credit investigation. There would be exceptions to the preservice interview for emergency care and, while no group would refuse care to the acutely ill patient, elective services can be postponed until the patient makes satisfactory arrangements for paying his account. Because a patient's financial situation is personal, information concerning it must be treated with sensitivity; the financial interview which may represent the patient's first contact with the group is merely a tool to enable the group to grant credit intelligently. According to the American Collectors Association in Minneapolis, knowledge of some details of a patient's financial circumstances can facilitate the collection process. A number of these items are:

1. Patient's full name, including middle initial
2. Patient's present address including length of time he has lived there; if for only a short period of time, patient's previous addresses and length of time at each
3. Homeowner or renter
4. Place of employment, length of time in present position, type of work
5. Spouse's employment, length of time in present position, type of work
6. Name of insurance policy underwriter and policy number if any
7. Name of relative other than spouse or children
8. Other credit references.

Financial Information

Estimate of Charges:

New patients are invited to request estimates of charges prior to laboratory and x-ray work. This will give you an opportunity to see what tests are scheduled and their estimated cost. You may request an estimate of charges at any time – – now or on future visits. Our cashiers are located on the first floor.

Insurance:

If you have insurance information to submit, our Insurance Department, basement floor, will assist you. We request that you pay us direct and allow the insurance to reimburse you.

Payment:

We ask new patients to start out with an understanding of their payment arrangement. If you are not in a position to pay the charges at the time the work is done, the balance will be payable within 10 days of receipt of your first statement.

Should you wish to discuss finances, please feel free to bring this to the attention of our cashier.

Figure 15-2. Patient Financial Information Card

If the financial interview discloses a potential or real collection problem, additional precautionary steps may contribute to its solution in advance or may remove it all together. For example, a patient may be asked to pay for his visit in cash at the conclusion of each office call; if this is not possible, the patient should be asked how he plans to pay the bill. The collector's request for a commitment to pay on a specific date probably will be sufficient to ensure payment. A third alternative, especially for the patient who expects a large bill, has no insurance, and is unable to determine how or when he will pay the account, may be for the group to request a third party signature on the payment agreement. This arrangement is similar to having a note co-signed and protects the group by establishing third party responsibility. A fourth alternative, in elective care cases, may be refusal to treat the patient.

A retail establishment granting credit usually requires that a finance charge be made on overdue accounts. While the American Medical Association's Judicial Council does not recommend the use of finance charges for patient accounts, for pressing financial reasons, more and more groups are instituting such charges. The aged analysis reports generated by the accounting system (see Chapter 8) can be used as a tool to identify and follow up credit problems. Other groups may indicate that a finance charge will be levied simply to encourage the patient to pay promptly—at least as promptly as he pays retail accounts having finance charges. According to a survey conducted in 1974, those groups charging an interest on overdue accounts had a collection percentage average of 97.0 percent while those using no interest charge had a collection percentage average of 93.7 percent.[1] If no financial interview is conducted prior to the patient-physician encounter, it is essential that the credit department or business office discuss the account with the patient before he leaves the center. This postservice interview can clarify credit policy and can assist personnel in obtaining a *definite* commitment from the patient concerning how he intends to pay his bill. It is unreasonable to expect that every patient will be able to pay the account in full upon receipt of an invoice. It is necessary, therefore, to be ready to offer the opportunity to make payments on a time or an installment basis. The amount of the payment should be determined according to established guidelines and preferably should be defined within the credit policy. Such guidelines might establish a minimum payment for a given balance—for example, 10 percent of the original balance each month or minimum of $50.00 a month on any account over $500.00. In establishing a time payment schedule, clarity and effective communication of the policy to the patient are of great importance.

Time payments can add significantly to the total of accounts receivable and some accounts may be paid over an extremely long period of time. It is essential that the group have a method for determining the aging of their accounts. As an account becomes older the value of the dollar paid decreases, especially during times of inflation. The age analysis chart shown below illustrates this principle.[2]

Account Age	*(Value Per Dollar)*
Current	$1.00
One Month	.90
Two Months	.86
Three Months	.81
Four Months	.75
Five Months	.71
Six Months	.67

Money paid on an account at the six-month interval is only 67 percent of the current market value. For any account over six months, the average value of one dollar paid is equal to fifty cents. The value of one dollar in accounts one year or more overdue is twenty-five cents. This scale serves to illustrate the necessity for establishing an aggressive yet fair collection policy to ensure financial stability.

Some health care providers report that the credit card concept has come to medicine. A major selling point of the credit or charge card is that credit card contracts assure the physician of immediate payment. In most cases, physicians switching to a credit card policy of payment will be forced to modernize their bookkeeping systems because quick conversion of accounts receivable to cash is dependent upon the group's making deposits as soon as possible. In addition, physicians should be aware of the cost associated with using the credit card method of billing, and these expenses should be weighed carefully against the expenses incurred through a collection program conducted by the group itself and against the decreasing value of the dollar over time.

Billing and Collections

A definite billing schedule should be established by the group. In some cases all accounts may be billed on the first or on the fifteenth of the month; most groups, however, will find that there is an advantage to billing some accounts on the first and others on different dates in the month to avoid concentrating a large portion of the clerical staff's activity within one relatively short span of time. Depending upon the charge system used, charges for patient care are generally accumulated either until the patient's period of care is completed or on a weekly or monthly basis. At that point, an itemized statement for charges is prepared and sent to the patient with regular cycle billings sent thereafter. Computer billing is a fast and efficient way of handling accounts, but care should be taken to ensure that it is cost effective. Certainly, a group should have a large volume of accounts receivable to justify the use of computer billing. This volume requirement could be reduced somewhat through time sharing with other organizations. Computer billing can be viewed as simply a mechanical tool for keeping track of accounts receivable and is only as effective as the credit policy of the group. A computer can automatically maintain the aged accounts analysis file and also can prepare follow-up notices and collection letters for overdue accounts. Regardless of the method used for billing, whether it be via computer or hand posting, billing should be prompt and fair with an accurate identification of potential collection problems.

If a group decides to bill on a monthly basis, the design of the monthly billing statement is critical. It should be easy to read and should readily identify for the patient the balance due and the amount owed. A method for quickly and accurately identifying a patient's payment when returned by mail includes incorporating a detachable return statement to be submitted with the payment. The billing statement itself can be used to encourage the patient to pay by reminding him of the terms prearranged for payment of the account. Short, concise messages such as "we missed your payment" or "please call our office immediately to discuss this account" can be added to the statement either automatically in computer billing, by the use of bright, eye catching stickers, or in some cases via handwritten messages. The method of writing in long-hand across the face of the billing statement may seem to be inefficient, but it does have the distinct advantage of letting the patient know that his account is receiving personal attention.

If the patient continues to be slow in his payment or does not pay as agreed, friendly reminders can be included as inserts with the monthly billing statement. Messages should be short, concise, and visually stimulating. A series of these inserts can be designed according to guidelines established by the group and can be sent in accordance with the patient's payment record. Inserts usually range from very friendly reminders to the threat of further collection action if the account is not paid promptly. In addition to the insert collection reminder, personalized collection letters also may be sent. Such letters should be concise and should clearly state the expectations of the group in regard to payment. A checklist for use in designing effective collection letters includes:

1. Setting a definite time schedule
2. Pressuring the debtor's anxiety without stifling goodwill
3. Always noting the amount due
4. Providing a motive for payment—a springboard to action
5. Expressing confidence that the debt will be paid
6. Keeping one foot in the door for follow-up methods

7. Making it easy for the debtor to make payment
8. Including all facts to permit debtor action without delay
9. Keeping letters simple and creative.

Another collection method commonly used is telephoning or telegraphing the patient in regard to payment, which often uncovers problems or potential difficulties that no letter or friendly reminder ever will. With the exercise of some degree of care and the establishment of policy guidelines, telephoning also can result in goodwill by putting the collection effort on a one-to-one, personal basis. As in the financial interview, telephone calls should be made by mature, sensitive people who can be firm but fair and who have a talent for asking the right questions in the right way. The telephone collector should receive guidance concerning what the group expects in the way of payment. The use of telegrams in collection efforts has been an effective tool for some groups for a number of reasons. A telegram commands individual attention and implies urgency and importance. It wastes no words in articulating the message quickly and usually will compel an individual to act. While a telegram should be commanding, it should always be courteous in tone.

When all collection methods have failed, a delinquent account may be referred to a legal adviser. A collection letter sent to the patient by an attorney may create a very different impression than that created by any other collection letter, telegram, or telephone call. Such letters should result in action by the patient and certainly must include the clinic's telephone number so that the patient has an opportunity to explain his circumstances. A collection letter also should explain what the patient can expect if he chooses to ignore the letter.

In some cases, the group can and should consider the use of a collection agency to secure overdue accounts. As in all collection efforts, however, collection agency methods should be fair to the patient and in compliance with medical ethics. Common procedures among less ethical collectors include intimidation, false representation as sheriff's deputies or process servers, and harrassment involving telephoning patients at their homes at odd hours and leaving "pay up or else" messages at their places of employment. It is especially important, therefore, to use care in choosing a collection agency. While most agencies are honest and reasonably efficient, the group should be cautious in its selection and should remember that most agencies do require a substantial fee, usually a specified percentage of the amounts collected.

Criteria for choosing a good medical collection agency include:[3]

1. *Medical credit bureau versus retail credit bureau.* A medical credit bureau serves only physicians and therefore is less likely to subject a patient to harsh commercial methods, or to violate confidentiality by sharing medical payment records with retail creditors.

2. *Location.* A location near the group practice enables group personnel and agency personnel to confer conveniently.

3. *Legal Aspects.* The agency should be licensed and bonded if state laws so require.

4. *References.* Agency management should be willing and able to furnish references from other medical and dental clients.

5. *Reports.* The agency should be willing to provide the group with itemized monthly reports and monthly remittances.

6. *Commissions.* The agency should charge commissions of approximately 30 percent to 50 percent of the *amounts collected*—not of the total amounts owed. It should allow the group to recall accounts without paying a penalty, and it should be willing to accept all the accounts that the group wishes to refer—not just those with high balances.

7. *Results.* The group should be able to expect the agency to collect between 30 percent and 60 percent of the accounts assigned to it. Less than 30 percent may indicate inefficiency; more than 60 percent is a sign that high pressure tactics may be in use. The manager of the agency should be willing to produce all form letters sent to the group's patients.

Sometimes the only recourse open to the group in collecting an account is to bring legal suit. Care should be exercised in this area because regulations will vary from state to state. In general, a suit establishes the existence of a debt and provides a remedy for collection. The group can bring suit through an attorney or the group's collection agency can bring suit. In the latter case the agency usually brings suit in its own name and the name of the group need never appear in print. Medical Group Management Association's *Clinic Manager's Manual* suggests that litigation in collection of an account is in order when:

1. Satisfactory results were obtained from the medical treatment
2. Payment can be made without producing a hardship
3. The medical and account records of the patient are accurate and complete
4. The fee for the service is reasonable
5. It has been established that the patient is legally liable
6. The patient is not judgment proof
7. The statute of limitations has ruled out a malpractice claim
8. All other reasonable means of collecting have failed.

Measurement of the Collection Effort

A group's collection percentage goal must be realistic in order to serve as a better tool for evaluating credit policies.

> The collection percentage is the ratio of net collections to adjusted gross bookings for a period of twelve consecutive months where: net collections shall include the payments and/or their third parties for services and supplies provided by the clinic excluding overpayments on accounts and collection on accounts turned over to collection agencies. And where: adjusted gross bookings will be charges for the same twelve month period for charges billed to patients and/or their third parties for services and supplies provided by the clinic excluding charges to be discounted as policy discounts, contractual adjustment or free service for which no bills will be sent.[4]

In most cases, the group will find that certain adjustments in the charges for professional services are necessary in order to formulate a realistic collection percentage. Some of these adjustments include:

1. Duplicate charges
2. Accounts of the medically indigent or uncollectable accounts
3. Settlements on accounts for third party payments.

In some cases, it is necessary to make a compromise on an account and to settle for less than the actual amount receivable. The difference between the amount due and the amount received should be deducted from the total charges for the period. Other adjustments are necessary because of the difference between billed amounts and insurance payments, welfare payments, Medicare payments, and special local and state program payments. These adjustments should be made against current charges. MGMA's *Cost Survey* (1975) reports an average collection percentage of 93.8 percent for existing 3-10 physician groups. Although the method of determining the collection percentage may vary from group to group, collection percentages of between 92 percent and 95 percent continue to be considered good for most groups.

Insurance Processing

On a percentage basis, more people are covered by some type of insurance protection against medical expense than ever before. Government insurance programs such as Medicare and Medicaid have contributed greatly to this increase. For example, in the fiscal year of 1966 and prior to the enactment of Medicare, local, state, and federal government insurance programs accounted for 26 percent of the 42.1 billion dollars spent on medical care in the country. In 1973, these same programs accounted for 40 percent of the 94.1 billion dollar health care bill. Federal programs accounted for 26 percent alone. Because so many people have insurance, either group or individual, federal or private, the group must be prepared to handle insurance claims in an efficient way. Unless the group is willing to establish a policy that does not require it to file insurance claims for the patient, it must face the fact that many patients will delay making payment until the insurance company has paid the claim. Should the group accept insurance assignments or prepaire claims for the patient to file, then it is essential to the management of accounts receivable that claims be filed quickly and accurately and in the form required by or easily understood by the insurance company. In some cases, particularly in handling Medicaid claims, it will be discovered that if a claim is not filed according to specific guidelines, it will receive no consideration. In general, however, the group has several options regarding insurance claim processing. It may:

1. Bill the patient, allowing him to file the claim
2. Bill the patient, and at the same time bill the third party on an assigned or not assigned basis
3. Bill the third party without billing the patient.

The group may find it advantageous to design its own insurance claim form, consisting of a combined itemized statement and medical report. It may be even less confusing to use one of the standard claim forms designed through the cooperative effort of the AMA and the Health Insurance Council. Still another option is to use the "superbill," a concept developed by the Medical Group Management Association which combines the bill and the insurance claim into one document in an effort to avoid duplication and costs. Even if the group does not file the insurance claim for the patient, it must provide a number of details before most third parties will make payment on the claim. The patient's name, address, sex, and date of birth must be reported. In addition, the report to be filed by the group should include an itemized list of services performed along with, in some cases, a standardized procedure code such as the AMA's Current Procedural Terminology. The report also should include any medical information necessary to document the services given, which may be in coded form according to a standardized diagnosis coding scheme such as *H-ICDA-2* of the Commission on Professional and Hospital Activities or *ICDA-8*, the *Eighth Revision of International Classification of Diseases, Adapted for Use in the United States*, by the American Hospital Association.

Because of the detail work involved, much of the insurance processing can be accomplished in a cost efficient manner by lay personnel. The collection of proper patient identification, the reporting of services, and the abstraction of proper medical data can be assigned to lay people trained in medical terminology and coding. This method of handling insurance usually is much more cost effective than one which relies on the physician and medical secretary to handle all paperwork associated with filing an insurance claim.

It seems as if every insurance company has a unique claim form, thus complicating an already complex situation and providing impetus to the standardization of claim forms. The advent of Professional Standard Review Organizations and utilization review of patient care provided to patients covered under Medicaid and Medicare also have contributed to the trend toward standardization of insurance reporting. As mentioned previously, many groups have proposed a standard claim form, and it is reasonably safe to assume that if a national health insurance bill is enacted it will require reporting of insurance claims in a specified, standard way. Presently, one of the advantages of HMO prepayment is that claims need not be processed to obtain the fee; fees are prepaid. The prepaid group, however, must bill for noncovered charges as well as for any co-payments and possibly may have to file with other organizations.

Some aspects of insurance claim processing require the establishment of policy guidelines. One such issue to be considered is the *assignment of benefits*, which involves the patient's assigning any benefit to be paid under his insurance coverage for direct payment to the physician or clinic. Other than immediate payment in full of the balance due by the patient, an assignment of benefits may be the best method for prompt collection of the account. Most insurance companies are very prompt and efficient in payment of their claims. The group should be aware, however, that under some third party arrangements, such as Medicare, if an assignment of benefits is taken, the group agrees to accept any amount paid on charges allowed by the third party as full settlement of the amount owed. In most cases, the assignment of benefits can be taken at the option of the physician. If the group is aware that the account may be a collection problem, it may be to its advantage to accept an assignment of benefits to ensure payment. The patient also may be better able to pay any balance not paid by his insurance than he is able to pay the balance in full. Under such programs as Medicaid and Medicare for patients with a chronic condition or disease, the group must bill only the third party and not the patient.

The group usually will want to keep a copy of any insurance claims filed for two reasons: to refile the claim should the original become lost and to maintain a record of when and where an insurance claim was filed. If for any reason there is a delay in the payment of the claim by the insurance company, the group has proof of when it filed the claim, and the patient can direct his complaint directly to the third party. If a delay is experienced in payment of the claim, the patient should be made aware of the fact that he remains personally responsible for payment of the account. The patient also should be advised of how long the group is willing to wait for payment. If payment by the third party is not made within a specified time frame, the patient should understand that he must pay the bill immediately. If the patient pays his bill and the group subsequently receives a check from the insurance company, the group must promptly refund the patient. This type of information should be included in the group's credit policy and should be explained to the patient during his financial interview.

An interesting concept that will not be explained in great detail here because of its variability due to individual circumstance is what is commonly referred to as *tape-to-tape insurance processing.* For groups having access to a computer for billing and insurance claim processing, insurance claims can be prepared in the standard form on magnetic computer tape which is sent to the insurance company for processing by its computer. It is then unnecessary to prepare a hard copy of the claim to initiate payment. This concept promises to have great potential in facilitating insurance payments and in processing data reported. If coverage is available for the service reported, claims payment should be made within a matter of days, thus contributing toward making the tape-to-tape method cost effective. Claims paid promptly create good will not only for the third party payor but also for the group because of the reduction in expense of handling accounts receivable.

In conclusion, it should be pointed out that the group's methods of handling insurance claims largely will be determined not only by the trend toward standardization but also by the methods of charging and fee setting. As the federal government becomes more and more active in the medical field through Medicare and Medicaid programs and eventually through national health insurance, medical care expenditures covered by such programs will designate by law and regulation not only what data must be reported but also in what form data must be placed. It would be in the best interest of the group, therefore, to keep the patient accounting system as simple as possible while still maintaining the financial stability of the group. The group should not allow paperwork generated by the system to interfere with the efficient and effective delivery of quality health care.

Chapter 16

Purchasing, Supply Inventory, and Maintenance

ESTABLISHING PURCHASING, SUPPLY INVENTORY, AND MAINTENANCE SYSTEMS

Physicians, especially those in private practice, do not have a reputation for good business management.[1] Whether or not this estimation is well-founded, it is logical to assume that a physician's degree of productivity generally will be related to the time he actually spends with his patients. The thoughtful physician, therefore, may conclude that physician time spent pursuing the art of good purchasing and inventory control would soon reach a point of diminishing economic returns. For example, time spent in the generation of income as a medical practitioner at the rate of from $50.00 to $300.00 per hour would produce better economic results than would time spent in negotiating a price for examination table paper which results in a reduction from $14.00 to $13.50 per roll, at a consumption rate of two rolls per day.

Regardless of group size, the physician's time is better spent in providing professional services; however, no state or national legislation or AMA guidelines prohibit the use of business acumen together with efficient and effective use of physician time. The point is that physicians can strive toward good business procedures in their medical practices. The delegation of authority to purchase required supplies and equipment to a specific person or persons on the clinic staff should prove to be a step toward increased productivity for the group. As an aid to the newly forming group, several companies offer inventory/purchasing systems which can be purchased as a package and may save the inexperienced group considerable time and money.

The Department of Health, Education and Welfare, which will be playing an increasing role in the medical economic picture, leaves no doubt about its attitude toward cost controls and toward buying performance and purchasing behavior as a means of controlling costs.

> The prudent and cost-conscious buyer not only refuses to pay more than the going price for an item or service, he also seeks to economize by minimizing cost. This is especially so when that buyer is an institution or organization which makes bulk purchases and can therefore gain economies because of the size of its purchases. It is quite common that discounts are given in these instances. In addition, bulk purchases of items or services often gives that buyer leverage in bargaining with suppliers for other items or services. These are advantages which any alert and cost-conscious buyer seeks, and it is to be expected that providers of services under the Medicare Program will also seek them.[2]

The quotation illustrates that not only is it prudent to seek the best price for a particular item purchased in connection with the physician-patient service, but also that adherence to this practice already constitutes a Medicare guideline and certainly could be anticipated to be part of any National Health Insurance Program that might be enacted by the Congress. As the federal government becomes the major purchaser of health care services, undoubtedly it will not look with particular favor on requests for fee or contract increases without corresponding evidence that purchasing, as one aspect of the total system, is being performed at reasonable plateaus of efficiency.

PURCHASING POLICY

The forming group should consider the development of written policies representing the attitude of and defining the procedures endorsed by the group physicians with regard to who can buy what, and under what circumstances. Contrary to good business management and effective systems development, all too often there is a customer-friend relationship between either the physician and/or his designated agent within the clinic and the supply representative. This may result in preferential vendor selection based on friendship rather than on item quality or price. Regardless of friendship, however, when dealing with any supplier, sound business procedures should be prescribed and followed.

Generally, purchasing activities can be divided into two processes: those involving the acquisition of capital items and those involving the acquisition of expendable items. Capital items are represented by equipment having an expected life of more than one year, such as a microscope, an electrocardiogram machine, or a set of surgical instruments. Capital equipment items cannot be deducted as ordinary business expenses. They must be capitalized first, then depreciated according to their reasonably anticipated useful life. Very small cost items, however, such as an instrument purchased separately at a cost of less than $50–$200, may be essentially capital in nature but nevertheless may be deducted as ordinary business expense items.

Establishing an explicit purchasing policy is essential whether the authority to commit the group for capital equipment items is given to a physician committee or to a member of the staff, such as the group's administrator. For example, authority to replace existing equipment by purchasing capital items costing under a predetermined amount, such as $200–$500 could be given to the group administrator, or to an appropriate department head. On the other hand, new items of capital equipment or replacement items expected to cost over the predetermined amount, could be approved by the group's executive committee or purchasing committee, and subsequently ordered through the group's administrator or a department head. If policy is not enforced with respect to this type of high cost equipment, the group may find itself obligated to pay for a piece of equipment which may have been ordered under pressure at a recent medical meeting where persuasive manufacturers' representatives were soliciting orders. Written policy can provide the physicians with an available rationale to defer judgment on purchase of equipment until a group decision can be made. The group should be very careful in acquiring any equipment which cannot be amortized in four years or less. Often, equipment may become obsolete before it can return the purchase price. The potential for continued service capability should be a deciding factor when choosing between comparable brands. Second generation models of new equipment usually represent an improved version. In addition, group members should be wary of gadget and gimmick purchases of medical equipment or devices.

Unlike capital items, expendable items usually are expected to be consumed in a reasonably short period of time. Items in this category include dressings, drugs, and business office supplies. Expendable items should not be purchased in large quantities in advance of anticipated need; often, group preferences in this area may change. Because expendable items have accounted for as much as 7 percent of the total expense in medical groups in the past, this area should not be neglected during policy formation.[3] It is essential to provide appropriate persons with the explicit authority for purchasing such items. If individual physicians or employees without proper authority continue to buy small items, the amounts of these purchases may become unwieldy and there may be needless duplication of items.[4] The group administrator, however, whose experience and judgment the group physicians rely upon, could be given the authority to purchase reasonable amounts of expendable supplies without regard to dollar limits. In the smaller medical group, purchasing of expendable items may be the responsibility of the various department heads or of experienced office personnel. In this case, cost control might be improved if a limit, such as $200, were placed on the purchase of expendable supplies acquired without the written approval of the group manager. Medical forms and other printed materials are included in the category of expendable items. In general, the purchasing and maintenance of the clinic's supply of printed materials may be regulated by the same guidelines as are other expendable items. Usually, only a six-month supply of such items should be accumulated.

Purchasing Responsibilities

In medical groups consisting of three to ten physicians, the delegation of authority for purchasing and general inventory control can be somewhat variable. In a recent survey conducted by the author, fifty-seven questionnaires were sent to physician groups of from three to ten physicians in forty-one states. Thirty-five replies (61 percent) were received and of those responding, none had a full-time purchasing agent; however, four groups did report that they employ a part-time purchasing agent. Figure 16-1 indicates the range of purchasing responsibilities in the responding groups.

Response to the questionnaire also indicates that in general the groups polled allow their laboratory and X-ray technicians to purchase more technical supplies. This also is true, although to a somewhat lesser degree, of drugs and medical and surgical equipment. While this policy may be satisfactory, if the group administrator (or in his absence a responsible physician) reviews and countersigns each requisition, he can remain aware of what is purchased and can be certain that the group's established guidelines are being followed. The administrator also may find it helpful in monitoring the purchasing activities of the departments to assume responsibility for approving all invoice payments and distributing them to the appropriate accounts.

Quality or Price

The group physicians will find it beneficial to develop a general purchasing philosophy concerning quality and price. The security and confidence generated by a familiar brand of supplies may result in the group's overlooking new and better items on the market. Physicians, as well as those individuals actually involved in purchasing for physicians, should know that cost awareness contributes to productivity, and that a balance between all components of production will yield the greatest output for the least effort.[5] There may be sufficient reason for a physician to pay a higher price for a particular item, and this is especially true in the area of drug purchase. Contrary to popular opinion, the primary criterion for the purchase of drugs should not be lower price. This is not to suggest, however, that brand name drugs should be considered as inherently superior to generic prescriptions. Physician satisfaction with the drug's results and patient response to the medication carry high priorities in the determination of the types of drugs to be purchased.

INVENTORY

An inventory, as an itemized list of goods, is a catalog or schedule of the property of a person or a business. When establishing a formal inventory system, group size is not particularly important; the principles and practices of effective inventory and purchasing are applicable to small as well as larger groups.[6] A relatively uncomplicated method for establishing a perpetual inventory system involves the use of 3 × 5 cards. Even the smallest group practice operation can benefit from this type of inventory card system. A standardized card, such as displayed in figure 16-2, may be purchased from numerous standard form producers, and usually at a cost which is less than if the cards were designed and printed by a local company.

The inventory card should contain: the name of the vendors from whom the product ordinarily is ordered; the date merchandise is received; the quantity of merchandise received; and if convenient, the cost per unit of the merchandise. Inventory cards may be filed in the general supply storage area or in the accounts payable area where they can be updated after a receiving report has been forwarded there. Over a period of time, usually not exceeding six months, a pattern of purchasing develops which enables the individuals responsible for purchasing to determine more accurately the usable quantity of the item

Authorized Person	*Office Supplies*	*Med & Surg Supplies*	*Lab Supplies*	*X-Ray Supplies*	*Hskpg Supplies*	*Drugs*
	Items Purchased					
Group Administrator	24	13	6	6	16	12
Department Head	8	16	24	24	15	18
Purchasing Agent Part-time	1	3	2	3	2	2
Others	2	3	3	2	2	3

Figure 16-1. Range of Purchasing Responsibilities

needed. This pattern, however, depends not only on the availability of the item, but also on the quantity used and the price. Many readily available items do not warrant the clerical work involved in keeping a perpetual inventory card by amount issued and balance. The perpetual inventory record can be reserved for critical items which require substantial lead time for reordering. For many items a low limit card can be utilized, or if the item is stocked by local suppliers, it may be necessary to reorder when the last item on the shelf is issued. It also is possible to assemble a package of expendables which will fill clinic needs for the period of time necessary to order and receive a new supply. When

PERPETUAL INVENTORY AND PRICE RECORD

VENDOR 1 | VENDOR 2 | VENDOR 3

FORM P-492 PHYSICIANS' RECORD CO., BERWYN, ILLINOIS - PRINTED IN U.S.A.

DATE 19	FROM VEN-DOR	QUANTITY	COST PER UNIT	DATE 19	NUMBER OF UNITS RECEIVED	ISSUED	BALANCE	DATE 19	NUMBER OF UNITS RECEIVED	ISSUED	BALANCE

DESCRIPTION	UNIT	DATE	MAXIMUM QUANTITY	MINIMUM QUANTITY
ITEM		LOCATION		

Figure 16-2. Perpetual Inventory and Price Record List

all items have been issued except for those in the package, the package may be opened, thereby signaling that it is time to reorder. Care should be taken to discourage clinic personnel from accumulating unnecessarily large amounts of supplies in their individual departments. Such practices make an accurate inventory count difficult to maintain.

Training of personnel in procedural methods associated with effective purchasing will prove to be beneficial to the overall operation of the clinic. In addition, there are a number of clerical tasks which can improve ordering efficiency. The group may want to establish a policy regulating quantities purchased according to the item's usual rate of consumption.[7] A supply list or catalog may be developed by duplicating items listed on the inventory cards. Distributing this catalog to departments that regularly order supplies can result in a systematic method for maintaining inventory. Purchasing practices also can be improved through the use of exact terminology and descriptions, since consistency in order descriptions will ensure replacement of the same stock.

Storage Space

When a storeroom is available, the supply inventory can be kept under key control. The assignment of responsibility for storage, issue, and receipt of supplies to *one* person facilitates better inventory control.[8] Initially, the group may not have a storage room. As the professional staff increases, however, the need for this type of space will develop rapidly. Regardless of the size of the medical group, one area or room should be especially designated for the storage of bulk supplies.

Stocking a store room requires careful planning. If a group practice is in the initial forming stage, doctors might be asked to list the supplies they feel they ordinarily will be using in their specific type of practice. One method which can be used in the initial purchasing of supplies involves contacting local supply companies which have a representative line of the franchise items necessary to fulfill the group's needs adequately. Usually, surgical supply or physicians' supply companies are willing to provide initial stocking on a cost-plus arrangement. Costs should be clearly ascertained, however, before a group enters into any such agreement. If treated as a cost-plus arrangement, the initial stocking agreement should be in writing and should include the dates of delivery, the procedure for handling shipping charges, and the clearly defined terms for cash payment within a specified length of time. A local supply company may exchange supplies already purchased but subsequently found not to have filled the need. This return contingency also should be included in any written agreement.

The availability of a central storeroom area and the amount of supplies stocked will determine the time necessary for completion of ongoing inventories. If, for control and convenience, supplies are kept in a central store area, occasional random inspection of the item quantity may be conducted to verify that the amount of supplies on the shelves corresponds with the amount listed on the inventory cards. Assuming that the group operates on a cash accounting basis, there is no particular advantage inherent in computing the total worth of the supply inventory on a daily basis, because items purchased are expended during and following the month in which they are purchased. The primary consideration in maintaining an accurate knowledge of the inventory is to guarantee the availability of required supplies for the patient and for the physician.

Ordering Supplies by Department

Clinic departments requiring supplies can use printed forms to requisition the required items from the central supply area. The traditional type of supply requisition form shown in figure 16-3 is readily available from numerous suppliers. An alternative ordering system employs a completely preprinted form which eliminates both the need for a catalog and the entering of an item description. Another more advanced system uses IBM-type cards as requisition forms. Regardless of the ordering form chosen, the important consideration is that information concerning the type as well as the quantity of items needed is effectively conveyed and that the ordering system interfaces efficiently with both the purchasing and inventory systems.

When the traditional type of ordering form is used, the various departments within the clinic should have a supply catalog available for reference so that the exact terminology and descriptions listed in the catalog or supply list appear on the form. One efficient way for departments to requisition supplies is to send completed requisition forms to the supply store room each Friday morning. A requisition list is completed after the area to be supplied has been appraised, thereby determining the anticipated need for the coming week. Individuals responsible for issuing supplies then have the entire weekend to retrieve and deliver the items and, as a result, the various departments can begin each week with full supplies.

As items are removed from central storage, inventory cards must be adjusted. If at this time it is apparent that the supply of a particular item is either exhausted or is being used at a rate which indicates that the supply soon will be diminished, a want-list or items to be purchased list could be developed. This type of list is helpful for systematically determining and then recording those items required and eliminates the need to rely upon memory or guesswork when placing orders for supplies.

Supply vendors usually have a specific route and ordinarily visit the clinic on a regular basis, varying from once a week to once a month. For items needed on an emergency basis, phone orders can be placed with vendors approved for a particular product. In order to be systematic, a purchase order always should be used. A note on the inventory card indicating both the name of the vendor's representative who solicits the group and the day on which he usually appears also will clarify the purchasing system and will help to establish a sound business relationship. Some clinics may wish to implement open purchase orders to cover certain items purchased regularly. These orders should span a specific time period and should stipulate a specific dollar amount not to be exceeded.

The individual responsible for procurement should be totally aware of the purchasing policy of the group. Consideration should be given to the possibility that vendors may offer gratuities as well as token gift items at special times, such as Christmas or other holidays. Most existing groups have established policies which discourage such practices. Purchasing personnel also should be wary of the vendor who professes to cut prices. Often a time-consuming study is required to determine if discounted items differ from the products of other

STORES REQUISITION REQUISITION NO.__________

DEPARTMENT__________ DATE__________ 19____

FLOOR OR DIVISION__________ DATE REQUIRED__________ 19____

QUANTITY		DESCRIPTION OF SUPPLIES NEEDED	TO BE USED IF PERPETUAL INVENTORIES ARE KEPT			
WANTED	DELIVERED		PRICE	PER	AMOUNT	ACCT. NO.

REQUESTED BY	APPROVED BY

SEND ORIGINAL TO STORE ROOM CLERK. DUPLICATE IS RETAINED BY DEPARTMENT HEAD.

FORM P-452 STORES REQUISITION
PHYSICIANS' RECORD CO., BERWYN, ILLINOIS - PRINTED IN U.S.A.

Figure 16–3. Central Stores Requisition Form

manufacturers and if the same number of items are in a package of the discounted product as are in a packaged unit of the regularly priced item. Dealing with a reputable vendor, whose representative has a reputation for efficient, good service as well as a thorough knowledge of the medical supply field, yields results which offset the possible monetary savings realized by purchasing from less reliable vendors who may be difficult to locate when there is a need for items to be exchanged or serviced.

If the group is reasonably sure that the vendor it has chosen will have available the items which are needed, purchase orders may be prepared prior to the representative's visit to the clinic. A more efficient way to order supplies, however, might be to develop a want-list which is retained at the purchasing location. A form combining the want-list and purchase order form may result in a more efficient use of clerical time. Nevertheless, before any order is placed, the group's purchasing agent should enter the vendor's price for each item on the purchase order form.

The Purchase Order

The use of prenumbered, multi-copy purchase order forms contributes to effective purchasing practices. The written purchase order system eliminates guesswork in paying invoices and statements, and assures both the supplier and the group that the item requested has been received at the quoted price. Purchase order forms should be prepared in duplicate and often in triplicate or more, depending upon their use. For control purposes, forms can be prenumbered sequentially and can contain the name of the medical group as part of the preprinted data. For items ordered by specific individuals within the clinic, purchase orders should contain the individual's name or telephone extension number. This additional information prevents delay and confusion in routing the ordered item(s) to the proper individual. Should the organization be tax exempt, the tax exemption number also may be preprinted. A sample order form is shown in figure 16-4.

Bids or Quotations

Another method of purchasing supplies is through the solicitation of bids or quotations. When using this particular system, the administrator or purchasing agent accumulates a list of items to be purchased. Usually, in order to obtain any real advantages from inviting bids, the total cost anticipated probably should be in excess of $500. The bid or quotation sheet should carry an introductory paragraph indicating any general conditions of the bid or quotation. Comments appearing under the general conditions might include: the name of the catalog used for identification of special items; whether or not substitutions will be allowed and, if so, under what conditions; whether or not the bid or quotation includes shipping charges or FOB shipping point; and any other special conditions that the purchaser might desire. After the general conditions are listed, each item either should be described fully or should carry a product identification number. Space on the form should be designed for the vendor to enter the price, the terms, the shipping information, and his signature. Figure 16-5 is a sample bid or quote sheet.

While often it is a good practice to obtain a price quote on individual items, it also may be advantageous for the purchaser to offer the total bid or quotation package to a vendor on an all-or-none basis. Some states allow franchised items to be priced only by the manufacturer and any vendor selling that particular item for less than the franchise or fair trade price is subject to losing his franchise and therefore becomes unable to sell that particular item. By including fair trade items along with non-fair trade items in a bid or quotation request, a supplier is better able to bid the fair trade items at the franchised price and to lower the price on nonfranchised items. In effect, this package approach also results in a discount on the franchised fair trade items as well.

One difficulty in bid or quotation buying is the possibility of purchasing items that are substandard. The description of each item, therefore, should be considered carefully, and only reputable, well-known, and dependable vendors should be invited to bid or to quote on items.[9] The possibility of receiving items of inferior quality increases when vendors do not anticipate continued business relationships with the medical group. A purchasing system is effective if (1) control is held by one person, (2) if convenience is not the sole criterion for selecting suppliers, (3) if prices, quality, and delivery are reviewed on a regular basis, and (4) if quotations are obtained from several suppliers for major items and large contracts (over $500).[10] Dealing with reputable companies with whom the group maintains certain understandings, such as concerning substitutions and returns, remains the best policy to follow. Purchasing through means other than the use of purchase order forms also should be controlled by policy determinations and in fact may be prohibited.

Drug Purchasing

The purchasing of injectable medications and narcotics requires special consideration. When possible, these items should be purchased through a licensed

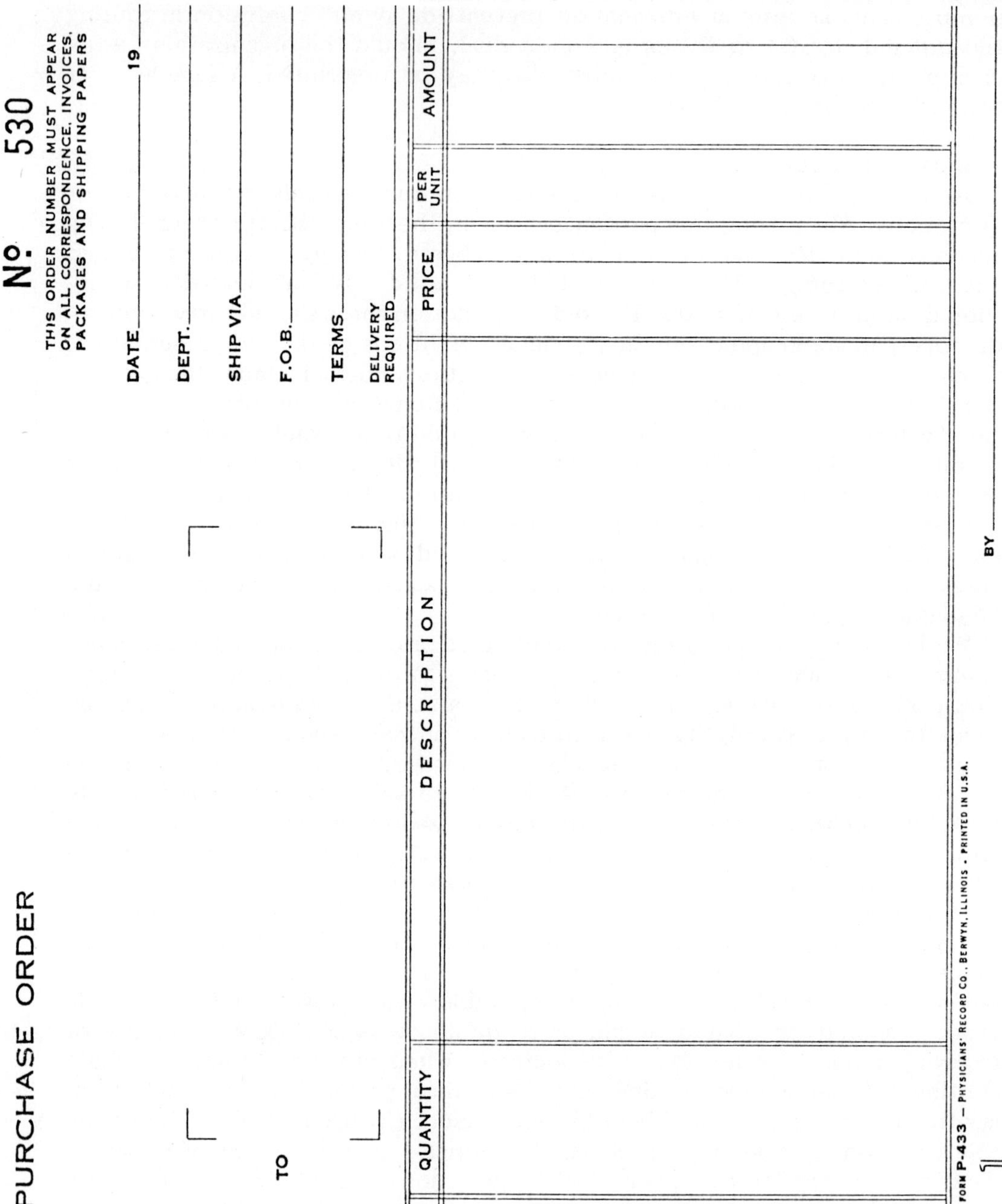

PURCHASE ORDER

No. 530

THIS ORDER NUMBER MUST APPEAR ON ALL CORRESPONDENCE, INVOICES, PACKAGES AND SHIPPING PAPERS

DATE ________ 19 ___

DEPT. ________

SHIP VIA ________

F.O.B. ________

TERMS ________

DELIVERY REQUIRED ________

TO

QUANTITY	DESCRIPTION	PRICE	PER UNIT	AMOUNT

BY ________

FORM P-433 — PHYSICIANS' RECORD CO., BERWYN, ILLINOIS - PRINTED IN U.S.A.

Figure 16-4. Purchase Order Form

Request for Quotations

General Conditions: Please quote on the below listed items. Sklar Mfg. Co. numbers for identification only. You may quote on either Sklar or equal quality. If quoting on other than Sklar, please furnish name of manufacturer and indicate warranty or guarantee. Please quote all items FOB destination. Owner reserves the right to reject all quotations. Award will be made on basis of quality as well as price, and in an all or none basis. Please return completed quotation prior to July 1, 1975.

	Number	Description	Per ea.	Total
1)	1 each	Ralks Treatment Unit, Sklar #100-90 complete. Two inch casters.	________	________
2)	4 each	Blake gallstone forceps, straight, 8¼", box lock, stainless steele, #205-140	________	________
3)	3 each	Sarot cardiovascular needle holders, very light, 7 1/8", stainless steele #280-65	________	________
		TOTAL:		________

Terms ________________ Delivery Date ________________

Firm Name ________________________________

Address ________________________________

By ________________

Title ________________

Figure 16-5. Quotation Request Form

pharmacy; if the group does not include a pharmacist, an arrangement might be made with a local pharmacist to purchase injectable medications on a cost-plus basis. Occasionally, direct sales contracts are available from pharmaceutical manufacturers, and in these special areas the medical group could deal directly with the manufacturer. Certain pharmaceutical items, however, are available only through a jobber and consequently direct purchase would not result in any financial advantage for a medical group. The numerous small drug items that usually are required on short notice also could be supplied by a clinic pharmacist or local pharmacy, or could be included in any type of special purchasing agreement between an independent pharmacy and the medical group. There also may be occasions when the pharmacist asks the medical group purchaser to obtain certain medical items for him, and this reciprocal service can be established on a basis identical to the procedure through which he sells supplies to the medical group.

In order to obtain the best price for the required quantity and also to prevent duplication of medicines under various brand names, the purchase of standard injectable medications requires careful study by the individual responsible for purchasing. There are a number of injectable medications that are exactly the same or very nearly duplicate one another, yet are packaged under different trade names. While doctors generally prescribe medication by brand name, the person responsible for purchasing can receive valuable assistance in purchasing drugs generically either from a pharmacy committee composed of group physicians or through consultation with the clinic pharmacist or an outside pharmacist. Determination of the type of medication to be used should rest solely with the medical staff, and standards of quality should not be sacrificed. In addition, the maintenance of a drug inventory that does not include a number of duplications will help to prevent unnecessary or unproductive expenditures.

Some medications are packaged in multiple-dose vials, others in single-dose units, and others in prepackaged, ready to use syringe units. There may be use for all three types of packaging within the drug inventory of the group. The multiple-dose vial generally provides a less expensive unit dose than either the single-dose vial or the syringe unit; however, date expiration and possible contamination must be considered. When using the single or syringe unit, dispensing of the mediane is perhaps more accurate. Use of the prefilled syringe unit reduces the needed stock of separate syringe and needle units and will reduce the time spent by a medical assistant or nurse in the preparation of an injection for the patient. A large variety of medications, as well as most narcotics, are available in prefilled syringe units. A widely known type of prefilled syringe unit uses a cartridge with a cartridge carrier. This product usually is packaged in lots of ten. Cartridges are available in various sizes, and each cartridge has an attached needle. It is not difficult for the assistant to choose the proper medication based on the doctor's order, and then in a relatively short time to prepare the syringe cartridge and the carrier with a controlled dose.

Regardless of the type of medications used, consideration should be given to purchasing the optimum quantity of the drugs needed, while at the same time taking advantage of quantity discounts when available without overstocking and risking lapse in drug expiration dates. Checking drug manufacturers' price lists or consulting a pharmacist will enable the individuals responsible for drug purchasing to obtain the best price for the required quantity.

Narcotics

The purchase of narcotics for the medical group requires special control and well-defined policy determinations. If the medical group decides to purchase narcotics, a special application must be completed and signed by the authorized person. The medical group must obtain a Drug Enforcement Administration (DEA) license from the United States Department of Justice, Drug Enforcement Administration, Washington, D.C., 20005. The license registration number will appear on narcotic order forms provided by the DEA. The official order form (Form BND-222C) must be completed accurately for orders of narcotics and selected amphetamines and barbiturates. A sample order form is shown in figure 16-6.

The DEA license requires an annual renewal; failure to renew will result in the group's being unable to purchase narcotics. A centrally administered procedure for the purchase of narcotics enables physicians to order narcotics for

U.S. DEPARTMENT OF JUSTICE
BUREAU OF NARCOTICS AND DANGEROUS DRUGS
OFFICIAL ORDER FORM
FOR SCHEDULE I AND II CONTROLLED SUBSTANCES

BOTH PURCHASER AND SUPPLIER MUST BE PROPERLY REGISTERED BEFORE USING THIS FORM. THIS IS AN ORDER TO SUPPLY DRUGS SPECIFIED BELOW.

NAME AND ADDRESS OF REGISTRANT

JOHN E. INGERSOLL
DIRECTOR, BNDD

BNDD REGISTRATION NO.

SCHEDULES

REGISTERED AS A

NO. OF THIS ODER FORM

TO (SUPPLIER) | STREET ADDRESS

CITY AND STATE | DATE

ITEM	NUMBER OF PACKAGES	SIZE OF PACKAGE	NAME OF ITEM		NO. OF PACKAGES RECEIVED	DATE RECEIVED
	TO BE FILLED IN BY PURCHASER				TO BE FILLED IN BY PURCHASER	
1						
2						
3						
4						
5						

THIS ORDER IS FOR EXACTLY ____ ITEMS (NUMBER OF ITEMS MUST BE SPECIFIED)

NAME OF FIRM IF NOT AN INDIVIDUAL

SIGNATURE OF PURCHASER OR HIS ATTORNEY OR AGENT

3
PURCHASER'S COPY

Figure 16-6. Controlled Substances Order Form

patient use within the clinic, as well as for use by the physician for out-of-clinic calls. It is a requirement that each physician have his own DEA license and number, also renewable annually, to be qualified to write narcotic prescription items. The physician's DEA license number also must appear on every controlled substance prescription. In addition, there may be state regulations requiring a license for the dispensing or use of other controlled substances. Information concerning this requirement may be obtained from the appropriate state medical association.

Narcotics Inventory

Narcotics inventory presents special problems for the medical group. These controlled items must be maintained in strict security and a running inventory which is checked periodically must be maintained. One possible inventory method is to retain the general supply of narcotics in a central location, preferably a safe, accessible to only one person. A smaller, day-to-day supply of narcotics could be kept in various areas as needed within the clinic, either in a locked drawer or locked box. Due to the sensitivity of the drug inventory procedures and the regulations concerning drug storage and use, a running inventory in these drawers or locked boxes also should be maintained. The inventory journal should indicate the amount of narcotics received and the date of receipt, as well as any dispensing of the narcotics. The book should list the patient's name, along with the date and dosage administered, or should contain a notation that the narcotics have been dispensed directly to a physician's bag. Narcotics do not necessarily represent a large monetary item in the inventory, but very strict federal regulations regarding controlled drugs necessitate that the best possible controls and inventory be maintained. Furthermore, the clinic administrator could take the responsibility for an occasional spot check of the narcotics inventory to determine if the amount present equals the number indicated in the inventory book. Any unusual usage or inventory discrepancy of narcotics should be reported to the clinic administrator or to the chief medical officer.

Receiving

After ordinary supplies or drugs have been ordered, the next step in the purchasing, inventory, and control process is documenting receipt of the goods. All goods received by a medical group should pass through a central point where certain items can be marked, or etched if possible, with a clinic identification number. In the receiving area, a stockroom record should be maintained giving a general indication of the material received. One possibility involves maintaining this record in a log book at the central receiving area. If there is a copy of the purchase order at the receiving location, it should be checked against the packing slip and the material received. If the order is complete, the storeroom copy of the purchasse order should be so marked and can be forwarded to accounts payable where it eventually will be verified against the itemized bill.

The use of a receiving report can be of even greater assistance in facilitating the communication necessary between the area receiving goods and accounts payable. Upon receipt of goods, a receiving report can be completed in duplicate, the original sent to accounts payable, and one copy maintained in the receiving area. A sample stockroom receiving record is shown in figure 16-7. This procedure allows accounts payable personnel to process itemized bills more rapidly, especially if the complete order has not been received. When items are back ordered, it is not possible to use the receiving area's copy of the purchase order for verification by accounts payable because the receiving area's purchase order is needed for checking future completion of the back orders. Use of a purchase order duplicate or of a receiving report, therefore, enables receiving personnel to maintain a copy of the purchase order as well as to advise accounts payable of the material received.

If a perpetual inventory card is being maintained in the receiving area, the appropriate notation indicating the change in inventory could be made on the card as items are checked in. Alternatively, the perpetual inventory card may be kept in the accounts payable section where the unit cost may be added, thus giving the group additional control on the pricing of goods. Another reason for maintaining perpetual inventory away from the receiving area is that individuals other than those who receive the goods keep the inventory, thereby providing better control against theft and unexplained losses. Duplicate inventory cards can be maintained in both receiving and accounts payable; however, each set must be continuously updated against the other.

STOCK ROOM RECEIVING RECORD

Date	No. of Pieces	Cartons Boxes Bales, Bdls.	Article	Name of Shipper	Our Order No.	Remarks

FORM A-662 PHYSICIANS' RECORD CO., BERWYN, ILLINOIS PRINTED IN U.S.A.

Figure 16–7. Stockroom Receiving Record Form

Either by use of a copy of the purchase order or through some other type of file, the receiving area should maintain a record of back orders. Routine checking of the back order file and notification of purchasing personnel will help to create flexibility in cancelling certain back orders, in reordering from a different company, or in ordering a substitute item if this is in the best interest of the group. Without proper information on the status of back orders, the purchaser may inadvertently reorder from several companies without canceling earlier orders, and after all orders have been filled he may find an excess of goods. In this situation a return agreement between the group and the supply representative would be beneficial. The practice of returning goods, however, should be kept to a minimum; the process involved takes time and is costly to both the group and the supplier. Whenever goods must be returned, a record of the return should be kept in the department initiating the return and an accurate description of the item should be listed on a returned goods credit form which is forwarded to accounts payable. The individual responsible for checking and paying bills then is aware that some supplies have been returned and that a credit memorandum is required to offset the charge that will appear on an itemized bill. A sample returned goods credit form is shown in figure 16-8. In addition, if items have been listed on the perpetual inventory and later returned, a corresponding adjustment in the perpetual inventory must be made in order to reflect the correct balance of the number of supplies on hand with the number indicated in perpetual inventory.

Paying the Bills

After a vendor has billed an order partially or completely, the shipment is usually sent to the group with a packing slip either attached or enclosed, and subsequently an invoice is mailed to the purchaser. A package slip normally contains a notation of the items enclosed, but does not itemize the prices. To minimize confusion and error, the responsibility for the receipt of invoices might be assigned to one person. If invoices are received at the accounts payable department, they can be compared to information sent from the receiving area. Each item could be checked for price and description and subsequently approved or disapproved along with an explanatory notation. At the end of the month or on a cyclical basis, the vendor usually will provide the purchaser with a statement which is an itemized list of invoice charges. At this point accounts payable could reconcile the individual invoices with those listed on the statement. If the statement is correct, the statement and invoices are attached and placed in an appropriate file for payment. Some supply companies allow a discount against the statement if the account is paid within a certain number of days. It is a good business practice to request this type of discount and to take advantage of it.

Accountability

While accountability for supplies can be managed well through the use of perpetual inventory records, accountability for clinic equipment and major items not kept in a central storage area presents a different problem. To enable a group administrator to have the best possible knowledge of the amount of money involved in equipment and major items, an inventory book could be maintained for this specific purpose. This type of record not only bears appli-

RETURNED GOODS CREDIT

Date____________________

Returned To____

____

____

____

Received By__________________________

FORM A-661 PHYSICIANS' RECORD CO., BERWYN, ILLINOIS PRINTED IN U.S.A.

Figure 16-8. Returned Goods Credit Form

cation to the group's balance sheet where such items would be listed as assets, but also is a useful tool for measuring insurance needs and a convenient method of checking for loss of equipment.

The group administrator may find an equipment and major item inventory book useful in evaluations for insurance purposes. In establishing the inventory book system, each room within the clinic could be assigned a number and could be represented by a specific inventory page. An equipment and inventory form is shown in figure 16-9. To put this plan into action a responsible individual who works in each room could complete the inventory of equipment and major items for that room. The inventory list then is incorporated into the equipment and major item inventory book located in the administrator's or comptroller's office. A copy of each room list could be maintained in the individual room to which it applies, where it could be posted and periodically checked for accuracy. This particular plan, however, does not permit easy relocation of furniture items. Some type of card file with a card for each major item of furniture or equipment should be maintained at a central location with a duplicate file maintained off the clinic premises. Each major equipment item also should carry an inventory identification number which should be recorded on the inventory card along with the series number, model number, make, and description of the item.

MAINTENANCE

Maintenance responsibilities may vary according to whether the group owns or leases the building. Maintenance may be provided by the building owner as part of a rental or lease agreement. When the medical group owns its own building, however, maintenance usually is provided either by the group's own maintenance staff or by an outside contractor. Maintenance, like purchasing, should be under the direct supervision of the group administrator, who delegates authority to the proper individual on the maintenance staff. If the medical group is renting or leasing space, the rent or lease agreement should state clearly who is responsible for major repairs and/or building modifications. The agreement also should state whether or not the approval of the owner is required for building modification.

Equipment and Instrument Inventory

Room No. ________ Date ______________

Item Number	Description	Required	Inventory	Value
1	Exam table	1	1	$ 525.00
2	Exam stool	1	1	85.00
3	Chairs, fibre glass	1	2	90.00
4	Suture scissors, 5", st.	2	2	24.00
5	Forceps, thumb, 5"	2	2	18.00
6	Forceps, Mosquito, cvd.	4	4	36.00
7	Forceps, Mosquito, st.	4	4	36.00
			Total	$1162.00

Figure 16-9. Room Equipment and Instrument Inventory Form

It would be unusual for groups of ten physicians or less to be able to employ qualified maintenance personnel who are expert in all required areas. An effective alternative is to rely upon skilled local people on an as-needed basis. When employing outside workers, however, the group should secure in writing an estimate of the cost of the anticipated repairs or modifications. In the event that the estimates exceed a nominal amount, such as $100, a contract calling for an itemized bill for labor and materials should be requested. Workers should not be engaged for repairs or modifications without a prior agreement regarding cost of completion and time requirements of the project. The group, however, may choose to contract on a cost-plus, guaranteed maximum, or other basis. The time of day during which the work will be carried on also must be ascertained and, if possible, suited to the convenience of the group's schedule.

A medical group should be familiar with building safety and fire regulations covered not only by local and state rules, but also under the Occupational

Safety and Health Act (OSHA). OSHA regulations are necessarily strict and building construction or modification of any size should not be planned without first determining the OSHA regulations. The group administrator can make periodic inspections, both scheduled and unscheduled, of the group's facility in order to determine whether or not the safety and fire regulations are being followed. Such inspections would include monitoring compliance with the requirement that fire extinguishers be checked annually for convenience, adequacy, and proper tagging.

Major equipment purchased by the group usually carries a specified guarantee or warranty, a written copy of which should be maintained in case of future need. The medical group usually will have an option concerning whether preventive maintenance and repairs on major equipment items is to be provided by the group itself or arranged through a contract maintenance agreement. As technology contributes to the sophistication of equipment, it is often economically more advantageous to allow the manufacturer to provide contract maintenance, which usually includes preventive as well as repair maintenance. As equipment is purchased, availability of such maintenance contracts should be explored and needs and responsibilities should be determined.

Housekeeping

Housekeeping, or the general upkeep of the clinic facility, may be the responsibility of the owner of the building or of the group itself. The purchase of housekeeping supplies may be delegated either to the head housekeeper, to the maintenance supervisor, or to the individual responsible for purchasing for the group. Purchasing for housekeeping should have the same guidelines that apply to purchasing in general. Good housekeeping is an essential consideration to the group, because of the degree of cleanliness required in a medical facility and because of the public relations impact of a clean, orderly building. While patients may not always be capable of evaluating their medical service, they are perfectly capable of making a judgment on the cleanliness of their surroundings—and they will make this judgment whether or not it is solicited. Routine housekeeping activities usually are conducted after clinic hours, but emergencies during daily operating hours necessitate the capability for continuous housekeeping. The group may contract with an outside agency to perform the routine housekeeping activities, and for housekeeping requirements which occur during the day, responsibility may need to be delegated to personnel in maintenance, purchasing, etc.

When the group employs contract housekeepers, the group administrator contracts with either an individual or a company for certain specific jobs. The group may elect to employ its own housekeeping staff but periodically may require a contract housekeeper to clean carpets, walls, etc. The need for contract housekeepers will vary among groups, and group administrators should consider some of the advantages resulting from the contract arrangement. Usually such an arrangement eliminates the need to buy expensive housekeeping equipment, such as buffing machines, carpet cleaners, and other capital items. In addition, while the group does not have to pay directly the employer portion of Social Security taxes for the work done and does not make contributions to pension plans, contract housekeeping services do take these benefits into account when determining their fees.

Grounds

The upkeep of medical facility grounds represents no special problem if responsibilities are effectively delegated. The grounds, especially the parking lots, must be kept litter free. In addition, designating parking slots by striping the parking lot will result in better utilization of the lot. Contract groundskeeping can provide a means of conserving capital required for grounds equipment because such services usually maintain costly equipment such as sidewalk vacuums and striping machines. If competent groundskeepers are contracted on a seasonal basis as needed, unnecessary overstaffing can be avoided. For example, although the clinic maintains the outside facilities, special jobs such as seasonal spraying of shrubs and trees and/or extensive snow removal may be contracted with a special service organization. Such contracts should be negotiated before the actual need arises.

Security

Security needs for the medical group facility will vary by community and according to the various segments served within the community. In smaller communities, security may be delegated primarily to the local police department. In a high risk area, however, a group may employ its own security guard or night watchman or may contract for a guard. As in the case of housekeeping and groundskeeping, contracting an outside security agent may provide the best answer for security needs. Regardless of the guard arrangements, the medical facility should be well-illuminated. Because a large number of clinic employees may be female it is especially important that the parking lot be lighted adequately. In addition, the group will want to make certain that the building is secure during nonworking hours. This responsibility may be delegated to the maintenance supervisor and may be augmented by burglar-alarm systems tied into the neighborhood police switch board. Effective security can result in reduced insurance premiums.

Vehicles

Some medical groups may require a motor vehicle for delivery, pickups, or other purposes. If the group does own or lease some type of vehicle, responsibility for its maintenance may be assigned to the maintenance department. The group should consider and determine policy guidelines for the personal use of clinic-owned motor vehicles, and it may be wise to indicate that under no circumstances should a vehicle be used for personal reasons without the express permission or notification of the group administrator. The administrator also should consider securing *liability* insurance coverage in an amount of at least one million dollars, either under the group's basic or umbrella policy. Liability insurance is important regardless of the group's organizational form or attitude toward insuring the vehicle itself.

The development of effective procedures and well-formulated policies in the areas of purchasing, supply inventory, and maintenance is important to the newly forming group so that physicians are able to pursue the practice of medicine in a group practice environment which is both orderly and economically viable.

Chapter 17

Personnel Systems

PERSONNEL ADMINISTRATION

In the delivery of health care, the importance and impact of human resources far outweigh the physical resources necessary to maintain a viable organization. The marketed product is a service delivered by human beings in accordance with goals and objectives established and agreed upon within the group of which they are a part. Personnel administration is the systematic management of human resources in which an effort should be made to initiate integration of individual employee goals with the objectives held to be important to the group practice. Personnel administration and the various systems which support and guide the administration of employee interrelationships has the twofold objective of ensuring the success of the group practice while maintaining the individual dignity of employees by seeking their contributions to the decision-making process. The group's particular value system will be reflected in the administration of personnel relations through a communication system which functions laterally and vertically within the organizational structure.

Critical to any discussion of employer-employee relationships is the designation of one person within the group who will be accountable for administration and control of personnel systems. A physician in the practice may be especially qualified for such responsibility, including personnel recruiting, job orientation, employee counseling, salary administration, discipline, and the assessment of personnel relationships. As the group grows, group members may not be able to devote sufficient time and effort to the management of personnel systems and may wish to consider hiring a clinic manager or administrator who is accountable on a full-time basis for all business and legal matters.

Personnel administration is complex. It will reflect not only the group's value system and the personalities of the group's members, but also the community's expectations and attitudes. It is wise to consult an attorney on a regular basis regarding changing state and federal laws which may affect employee relations. Law suits filed by disgruntled or terminated employees are nurtured in an environment of obsolete, illegal personnel practices. Larger groups may find an industrial psychologist in the community to be of assistance in recruiting and selecting personnel, in resolving conflicts, and in implementing human relations practices and procedures. Consulting regularly with hospital departments of personnel and employee relations concerning changing wage and salary administration, changing legal requirements, and employee relations precedents and practices also may be helpful. State hospital associations and city personnel administrator associations are additional information sources. Finally, it is possible that the group itself may have a psychologist on the staff who is willing to provide assistance.

Personnel administration also demands time and continuous attention. Attrition and changing attitudes contribute to this state of flux. As the objectives and mission of the group change, the types of employee skills necessary and possibly the types of employee personalities required may differ. Systems become obsolete and as a result personnel practices can become chaotic.

The impact of sensitive personnel policies and practices is of even greater significance. As colleague physicians work together and as physicians supervise paraprofessionals and clerical employees in group practice, everyone in the clinic may become immediately aware of omissions in guidelines for covering individual requests and personal needs. It is helpful to develop a personnel manual specifically designed for a particular group practice, the purpose of which is not to encourage bureaucracy or organizational rigidity, but to provide a mutually acceptable framework for working and operating together. A personnel manual or handbook should be a dynamic document, not an archeological relic to be placed on a dusty shelf and forgotten. Its usefulness depends upon maintaining its currency as an up-to-date reflection of the group's changing requirements and the needs of everyone within the organization. Employee enthusiasm and commitment will be inhibited by antiquated, punishing, and insensitive policies and procedures.

Dissatisfaction also may develop from perceived inadequacies in status, salary, and security, from ineffectual supervision and relations, and from restrictive working conditions. When the importance of such factors is not heeded, job dissatisfaction accelerates. The failure on the part of an employee to identify with his job, costly employee turnover, poor morale, friction, and in-fighting are obvious results. Job identification and productivity also can be influenced by the job itself, by job responsibility and recognition, by authority and influence, by the opportunity to learn and develop, and by achievement and advancement opportunities. Committed group employees are generally those who have been granted these intrinsic rewards.

Employee Motivation and Job Commitment

Studies reveal that many employees in the health care field are dissatisfied with their jobs and that, as a result, group medical practices unnecessarily lose a visible percentage of talented people. Less obvious than these problems, however, is the costly incidence of on-the-job retirement. Some unmotivated group employees have almost no capability yet continue to remain on the payroll. In terms of human potential and worth to the group, there probably are even more instances in which a person's talents are used restrictively. Such a waste of personnel is especially debilitating for a health organization whose prime objective is the achievement of performance objectives in the field of patient care. These problems might be partially alleviated by a pragmatic understanding of the nature of motivation which comes from *within* the employee, rather than that which is generated externally by management. The personnel administrator's awareness of the nuances and complexities of task identification will result in more involved and committed employees and fellow physicians.

Many group practice administrators believe that their approach is effective and cannot understand why employees are unresponsive to attempts to instill motivation. A number of fallacies exist in current thinking on motivation. For example, in order to save his clerical staff the "embarrassment" incurred or the time lost because of an assignment's being done incorrectly, a group practice manager may insist that all details, no matter how small, be prescribed and resolved by him. By understanding that an integral part of a person's job motivation is the pride inherent in self-initiated responsibility, this group practice manager might discover that his personnel are adept and eager to handle assignments, that they can monitor their projects through self-direction, and that they enjoy reporting, "That was *my* decision," when an action is questioned. A second widely-held belief concerning motivation is that employees work primarily to receive money. Money does not have the sustaining effect of motivating performance; its effect usually is short-lived. Above a certain level of remuneration, pecuniary motivation is of secondary interest. Sufficient pay can temporarily guarantee that an individual appear on the job, but it cannot induce job interest.

Some supervisors direct their staffs in much the same way that a manipulative kindergarten teacher would control a rambunctious group of five year olds. Strategies such as granting personal favors and soliciting through personality appeals often are ineffective. Another approach involves creating a competitive environment. When these tactics fail, supervisors may resort to exercising authority by speaking from a stance of power and control. An insensitive manager may try to induce fear and threaten his employees, with his own fear of humiliation as the impetus underlying his action. Implicit in this type of behavior is an authoritarian management attitude of superiority. An administrator who confuses extrinsic pressure with the self-released, internal elements constituting motivation is handicapped in his managerial perceptions. Such an approach breeds distrust, disunity, and resentment in an organization. Performance commitment begins with the employees' internal desire to work because of the inherent meaningfulness of the work itself. An effective manager will be aware that there may be a number of ways to motivate each individual, that no two people are ever alike, and that coping with life and job events differs with each person. Individual employees will differ according to:

1. *Job Expectations.* Individual job expectations will depend on the employee's maturity, age, and past job and employer experiences. Whereas one person may approach with interest and enjoyment a position requiring patient contact, another employee may be happier in a clerical position with central supply. The effective manager evaluates individual interests, job expectations, and different personality needs before assigning responsibilities and thereby avoids creating an inappropriate job situation and climate which results in poor self-initiating behavior and job discomfort.

2. *Skills and Abilities.* By recognizing and reinforcing employee talents, a manager is able to match a person's interest with his work assignments and can increase an individual's job identification.

3. *Individual Work Values.* What constitutes worth in any employee's work life is as varied as people's expertise. An effective manager considers different work values in assigning tasks and is aware of his employees' basic attitudes toward vocation and life style. For example, some individuals may be frustrated and unproductive in a position where they can see no beneficial outcome from their endeavors.

4. *Past Job Experience.* An ingredient which shapes a person's present job motivation is his past, work-related experience. It is unwise to assign a project requiring a certain expertise in human relations to an employee who has experienced failures in similar situations in the past. He may be unsure of his own ability and, lacking self-confidence, may be preparing psychologically for another failure. Being aware of and sensitive to individual differences of employees and their perceptions of their jobs are important factors in hiring and motivating personnel.

Prior to beginning group practice employment, each applicant has certain preconceptions and expectations related to job satisfaction. Often, when prior conceptions are not consistent with actual job experiences, a lack of compatibility between expectations and job realities results for both employer and employee. If an employer makes a conscientious effort to inform an employee exactly what is expected of him, the employee is not as likely to make false inferences about the purpose of his work, his position in the group, or his required contribution. It should be remembered that constructive interest, together with helpful counseling, can in itself contribute support for mutual understanding.

Motivation is directly related to the amount of purpose the employee sees in his work. That work should fulfill his desire to make a significant contribution and should be integrated with his concept of self. In other words, to be motivated, an employee needs to feel a sense of importance. A temporary person, employed through a manpower rental agency and assigned to different organizations every week, will not have the commitment to a job that a full-time employee may have. Some permanent employees, however, may seem detached, uninterested, and dissatisfied with their work. In addition to reexamining such individuals' particular interests, skills, work values and personality needs, the group should try to stimulate job identification. Personal recognition is vital and meaningful, but group acceptance of an individual's work also is important for motivational release. For a clinic administrator to try to change employees' personalities is most difficult. It is far better to approach the managerial challenge from a different perspective and to gear assignments to the individual's personality.

Each person also has a desire to develop and to grow, thereby reinforcing his self-worth. The German poet Goethe expressed how the need to become can be released: "If you treat a man as he is, he will remain as he is; if you treat him as if he were what he could be, he will become what he could be." Such a motivational prescription seems obvious, yet it is one that too few managers put into practice. A person's sense of status also is directly related to the influence he believes he has in his work. By establishing opportunities for a person to exercise influence and to make decisions on his own, a clinic manager is helping the individual to *be* important, not just to feel important. An administrator can create a sense of job and personal importance by being receptive to suggestions from employees and by giving them a chance to communicate with management. An administrator's actual willingness to spend time intently listening to an employee is an indication of the importance he assigns first to this person as a human being and, secondly, to the employee's ideas. True job motivation includes not only the opportunity to initiate new ideas and to make decisions, but also to profit from errors as well. The motivated employee who has been given the freedom and managerial support to commit himself can learn from occasional mistakes and will feel a responsibility for his errors. He also will feel committed to the job because of the responsibility and trust he has been given.

Establishing a climate for real achievement and responsibility is another means of stimulating drive and commitment. Ultimately, individual goals are integrated with the long-term goals and mission of the group practice. One mark of a climate conducive to achievement is the existence of clear lines of authority for decision-making. Taking into consideration an employee's particular talents, job interests, and goals, he and the administrator must determine how various potential can best be put to use. A motivational environment depends upon shared authority (see Chapter 6) together with a bond of trust between supervisor and employee. The administrator, however, is entitled to be kept informed when the employee decides on a course of action. A second characteristic of an achievement-oriented environment is the mutual determination of goals on a bimonthly or trimonthly basis. When this approach is combined with the administrator's awareness of each individual's personality needs and need to participate and to influence, job objectives become alive and relevant to the employee. A clinic administrator should develop with his employees well-defined tasks which call for significant contributions. The atmosphere must be open, with no hidden expectations on either side.

Terms of Employment

Most people accept a position according to the employment terms as described in an interview or in casual conversation with the interviewer. When employing professional or paraprofessional people, however, there are times when a formal employment letter/contract is advisable. This contract usually outlines employer expectations, conditions of employment, salary quoted on a weekly/monthly basis, reasons for separation or termination, and, possibly, conditions under which investment in ownership may be merited. An attorney should assist with the details of this agreement. Whether formal or informal, the agreement between group and employee is based largely upon goodwill and a desire to understand the other person's position. An employment agreement should be a flexible understanding between employer and employee which may be modified at any time depending upon the demands of the group practice organization, health industry concerns, or the needs of the individuals involved. Job climate will be established by the terms of employment. Individual dedication as well as group spirit result from management policies which reflect a genuine interest in people, patients as well as employees.

It is most important that any unusual or irregular conditions of employment be spelled out clearly in the employment agreement. For example, part-time employees may not be eligible for certain benefits received by permanent employees. Eligibility for pension plans, profit plans, medical services, or other fringe benefits also should be made clear. In addition, any unusual requisites for temporary, part-time, or permanent employment should be indicated. If permanent employment is dependent upon successful completion of a probationary period, a physical exam, and/or positive reference checks, these requirements should be communicated to the individual before he makes a commitment to the group. Under Occupational Safety and Health Act (OSHA) legislation, the employer is obligated to provide a safe and healthful environment for employees. Preemployment physical examinations contribute to the maintenance of a healthful environment, and not hiring personnel with health hazards helps to protect the premium structure of group insurance programs. If the hiring clinic is to be responsible for conducting preemployment physicals, it must be determined how these examinations will be divided among group physicians. If each prospective employee's own physician will perform the employment physical, payment for the service must be assigned. Responsibility for notification of results also must be delegated. To maintain a healthful environment and the stability of the benefits program, criteria for possible follow-up physicals for correctible ailments must be established and arrangements for annual physicals and periodic immunizations for present employees also must be made.

ORIENTATION

The purpose of orientation is to familiarize new personnel with the systems and procedures adopted by the group, to help new employees become acquainted with current staff members, and to improve service to patients through a well-informed staff. Instituting an orientation program first involves delegating to the personnel director or to the departmental supervisors responsibility for presenting the program. Or the group may rely on audio/visual presentations for part of the program. Areas of emphasis in the orientation program might include:

1. Tour of the facility
2. Fire drill demonstration and location of fire-fighting equipment
3. Organization's history
4. Understanding key systems, policies, and benefits

5. Management and organizational structure
6. Recognition (by sight) of key personnel.

In addition, the individual supervisor may wish to provide the new employee with more specific orientation information.

Position Definition and Descriptions

A job description is based upon the definition and analysis of job functions, the limits of authority for decision making, the assignment of specific responsibilities, and the activities that comprise a job or series of tasks. The greatest single source of job descriptions is the United States Labor Department's *Dictionary of Occupational Titles*. Specifically, group practice job definitions should state what is to be done, the results expected, how the job is to be done, and why it is to be done. Job descriptions also should provide information on significant aptitudes, interests, and temperaments required for adequate performance. No job description can be exhaustive, partially because no job remains static. If, for example, 75 percent of the nursing jobs in a medical group practice have elements in common, responsibilities involved in the remaining 25 percent should be delineated clearly. A job description or position definition should be as explicit and as operational as possible. It should be dated and should indicate the clinic section for which it was written. Routinely, job descriptions should include the following types of information:

1. Occupational title and any other names by which the position is known
2. Organizational relationships
   a. Title of the person to whom the employee reports
   b. Supervision, if any, of other personnel
   c. Responsibility for coordinating the job with others
3. A brief, written summary of the primary functions or responsibilities of the position
4. An enumeration of tasks to be performed, such as a listing of specific duties perhaps with percentage or indications of how time might be spent per week/day
   a. Principal duties and decision making areas
   b. Tasks/activities which might be delegated (but controlled)
   c. Combination tasks such as working/coordinating with other people in joint activities or functions.

A job description and the analysis which precedes it is intended to ensure that an employee understands the primary accountabilities of his job. On the basis of an appropriate job description, differentiations can be made in terms of responsibilities, and both salary ranges and levels of authority can be determined. Job descriptions also contribute in the interviewing and employee selection process by providing a basis for understanding how the organization works and what is expected from the potential employee. Well-written job descriptions can be most helpful in:

1. Hiring, orienting, and inducting new employees
2. Follow-up and training
3. Reviewing performance

4. Preventing dissatisfaction or settling complaints
5. Transferring, upgrading, promoting, or downgrading/termination.

Job descriptions should be related to the organizational structure of the group (see Chapter 6) and may be centralized and general; for example, all clerical personnel fall within the same job category. On the other hand, job descriptions may be departmental and specific, such as that of the medical records secretary, which differs from that of the appointments secretary. It also is possible for the group to utilize a hybrid approach which could result in job descriptions for the nursing staff being stated generally for all nurses, while job descriptions for clerical personnel would be delineated specifically for each position. Lastly, as a practical rule-of-thumb, position descriptions should be reviewed and, if necessary, revised, at least every two to three years.

Because a small group practice is not likely to have the resources to devote to job analysis and job description, descriptions may be borrowed from other health care institutions and may be used as a guide. It is important, however, that any borrowed job description be modified and adapted to the particular situation and that it clearly spell out the differences between the way the group expects to operate and the ways in which the group may differ from the traditional process of placement found in other health institutions.

Salary Administration

In any discussion of wage and salary administration it is important to emphasize that the purpose of such a program is not necessarily motivational. It may be only supportive with the basic purpose being to provide fair treatment and adequate reward for comparable job responsibilities, efforts, and achievement. While salaries should be competitive with those in the recruiting market place, many other factors make a job rewarding or satisfying. Money should not be thought of as the most important factor, particularly in the health field.

Because salary schedules have so many legal implications, it is mandatory that any program be discussed thoroughly with an attorney. Both the federal government and the state governments have provisions concerning age and sex discrimination, minimum wages and overtime, length of the work week, and exemptions based upon a number of employment factors. Recruiting success and attrition rates are indicative of adequacy of wage and salary structures. The group's wage structure should be reviewed at least annually to ensure conformance with changing conditions, both internal and external. Each employee's performance and wage/salary should be reviewed at least annually; for newer employees or for those on probation, thirty- or ninety-day review periods could be instituted.

A salary program should provide ranges for each job category or for closely related families of jobs. Jobs may be ranked in a hierarchy from most to least complex, or according to the degree of complexity of various factors which enter into the jobs. A narrow wage range can be provided for jobs classified at a lower level and a broader range for jobs classified at higher levels. This system will produce a curve resulting in entry level jobs having only about 10 percent variation between the starting rate and ceiling rate, whereas the upper level jobs may have a 50 percent differential. Thus, growth, tenure, and merit differences, as well as other considerations, can be included. Generally, it is recommended that only wage/salary *ranges* be made known to the employees via job descriptions. This knowledge may create some stimulus for the employee to pursue additional training to increase his professional competence and financial growth. It is important that merit salary increases be based upon standards which are easily recognizable by the employees and which can be applied fairly across all jobs at the same level.

Length of service increases may cancel out the value of merit increases. In some cases, if an employee is not performing satisfactorily, he should be replaced or his responsibilities and wage level should be realigned with actual performance. It is possible, however, that the now unproductive, marginal employee was once a cornerstone of the organization. Some managers may feel that the organization has a responsibility to such people and, if so, it may be possible to freeze such a person's salary. In general, salary increases should reflect cost-of-living adjustments of between 4 percent and 8 percent, merit and recognition of performance excellence between 5 percent and 12 percent, and/or both. Increases usually are spaced between eight to eighteen months. It also must be decided if every employee will be evaluated at a time corresponding to the organization's fiscal year, or if each employee will be evaluated on his employment anniversary date. In addition, special evaluations may be possible at any time depending upon extenuating circumstances.

Performance Appraisal and Review

Clerical and paraprofessional medical employees should know how their performance is perceived by the administration. Stronger employees will demand to know if they are performing satisfactorily, what they can do to improve their performance, and how they can move up in the organization. Management should indicate to employees when their performance is excellent, satisfactory, or below standard. Formal employee evaluation is important for determination of salary increases and promotions as well as for counseling, communication, and rapport. Preprinted forms, narrative written descriptions, or a combination of both may be used in evaluation procedures (see Appendix 17A). Examples should be available from other health care institutions. Each group, however, will have unique requirements which must be reflected in the evaluation instrument chosen.

When developing a performance appraisal or rating form, it is important to maintain as much objectivity as possible. Generally, the fewer the number of factors being rated, the easier and simpler the evaluation is to administer. With a relatively small number of people under consideration, it might be easier to rank people in order, establishing satisfactory performance as the median point. A single, overall judgment, however, is not sufficient for a meaningful performance appraisal system, the purpose of which is not only to recognize acceptable behavior but also to stimulate performance in different task areas. It is necessary, therefore, to identify and record positive job behavior as well as performance deficiencies.

For long-term employees and for the new staff member, evaluations should be conducted annually and more often during the early months of employment. While standards for performance usually are stated in the job description, a great deal of performance review will be subjective. In a small group practice, some degree of objectivity can be maintained by having all managerial people rate individuals and pool the findings. Another alternative is to have only the supervisor rate employees, with the manager or personnel director reviewing the rating. For technical personnel in a group, the physician's input is valuable and can be combined with the administrator's analysis to produce an overall evaluation.

To effectively evaluate employees, a personnel record system should be established. Such records ensure continuity and relieve management of the task of remembering details concerning each employee. Records provide personal data, evaluations, consultations, pay history, recognitions, and documentation of personnel activities. In this area, confidentiality can be a key issue, and it is important to determine exactly who has access to such files. In addition, length of retention and active/inactive designations must be decided upon.

Employee Counseling

At times, every employee needs counseling, guidance, or job coaching. There is a distinction, however, between the need for professional therapy and the usual job related occasions when people become confused, uncertain, or preoccupied, thus affecting job performance. From management's viewpoint, it is important to be alert to such situations. A preoccupied or irritated employee can cause strained relationships between both patients and fellow staff members. Counseling may help to reduce such friction and also may help to provide direction and to maintain control, to correct deficiencies and misunderstandings, and to improve efficiency and effectiveness from both a business and a personal standpoint.

Personalities and individual differences can have a major impact upon small groups. The group should decide who in the organization will act as counselors—physicians, administrators, personnel supervisors, etc. The counseling process itself may be oral, written, or a combination of these, and always should be carried out discreetly so that confidentiality is maintained and embarrassment avoided. For additional guidance in dealing with a problem employee or employees with problems, the group may consult a local organizational psychologist. An example counseling plan is shown in figure 17-1.

The role of counselor is an unnatural one for many people. The counselor's own value system must be sublimated for him to be nonevaluative and nonjudgmental in dealing with an employee's problems. First and foremost, the counselor is attempting to facilitate *intra*personal communication. To initiate an employee counseling process in response to a specific situation, the employer can:

1. Help the employee to define the situation
2. Encourage the employee's free expression of feelings which usually are negative at first—for example, fear, anger, and anxiety
3. Help the employee to accept and recognize such hostile feelings as natural under the circumstances
4. Help the employee to clarify whatever insight he has about himself
5. Help the employee to clarify possible decisions and attendant courses of action.

This form should be used for organizing thoughts, and is not to be given to the employee.

Employee Name ____________________

1. How long has the employee worked at the clinic? ____________________
2. How has the employee improved his (her) performance during the past year?
____
____
3. What do you particularly like about this employee?
____
____
____
4. What would you like to change about this employee?
____
____
____
5. What can the employee do to improve his (her) performance?
____
____
____
6. What will the supervisor do to help the employee? ____________________
____
____
7. What work can the employee be complimented on? ____________________
____
____
8. How long since last salary increase? ____________________
Amount of increase? $ ____________.
9. Next salary increase? $ ____________. When? ____________
10. Is employee now at top of automatic increase schedule? ____________
Possible next increase date? ____________________

Comments of Supervisor (following counseling session): ____________________
____
____

____________________ Date ____________________ Supervisor

Figure 17-1. Employee Counseling Planning Outline

Situations to avoid in counseling employees include prying or probing, overly praising, criticizing or making negative evaluations, interpreting an employee's behavior, or giving advice and making suggestions.

Conditions of Work

Every employee should know under what conditions work is to be performed. Conditions should be stated clearly so that there is no doubt about business hours and unusual but anticipated demands such as overtime, Sunday work, or coverage during holidays. Fringe benefits, vacations, rest breaks, and time off for such things as sick leave, family death, or jury duty should be indicated as should guidelines for personal conduct.

Violation of office rules requires some type of constructive discipline and a definite and recognizable degree of reprimand if the rules or procedures are violated continually. Discipline need not be harsh but should be consistent, well defined and recorded and enforced without inequities. Personnel handbooks can be secured from a variety of medical institutions in order to ascertain the range of topic areas and the type of wording generally used. An elaborately printed handbook is not necessary; an inexpensive three-ring binder with pages divided into various sections should suffice. If the group's facility is close to or furnishes services to a larger health care institution, such as a hospital, it is mandatory that the personnel policies of that institution be kept firmly in mind when stipulating group working conditions. The list below indicates areas that should be covered in describing the expectations which management has of its employees:

1. Absence and tardiness
2. The reporting of accidents and injuries
3. Appearance, courtesy, and office dress code
4. Confidential information (business, employee, and patient)
5. Discipline
6. Employee record changes
7. Fire prevention and fire drills (disaster planning)
8. Identification and office security
9. Lunch and coffee breaks
10. Time cards or recording of attendance
11. Personal mail and phone calls
12. Physical examinations
13. Problems and complaints
14. Safety
15. Smoking
16. Soliciting for contributions, drives, causes, etc.
17. Termination—voluntary and involuntary
18. Grievances and employee suggestions.

Discipline and Termination

Termination of employment should be considered only after all other avenues have been exhausted. The courts have ruled that in order to discharge an employee, the employer must document the employee's violation of published rules and procedures of the organization. It is incumbent upon the employer to show that management has followed its prescribed disciplinary procedures before bringing about a termination and that the employee continued to violate rules after being given an explicit warning. Most termination procedures involve a written disciplinary notice to the employee, with a copy placed on file. An attorney can advise a group on exact procedures to be followed in instances of involuntary termination.

Some serious offenses, such as stealing, a drinking problem which interferes with job completion, or direct insubordination can contribute to immediate dismissal. Grievance procedures or legal hearings are apt to be unpleasant. If employees know the rules and the procedures which are to be followed and know that such rules are enforced impartially and without favoritism, employers are less likely to be brought into court. It should be stated to all employees that during a probationary period of from thirty to ninety days, a new employee may be terminated for any cause whatsoever. During this period, irritating personal habits and marginal performance characteristics can be the basis for discharge. After the probationary period, however, whatever cause may exist must be based solidly on marginal performance or violations of stated rules or procedures. There will be times when misunderstandings arise, when people are unhappy with their work, or when there are personality differences which make job performance somewhat difficult. Such conditions may call more for counseling than for discipline. If a job performance situation grows more serious, however, decisive action must be taken.

It must be decided who in the group will carry out involuntary terminations—supervisor, personnel director, or administrator. The terms for such terminations as well as requirements of notice—usually two weeks for both clinic and employee—also should be clearly delineated. Often, a group physician is involved in the circumstances leading to the involuntary termination of an employee. At such times, it is helpful if the group has already established a firm policy stipulating the *degree* of his involvement. Policies may differ as to what is owed the discharged employee. At the low end of the scale, accrued pay may be the only compensation due an employee. Group policy, however, might dictate the payment of accrued pay plus accrued vacation with a week's pay for each year of service. How generous or conservative the group may be should be consistent with the rest of its personnel policies and its attitude toward employees.

At the point of termination, it should be clear to the employee what references, if any, he may expect from the group. Termination may not reflect a personal failure on the employee's part but rather a divergence between his desires and motivations and the circumstances of the job. If so, this fact should be communicated to the individual. Employees appreciate firmness and honesty from management. It has been shown that severity is not intolerable as long as all the published rules are enforced equally. It is when management is arbitrary—acting leniently and then tightening the rules—that employees become dissatisfied.

Benefits

As an area of financial concern for clinic management, benefits should be established only after careful thought and cost projecting. Benefits emanate from several sources (see Chapter 9). Traditionally, hospitals and other major health care institutions have not paid high wages, but have compensated by giving more benefits in lieu of higher wages or salary. In establishing a benefit program, the group should investigate the benefit structure of other local organizations. When recruiting personnel, those benefits which are based upon results, productivity, or efficiency should be emphasized. Nurses and technicians usually prefer a clinic environment rather than a hospital environment;

nevertheless, the cost of living dictates that acceptable wages and benefits must be competitive. The organization should provide benefits for its personnel that individually they would or could not provide for themselves. For example, insurance coverage, whether individual or group, means little until it becomes necessary to use it. If benefits constituted 8 percent of salaries and in lieu of the benefits the employer increased wages by 8 percent, the individual employees still could not purchase the same amount of benefits as were available through the purchasing power of the group as a whole. While the amount and scope of benefits will vary from group to group, some benefits, such as workmen's compensation, are mandatory in most states. Other insurance covering major medical, hospitalization, life and disability, or the providing of health services and medical care should be discussed with an insurance agent or consultant. Many of these programs are necessary under law and, therefore, have become so standardized that legal aid is probably not required.

As a rule of sound business practice, it is much better to draft a policy statement concerning available benefits before the actual need for such a statement arises. As situations occur, hasty and inconsistent decisions often are made which later cause difficulty or set a poor precedent. Almost any hasty decision may be interpreted by the employee as in the best interest of management and against the interest of the employee. The list below indicates some of the major benefit areas:

1. Insurance
   a. Basic hospitalization and major medical coverage
   b. Life
   c. Short- and long-term disability coverage
   d. Malpractice (both paramedical and physicians)
2. Health services, medical, and dental care
3. Vacations and vacation pay
4. Paid holidays and allowable personal time off
   a. Leave of absence
   b. Sickness
   c. Emergency time off
   d. Maternity
   e. Jury duty
   f. National Guard or military
   g. Voting or political activity
5. Retirement and pension plan
6. Workmen's compensation
7. Profit sharing or bonus arrangements
8. Educational allowances and reimbursement policies
9. Employee facilities
   a. Lunchroom
   b. Locker space or personal storage
   c. Parking
10. Extra pay provisions
    a. Shift premium
    b. Overtime
    c. Holiday pay

d. Bereavement pay, etc.
e. Allowance for uniform cleaning or clinic-provided uniforms.

Employee benefits may be rights or they may be privileges. Today many benefits have become routine expectations. Although it is more likely that benefits will be meaningful when they are evaluated on a local basis, the results of a 1973 national survey of seventy-two group practices and hospitals (see pages 8-9 of the January/February 1975 issue of *Medical Group Management* can provide guidelines to forming groups. The key results of that, *Journal of the MGMA*) survey are summarized below:

1. *Holidays*—Thirty-one different holidays were provided for, but the average number of total holidays was 7.1 days.
2. *Vacations* varied according to length of employment:
   a. Less than one year—average of 6.4 days
   b. One to five years—average of 10.6 days
   c. Six to ten years—average of 14 days
   d. Ten plus years—average of 16.1 days.
3. *Sick leave* averaged 11.4 days per year.
4. *Leave of absence* averaged a maximum of 159 days.
5. *Insurance benefits:*
   a. Medical insurance benefits were provided by 87 percent of the organizations.
   b. Life insurance was provided by 84.2 percent of the organizations; benefits ranged from $1,000-$50,000, and 92.5 percent of the organizations paid the total employee premium.
   c. Disability insurance was provided by 50 percent of the organizations; 90 percent of the organizations paid the entire premium, and benefits averaged: elimination period—103 days; benefit percentage—59.3 percent of gross salary; maximum monthly benefit amount—$1,117.00.
6. *Retirement plan* was provided for by 96.3 percent of the survey organizations.

RECRUITING, SELECTING, AND INTERVIEWING APPLICANTS

In a small health organization, recruitment, selection, and placement may be a somewhat haphazard process. In larger organizations, however, responsibility for each of these functions may be assumed by a specialist. The small group may fail to conduct a planned and systematic recruitment and may think only in terms of filling a vacancy. It may be that there are not enough candidates from whom to choose; consequently, recruiters should have a clear understanding of the job description and efforts should be extended to produce many candidates from a number of sources. Present employees are a good source. Registries for professional and technical people are another source. Advertisements in local newspapers have both advantages and disadvantages. It may be better to use blind box ads which do not identify your clinic. Graduates and those in training in local educational institutions are yet another source. General business sources may be able to suggest people who are interested in careers in the medical field and who can begin in clinic support functions and move into more responsible positions. There also are executive search organizations and employment agencies who will provide job candidates. For a fee, most temporary manpower agencies will permit the hiring of their part-time people who prove satisfactory.

Recruiters should know exactly what they are looking for before the selection screening process is begun. Interviewing can be divided into two steps. The first step is a brief, screening interview to eliminate obvious disqualifiers such as unacceptable salary demands or the inability to work certain hours. This portion of the interview can be handled by a receptionist. For those applicants who qualify, the second interview should be in depth. It cannot be emphasized too strongly that a definite time should be set aside for this encounter. If sufficient time is not provided, it is possible that the interviewer cannot communicate enough information to the potential employee so that he can evaluate the job properly. It also is possible that the applicant will not have had the chance to communicate enough to the interviewer for him to judge whether the individual is qualified for the job. When interviewing is completed in a cursory or perfunctory manner, the group may become trapped in an endless cycle of recruiting, interviewing, selection, and termination. Because recruitment and retraining are significant cost factors and because job efficiency and effectiveness mean greater productivity, long-tenured, well-qualified people are important to the practice.

The clinic administrator should have access to a comprehensive personal history form as a part of the selection process which elicits from the applicant fairly specific information regarding education and work experience, family circumstances, wage and hour requirements, and types of responsibilities desired (see figure 17-2). It is important that any form used does not have items that could be construed as prejudicial or discriminatory. After the preliminary or screening interview in which various applicants are judged as acceptable, appointment times should be established and the candidate should be given a personal history form to take home, complete, and return at the time of the final review.

Some groups choose to have their job applicants evaluated through assessment and testing by psychologists who are familiar with health care facilities and systems. Such tests do not reveal a person's technical competence, but they do provide a measure for intelligence and other broadly based problem solving capabilities, and they supply hiring information regarding the suitability of the person for types of work as well as evidences of motivation and personality. Testing applicants for employment has some legal implications, and often it is wise to consult an industrial or organizational psychologist. A properly conducted psychological evaluation program should make available additional information about candidates which can lessen the element of risk in hiring; however, a testing program may be expensive and out of the realm of possibility for a small, newly-forming group.

Interviewing

Before starting an in-depth interview, the data on the application blank should be analyzed. As items are reviewed, the interviewer may be able to con-

Employment Application

Date____________________ 19_______

Name____ Social Security No.____________________
(Last) (First) (Middle)

Address:____________________________ City____________________ Phone ____________

Previous Address ____

Position Applied For____________________ Salary Expected____________________ ☐ Part-time ☐ Full-time

How long do you expect to work?________________ Are you available to work overtime, if needed?________________

PERSONAL DATA

Date of Birth____________________ Age__________ Height __________ Weight __________

Health: Excellent ☐ Fair ☐ Poor ☐ Physical Handicaps____________________________

Name of Spouse____________________________ Occupation of Spouse____________________

Number of Dependents__________ Ages of Dependents________________ Convictions other than traffic violations (specify)____________________

EDUCATION

School - Draw circle Around Highest Grade Completed: 1 2 3 4 5 6 7 8 9 10 11 12 13 14 15 16 17 18 19

NAME AND LOCATION OF HIGH SCHOOL OR COLLEGE	ATTENDANCE		DEGREE OR DIPLOMA	MAJOR SUBJECT	GRADE AV.
	From	To			
High School					
College or University					
Technical Business or Professional Training				License or Registration	

EXPERIENCE - Position Held, including Military Service (List Last Position First)

COMPANY	PERIOD		SALARY	JOB TITLE AND BRIEF DESCRIPTION	REASON FOR LEAVING
	From	To			
(1) Name________				(1)________	
Supervisor________					
Company Address________					
(2) Name________				(2)________	
Supervisor________					
Company Address________					
(3) Name________				(3)________	
Supervisor________					
Company Address________					

May we request references from the above?________________ Has notice been given present employer?________________

Do you type?______ Approximate speed________ Do you take shorthand?______ System__________ Approximate speed________

Other special skills____

In an emergency notify____________________________ Relationship____________________

Address____________________________ Phone____________________

Figure 17-2. Employment Application

CHARACTER REFERENCES

Do not refer to mere acquaintances, previous employers or relatives. Refer to people who know you well, either personally or in business.

Name Occupation Address

1. ______________________________

2. ______________________________

3. ______________________________

May we request references from the above? ____________

Use of Alcohol - Abstain______ Socially______ Other (explain)____________

Referred by____________________ Are you personally acquainted with or related to any present or former employee of the clinic? Yes ☐ No ☐ Name of such employee ____________

Use this space for any additional information you would like us to have to help judge your qualifications.

I understand that the information on this employment application has been requested for purposes of evaluating my qualifications in regard to the requirements of the specified position and that the information will not be used to unlawfully discriminate.

I understand and expressly agree that the clinic may make or employ an agency to make such pre-employment investigation of my competence, character, general reputation, personal characteristics and mode of living as it may choose and that information concerning such matters may be obtained through contacts or interviews with former employers, neighbors, friends, associates or any other person with whom I am acquainted or who may have knowledge concerning the attributes referred to. I expressly consent to and acquiesce in such investigation. I also understand and have been informed that I have the right to make a written request within a reasonable period of time for a complete and accurate disclosure of the nature and scope of the investigation made.

Should I desire to leave the employ of the Clinic, I promise to deliver my resignation to my supervisor two weeks prior to the date it is to go into effect. I understand and agree that at no time, whether I am an employee of the Clinic or not, will any information regarding patients of the Clinic be revealed to anyone other than those authorized to receive it. I understand that the giving of information concerning a patient to those not authorized to receive such information is unlawful and shall be sufficient cause for my immediate dismissal.

I certify that all information given on this form is true to the best of my knowledge, information and belief and I understand that I will be subject to dismissal if I have made any misrepresentation herein. I also give my consent to any pre-employment medical and physical examination required by the Clinic.

____________________ Applicant

APPLICANT—DO NOT WRITE BELOW

Interviewer ____________________ Date ____________

	Excellent	Good	Average	Below
Speech				
Neat and Clean				
Interest in Clinic				
Job Knowledge				

To replace____________

Position____________

Dept.________ Sal. Sched.________

Salary discussed ____________

Employment Agreement:

To start________ Salary________

Hours and Days: ____________________

Special conditions of Employment: ____________________

COMMENTS:

Revised 5/74 by the Medical Group Management, 4101 E. Louisiana Ave., Denver, Colorado 80222

Figure 17-2. (Cont.)

struct a picture of the applicant and make an estimation of his potential. Consistency among areas of education, work, home life and play is important, as are problem areas, such as health or unemployment. Any areas which are not clear should be noted so they may be investigated.

The applicant's vocational interests, his relationships with others, the quantity and quality of his ambitions, his general and specific abilities, and his immediate and long-range goals are categories that should be explored. The interviewer should be friendly, interested, and understanding, and the interview should be conducted privately. The first question in any area should be general and open-ended, leaving the applicant the widest latitude possible for response. As the interview continues, questions can be more specific. The applicant should be encouraged to do most of the talking and the interview should be continued until there is enough information accumulated for an accurate evaluation of the applicant's potential. After this point, the interviewer can proceed to discuss the position. If he describes the requirements of the job at the outset, he may receive from the applicant only what the applicant thinks he wants to hear.

If the applicant is allowed to speak freely, he will reveal things of great importance to him which will also be of significance to the interviewer. Inconsistencies should be easy to identify. The interviewer should not interrupt or argue with the applicant nor should he let the applicant feel that he is in any way judgmental. The interviewer should pay attention to the feelings and attitudes expressed by the applicant as well as to the intellectual content of the applicant's comments. Emotional needs and attitudes can be very important in ascertaining future behavior.

As the interviewee produces information in response to questioning and encouragement, the interviewer should keep the responsibilities of the position in mind. The most common standard is a well written job description. During the interview the interviewer can form hypotheses about how the applicant would act and can ask questions to test the hypotheses. As soon as the interview is completed, the interviewer should make objective notes concerning what he has seen and heard from the applicant.

In one sense, the interview is never completed. The data produced through the interview, in addition to what is gained from other sources, have to be integrated—a process which may take a considerable period of time and thought. To a large extent, practical considerations will determine the amount of time available for the candidate's interview. If it becomes apparent that a second in-depth interview may be necessary, detailed information about the job need not be disclosed until then. When this information is consistent with what the applicant has revealed about himself, the job will be highly attractive. When the job demands are at odds with the expressed attitudes of the candidate, however, the groundwork will have been laid for a rejection that can be more easily accepted. The accept/reject decision should be communicated to the applicant as early as possible.

After recruiting, interviewing, and arriving at a selection of one or two candidates for the job available, it is mandatory to check their references carefully. If a person has been employed at another clinic, or hospital, a relatively good picture of how he is likely to perform should be available. Checking references should include asking specific questions concerning the person's strengths on the job, his weaknesses, and in what capacities he performed in an average fashion. Objective data should be sought. If a former employer has reached a conclusion or judgment about the candidate, the basis for that attitude should be sought. Attendance, willingness to conform to working odd hours, as well as any other kinds of conditions which might exist in the group's particular situation should be included in questions directed toward the references. In addition, the personal history form and dates given for occupations should be checked against actual time on the job. Large hospitals sometimes seem uncooperative in checking references. When interviewing a person formerly employed by a hospital, the interviewer should secure the names of those people who directly supervised the applicant. The personnel department may be able to supply only a written record which is far from complete. The group may wish to check as many as five references. If people are concerned about who is calling for reference checks, the interviewer may have to provide his name and telephone number and ask that he be called back in order to substantiate that the inquiry for information is legitimate. If the opening is for an important position, a personal visit to a previous reference would be recommended.

In addition to developing interviewing and selection techniques, the group also must decide exactly who will be responsible for recruiting and interviewing. Various possibilities include supervisors, the personnel director, the administrator, or a committee of these individuals. The role of the group physicians in these processes also must be defined, especially in terms of hiring other physicians and various paramedical personnel. Formal procedures must be established for handling drop-in applicants. Even when no formal position opening exists, the proper treatment of drop-in applicants can have a favorable public relations impact and may be beneficial to the group in searching for suitable applicants for future job openings. Group members should bear in mind that physician recruitment may differ substantially from employee recruitment. Special interviewing procedures may be required, and drop-ins may be treated according to specially defined guidelines.

Finally, the group must consider employment contracts and commitments. Who can make commitments, whether verbal or written, the period covered by the contracts, contract conditions, and the intent of such contracts are areas requiring procedural limitations. Equal Employment Opportunity (EEO) as well as other government regulations may necessitate interpretation by the group's attorney. The Medical Group Management Association publication *MGMA Digest of Medical Group Employment Contracts and Income Distribution Plans* (1974) is an excellent resource for the forming medical group.

Training and Development

The clinic manager as well as the group physicians will have the responsibility for employee training and development. Development is a process involving planned learning experiences to stimulate the performance of the individual. Through these experiences, effectiveness of job performance can be increased and the employee can be prepared for a broader scope of responsibility. When a well-trained replacement can step into a situation, both management and employee anxiety is minimzed. Such continuity is important to the clinic, to the patient, and to the employees. A clinic invests in training employees whom it wants to retain, and such development allows employees to perform in a number of different capacities. Reserves and interchangeability are critical for effective succession. Many people have anxiety concerning their careers and when management does not give attention to this anxiety, it may lose productive, responsible employees.

Employee development primarily occurs through on-the-job experiences in a supervisor-subordinate relationship of mutual trust. People grow in a climate of challenge, change, and encouragement. In an environment that offers diversified experiences and opportunities, the employee matures as a result of learning from mistakes and supportive counseling. If one is not held accountable for results, is not asked to take decision risk in proposing new action, and is not given responsibility for results, one will not grow; however, goals which include areas outside the employees' present level of performance must be realistic. On the other hand, employees may want to pursue certain goals for self development, but it may not be expedient for management to allow them to do so.

The discussion in this chapter has focused upon the elements of personnel management. The actual management structures available to implement the procedures presented here are dealt with in other chapters of the text. It should be pointed out, however, that organizational configurations as well as channels of authority can be varied greatly yet still allow employees to fulfill their basic vocational needs such as job recognition, two-way communication, a sense of belonging, and emotional security. The criteria for ensuring such results are consistency and predictability of management's expectations, integration of employee goals with those of the group practice, and an effective climate for maintaining upward and downward communication.

Appendix 17A

Employee Evaluation Form

NAME: ______________________________ DATE: ______________________

DEPARTMENT: ________________________ JOB TITLE: __________________

Purposes of this Employee Evaluation:

To take a personal inventory, to pin-point weaknesses and strengths and to outline and agree upon a practical improvement program. Periodically conducted, these Evaluations will provide a history of development and progress.

Instructions:

Listed below are a number of traits, abilities and characteristics that are important for success in business. Place an "X" mark on each rating scale, over the descriptive phrase which most nearly describes the person being rated. (If this form is being used for self-evaluation, you will be describing yourself.)

Carefully evaluate each of the qualities separately.

Two common mistakes in rating are: (1) A tendency to rate nearly everyone as "average" on every trait instead of being more critical in judgment. The rater should use the ends of the scale as well as the middle, and (2) The "Halo Effect," i.e., a tendency to rate the same individual "excellent" on every trait or "poor" on every trait based on the *overall* picture one has of the person being rated. However, each person has strong points and weak points and these should be indicated on the rating scale.

ACCURACY is the correctness of work duties performed.

______	______	______	______	______
Makes frequent errors.	Careless; makes recurrent errors.	Usually accurate; makes only average number of mistakes.	Requires little supervision; is exact and precise most of the time.	Requires absolute minimum of supervision; is almost always accurate.

ALERTNESS is the ability to grasp instructions, to meet changing conditions and to solve novel or problem situations.

Slow to "catch on."	Requires more than average instructions and explanations.	Grasps instructions with average ability.	Usually quick to understand and learn.	Exceptionally keen and alert.

CREATIVITY is talent for having new ideas, for finding new and better ways of doing things and for being imaginative.

Rarely has a new idea; is unimaginative.	Occasionally comes up with a new idea.	Has average imagination; has reasonable number of new ideas.	Frequently suggests new ways of doing things; is very imaginative.	Continually seeks new and better ways of doing things, is extremely imaginative.

FRIENDLINESS is the sociability and warmth which an individual imparts in his attitude toward customers, other employees, his supervisor and the persons he may supervise.

Very distant and aloof.	Approachable; friendly once known by others.	Warm; friendly; sociable.	Very sociable and out-going.	Extremely sociable; excellent at establishing good will.

PERSONALITY is an individual's behavior characteristics or his personal suitability for the job.

Personality unsatisfactory for this job.	Personality questionable for this job.	Personality satisfactory for this job.	Very desirable personality for this job.	Outstanding personality for this job.

PERSONAL APPEARANCE is the personal impression an individual makes on others. (Consider cleanliness, grooming, neatness and appropriateness of dress on the job.)

Very untidy; poor taste in dress.	Sometimes untidy and careless about personal appearance.	Generally neat and clean; satisfactory personal appearance.	Careful about personal appearance; good taste in dress.	Unusually well groomed; very neat; excellent taste in dress.

PHYSICAL FITNESS is the ability to work consistently and with only moderate fatigue. (Consider physical alertness and energy.)

Tires easily; is weak and frail.	Frequently tires and is slow.	Meets physical and energy job requirements.	Energetic; seldom tires.	Excellent health; no fatigue.

ATTENDANCE is faithfulness in coming to work daily and conforming to work hours.

Often absent without good excuse and/or frequently reports for work late.	Lax in attendance and/or reporting for work on time.	Usually present and on time.	Very prompt; regular in attendance.	Always regular and prompt; volunteers for overtime when needed.

HOUSEKEEPING is the orderliness and cleanliness in which an individual keeps his work area.

Disorderly or untidy.	Some tendency to be careless and untidy.	Ordinarily keeps work area fairly neat.	Quite conscientious about neatness and cleanliness.	Unusually neat, clean and orderly.

DEPENDABILITY is the ability to do required jobs well with a minimum of supervision.

Requires close supervision; is unreliable.	Sometimes requires prompting.	Usually takes care of necessary tasks and completes with reasonable promptness.	Requires little supervision; is reliable.	Requires absolute minimum of supervision.

DRIVE is the desire to attain goals, to achieve.

Has poorly defined goals and acts without purpose; puts forth practically no effort.	Sets goals too low; puts forth little effort to achieve.	Has average goals and usually puts forth effort to reach these.	Strives hard; has high desire to achieve.	Sets high goals and strives incessantly to reach these.

JOB KNOWLEDGE is the information concerning work duties which an individual should know for a satisfactory job performance.

Poorly informed about work duties.	Lacks knowledge of some phases of work.	Moderately informed; can answer most common questions.	Understands all phases of work.	Has complete mastery of all phases of job.

QUANTITY OF WORK is the amount of work an individual does in a work day.

Does not meet minimum requirements.	Does just enough to get by.	Volume of work is satisfactory.	Very industrious; does more than is required.	Superior work production record.

STABILITY is the ability to withstand pressure and to remain calm in crisis situations.

______	______	______	______	______
Goes "to pieces" under pressure; is "jumpy" and nervous.	Occasionally "blows up" under pressure; is easily irritated.	Has average tolerance for crises; usually remains calm.	Tolerates most pressure; likes crises more than the average person.	Thrives under pressure; really enjoys solving crises.

COURTESY is the polite attention an individual gives other people.

______	______	______	______	______
Blunt; discourteous; antagonistic.	Sometimes tactless.	Agreeable and pleasant.	Always very polite and willing to help.	Inspiring to others in being courteous and very pleasant.

OVERALL EVALUATION **in comparison with other employees with the same length of service on this job:**

______	______	______	______	______
Definitely unsatisfactory.	Substandard but making progress.	Doing an average job.	Definitely above average.	Outstanding.

COMMENTS

Major weak points are—

1. ______
2. ______
3. ______

and these can be strengthened by doing the following:

______

Major strong points are—

1. ______
2. ______
3. ______

and these can be used more effectively by doing the following:

______

Rated by ____
(Name) *(Title)*

(If not used as a self-evaluation form, the employee should sign below)

A copy of this Report has been given to me and has been discussed with me.

______________________________ ______________
(Employee's Signature) *(Date)*

Form 102

Chapter 18

Systems Automation

DETERMINATION OF THE NEED FOR AUTOMATION

During the middle of this century, the information explosion together with the communications revolution contributed greatly to methods of problem-solving associated with the scientific method. In every field, individuals became concerned with gathering information and applying the results of this accumulation of data to the evaluation of business endeavors and industrial production. Often, the collection of such information was stimulated by the need to bill large numbers of individuals for services, while supplying documented evidence from a number of different sources concerning the extent of those services. The health care field is such an industry and has undergone a metamorphosis in methods of health care delivery and payment mechanisms. In many cases, third parties are responsible for making payment. One of these third parties in particular, the federal government, has been responsible for a large percentage of the requests for detailed information related to the treatment of patients under its payment jurisdiction. The problem created is twofold—how to store the medical information economically and efficiently and how to retrieve particular portions of it quickly and accurately. In addition, there appears to be an absence of an industrywide knowledge of what data processing hardware and software are available, and an absence of industrywide guidelines defining acceptable levels of performance for data processing systems. Department of Health, Education and Welfare statistics show that 60 percent of the hospitals in the United States are using some form of data processing, but many of these data processing activities have been disappointing to management because of a failure on the part of the organization to formulate sound objectives, to communicate them to planners and programmers, and to resist pressures imposed by vendors. The need for automation is ever present and growing, and modern day computers have come a long way from the University of Pennsylvania's ENIAC that had a half million soldered joints, 18,000 vacuum tubes, 6,000 switches, and 500 electric terminals.[1] In group practice facilities and in hospitals, objectives to be considered in systems automation might include:

1. Better service to the community
2. Better patient care
3. Shorter patient stay
4. Better financial management and control
5. Increased facility utilization
6. Reduction of the rate of increasing costs
7. Better personnel utilization
8. Reduction of lost charges
9. Faster collection of accounts receivable
10. Reduction of capital tied up in inventory
11. Discounts on faster payments of accounts payable
12. More accurate accounting
13. Faster payments from third parties
14. Accurate data for amortization
15. Statistical data for decisions on procurement
16. Better medical records for medical audits and accreditation
17. Schedule preventive maintenance of plant.

The predispositions of group members, administrative philosophy, and cost factors, as well as the results of strategic planning will contribute to decisions regarding the implementation of data processing systems. This chapter will serve as a source of technical information to be applied after such groundwork has been established by the group.

Electronic Data Processing

Modern electronic data processing technology makes available sophisticated information systems which only a few years ago were not available at any cost. Developing effective systems is a complex task involving objectives, people, equipment procedures, data base, input, output, control, limitations, communications, dynamics, and careful weighing of potential costs and benefits. What kinds of information are needed and how often such information should be reported will vary from organization to organization. Information systems characteristics fall into three general categories: control information, planning information, and planning and control information. Control information usually is financial data which are very detailed and oriented to past activities. In composition, it follows organizational lines and covers short time periods. Planning information usually is not financial in nature, is not too detailed, and is oriented to the future. It transcends organizational lines, shows trends, and covers long time periods. Planning and control information also usually is nonfinancial data, can move from the very detailed to the very general, and is both past and future oriented. Such information transcends organizational lines, shows trends, and covers both long and short time periods. There are times when information is most usable in its original form; at other times, it should be related to a standard of comparison, such as past performance. Most individuals feel that any data collected should be 100 percent accurate and therefore spend a great deal of money trying to accumulate data which are flawless; however, many productive decisions can and have been made on summaries and averages of incomplete and less than accurate information.

The computer has been described as an information machine. Just twenty-five years ago, there were less than twenty computers in the United States. Today there are over one hundred thousand, and computer users are beginning to realize that they are dealing with a powerful tool capable of handling vastly differing types of data such as those characteristic of economic, social, and political information. According to Dr. Carl Hammer, director of Computer Sciences at the UNIVAC Corporation, in a speech delivered in Moscow on May 30, 1974, "the data processing and computational work done by approximately one hundred thousand machines in the United States alone could no longer be carried out by hand. It would take approximately four hundred billion people (one hundred times the world population) to tackle this work load in our complex mind amplifying society."

Effective data processing appropriate to the organization's needs and resources can reduce operating costs, clerical costs, and overhead expenses. Groups who are considering some form of electronic data processing can begin by conducting a systems analysis of their day-to-day operations. Flow charts which indicate information transfer within the clinic will help to identify sets of procedures whose speed and efficiency could be markedly improved through automation. In many cases, especially in small organizations, an analysis of this sort is an end in itself for improving and streamlining routine operations. In the meantime, procedures can be standardized for possible conversion to automated methods in the future. In other instances, however, inefficiencies are identified which often can be corrected or improved through automation.

Billing and Accounts Receivable. Billing and accounting procedures are apt to be fairly routine once certain initial choices are made relating to methods of reporting, and procedures consequently become amenable to programming for computerized processing. A number of such computer programs for billing and accounts receivable are available from vendors or from other health care institutions and can be adopted for use by individual group practices. Applicability and availability of programming techniques make this area usually one of the first to be automated. The biggest problem in any manual or automated billing and receivable system is developing an accurate and fast method for capturing charge and cash information and entering this information into a system for the proper charging or crediting of a patient's account. Usually this task is accomplished by employing a service sheet and batch processing. While data gathering at the point of the transaction is more desirable, at the present time it is a very expensive technique. An effective billing and accounts receivable system should have included within it a financial screening technique. Basic to this system are detail and balance forward capabilities, dunning letters, trial balances by insurance type, and account age. Collection agency data also should be available and should indicate how much money has been turned over to an agency and how much of the amount has been recovered.

Several information, billing, and receivable package services are available from vendors or are available on a shared basis. Most have been developed for hospitals but in some cases might be modified for a group practice operation. Some of these are:

1. Medinet—Information service business, a division of the General Electric Company
2. Medelco—Total Hospital Information System (T.H.I.S.), a subsidiary of Reley Corporation
3. Reach Corporation—A subsidiary of National Data Communications Incorporated
4. Technicon Medical Information Systems Corporation
5. MediData—Combined efforts of Charlotte Memorial, Presbyterian, and Mercy Hospitals of Charlotte, N.C.
6. IBM—Medical Information System Program (M.I.S.P.) and Shared Hospital Accounting System (S.H.A.S.)
7. Shared Medical Systems—They use the IBM S.H.A.S. package and others.

General Ledger, Budget, and Payroll. Many vendors also offer package payroll programs which can be simple or extremely complex, including only basic tax calculations or numerous sophisticated management reports. At a minimum, an effective payroll system should include:

1. Check writing
2. Check reconciliation
3. Payroll register
4. Outstanding check register
5. Labor distribution reporting
6. W-2 reporting
7. Labor statistics by reporting period with year-to-date figures.

After billing, accounts receivable, and payroll have been automated, automation of the general ledger and budgeting processes often follows. Accounting systems contain much of the same basic data although they are presented in differing formats. As a continuation of the automating process, computerization of the accounting functions logically follows, providing more timely information, greater accuracy, and the removal of much of the clerical drudgery that accompanies this type of activity.

Accounts Payable and Purchasing and Inventory. Accounts payable is another accounting system that is repetitive in nature and uses the same data to produce several different reports. An effective system should allow for discounting and accruals and should be capable of keeping track of obligations, even though payments have not been made.

The purchasing and accounting departments usually have a joint responsibility for inventory. The concern in accounting is with the inventory's worth in purchasing and with maintaining an inventory record by additions and deletions. Accounting procedures should establish the method for determining worth, and the purchasing department should endeavor to buy at the best price. If it is purchasing's responsibility to maintain stores, it must establish accurate check in and out procedures. In hospitals, automation often brings about centralization of purchasing responsibility. Much hospital purchasing is carried out by pharmacy, dietary, maintenance, and often central supply, in addition to the purchasing department. The wide variety of items involved make this method of purchasing difficult but not impossible to automate. A good system should include not only present inventory but also items on order, back orders, and substitutions. Automated purchase order initiation can relieve purchasing personnel of a good deal of typing and can offer management more control over the purchasing function.

Medical Records. A number of excellent methods for computerized storage of information contained in patient medical records have been designed. Due to the nature of the data, however, numerous problems still exist and currently there is no widespread usage of these programs. In order for the information to be useful it must be readily retrieved, and this fact, among others, makes the computerized medical record financially feasible only to hospitals and large group practices at the present time. Data contained in the record must be summarized and coded for computer storage. Certain portions of the record are more easily coded and stored than others. Universal acceptance and use of the problem oriented record should provide more easily codable information and should provide an impetus to future computerization. The amount of narrative information alone makes computerization of the record in its present form prohibitive. Some of the institutions that have worked on a computerized medical record are:

1. King's College Hospital, London
2. Karolinski, Seraphimer, and Danderyd Hospitals, Stockholm; Karolinski has 2,000 beds and Danderyd reports 1.5 million patients
3. Kaiser Permanente Medical Data Base System, San Francisco
4. Massachusetts General Hospital, Boston; this hospital has an outpatient clinic ambulatory medical system for the Harvard Community Health Plan. Their system has been functioning for approximately three years and is the primary medical record for over thirty thousand members with over one hundred thousand visits annually.

Dietary Service. The best known set of computer programs available in this area is the computer assisted menu planning or CAMP program, which provides the dietician with a system for planning menus that meet predetermined nutrition and variety requirements. The system also provides information for the purchasing of raw foods.

Maintenance/Engineering Department. In the engineering department, there are three activities that can be computerized easily—personnel scheduling, preventive maintenance scheduling, and work order request control. A current idea in this area is facilities management using computerized building automation.

Companies such as Johnson Controls, Powers, and Honeywell, who have been in the building control business for years, are being joined by IBM as energy conservation becomes more important. These building systems are designed to:

1. Provide occupants with comfort and safety
2. Protect against fire
3. Provide communication
4. Control lighting
5. Coordinate and operate machinery for optimum energy use.

Laboratory. For laboratories with a sizable volume of testing, such as three hundred thousand tests per year, a number of successful systems are available. The primary objective of the laboratory system should be to report test results, reduce errors of transcription, and reduce clerical work. The system also should provide better management tools, particularly in the area of load status, quality control, and cost. Within the laboratory, a variety of communication problems is presented as a result of terminology used by the separate laboratory science disciplines and the very nature of the technical data emanating from each. Methods of coding for automation and for the collecting of batched, processed, numerical dated clinical chemistries differ from those used to encode the prose descriptive results of tissue pathology, the mixed numeric and descriptive data of hematology and microbiology, and the binary data of blood types. It is necessary, therefore, to approach each of the laboratory's specialties of chemistry, hematology, blood banks, serology, microbiology, urinalysis, cytology, and tissue pathology as separate systems rather than to attempt to impose a standard pattern of record keeping upon all.

Pharmacy. Several systems which will do specific tasks for the pharmacy are being marketed. Such systems can reduce both the number of late charges and errors in pricing and can automatically produce typed medication labels, thereby reducing clerical work load. Some systems include pricing, charging, inventory control, formulary listing, and purchase order preparation, and can result in inventory reduction, cost reduction of formulary preparation, and a reduction in time spent on inventory and narcotic control.

Radiology. Computers are used in radiology for diagnostic, information, and administrative systems. In addition, special computer techniques and programs have been developed as aids in teaching programs. For diagnostic evaluation, several programs are available which use various statistical methods to develop a diagnosis. The information systems store, retrieve, and transmit reports. The objective of administrative systems is to allow for the orderly management of patients, timely test reporting, file room control, billing, and statistical compilation. An example is the Missouri automated radiology system which is a time sharing, teleprocessing information system developed by the University of Missouri.

Electroencephalogram. Considering the relatively small number of EEG tests performed, the amount of developmental work completed in this area has met with little or no general acceptance. Although the activity of the human brain was first recorded over forty years ago, the EEG analysis constitutes a formidable problem in pattern recognition. EEG recordings represent the difference in electrical potential between pairs of electrodes inserted in the scalp. The voltage measured is approximately one hundred times less in amplitude than the recordings of the EKG. Computer programs have not yet been developed which can interpret successfully the sixteen channel strip chart that is produced from twenty-one electrodes providing signals from frontal, central, parietal, temporal, and occipital regions of the brain. A new concept, however, based on statistical probability offers some promise.

Electrocardiogram. As a diagnostic procedure, the EKG is one of the most widely used in the daily practice of medicine. Fifty million EKGs are performed annually in the United States. The electrical signals generated by the heart are repetitive and can be translated relatively easily into a medium appropriate for objective mathematical treatment. Analysis methods have been developed in which pattern recognition, wave form measurement, and interpretation are performed by the computer. Five computer programs are being used presently for EKG interpretation. The companies who sell or lease these turnkey systems include: Digital Equipment, Hewlett-Packard, Market, MedLab, and Varian.

Respiratory Therapy. The most common computer applications used by respiratory therapy, other than for administrative tasks, are included in physiological monitoring systems and multiphasic screening and are for the collection and evaluation of spirometry data with limited blood gas analysis. There are several diagnostic systems in operation, both in pulmonary function and cardiopulmonary laboratories.

Multiphasic Screening. Multiphasic screening refers to the combining of multiple tests to screen for a number of diseases. Automated multiphasic screening is the expanded concept of utilizing automated and semi-automated electronic and mechanical equipment to determine whether the likelihood of disease being present is enough to warrant further specific testing. Automated and computer techniques offer the advantages of:

1. Decreasing unit cost per test
2. Improving accuracy and standardization of tests and procedures
3. Improving efficiency of service to the patient through close integration of a large number of test procedures
4. Facilitating early detection of a wider range and greater number of unsuspected disease among apparently healthy people
5. Relieving medical personnel of the burden of routinely screening large numbers of relatively healthy people.

Kaiser Permanente uses automated multiphasic health testing (AMHT) and provides multiphasic health checkups for more than two thousand patients each month. IBM has an AMHT computer package available for sale or for lease.

Personnel Resources

When planning or operating even the smallest data processing installation, a great deal of personnel expertise is necessary. A large number of capabilities often must be centered in a small number of individuals or realized through use of consultants who can be called in when needed. The data processing manager often assumes the role of operations and computer science specialist, behavioral scientist, and facility engineer. The programmer becomes a software specialist, data base engineer, and programming training analyst and instructor; the systems analyst becomes a method and procedure specialist, statistician, and human factor specialist. With demand for this type of talent, it becomes obvious that selection of proper personnel to fill data processing positions is vitally important. It also is obvious that individuals possessing many of the talents and skills needed in data processing are difficult to find.

Operations. The position of computer operator can be filled by an individual with a high school education or less. Education, or the lack of it, has not been an important factor for success in this position. For the group having a policy of promoting from within, education could become a criterion if an operator's next step is into a systems programmer or management position. The person chosen for this job should be conscientious, accurate, and very thorough concerning details. He should be capable of following instructions, able to learn simple tasks quickly, and manually dexterous. Manufacturers of computing equipment often can provide the formal education necessary for systems management and programming, but most computer operator training courses are conducted on the job and are the responsibility of the equipment user. Because of the importance of this job, the courses must be planned carefully and should include the following subject areas:

1. Introduction to data processing for operators
2. "Hands on" machine operation
3. Operating system concepts for operators
4. Operating system job control for operators
5. Installation standards and procedures.

Auditors. Whether auditing is conducted internally or by an outside firm retained by the group, auditors should play an important role in helping to correct or to prevent unproductive data processing practices. They should be concerned with:

1. The organization of the data processing department
2. The method, systems, and procedure standards
3. Documentation and documentation standards
4. Security
5. Facilities.

Administrative Personnel. The data processing director or manager should be a computer scientist with sufficient experience or training in the biological sciences to enable him to communicate with the medical and paramedical staff. It is the responsibility of the person in this position to plan, administer, and control all data processing activities of the organization; to interpret and apply organizational policies and objectives across all data processing activities; and to provide professional services for feasibility studies, systems analysis, design, hardware and software selection, programming, and the data center operation.

Systems Analyst. This position demands a business orientation and data processing education and experience, as well as an ability to visualize, to integrate, to plan, and to anticipate future business needs. The systems analyst is responsible for carrying out feasibility studies, recommending courses of action for systems under consideration, investigating potential new uses for the computer in the organization, and preparing work plans for systems development.

Programmer/Analyst. This individual should have an undergraduate degree in mathematics, science, or engineering. The position calls for a person with a logical, analytical mind able to define problems. The ability to communicate verbally and in writing also is essential, as is the ability to work with others. Responsibilities of this position include:

1. Analyzing job requirements
2. Preparing specifications
3. Evaluating hardware/software
4. Preparing time and cost estimates
5. Programming.

Information Requirements and Evaluation

Information and information systems as they apply to modern data processing and computers consist of much more than methods for the manipulation of numbers. Information systems deal with action, human behavior, and complex interrelationships improving communication between individuals and departments and providing consistency necessary to the effective interfacing of all operating systems. Job descriptions often are predicated upon the types of information processed by the employee. Levels of position and kinds of management also can be defined by classes of information dealt with as a part of the job. As information systems are installed or modified, management structure may change due to faster access to information.

Various data gathering instruments are necessary to capture information for processing, including questionnaries used with and without prompters, automatic recording devices, machine and computer printouts, photographic and X-ray film, tabular forms, teletype transmissions, mark sense or optical character recognition documents, and audio and digital magnetic recordings. Data processing systems now offer a wide variety of devices that allow data to be directly entered into a computer or into an intermediate medium for subsequent entry into a computer. Many of these data entry devices create an audit trail which is a printed record of the data actually received by the entry device. Data entry or input devices fall into the following categories.

Keypunch and Verifying Machines. In spite of the wide spectrum of technologies available for data input, keypunch machines have been and still are the most standard means of data entry. The punch card is a very practical document and can be used and interpreted by people as well as by machines. Some of its limitations include size of card available for data, and operator idle time due to the time interval between cards in the keypunch machines. In addition, errors often can be costly and difficult to correct. Unfortunately, current keyboard entry devices are only 50 percent more efficient than throughput of the original keypunch machine, and keypunch direct costs for operators, wages, and equipment have doubled in the last two decades.[2]

Punched Paper Tape. Keyboard to paper tape is not a new technique. The most common form of such devices is similar to a typewriter or teletypewriter which produces punched paper tape as copy. Paper tape also can be produced as output by a variety of business oriented devices, including adding machines and cash registers. Low speed is the major drawback, while low cost is a major advantage.

Magnetic Character Readers. This system is used primarily by the banking industry, which has played a major role in developing technology to replace the keypunching of check transactions. The system calls for certain pertinent information, such as bank transit number, amount, account number of the depositor, and transaction code to be recorded in a specific area of the check in magnetic ink. Machines read the information electronically, sort the checks, and at the same time, translate the data into a computer readable form. Other applications that have been developed are point of sale recording and credit card data entry.

Mark Sense Readers. These devices optically read marks on documents and, therefore, are able to enter data directly into a computer without any intermediate form of data transcription. Mark sense reading has been used widely in the educational field and was used in the 1970 Census. It does have a place in the data entry field, particularly with turnaround document systems. In many of the clinical laboratory systems, mark sense units are becoming prominent and seem to have potential for success in the medical environment. The greatest advantage of mark sense readers is their simplicity. Their disadvantages are high error factors due to improper marking and generally slow processing since equipment is not completely electronic.

Optical Character Recognition (OCR). In the late 1950s and into the 1960s, a very exciting technology was announced involving devices that could read printed or handwritten alpha numeric information from specially sized documents, tapes, and standard pages. The information then could be recorded on magnetic tape or transferred directly into a computer for processing. The actual development of this technology, however, has been very slow and consistently below industry forecasts. The major advantage to OCR is its ability to enter data by machine, thus bypassing other entry methods such as keypunch and key tape. As an example, the proper OCR font can be installed on IBM Selectric typewriters, thus expanding the scope of data entry to stenographers, secretaries, and clerks. Disadvantages to the system are high equipment cost and limited adaptability relative to various applications.

Key to Tape Devices. These devices consist of one or more keypunch style keyboards and a computer compatible magnetic tape drive. Data is keyed in through the keyboard from the source document, and rather than being punched into a card as in the case of a keypunch, it is read onto magnetic tape which then can be read into a computer. The advantages of this system are that it provides for variable record lengths of greater size than does the punch card, and that the process is electronic, resulting in better "uptime." In addition, it is quieter and thereby is more conducive to the promotion of a pleasant work environment. This type of system provides a fast means for input into the main computer and eliminates the use of cards, which results in cost savings and a space requirement reduction. Some disadvantages are that correcting entry errors takes longer and that training time for data entry operations is more extensive than for keypunch operators.

Source Data Automation (SDA). This system collects data concerning an event or a transaction into machinery in real time (the time it is actually happening) and at the location where the event occurs. Uses for this type of system include the monitoring of mechanical and electrical systems which usually consume almost one-half of the cost of maintaining a building. With building automation, one individual from a central console can operate and control all the mechanical and electrical systems in the building, thereby permitting effective scheduling and adjustments of energy consuming equipment. SDA also can monitor employee attendance and record labor distribution and can serve as a basis for production and inventory control. Other uses include monitoring safety and security functions, including the locking and unlocking of doors and the operation of sprinkler systems.

Point-of-sale recording devices come under the general SDA category. Examples of this type of system are cash registers equipped with computer compatible tapes (magnetic or paper) and standard register source record punches used in many of today's hospitals. The capturing and recording of analog signals also fall into the category of SDA. Such systems offer the recording of various types of measurements, such as pressure, rate, temperature, and sound through several types of transducers including microphones, electrodes, pressure transducers and gauges, potentiometers, temperature probes, and pumps. In medical facilities in which full cycle data acquisition capabilities are becoming a requirement, analog signal sensing is becoming more important. Patient monitoring in operating rooms, intensive care units, coronary care units, and catheterization labs, and multiphasic screening are among the major challenges for the future. The monitoring of pathology laboratories and X-ray equipment also is considered in this group.

Key to Disc. Key to disc systems are similar to key to tape. The shared processor or keyboard to disc system is designed for a five to 128 multikeyboard arrangement. This system allows multiple key stage stations for the simultaneous imputting of data to one central disc storage. The keyboards are controlled by a minicomputer that places keyed data temporarily into a disc prior to transmission to a computer compatible magnetic tape. The system, rather than the operator, reformats the data. The system also performs error checks and editing and allows random accessing of data. When compared to keypunch equipment, key to disc has almost the same profile as key to tape. In addition, other advantages include the capability for a number of key input units to be placed at remote locations and the deleting or inserting of a record held on disc prior to writing it onto a magnetic tape. The measurement of operator productivity indicates a 15 percent increase over key to tape systems. The arithmetic capability inherent in key to disc permits balancing of predetermined audit controls; thus, no verification is required. Disadvantages include the hardware's being more expensive and the requirement for greater operator sophistication. Salaries, therefore, are more prone to increase for key to disc systems than they are for keypunch or key to tape systems.

Computer Terminals. The combination of low cost peripherals, communication equipment, and minicomputers have led to cost effective terminals that are beginning to offer one more means of data entry. With cost reductions, the use of remote terminals for batch inputting becomes attractive to small data processing users who cannot justify their own data processing equipment. The basic function of the terminal is to provide interface between the operator element and a data processing system, usually via a telecommunication network. To enter data into the system, most terminals employ a keyboard which may be as simple as a twelve key, touch tone phone or as complex as an accounting machine keyboard. Other terminals include CRT displays which are television-like screens with a cathode-ray tube (CRT) for output and a keyboard for input. At the present time, there are at least 110 different CRT display terminals offered by fifty manufacturers. Also available are graphic terminals in which graphic displays are produced by illuminating random or sequential points on vectors or on a fixed matrix. For the input of graphic data, a device such as a light pen can be used to provide the user capability to manipulate input data.

In a different class are terminals known as intelligent or programmable terminals which represent a growing class of data communication equipment. This type of system usually is built around a minicomputer, may possess impressive ability to format data, and also may have processing capabilities of its own. These devices almost always produce output tape and can transmit the recording data to a central or remote computer. After information has been input to a computer, the choice of storage methods must be made. Storage can be internal or external to the processing unit of the computer. Internal storage often is referred to as working storage and is the part of the main computer where data is processed and where calculations and comparisons are made. It also houses the program that gives instructions to the computer. External storage allows data to be put on media that can be removed from the computer and stored off line or outside the working area until needed. The most common storage devices are magnetic tape and magnetic disc. Computer tape is the same format as audio recording and playback tape. The tape is wound onto reels that are mounted on devices known as disc drives. Discs are the shape of ordinary flat phonograph records, each side containing concentric tracks in which information may be stored. Recording and reading heads are mounted on an access arm that can reach any track on any disc, thus making any piece of information recorded on the disc available to the computer. Retrieval of information from magnetic disc is faster than tape and allows for random accessing. Because it is wound on reels, magnetic tape is sequential; therefore, the tape must be read sequentially until the required data is found. Other types of storage include film, magnetic drum, and photographic storage, but none of these techniques is found in great numbers in the medical environment.

Data formatting of information on a computer printout should be given a great deal of attention when planning any computer system. The layout must be designed for the user. Even though the information displayed is the same, whether it is printed vertically or horizontally can make a significant difference to the user. Size of paper is another consideration. First time computer users find themselves buying new, oversized folders and file cabinets to accommodate computer printouts. Forms of different color and the use of shading also should be investigated. The dissemination of computer reports is a subject that is usually given little or no attention until the time reports are not delivered as required. Usually this delay is the result of the computer operator's having machine problems or becoming too busy. When planning a computer installation, some attention should be given to this problem. It is unwise to use the computer operator as a messenger, for when he is away the computer is nonproductive. This problem is intensified during evening and night shifts.

Accuracy, Timeliness, and Understandability of Information Processing System. Forms design plays a key role in the accuracy of the recorded data. The form designed should allow for the logical and orderly entering of information and should give the person responsible for completing the form every advantage to record data accurately. Ease of data entry into an automated system and coding must be taken into consideration. Some of the more prominent items requiring coding include a physician number, patient identification, a family account number, *ICDA* or *H-ICDA*, and Blue Cross/Blue Shield diagnosis or procedure coding. Poor forms design can result in a large error factor in recording, coding, and transcribing data into a computer system. Schedules must be established for data being entered into an automated system and for output reports. Without clear cutoff dates, financial and statistical information will be useless. Control over charge slips and appointments, both new and return, will allow management to make intelligent decisions regarding the direction of the operation. Without this control, it becomes impossible to make comparisons with any degree of accuracy.

The major factor in the understanding of reports generated from information processing systems is the adoption of a set of uniform terms for which explicit meaning is stipulated. As an example, there should be a clear definition of the term "new" and the term "return" in reference to patients. It should be decided whether visits to the laboratory and X-ray departments after an examination with the physician are to be counted as separate visits or as one visit. No two group practices will be identical in their functional requirements or their methods for implementing data processing systems to meet those requirements. When developing a data processing system, emphasis should be placed on collecting, recording, storing, correlating, formatting, and disseminating data. Most administrators will agree that one of the major deficiencies in the health care field is an inadequate amount of information on possible methods of data processing and the lack of quick access to that information at all levels. Currently available information frequently is insufficient, inaccurate, or untimely in relation to decision making needs.

SYSTEMS DEVELOPMENT PLANNING

The word systems has been defined as, "a set of related things, organized data, etc." Systems development is a process for implementing change. The process for developing any system should follow a logical pattern: (1) the formation of objectives; (2) a definition phase; (3) a preliminary design phase; (4) a detailed design; (5) testing; (6) conversion; (7) an operational phase; (8) evaluation phase; (9) support and maintenance. It is extremely important to effectively manage these activities so that objectives can be met. Sometimes there is a tendency to develop systems that serve the needs of the computer rather than of people. One of the reasons that many organizations elect to rent data processing equipment rather than buy it is that equipment soon becomes obsolete and equipment manufacturers discontinue support of hardware and software. New and improved technology does account for a good portion of the obsolescence problem. Systems obsolescence presents a problem different from hardware obsolescence; systems begin to become obsolete the day they are installed. This obsolescence is caused by items being overlooked in the original systems design, by changing management philosophy and policy, by new or changed government regulations, and by social or economic change.

The decision to acquire data processing equipment usually is an economic one. Often, financial considerations are overridden by other factors such as management philosophy, laws and government regulations, the general economy, or in some cases, even personalities. In acquiring equipment, there are five financing alternatives:

1. *Rent from Vendor.* This is the most popular method. The equipment belongs to the manufacturer and rental usually includes prime shift maintenance. In most cases, the vendor insures the hardware and no coverage is necessary on the part of the renter.

2. *Cash Purchase.* If cash is paid, the group, of course, owns the equipment and benefits from investment tax credit (profit group only), residuals, and depreciation. In addition, the equipment is a capital asset. In the case of computers, residuals take the form of resale value, and there is a market for used computers. Other considerations in regard to purchasing equipment involve the loss of money that possibly could be used for income producing opportunities. Inflation trends also should be weighed.

3. *Bank Loan.* Financing a purchase through a third party's money plus interest results in all of the advantages and disadvantages of an outright purchase.

4. *Time Purchase Agreement.* Time purchases result in outright ownership, but usually require large initial cash outlays.

5. *Third Party Leasing.* This type of financing conserves working capital and results in less bookkeeping and paper work. There are several types of leases that should be explored: (a) finance lease, (b) true lease, (c) master lease,

(d) leverage lease, (e) equipment risk programs, (f) sale and lease back, (g) vendor finance programs, (h) portfolio acquisition, (i) industrial time sales, and (j) lease-purchase.[3]

Ninety-seven percent of data processing budgets cover expenses generated for personnel, hardware, and supplies. The percentage of dollars spent on each of these items will vary depending upon the yearly data processing costs.[4]

Yearly Data Processing Costs:	*$25K*	*$25K–200K*	*$100K–250K*	*$250K–500K*
Hardware	26.13%	36.31%	34.51%	39.48%
Personnel	51.82%	52.79%	55.84%	49.60%
Other	22.05%	10.90%	9.65%	10.92%

In industry, data processing costs can run from 3 percent to 5 percent of an organization's yearly budget. In medical institutions, the cost to date has been less—somewhere between 1 percent and 3 percent.

In industry fifteen years ago, data processing was an adjunct of the controller's department. Top management took it for granted that data processing was merely a faster method for bookkeeping and accounting and actually gave it little attention as long as payroll and other basic accounting functions were completed on time. As computers became more sophisticated, attitudes changed. Today, systems and data processing managers commonly are within the purview of vice presidents. Some are vice presidents themselves while others are presidents of newly created data and consulting service divisions. By nature, accounting is an after-the-fact postscriptive type of activity. Systems development is prescriptive in nature and this should be taken into consideration when organizing a data processing activity. Business problems do not respect organizational lines and departmental jurisdiction. If, therefore, systems development is intended to solve those business problems, data processing activities must be authorized across organizational lines. Successful data processing organizations have been given the freedom to search for opportunities to approach such problems. Any successful systems project team must understand that organizational problems are one of the most critical areas it will encounter and, therefore, must have the skill necessary to cope with such problems. The organization chart for the data center itself can include the following five functions:

1. *Data Control.* The control of input to the center and output from the center
2. *Data Preparation.* The batching and coding function before data are entered into a computer system
3. *Operations.* Data entry clerks or keypunch operators and the computer operators
4. *Scheduling.* The control of the day-to-day operation
5. *Systems Programming.* The systems development team.

Legal problems with data processing installations can be almost nonexistent if, when negotiating a contract for hardware and software, care is taken to obtain a detailed proposal of equipment, programs, and technical support stating the responsibilities of the buyer and seller, including the length of the contract and cost. The responsibilities for insurance coverage of equipment must be clear. Who will be responsible for the equipment in transit from the factory to the installation, on the loading dock, during installation, and after installation must be established. Who will be responsible if the equipment must be moved also should be determined.

The safeguarding of data has not been a problem in the past but can be a legal consideration in the future. Protection of medical data has become more important because of the greater use of computers by medical facilities, planning agencies, research groups, and third party payors. Good management practices are the controlling factors determining who has authorized access to specific data, who will see it, and who may add or delete information. To meet these safeguard requirements, the group should consider: (1) selecting one person to be immediately responsible; (2) informing each employee about the safeguard requirements; (3) specifying penalties to employees who violate the safeguard; (4) taking reasonable precautions to protect the data in the system from anticipated threats or hazards; and (5) transferring no identifiable personal data to another system unless such other system also fulfills safeguard requirements.[5]

In recent years, the value of systems theory has received increased recognition. In order to utilize systems theory, however, objectives must be stated; the more precisely objectives are stated, the more effectively they will be implemented. When objectives are stated vaguely, a great number of assumptions must be made and it is less likely that a systems program will be successful in meeting the group needs. Systems objectives, similar to overall group objectives, are established goals; a systems development program is the strategy employed to achieve those goals. Objective setting is a process of relating expectations to resources. Usable objectives are best established jointly by the supervisor and the supervised. Frederick G. Withington predicts that computers developed from 1982 on will be magnetic, bubble, and/or laser, holographic technology distributed systems. In addition, he predicts that the systems will be working with simulation, forecasting models, and decision trees.[6] Even today the Systems Dynamic Laboratory at the Massachusetts Institute of Technology has developed mathematical models of world systems in which computers project data as far ahead as two hundred years. Real time systems and time sharing will make the power of the computer available to workers at their desks and even to homemakers in their homes. Whether Mr. Withington is correct or not, there is no doubt that scientific and technical innovations will markedly affect systems development planning.

Elements of the System

Systems design is the marriage of people, methods, and equipment in a fully planned program for accomplishing certain objectives. A successful data processing team requires a blending of managerial and technical abilities. The *administrator* responsible for the data processing activities should have a background in systems design, data processing, and management. His goals should include knowledgeable, responsible leadership aimed at a profitable data processing operation. Education, communications, staffing, planning, ongoing evaluation, and operational economy should be among his major concerns. The *data proc-*

essing manager should be well versed in the problems of programming and computer operations. His goal is to run day-to-day operations smoothly, to develop new applications, and to maintain liaison with management through establishing schedules, revising schedules, conducting programmers' meetings, investigating errors, developing applications, and acting as a liaison to management. The *systems programmers* are faced with two major requirements that are somewhat in opposition. One is the need to develop continually new applications, and the other is to keep and to modify applications already in service. In meeting these requirements, often it is necessary to balance the staff with programmers who are innovative and creative and those who are content to work day after day with existing programs. A programmer's activities include keeping track of data and programs, creating test data, documenting programs, writing run books, creating new programs, and changing and maintaining existing programs. Thirty percent of programmers' time may be devoted to systems design, 20 percent to coding, 2 percent to clerical, 30 percent to debugging (testing and correction), and 18 percent to documentation. *Computer operators* are expected to follow programmer instructions, handle computer loops and programming halts, anticipate computer setups, select and maintain correct tape and disc files, minimize wait time between jobs, and maintain schedules.

The selection of a *computer* depends upon its ability to meet group objectives within the financial range the group can afford. Other considerations include group personnel's ability to operate and to program the system. Whatever equipment is chosen, backup and reliability must be considered. The duplication of certain critical equipment may have significant impact in reducing computer downtime. In addition, each major application should have a backup procedure to follow when the system is down. Backup can be manual or can involve the use of someone else's computer equipment. An ample spare parts inventory also should be available. When negotiating a computer contract with a vendor, the group should insist on rapid vendor response to correct unanticipated failures in equipment. A strong preventive maintenance program to reduce unanticipated failures will be helpful. An effective program will disclose many problems before they become serious enough to bring operations to a halt. Such programs should be performed on "off hours" whenever possible. Housing the computer should be given a good deal of attention when planning an installation, and vendors can be helpful in this area. Considerations should include computer layout, power requirements, air conditioning, lighting, and the need for a raised floor.

The composite data to which a computer system has access in the performance of its duty is known as its *data base.* Information contained in the data base will depend upon group objectives and needs. A patient billing system requires patient's or responsible party's name and address, charges, payments, and the amount of insurance filed. When applications are expanded the data base also will grow. Over the years it has become apparent that individual application files are difficult to control and to update. This duplication of information is expensive and often inaccurate. In recent years, there has been a trend towards common data bases that serve many of the application areas within an organization, thus eliminating many of the problems encountered with multiple files. Data base management for a computer system is a complex series of linkages that allow access to related data for retrieval and updating. Data base management programs are available from vendors, software houses, and sofware brokers. Due to the complexity of this type of software, it would be very difficult to develop this type of computer program in-house. Systems development planning should include rules and procedures for data handling. No job should be assigned to the data center until it has been tested completely and has been proven to operate successfully by the programming staff. Every transaction put into the system should be verified in total or in part. Data input clerks should not be allowed to verify their own work and production standards can be used to assure optimum efficiency. At a minimum, the data center should have:

1. A workable schedule (manual or automatic)
2. A schedule for cleaning tapes and discs
3. A log of tape and disc identification labels
4. A console log documenting downtime and reasons for reruns and preventive maintenance
5. Run books that describe application, files, the job flow, and restart procedures
6. A procedure for externally labeling tapes and discs
7. A procedure for hardware and software errors
8. A hardware preventive maintenance plan
9. A policy to allow only people necessary to the operation into the computer room.

It should be recognized that not all applications or problems can be solved by the computer. In many cases, particularly with small volume jobs, the pen may be mightier than the computer, and this fact must be taken into consideration in systems development planning. No hard and fast rules separate applicants for computer or manual processing, but some questions that may be asked include: What is the estimated number of manhours that would be saved if the project were computerized? What are the estimated savings in personnel salaries, materials, and floor space? Can any scientific or research value be realized? Can any patient benefits be realized? As control for any computer system, input batches should be logged and time stamped and there should be a clear system for tracking transactions through the data center. A corrective routine should be present for input errors and there should be computer controlled totals as well as a distribution list for periodic reports.

Subsystems

An important part of systems development planning is the process of reviewing in detail each major application area and further defining each one in terms of identifiable subsystems. Each of these subsystems also should be analyzed and documented. Tasks that must be performed can then be identified and realistic completion dates can be assigned to those tasks and the subsystems. For illustrative purposes, when developing a payroll system, the subsystem might include:

1. Time sheets
2. Calculations involved in withholding deductions, etc.
3. Check writing, signing, and controlling
4. Check reconciliation
5. Year-end W-2 processing
6. Weekly, monthly, and yearly statistical reports.

OPERATIONALIZING THE SYSTEM

When operationalizing a system, the major objective is, of course, to move from the present system (manual or automated) to the new system. Subsystems involved in this process are: design testing, conversion, operating procedures, evaluation, and a plan for support and maintenance. Operationalizing is a system within itself, separate and apart from the desired operating system after conversion. Few organizations find themselves in a position to move directly to a new system without extensive and rigorous testing. The danger of not testing can be very serious and it almost always is certain that such shortcuts will lead to critical problems. Two phases of testing usually are necessary—continuity testing and final or parallel testing. Continuity testing should occur after all major subsystems have been completed and have been tested individually and should result in the assurance that all programs work as part of the complete system. To perform this type of testing, a representative sample of all of the various kinds of input data, both valid and invalid, are processed by the system and the results are checked and verified in every respect. The time necessary to perform continuity testing will vary depending upon the complexity of the system. While a complex system may be very expensive to test, such testing can prevent many serious problems that could occur later, after the system is in operation.

Final testing is similar to continuity testing except that it is performed when there is no existing system from which to convert. In this case, actual "live" data are used to test the system. Parallel testing is used when an existing manual, semi-automated, or automated system is to be converted to a new system and is performed by processing identical data through both the existing and the new system. Results from the two systems are compared, when possible. New procedures must be incorporated in those areas where the new system produces results or handles conditions not presently incorporated in existing systems. After a parallel test which has proven the workability of the system, conversion may be accomplished by continuing to run under the new system, gradually adding the remainder of the work and dropping operations under the old system; or by dropping parallel operations completely and by converting all work at one time, thus operating fully under the new system with the old system no longer in operation.

Anyone who has implemented a new system may remember the conversion as a critical time. Conversions usually are performed on tight schedules and on weekends or "off hours" so that daily work patterns are not interrupted. At this time, clerical errors appear, controls break down, programming problems surface, and operating personnel and clerks are apt to make mistakes. A great deal of attention should be given to planning targets and clearly defined schedules when converting to a new system. The assignment of responsibility concerning who will assemble the data, correct the errors, validate the controls, and solve the problems in systems design and programming must be made clear.

When the system is ready to become operational, at least three basic kinds of documentation should be available for operating procedures. The first is a general information manual describing the system and its important features for high level administration, department heads, and supervisors. In addition, a users' manual should indicate the department for whom the system was developed and what personnel must do to ensure that the system performs as required. If possible, this documentation should be written by the user. Lastly, an operating manual should be prepared for computer operations personnel to instruct them in running the system. Once a system is in operation, continued evaluation of its performance is necessary to ascertain whether it meets the basic requirements it was designed for and whether it is controllable. Such an evaluation should include investigation of ways the system can be improved. The programming section of the data processing unit should be charged with improving the performance of existing programs, correcting deficiencies, and making systems extensions to comply with new or changing requirements. Data processing units find that maintenance of existing programs is a major activity, the costs of which increase each time the department adds a new system.

INFORMATION PROCESSING PROCEDURES

Forms play a major role in developing data processing systems and in maintaining ongoing data processing applications. As an administrative tool, therefore, forms should be clear, capable of being easily understood, concise, limited to essential words, complete, and appropriate. A good form provides a pattern for thinking and should serve as a mental checklist. The prime purpose for many clerical procedures is to explain the use of various forms. With this in mind, a great deal of attention must be given to the information printed on forms and to the purpose such information fulfills in the system and in the organization. Thought must be given to the accuracy, cost, and speed of processing. Because forms in their first design are never 100 percent efficient, suggestions for improvement should be elicited from individuals who use them.

It also is important that forms be properly identified. For purposes of control, forms should be numbered and dated with the last revision. When designing computer input forms, all-purpose or three/five spacing should be considered. Three/five spacing is represented by three horizontal lines to the inch and five digits to the inch between each vertical rule. This type of spacing is satisfactory for both handwritten and/or typewritten material. The ease with which a computer can input data recorded on such a form also should be weighed. The first consideration, however, should be for persons completing the forms.

A printed rule is used to separate data groups into different zones and to guide the writer or reader's eye as he uses the form. Only lightly printed rules are necessary; people who read forms attend to the filled-in information, not the rules. The same philosophy should apply to captions. Small typeface should be used throughout the form unless there is a definite reason for a larger typeface. In addition, box designs can make the form attractive, and for the typist can result in a 15 percent to 30 percent savings in keystrokes.[7] Forms should not be designed to cover a page of paper and extend to its edge. The printer will need at least one-fourth inch to one-half inch for the gripper margin for the presses. Due to additional requirements for filing and storage, forms should be standardized in size. Forms should be designed to be self-instructing. A well-designed form will assist in procedural work, will delineate responsibilities involved in completing the form, and will help to control the system. Choosing the proper carbon also is important. Carbons for handwriting differ from those designed for a typewriter or a computer printer. Hardness of the platen and the weight of the paper are additional factors. Sensitized paper for which carbons are unnecessary represents yet another option.

It is necessary to establish guidelines in two areas for the control of waste. The first involves forms ordering. Because of bulk pricing, it is tempting to order in large volumes. If, however, the form is redesigned before the complete stock is used, all remaining stock becomes useless. Forms waste also occurs in the data section. If not instructed properly on the loading and unloading of printers and if not requested to use stock paper for as many internal jobs as possible, computer operators may waste expensive forms. Data processing forms fall into two categories. Input forms are action oriented, while output forms are records and reports generated by the computer. In controlling input or action forms, it is necessary to know who initiates each form, where it goes, and where it finally stops. In monitoring computer output forms, personnel must know the purpose of each form, who looks at it, if additional information is added, and how often it is used. Because of multiple requests, copies of many forms will need to be duplicated and it is important to know the reason for each copy. Multiple copies of data processing forms are expensive.

Information Storage

The first and most obvious requirement of information storage systems is that they must be of sufficient scope to store the data and must permit ready access to the information quickly. Two goals of efficient information storage are to maintain clinically and administratively relevant data readily accessible for each patient served in the health care delivery system and to provide a source for the systematic retrieval of medical data across large numbers of patients for any desired retrospective administrative and research study. In electronic data processing several types of storage media are available to accomplish these two goals. The most commonly used are disc direct access storage and magnetic tape. Decisions regarding the combination of these storage devices are easy to make in some instances such as for program instructions, tables, and work space but not as easy to make for storage of patients' records, which may need to be readily accessed. The selection of magnetic tape for relatively slow serial retrieval versus disc files for direct access is a straightforward decision if retrieval requirements are predictable. When choosing peripheral equipment such as tape and disc drive units, the group should consider plug compatible discs and tape systems from vendors other than the central processing unit vendor. A number of firms now manufacture plug compatible equipment which is more economical than that produced by the central unit vendor and which may serve the group's needs more efficiently. Vendors who sell plug compatible equipment are:

Ampex	Control Data	Memorex	STC
Cal Comp	IBM	Mohawk	Telex
CIG	Itel	Potter	

The following features should be considered when investigating disc storage:

1. Configuration (maximum number of spindles on-line)
2. Storage capacity (recording surfaces per disc pack)
3. Performance (head movement time, average access time, start-up time, and stop time)
4. Price and maintenance.

Magnetic tapes are manufactured in several different formats, and compatibility should be the criterion for selection. Tapes usually are one-half inch in width and may be as much as twenty-four hundred feet long. Information can be stored on seven or nine tracks and at various densities including 200, 556, 800, 1,600, and 6,250 bits per inch. Tape speed and transfer rate, rewind time, read backwards, and price and maintenance are general features of a tape storage system which should be adaptable to the group's needs. An operational consideration is that tape drives must be cleaned after every six to eight hours of use.

When designing a storage system, policies involving data independence, data integrity, performance, compatibility, and security should be established. When possible, data should be discrete; relationships require extensive manipulation for evaluation. The physical structure of data within the data processing system is complex, and changing relationships require extensive reprogramming to process data. Data must be protected against accidental or deliberate destruction. Rules should be established for right of entry, correction, and removal of data. When possible, such control should be programmed into the computer's logic. In addition, performance must be consistent, measurable, and adjustable to satisfy changing needs. Data that has low priority without need for real time access can be stored on slower and less expensive equipment. Future hardware and software technology should be kept in mind to minimize the need for reprogramming. Finally, data processing personnel who have access to clinic records must share responsibility for protecting the confidentiality of that information. Accidental disclosures, however, may happen through instances of hardware, software, or human failure. Such situations sometimes occur due to nondiscretionary disposal of computer printout or the routing of privileged information to inappropriate individuals.

Information Display

Information generated by a computer may be displayed either on a cathode ray tube or on hard copy from a computer printer. The alpha numeric characters displayed on a cathode ray tube are generated in a five by seven point dot matrix or by a stroke system which forms symbols by drawing short straight lines between specified coordinates. The usual screen size is four to six inches by eight to nine inches; it may be horizontally or vertically oriented, and also may be interfaced with a television monitor. The capacity of a display may vary from 240 to 2,080 characters. Colored television monitors are available for special functions and are being used in a medical setting to provide red colored error or warning messages. Search or response time can present a problem and is a function of types of storage and availability of the computer. People waiting for a computer to respond to their inquiries usually are unhappy if made to wait more than five seconds. Associated printers are available together with cathode ray tubes to provide the user with hard copy of data shown on the tube. Electric, on-line typewriters are one example of this type of printer, but such devices are slow and noisy. An alternative is an impact printer which is quieter and prints 30 to 100 characters per second. Electrostatic printers also are quiet but require special paper that is very expensive. Yet another type of printer, the ink jet, is fast and quiet, but requires frequent servicing. Vendors can offer a wide range of computer printers with all kinds of typeface, and upper and lower case, alphabetic, numeric, and special characters. The speeds of these printers range from 300 to 1,800 lines per minute. The usual number of horizontal print positions is 120 or 132 per line, and vertical spacing is six or eight lines to the inch.

Documentation

The weakest element in most data processing systems and also in most clerical systems is documentation. By its very nature, data processing implies an ordered approach to problem solving. Documentation, therefore, must be an integral part of any computer installation. The lack of operating, user, and manager documentation for a system can lead to costly errors because of misused or unused program features. In order to overcome this, management must motivate systems analysts, programmers, and users to document the operating systems adequately. Such documentation includes the use of flow charts, block diagrams, final compilation or assembly listings, operating instruction, user instructions, and a record of each change made after the system was installed. Documentation standards should be established and compiled in a standards manual. Failure to formulate and use standards frequently has resulted in the inability to follow and comprehend systems and programming design. This is particularly true when the systems analyst or programmer who designed the system no longer works for the organization. The backbone of good documentation is flow charting, the purpose of which is to present a graphic display of a system. Specific symbols are used to represent different types of action. Actual symbols used may differ from organization to organization but should be standardized within a single institution. Computer and form vendors have available plastic templates with standard symbols. As in all documentation, forms play an important role. Some of the more common forms which can be procured from computer vendors at a nominal charge are:

1. Card layout sheets
2. Multiple card layout forms
3. Record layout (tape and disc) sheets
4. File maintenance forms
5. Printer spacing charts

6. Run specification sheets
7. Computer run sheets
8. Decision tables.

There are two categories of documentation for an operational system, one for the computer user and the other for the computer operators. The user should have documentation that explains from his standpoint the system's functional requirements as well as a users' manual explaining the proper use of the system. The computer operator should have an operations manual, explaining in detail how the system is run. Such documentation, often called a runbook, details what actions are to be taken on operating systems or input/output control systems messages and indicator lights. Also included should be console procedures in the event of machine or software malfunction and procedures for job starts and completions. In addition to the runbook, there should be written procedures for emergency and security. The computer operator also generates documentation by keeping various logs which, at minimum, should include:

1. Recording computer time and logging in jobs (some computers do this through their operating systems software)
2. Logging machine problems
3. Recording control information.

In order that programs can be maintained, system specifications must be documented. Such documentation is oriented to programmers and includes:

1. A description of how the program fits into the total system
2. A print format or other display formats required for each type of output
3. Flow chart showing inputs and outputs
4. Layout of input and output records (magnetic tape or disc)
5. Transaction coding
6. Information that pertains to controls.

Program documentation also is vital to maintenance of a system and contains details concerning the computer processing logic, including overall systems flow charts, block diagrams, and assembler listings. For each system there also should be a general information manual which includes a general, overall systems flow chart, exhibits of input forms and output reports, and a narrative of the system and its important features.

Comparison of Information Processing Systems: EDP and EAM

Electronic Data Processing (EDP) and general purpose computing systems range from $5,000 per month rental to almost any amount imaginable. Equipment is available from several different manufacturers, including:

Burroughs	Honeywell Information Systems	NCR
Control Data	IBM	Siemens Corporation

Digital Equipment	International Computing Ltd.	Singer Company
Greyhound Computer	Memorex	UNIVAC-Sperry Rand Corp.
		Xerox Corporation

Electronic Accounting Machines (EAM) and small accounting computers are available from most of the above manufacturers at purchase prices of $5,000 to $75,000. Clinics and hospitals along with more than a half-million businesses or other organizations, employing fewer than 150 employees, are marketing targets for this type equipment.

EDP equipment is very flexible and can be expanded to almost any size desirable. Limiting factors are cost and the personnel necessary to operate and program this complex equipment. EAM equipment, however, is limited in its expandability and flexibility. Most applications are limited to billing, payroll, general ledger, accounts receivable, accounts payable, and inventory management. The processing speed of all general purpose computers, even small ones, is extremely fast. The important thing to remember is that the data must be accurately acquired and read into the computer. Retrieval time often is the same for both EDP and EAM equipment. The significant measurement is the total throughput time—i.e., the total time necessary to process data from beginning to end. EAM equipment is slow compared to EDP hardware. Its characteristics include direct key input and low speed printed output.

EDP languages are codes used to provide instructions to the computer in the framework of a program. Software can be defined as programs that direct computers to perform specific functions. The term software also may include the complete process of designing, coding (languages), testing, and installing those programs. The term software package refers to a specific computer program or sets of programs designed to perform one or more functions. If such packages are bought or rented, they are available in "canned" form as a systems package with associated documentation and maintenance. Application packages are programs written for specific processes such as payroll, accounts receivable, accounts payable, etc. Software is generated as a result by in-house personnel, computer manufacturers, user groups, software houses, and software brokers.

An important decision concerning software is whether to develop the program in-house or to purchase. If the decision is to accomplish the job in-house, some of the obstacles confronting the group include the high cost of development and the fact that it is difficult to recruit competent programmers. In-house development may require a few months or several years, depending upon the complexity of the programs and the competency of the programmers. Costs are almost impossible to predict accurately and some planned programs never reach completion. In addition, comprehensive documentation, so necessary to smooth running operations, often is not accomplished. If the decision is to buy, the following major steps should be taken:

1. Determine the systems requirements.
2. Gather data about available software packages.
3. Narrow the field by selecting two or three of the best packages.

4. Evaluate and compare in terms of computer compatibility, feasibility, performance, installation, documentation, and cost.
5. Determine the form in which it will be developed (cards, tapes, paper documentation).

EAM equipment often comes with programs complete; therefore, software and language considerations are not necessary. If the system does not have software as part of the arrangement, the process of appraisal suggested for EDP equipment can be employed.

For both EDP and EAM equipment, if the group has had past experience with a particular manufacturer, such knowledge should be applied when deciding on a data processing system, and in all cases the following steps should be applied before buying or renting any equipment:

1. Prepare or have prepared detailed specifications on all hardware and software.
2. Observe a full-scale demonstration on the equipment, and for EAM equipment with at least one principal application demonstrated.
3. Obtain a detailed proposal of equipment, software, and technical support.
4. Determine processing time for the application.
5. Define the responsibilities of buyer and seller.
6. Negotiate total purchase price or monthly rental.
7. Obtain a list of other users.

Systems and Equipment Selection

The group's bid specification for vendors should include:

1. The organization's overall objectives
2. The objectives of the data processing department
3. An inventory of present data processing equipment (if any)
4. A narrative of proposed applications and their input volume and output reports
5. A request for proof of vendor's commitment to the medical industry
6. A request for specifics on:
   a. Proposed equipment and software
   b. Maintenance
   c. Education
   d. Testing
   e. Application implementation schedule
   f. Growth capability
   g. Cost and contract offerings
   h. Equipment availability
   i. Systems support
7. Any special requirements (such as interfacing with existing equipment).

Specifications should be approved by high level management before being released to any vendor. After release has been made, all requests for additional information should be answered in writing. The vendors should be told when their proposals are due and when a decision can be expected. As vendors submit proposals, the group should narrow the field to no more than three vendors by checking for basic compliance with bid specifications. After the field has been narrowed, on site visits should be made to other data processing installations that have the proposed equipment. It is desirable, but not absolutely necessary, that the visited installations be medical facilities.

A technique for evaluating computer speeds and output is referred to as a "benchmark." Benchmark programs are used to arrive at running times for a given volume of work. To accomplish this, identical jobs or series of jobs are run on two or more different types of computers and the times and output are compared. While this technique is not as valuable with modern computers as it once was, it does give the potential computer customer an opportunity to see the proposed equipment running one of his jobs. If for some reason there is a problem, it allows the customer to see the vendor's reaction to that problem. Comparing various models of printers, card punches, tape drives, and disc drives has less relevance today than ten years ago. Almost all vendors make such types of equipment that are both reliable and fast. Some of the more critical points to evaluate in hardware and software selection are:

1. Compliance with the bid specification
2. Cost and price performance, including maintenance costs
3. Contracts—length, cancellation provisions, etc.
4. Capacity and ability to add memory, input/output devices, and features once the computer is installed
5. Variety, speed, and cost of input/output devices available and the programmed support available for them
6. Reliability and availability of backup equipment
7. Delivery schedules
8. Physical requirements, such as power, floor space, air conditioning, and floor loading
9. Programs and programming aids:
   a. Applications, utility, and diagnostic programs
   b. Special sub-routines
   c. Programming language support, features, and efficiency
   d. Operating systems features
   e. Operating repertoire and power
   f. Systems and procedure assistance
10. Testing arrangements (amount of free testing time will vary from vendor to vendor)
11. Vendor educational facilities, location, and cost
12. Maintenance of equipment—response time and spare parts
13. Conversion assistance
14. Reliability of service—company backing and company experience
15. Experience in the heath care field.

Shared or Service Bureau

Shared or service bureau computing services are commercial organizations that provide computer base services to users at remote locations through a telephone hookup, making use of teletypewriters or other data terminals. Evaluating shared or service bureau arrangements differs somewhat from the evaluation procedure used when buying or leasing a computer. The service bureau contract should contain a guarantee; any shared system may become overloaded by too many users, thereby resulting in a slower response time that will downgrade service. Various item costs should be investigated. For terminal rental, a flat monthly rate usually is required. Usage time may be calculated as either clock time from hookup to sign off, as actual computer time used, or as a flat rate or combination of these. Often, there is a flat rate connection charge each time the computer is used. Other cost items include telephone line or toll charge, data set or acoustic coupler rental, and basic telephone service rates. When service will be available is another important factor to check. Computers usually are available only at certain times, and the group should be sure to inquire about night, Saturday, Sunday, and holiday availability. A provision should be made for consulting, training, and troubleshooting by the shared or service bureau company. Other points to be investigated are:

1. Programming languages
2. Maximum program size per user
3. Maximum storage device space
4. Application packages offered.

Some of the advantages of shared or service bureau systems are:

1. Flexibility—the group can buy only what it needs
2. Ease of use—the operations usually are straightforward and the terminals simple to use
3. Instant communication
4. Fast turnaround
5. Usually a wide variety of languages, application programs, networks, and data bases are available.

Some of the disadvantages of shared or service bureau systems include:

1. Questionable reliability
2. Slow input and output
3. Low computerizational efficiency
4. Questionable data security
5. Systems loading problems when the computer is down or the system busy
6. Communication costs
7. High on-line data storage cost
8. Loss of control.

Turnkey Systems

A turnkey system is one in which a vendor assumes all responsibility for installing a computer, which includes the analysis, equipment selection, installation, maintenance, training, and documentation. When the vendor has completed these activities, the user has only, figuratively, to turn the key to have an operational system. Although this approach requires only a minimum expenditure of time and effort by the purchaser, several points should be considered:

1. There is an initial cost involved in all turnkey systems, and there also will be ongoing operational costs.
2. Even if the system performs as promised, it will take a long time to amortize the initial capital investment.
3. The system must meet not only the present needs but also future requirements.
4. The choice of a turnkey system permanently locks the user with the vendor.
5. The rapidly changing state of the art could make today's system outdated in a short period of time.
6. Any modification or addition to the system after installation can be expensive.
7. Before choosing a turnkey approach, if the user does not have a data processing expert on the staff, advice should be sought from a consultant.
8. An attorney familiar with automation contracts should review the agreement before it is signed by the group.

Minicomputers

Minicomputer technology has advanced to the stage of offering management, economic, and organizational potential. Today's minis cost approximately one-fortieth as much as large computers but they can do a great deal more than one-fortieth of the work. Many small companies who formerly used service bureaus are beginning to use general purpose minis. This also is true of medical centers and hospitals, as well as:

1. Equipment manufacturers who incorporate minis into their own product line
2. Seasonal data processing users to supplement their present equipment
3. Unsophisticated and first time users who want complete systems programmed and installed on a turnkey basis.

Some minis are used as front-ends to larger computers. In this case, the mini usually handles communication between terminals and the central computer. Others are used to handle independent applications and require no link to a larger central computer, such as in pharmacies, radiology departments, and pulmonary function laboratories. In some cases, data is interchanged on a periodic basis. Minis also are being used in two or more departments and can be tied together in networks by telephone lines to permit the sharing of data and programs. Typically, minis are located nearer the user. When considering a minicomputer, potential buyers should ask:

1. Have the minis actually been installed at another location?
2. If so, what has been the user's experience?
3. What software support is available?
4. Who will provide services and under what conditions?

This chapter has presented material which should be helpful to small groups who wish to utilize electronic data processing on a shared basis and for larger groups who are engaged in long range planning and intend to expand. Each group will want to assess its needs carefully and reexamine its objectives while exploring the possibility of automation. In any case, conversion to automation should be gradual, perhaps one function at a time, with emphasis placed upon alerting and educating all group practice personnel and patients in relation to procedures and expectations of the automated systems.

Chapter 19

Statistical Analysis Systems

SOME GUIDELINES FOR SYSTEMS DESIGN

In the preceding chapters in this section, a variety of group practice operating systems has been discussed. All of these systems are vital to the successful operation of any group practice. While each system is discrete, with its own specific functions, the overall process of performance evaluation and control incorporates and makes use of the outputs of all such systems. This chapter is entitled "Statistical Analysis Systems" to highlight three aspects of the process of performance evaluation and control. First, the term "statistical" rather than the broader terms "data" or "information" is used because it connotes quantitative information—numbers. While health care delivery is obviously too complex an undertaking to be reduced to numbers and any attempt at describing or evaluating it exclusively in quantitative terms is likely to be inadequate, that very complexity creates a need to treat the most salient factors expeditiously. Maintaining and improving the health of patients underlies all group practice activities. Any time saved in the process can be used to great advantage. The translation of information—even qualitative information—into statistics can hasten the identification of inadequacies in program performance so that they may be corrected in a timely manner and can reinforce the rationale for using present methods of operation. Data other than numerical statistics should be available for purposes of refining an understanding of these problems.

"Analysis" implies the search for meaning through the application of judgment. There must be a reason for selecting a particular set of numbers, such as a need for illuminating some aspect of performance. Otherwise, one quickly is confronted by such an extensive array of undifferentiated facts that there is no way to absorb, integrate, and, ultimately, to make sense of them. Statistics must be structured so that they lend themselves to logical analysis. "Systems" is a term that has become quite fashionable over the past decade and, fortunately, one that has been generalized to the point that virtually every set of organizational activities—be they related or not—has come to be regarded as a system. A rather simple definition of what is meant by "system" in the context of the present discussion is "that set of elements interrelated to perform functions or to achieve goals."[1] The interrelatedness of the elements is a theme central to this discussion. The objective, then, is to describe how a system can be developed which enables a medical group to evaluate on an ongoing basis the effectiveness of the practice in achieving its missions and to translate the findings of that evaluation into terms which aid those who must make the day-to-day decisions that determine group practice performance.

There is no one best method for developing a good statistical analysis system, but there are pitfalls which many group practices have encountered that can be avoided if those charged with the responsibility of systems development adopt a certain perspective from the outset. This perspective might be characterized through the following guiding principles:

1. Statistical data should not be collected, aggregated, reduced, analyzed, or reported for their own sake.
2. Determination of a use for the end results should precede determination of the data to be gathered. These outputs must be perceived as necessary by group members either (a) for effective management of the group practice or (b) to meet reporting requirements of external agencies.
3. Both the administrative and professional staff members of the group must be actively involved in the process of system design and implementation.
4. The system once developed and operating should in no way interfere with the optimal provision of medical care.
5. The confidentiality of sensitive data—related either to individual patients or physicians—should be carefully protected and necessary safeguards built into the system.
6. Whether the system should operate either wholly or in part in an automated mode should be assessed only after the basic system requirements are determined.

This last point should be stressed. Because they exist—and in great numbers—automated data systems that make use of sophisticated hardware have a tendency to be viewed as ends in themselves rather than as means to a larger end. They seem to confer upon the organization that uses them a self-image of efficiency and a sense of being at the forefront of the science of group practice management. All too frequently these expensive systems do not achieve their full potential, because the basic criterion for acquiring them was hardware preference rather than systems requirement. Deciding upon a method of data processing—be it manual, mechanical, electronic, or some combination of all three—cannot be done intelligently without first deciding exactly what the system must accomplish. The other guidelines noted above are largely self-explanatory and will not be expanded here; however, in moving through the system development process observations can be made as to how these guidelines can influence the choices made.

SPECIFYING OUTPUTS

While beginning with anticipated outcomes might seem logical, doing so takes a considerable amount of self-restraint. There is a strong temptation to specify kinds of input first, in response to the requests of a rapidly increasing number of external agencies and organizations that require health care providers not only to produce data of a certain type but to collect particular items of data for entry into their data bases. Given such requirements, it is easy to understand the reaction: "What data are we compelled to collect and what use can we make of them?" The difficulty is in refraining from asking this question until after asking: "What decisions and evaluations do we need to make in the process of monitoring our program and planning for the future, and what data do we need to collect to produce statistics that will help us make these decisions?"

Internal Management Requirements

Articulating the group's statistical requirements for internal management purposes should begin with the group's mission statement. As explained in Chapter 3, this statement defines the group's reason for being; decisions of the group that do not reinforce these missions will tend to undermine them over time. For each mission selected, then, an effort should be made to develop a list of performance measures or evaluative indices which would inform the group on a regular basis as to whether that mission and the objectives defined in support of it are being achieved.

Earlier (Chapter 3, Table 3-1), reference was made to some examples of "criteria" presented in the *Self-Analysis Manual.*[2] These criteria and many more included in that manual show that there is a vast range of creative possibilities for performance measurement. Not all of these "criteria" are quantitative; many involve subjective evaluations derived from interviews, opinion polls, and the like. Not all are produced by an ongoing data collection system; many are based on periodic or ad hoc studies. Still others emerge from samples taken from existing records rather than complete tabulations. The following examples represent still other possibilities.

Mission or Prime Objective: To meet the health needs of the patient by providing comprehensive quality care.

Sub-objective: To provide fully acceptable episodic care.

Possible Criteria or Performance Measures:

1. Percentage of time episodic patients are forced to seek treatment elsewhere due to clinic's being closed or because of a delayed appointment (from patient interviews and emergency room records)
2. Average waiting time for walk-in patients to see a physician (from Patient Flow Analysis)
3. Thoroughness of examination and adequacy of management procedures initiated (from sampling chart audits)

Sub-objective: To provide comprehensive multidisciplinary care.

Possible Criteria:

1. Number of new patients given referrals to: (a) social services, (b) dentist, (c) nutritionist, (d) visiting nurse, (e) psychologist

2. Percentage of referrals completed and outcomes recorded in patients' records
3. Average number of patient encounters per day for each discipline
4. Percentage of nurse's time, social worker's time, etc., spent in direct patient contact (available from Work Sampling)
5. Average number of cases "team conferenced" weekly
6. Number of "team conferenced" patients from whom multidisciplinary "care plans" have been implemented.

Sub-Objective: To provide the patient with a continuity of care delivery consistent with recognized good practice.

Possible Criteria:

1. Percentage of time patient sees same physician for all visits related to single problem or set of problems
2. Degree to which the patient sees the same team of health professionals for all visits
3. Degree to which the patient's group physician follows through on hospitalizations
4. Percentage of patient's records that are: (a) available, (b) complete, and (c) accurate for all clinic visits (obtained from Information Sampling)
5. Availability of reports in patient's medical record folder for all lab tests, X-rays, and referrals to supportive disciplines.

Operationally, those responsible for the group's management are not likely to look at each of these performance measures singly or with an equal degree of attention. Most likely, several aspects of performance will be observed simultaneously and an attempt will be made to interrelate them. The following situation illustrates the interrelationships among several measures: The monthly actual fee-for-service revenue figures compared against the projected figures in the financial plan show an increasing negative variance of greater than 10 percent. This apparent discrepancy prompts the administrator to investigate further. When he looks at a profile of the program's patient load for the preceding several months, he notes that smaller than expected percentages occur in the age categories of the very young and the very old. Additional analysis shows that the figures are particularly low among patients from a certain group of census tracts in these age groups, and that their problems appear to be more acute than those of comparable patients from other areas who use the program more frequently on preventive health care visits. The waiting time before entering the physician's office is also greater for those patients who are from these lower encounter rate groups. Finally, an analysis of the history of those patients in the census tracts and age groups under study reveals that there is a higher frequency of first visits handled by nonphysician staff than for the rest of the patient population.

The administrator who confronts these facts is in a position to formulate several hypotheses. Answers are not immediately apparent but at least there is some basis upon which to improve the program's performance. First of all, one performance measure alerts the administrator to the fact that revenue has not been generated at the predicted rate. Another measure suggests that a distortion in the age profile may underlie this variance, since higher utilization is typically associated with the very young and the very old. A third measure reveals that this distortion is geographically-based. Other measures provide additional clues. Those patients from the low encounter groups do not utilize the program for preventive medicine as much as do other patients, and have a higher incidence of acute and serious illness. In addition, their waiting time at the facility is longer. Could it be that patients discouraged by longer waiting times do not return or, worse, spread the word in their communities that the program is unresponsive? The extent to which these patients are disproportionately handled by staff other than physicians on their first visit may contribute to their being discouraged from visiting again until they are acutely ill. Could it be that less than adequate care is being rendered at these initial visits, that the staff is impersonal, or that the problems have gone unnoticed?

All of these possibilities must be investigated and the actual causes of inadequate program performance pinpointed. It is then that corrective action may take place. In the above example, corrective action could take many forms: improving the transportation capability of the patients in certain census tracts, expanding a preventive medicine educational program in these areas, changing policies regarding level of professional staff who handle patients on first visits, reallocating patient loads, changing hours of operation or increasing the nursing staff to assume responsibility for certain routine tasks so that waiting times can be reduced, alerting staff to the probability of noncompliance with physician directives by patients in certain age and socioeconomic levels, and so on.

Measurement of Quality of Care. "Quality of care" is difficult to define, much less quantify. Yet without some sense of the effectiveness with which a program is providing health care to its patients, regardless of the amount of financial, marketing, or utilization data, a comprehensive analysis is not possible. Ultimately, all decisions—even those that relate to questions of financial viability—must be weighed against this question: "How will this affect the health of our patients?" Although the problem of measuring quality of care is a difficult one, there are approaches available which have been found to be quite insightful.

One indication of quality is measurement of the *impact* of health care rendered by the program on the patients who have used it. In other words, given an encounter or a series of encounters with a program, is the health of the patients better or worse? Of course, it is necessary to create some standard against which to measure improvement or deterioration. The standard can be derived internally: "We want to reduce our hospitalization rate for diagnoses X, Y, and Z by 50 percent." It also may be derived externally: "We want to reduce our hospitalization rate for diagnoses X, Y, and Z to a level at least equal to the best rate existing in similar programs elsewhere in the country." In both cases, the assumption is made that if hospitalization is required for these diagnoses, an inadequate level of care—presumably preventive care—has been rendered in the ambulatory setting. In this instance, rate of hospitalization may be an appropriate measure of health care impact. For other diagnoses or health conditions, it may be necessary to measure impact differently. For example, the rate of return visits for the same illness may be a useful indicator. So, too, may be the infant mortality rates among new mothers who received prenatal care as part of the program. Over a long period of time morbidity rates for a variety of diseases within the population served by the program may be good indices of the program's overall impact.

Since it is an exceedingly complex task to determine the role which one program's performance ultimately plays in the amelioration of a given community's health, performance often is evaluated in terms of the degree to which the practice of medicine is consistent with accepted standards. A very common set of quality measures, therefore, concerns the adequacy of *treatment*. While measures of impact attempt to assess the effects of a program's medical performance on its patient population, measures of treatment attempt to assess whether the approaches to treatment used by the program providers constitute "good medicine." On the basis of historical evidence, health care known as "good medicine" is assumed to have positive effects. Again, standards of performance may be internally or externally derived. In either event, the medical professionals themselves must be relied upon to develop these standards and to apply them to the program's practice. This "peer review" approach, if it is to be effective, must have the full support of the professional staff—and it must lead to corrective action when such action is indicated.

Frequency of Measurement. All performance measures selected for regular evaluation will not need to be reviewed with the same frequency. Several factors probably will need to be considered in assigning the appropriate reporting frequency to each performance measure. These are:

1. Importance of the measure (and the mission which it reflects) to overall group success
2. Implicit time frame of the performance measure
3. Built-in time lag due to the relative difficulty of producing the measure
4. Length of time anticipated for corrective action to take place once the measure is reported.

All but the first of these factors result from implicit characteristics of the performance measure and, as a result, may be somewhat beyond the control of the group. Management can have substantial influence, however, in terms of establishing priorities among missions and objectives, as was observed in Chapter 3. It is at this level that the relative value of a particular performance measure is determined, but establishing priorities among seemingly intangible items can be difficult. The authors of the *Self-Analysis Manual*[3] suggest that it is sometimes helpful to ask questions such as:

1. Can twice as much funding be justified to achieve this objective as in achieving another one?
2. Can dropping this goal be justified more readily than dropping one which involves reducing the staff?
3. How much more difficult (twice as difficult? three times as difficult?) would it be to defend this program as opposed to another one?
4. How much more serious are the consequences if this objective is poorly met rather than another one?

Internal Management Reports. To illustrate how pertinent information relating to operating systems can assist group practice management in evaluating performance and can aid both administrative and medical staffs in their decision-making, a sample set of internal management reports is presented here. This set is, of course, only one of many possible arrays of system outputs. Within comprehensible limits, a variety of uses has been combined into a single table. Although presented here as tabulations or contingency tables, each table could be translated into graphic displays resulting in far greater communicative power. For example, selected figures might be extracted from one of the reports and displayed in a bar chart or a time series together with comparable figures from prior reporting periods. Indeed, the raw data may be more meaningful when expressed in percentage terms or as rates related to some known population base. Later, in the discussion of report formats, some of these other possibilities will be explored.

T1: Chronological Encounter Summary (figure 19-1) and *T2: Current Caseload Summary* (figure 19-2) are *tabulations* representing information accumulated on a regular basis. The purpose of the *Chronological Encounter Summary* is to provide administrative and clerical staff with a running account of the program's activity. By reviewing the *Current Caseload Summary* a physician can determine the identity of his patients during a specific time period (e.g., his current caseload), the number of encounters each patient had and, if he so desires, the date of each encounter. Additionally, this tabulation reports the type of each patient's last encounter as well as its date. While this does not permit a physician to determine the character of *all* the encounters that each of his patients has had, it does indicate the length of time since any given patient has seen the physician as well as the purpose of the most recent visit. A physician might find this summary particularly useful if he wants to determine which patients should be contacted for new appointments.

Administrative Reports. Administrative reports are intended primarily to help the administrative staff monitor the overall utilization of the program and its services, to characterize the demography of the patient load, and to track the distribution of revenue among providers, payors, and types of encounter.

A1: Revenue Distribution by Payment Source (figure 19-3). On the basis of this report, it is possible to determine the relative proportion of total revenues derived from each of the major sources of payment. Moreover, these proportions can be ascertained by individual providers to determine whether there is an inordinate utilization of any providers by patients represented by any one particular third party payor. Even within a particular payment source category, the revenue per patient and per encounter figures can be compared from provider to provider in an effort to uncover instances of abnormally high or low charging. Although the example shown assumes a fee-for-service approach to charging for health services, with some modification a similar report could be generated in a prepaid setting or in a setting which combines both fee-for-service and prepayment.

A2: Revenue Distribution by Encounter Type (figure 19-4). From this report, characteristics of the encounters experienced in the program can be drawn. The extent to which the program has been utilized for acute illness versus injury or chronic illness, as well as the extent to which each of the physician and nonphysician providers has been utilized for each of these encounter types is readily apparent. It also is possible to observe the relationship between revenue and type of encounter both for the program as a whole as well as for

Date	Patient	History Number	Payor	Contract Number	Claim Number	Provider	Number Items	Total Charges	Credit	Balance

Figure 19-1. T1. Chronological Encounter Summary

Provider	Patient	History Number	Number of Encounters	Type of Last Encounter	Date of Last Encounter

Figure 19–2. T2. Current Caseload Summary

	Blue Shield					Medicare					Self Pay					Total				
Provider	Pat	Enc	Rev	Rev/Pat	Rev/Enc	Pat	Enc	Rev	Rev/Pat	Rev/Enc	Pat	Enc	Rev	Rev/Pat	Rev/Enc	Pat	Enc	Rev	Rev/Pat	Rev/Enc
Total																				

Figure 19-3. A1. Revenue Distribution by Payment Source

Provider	Acute Illness			Injury			Chronic Illness			Initial Assessment			Routine and Preventive			Non-Physician			Total		
	Rev	Enc	Rev/Enc	Rev	Enc	Rev/Enc	Rev	Enc	Rev/Enc	Enc	Rev	Rev/Enc	Enc	Rev	Rev/Enc	Enc	Rev	Rev/Enc	Enc	Rev	Rev/Enc
Total																					

Figure 19-4. A2. Revenue Distribution by Encounter Type

each of its providers. On the basis of this report, decision-making can be facilitated in the areas of pricing and new patient distribution.

A3: Revenue Distribution by Service (figure 19–5). In programs where there is no uniformly applied fee schedule, a report such as this is useful because it presents a current picture of the *de facto* fee schedule established either formally or informally by each physician within the program in the treatment of fee-for-service patients. Utilization of services by patients in a prepaid plan could be monitored in a report based on a similar format, with the difference that the only "service" generating revenue would be standard visits. Enrollment revenues associated with these patients would have to be checked via the accounting system, since such revenue is not generated directly by patient encounters.

Apart from identifying revenue sources this report also enables the quantification of items of service for each type rendered for the program as a whole and by each provider separately. Comparing this report with *A2: Revenue Distribution by Encounter Type* would permit the group to perceive relationships between the range of services rendered on a physician by physician basis and the patterns of encounter type also experienced during the same reporting period.

A4: Age and Sex Profile of Caseload (figure 19–6). This report illustrates a method for characterizing the total patient population in terms of its demographic and socioeconomic attributes. For the sake of simplification, age and sex are assumed to be the only demographic variables to be routinely collected by the system. This report links the number of encounters to the number of patients within each age and sex category for each physician. Trends in the number of encounters per patient in any particular age group can be noted and compared for both sexes. Other trends may be noted when one physician's patient load is compared with another's for the same age and sex category. While a report such as this does not contribute to understanding the reasons underlying any observed trends, it does describe the nature of the medical practice in simple demographic terms.

A5: Derivation of Caseload by Age and Sex (figure 19–7). Because there are additional socioeconomic and demographic data by census tract typically available from outside sources, inferences concerning other characteristics not directly available from internally derived data can be made from the census tract distribution of the caseload shown in this report. In addition, the known age and sex profile of the program's caseload can be broken down by census tract and can be compared with profiles developed independently for the same census tracts. This allows for the identification of population segments that are not being served by the program in proportion to their numbers in the community.

Resource Management Reports. System outputs defined as resource management reports focus on the utilization of manpower and physical resources within the program. Such reports serve the purpose of assisting the administrator in achieving a more efficient allocation and management of these resources by focusing on the duration, timing and manner of personnel, equipment, and facility utilization.

		Dr. Smith			Dr. Jones			Dr. Brown			Dr. White			Total		
Code	Service	No.	Rev	Av Fee	No.	Rev	Av Fee	No.	Rev	Av Fee	No.	Rev	Av Fee	No.	Rev	Av Fee
	Total															

Figure 19-5. A3. Revenue Distribution by Service

Provider	Under 34						35 to 64						Over 65						Total					
	Male			Female			Male			Female			Male			Female			Male			Female		
	Pat	Enc	Enc/Pat	Pat	Enc	Enc/Pat	Pat	Enc	Enc/Pat	Pat	Enc	Enc/Pat	Pat	Enc	Enc/Pat	Pat	Enc	Enc/Pat	Pat	Enc	Enc/Pat	Pat	Enc	Enc/Pat
Total																								

Figure 19-6. A4. Age and Sex Profile of Caseload

	Under 34						35 to 64						Over 65						Total					
	Male			Female			Male			Female			Male			Female			Male			Female		
Provider	CT 308	CT 309	Tot	CT 308	CT 309	Tot	CT 308	CT 309	Tot	CT 308	CT 309	Tot	CT 308	CT 309	Tot	CT 308	CT 309	Tot	CT 308	CT 309	Tot	CT 308	CT 309	Tot
Total																								

Figure 19-7. A5. Derivation of Caseload by Age and Sex

R1: Duration of Encounter Types by Day (figure 19-8). This report permits the comparison of the relative utilization of the program on specific days of the week not only in the aggregate but also in terms of the configuration of encounter types common to each day. Over time, trends in the types of encounter that take place can be monitored by observing whether certain days of the week are more typically associated with certain types of encounter. This report also reveals relationships between the number of encounters and their duration as well as differences in duration that appear to be specific to particular encounter types.

R2: Duration of Encounter Types by Time (figure 19-9). By combining the results of report R2 with those of R1, a rather complete understanding can be achieved of the pattern of encounter type by day and by time. It can also be determined whether the duration of these encounters follows predictable patterns which may be modified in the interest of operating efficiency.

R3: Distribution of Services by Day and Time (figure 19-10). This report facilitates the identification of trends as well as of changes in the pattern of service usage in the same manner as do reports R1 and R2. By focusing specifically on one category of service, such as X-rays or laboratory tests, but not in relation to various encounter types, usage can be more effectively scheduled during the day or week. It should be noted that totaling the number of services rendered for a given day or time period does not necessarily present an accurate picture of facilities or manpower utilization. An X-ray cannot be equated to a laboratory test. Each has its own characteristic workload. By appropriately weighing each unit of service through the application of properly developed relative value units, it may be possible to achieve more meaningful comparisons.

R4: Derivation and Status of Encounters by Type (figure 19-11). By analyzing data relating to facility usage, available program resources may be better allocated. In this case, it is possible to learn whether certain types of encounter are disproportionately generated by patients from a particular geographical location and/or whether they are generated by patients with a particular appointment status. For example, do patients who live closer to the program facilities tend to walk in on a nonemergency basis more frequently than do patients farther away whose encounters are typically the result of appointments? Are injury treatments more commonly associated with emergency walk-in situations as opposed to direct referrals?

R5: Status of Encounters by Day and Time (figure 19-12). This distribution indicates whether any relationship exists between how and when encounters take place. Are there more walk-ins on Monday than on other days? Are there more appointments in the morning than in the afternoon? Are nonemergency walk-in encounters more prevalent on weekdays than on weekends? Depending upon the answers that emerge, it may be necessary to implement changes in staff schedules or make other modifications in the configuration of program resources to better fit the appointment status patterns that are observed. Alternatively, steps might be taken to change the appointment status patterns in those areas that are amenable to change, such as shifting a portion of the appointment load to periods that are typically low in walk-ins or to direct referrals.

Day	Acute Illness			Injury			Chronic Illness			Initial Assessment			Routine and Preventive			Non-Physician			Total		
	<¼	¼-½	Tot	<¼	¼-½	Tot	<¼	¼-½	Tot	<¼	¼-½	Tot	<¼	¼-½	Tot	<¼	¼-½	Tot	<¼	¼-½	Tot
Monday																					
Tuesday																					
Wednesday																					
Thursday																					
Friday																					
Saturday																					
Sunday																					
Total																					

Figure 19–8. R1. Duration of Encounter Types by Day

	Acute Illness			Injury			Chronic Illness			Initial Assessment			Routine and Preventive			Non-Physician			Total		
Time	⟨¼	¼-½	Tot	⟨¼	¼-½	Tot	⟨¼	¼-½	Tot	⟨¼	¼-½	Tot	⟨¼	¼-½	Tot	⟨¼	¼-½	Tot	⟨¼	¼-½	Tot
6:00 - 7:59 a.m.																					
8:00 - 9:59 a.m.																					
10:00 - 11:59 a.m.																					
12:00 - 1:59 p.m.																					
2:00 - 3:59 p.m.																					
4:00 - 5:59 p.m.																					
6:00 - 7:59 p.m.																					
8:00 - 9:59 p.m.																					
10:00 - 11:59 p.m.																					
12:00 - 1:59 a.m.																					
2:00 - 5:59 a.m.																					
Total																					

Figure 19-9. R2. Duration of Encounter Types by Time

Code	Service	Tot	Monday			Tuesday			Wednesday			Thursday			Friday			Saturday			Sunday		
			AM	PM	Tot	AM	PM	Tot	AM	PM	Tot	AM	PM	Tot	AM	PM	Tot	AM	PM	Tot	AM	PM	Tot
	Total																						

Figure 19-10. R3. Distribution of Services by Day and Time

Appointment Status	Acute Illness			Injury			Chronic Illness			Initial Assessment			Routine and Preventive			Non-Physician			Total		
	CT 308	CT 309	Tot	CT 308	CT 309	Tot	CT 308	CT 309	Tot	CT 308	CT 309	Tot	CT 308	CT 309	Tot	CT 308	CT 309	Tot	CT 308	CT 309	Tot
Appointment																					
Telephone																					
Direct Referral																					
Walk-in Emergency																					
Walk-in Non-emergency																					
Total																					

Figure 19-11. R4. Derivation and Status of Encounters by Type

		Monday			Tuesday			Wednesday			Thursday			Friday			Saturday			Sunday		
Appointment Status	Tot	AM	PM	Tot	AM	PM	Tot	AM	PM	Tot	AM	PM	Tot	AM	PM	Tot	AM	PM	Tot	AM	PM	Tot
Appointment																						
Telephone																						
Direct Referral																						
Walk-in Emergency																						
Walk-in Non-emergency																						
Total																						

Figure 19-12. R5. Status of Encounters by Day and Time

Patient Management Reports. These reports share the common characteristic of relating utilization of the program's resources to variables which reflect the causes of utilization—namely encounter type and diagnosis. It is anticipated that the professional staff, having reviewed these aggregate data, will be in a better position to improve the ways in which patients are managed individually.

P1: Distribution of Services by Major Diagnosis (figure 19–13). This report serves a twofold purpose. First, it identifies those diagnoses which have had the highest frequency rate during the reporting period. Frequency is measured in terms of the number of patients (not the number of encounters) with the most common diagnoses. Over time, this report permits the determination of important trends in the kinds of diagnoses being treated. Secondly, the report displays a distribution of services rendered to the patients within the major diagnostic categories, which allows the professional staff to observe the patterns of treatment associated with these diagnoses and to note whether these patterns tend to deviate from the norm or vary with time. Another interesting feature of the report is that it allows for tracking the number of services per patient on the average. In the area of X-rays, for example, it may be helpful to stipulate as a general rule the number of X-rays per patient that would be acceptable within each of the major diagnostic categories during a particular time period so that excessive utilization would be immediately apparent.

P2: Distribution of Ancillary Procedures by Encounter Type (figure 19–14). This report is similar to P1 in that it relates the incidence of particular service items to the number of patients in certain categories. Here, the individual ancillary procedures within the laboratory test and X-ray categories represent the service items and are distributed across patients in the various encounter types. Although these services could be routinely related to diagnostic categories, these procedures probably should be the subject of a special report which quantifies gross utilization according to major encounter types so that it may be possible to gain some general insight into the rationale for their use.

P3: Drugs Prescribed by Diagnosis (figure 19–15). This report can be structured in two ways. First, interest may be focused on a specific subset of drugs to determine how often they have been prescribed and to how many patients, regardless of diagnosis. Alternatively, focusing on a specific subset of diagnoses would give an indication of the range of drugs that are prescribed to those patients in each diagnostic category. In the first instance, concern is directed at the possible overutilization of selected drugs; in the second, at the pattern of prescription that accompanies a particular diagnosis in an attempt to determine whether that pattern falls within some predetermined range considered good medical practice.

P4: Distribution of Dispositions by Diagnosis (figure 19–16). As in the preceding reports, the number of treatment events (dispositions) is related to the number of patients affected. By further stratifying the patient load into either some selected group of diagnoses or into the major diagnoses (per report P1), noteworthy patterns of disposition as they relate to diagnosis can be discerned. For example, should it appear that hospitalization is increasing in frequency for either a particular diagnosis or for the program overall, it may be of interest to carry out a special study which relates the frequency of hospitalization to the number of encounters, the availability of certain insurance

Code	Service	Acute Illness Encounters															Other Encounters			Total		
		Diagnosis A			Diagnosis B			Diagnosis C			Other			Total								
		Pat	No.	No./Pat	Pat	No.	No./Pat	Pat	No.	No./Pat	Pat	No.	No./Pat	Pat	No.	No./Pat	Pat	No.	No./Pat	Pat	No.	No./Pat
	Total																					

Figure 19–13. P1. Distribution of Services by Major Diagnosis

Code	Procedure	Acute Illness			Injury			Chronic Illness			Initial Assessment			Routine and Preventive			Non-Physician			Total		
		Pat	No.	No./Pat	Pat	No.	No./Pat	Pat	No.	No./Pat	Pat	No.	No./Pat	Pat	No.	No./Pat	Pat	No.	No./Pat	Pat	No.	No./Pat
	Total Lab Tests																					
	Total																					

Figure 19-14. P2. Distribution of Ancillary Services by Encounter Types

	Diagnosis A			Diagnosis B			Diagnosis C			Diagnosis D			Diagnosis E			Other			Total		
Drugs Prescribed	Pat	No.	No./Pat	Pat	No.	No./Pat	Pat	No.	No./Pat	Pat	No.	No./Pat	Pat	No.	No./Pat	Pat	No.	No./Pat	Pat	No.	No./Pat
Total																					

Figure 19-15. P3. Drugs Prescribed by Diagnosis

Disposition	Diagnosis A			Diagnosis B			Diagnosis C			Diagnosis D			Diagnosis E			Other			Total		
	Pat	No.	No./Pat	Pat	No.	No./Pat	Pat	No.	No./Pat	Pat	No.	No./Pat	Pat	No.	No./Pat	Pat	No.	No./Pat	Pat	No.	No./Pat
Home																					
Return																					
Patient Calls																					
Doctor Calls																					
Refer																					
Hospital																					
Total																					

Figure 19-16. P4. Distribution of Dispositions by Diagnosis

benefits, the time of day, the day of week, or for that matter, any of the variables previously cited in other reports.

External Reporting Requirements

Earlier it was noted that an increasing number of parties external to the group practice have requirements for data which must be accommodated if that practice is either to continue to function or to be reimbursed for services rendered. Having developed a clear understanding of what is needed for internal management purposes, the group can turn its attention to what various outside parties require and can attempt to integrate these requirements into the system. To the extent possible, it will be expedient to eliminate redundancies that arise between internal and external requirements, to strive at all times to satisfy both sets of requirements with the same performance measure or output datum.

Giebink highlighted the impact of these outside agencies on group practice data systems:

> Federal programs have great impact on recordkeeping. Medicare and Medicaid claim information, including personal data on the patient, medical information, and charges, must be submitted to the claims processor. Provider certification requirements for both programs hinge on documentation of financial, operational, and professional activities. Fee-for-service practices may use standard rate schedules for computing charges; prepaid practices must provide cost and service data as part of contract and rate negotiations with Medicare and Medicaid agencies.
>
> Practices receiving federal grants and other funds for services to the indigent or for categorical programs are subject to federal agency requirements for routine reports of population, utilization, and financial data. Programs such as family health centers, neighborhood health centers, health networks, and migrant health projects have elaborate reporting requirements. Child and youth projects and maternal and child health programs also have their own requirements. Federal guidelines will probably provide detailed guidance on routine reports, special studies, and evaluation systems required for Health Maintenance Organization projects financed through recent legislation. Practices intended to apply for HMO funds must comply with HMO requirements and, therefore, design records systems to be efficiently integrated with existing operations.
>
> PSRO's or other quality assurance and utilization review programs may eventually have profound impact on practice information systems.[4]

In an article prepared by the Executive Committee of the American Association of Health Data Systems, potential PSRO data requirements were discussed in relation to ambulatory care. These requirements fall into three areas: Establishment of Standards, Ongoing Surveillance, and Investigation of Variation from Standards.[5] A central feature in all of these areas is the probable use by the PSRO of a minimum basic data set consisting of provider, patient, and encounter data that is consistent with the recommendations of the National Committee on Vital and Health Statistics. This minimum data set which is discussed in detail below will in all likelihood become a standard requirement not only for PSROs but for a wide variety of other governmental programs.

Internal Reporting. The examples of system outputs presented in the foregoing discussion are in the form of tabulations and contingency tables. Although structured beyond the level of raw data, they can be improved upon in terms of communicative effectiveness. As tools for the analyst, each provides on a single page a considerable amount of information; however, as interpretive documents for the manager or health care professional, they do not necessarily convey quickly and dramatically the salient information they contain. It is up to the individuals charged with the analysis of these reports to carry the process of interpretation one step further and to recast selectively those elements within the basic report documents into more meaningful numerical terms or into more effective graphic displays.

Numerical Manipulation. One of the most useful steps that can be taken to enhance the interpretive value of the data is simply to express them in terms that permit more insightful comparison from one reporting period to another. Figure 19-17 is an example of one such way to manipulate the output data. Report R3 has been recast in percentage terms. The total number of services rendered during the reporting period has been taken as the base and all other figures in the report are expressed as percentages of this base. While the report itself has not been changed in format, its content is more meaningful to someone who is concerned less with the absolute number of services rendered during the period, and more with the proportion of total services rendered falling into each of the service day and/or time categories.

Another manipulation is illustrated in figure 19-18. Here the data in report R4 are reported in terms of the "rate per 100 patients." Since the total number of hypothetical patients during the reporting period is seventy-five, each of the figures in R4 has been divided by seventy-five and multiplied by 100 to establish the rate per 100 patients. Had there been 100 patients, the resulting rate would be identical with the figures shown in R4 and had there been 200 patients the rate would be one-half. The utility of converting absolute numbers into rates per some base population is most clearly evident when investigators want to identify trends in utilization even though the size of the base population is changing over time. The base population need not be the patient population; if the group is a prepaid program, or has a prepaid component, it could be the enrollment population; or it could be the population of the catchment area.

Graphic Displays. By selecting certain summary figures from the basic reports and displaying them graphically, outputs become much more comprehensible. For example, in figure 19-19, the day-specific totals from report R1 are displayed in a bar chart. As a result, the day-to-day variations are immediately observable as are the number of encounters involved. A variation of this display technique is shown in figure 19-20 where a numerical manipulation is performed by taking each day's total encounters as the base. Although the visibility of the day-to-day fluctuations in total encounters is lost, day-to-day encounter type mix can be seen readily.

In figure 19-21 the outputs of report A2 are adapted and augmented by additional data underlying but not reported in A2. The result is a chart that shows the range in revenue per encounter values by type of encounter for the program overall, together with the average revenue per encounter figure within each encounter type. This is the familiar Dow Jones stock price format, high-

			Monday			Tuesday			Wednesday			Thursday			Friday			Saturday			Sunday		
Code	Service	Tot.	AM	PM	Tot	AM	PM	Tot	AM	PM	Tot	AM	PM	Tot	AM	PM	Tot	AM	PM	Tot	AM	PM	Tot
19	EKG	13.0	.6	1.1	1.7	1.7	1.1	2.8	1.1	1.1	2.3	1.1	1.7	2.8	.6	1.7	2.3	.6	.6	1.1	–	–	–
23	Cast Application	7.9	–	–	–	–	1.1	1.1	–	–	–	–	.6	.6	–	–	–	–	2.3	2.3	1.7	2.3	3.9
24	Minor Surgery	1.1	–	–	–	.6	–	.6	–	–	–	–	–	–	–	.6	.6	–	–	–	–	–	–
25	Injection	6.8	.6	.6	1.1	–	.6	.6	.6	1.1	1.7	–	–	–	1.1	–	1.1	1.1	.6	1.7	–	.6	.6
27	Sigmoidoscopy	2.8	–	.6	.6	.6	1.1	1.7	–	–	–	–	.6	.6	–	–	–	–	–	–	–	–	–
29	History and Physical	2.3	.6	–	.6	.6	.6	1.1	–	–	–	–	–	–	.6	–	.6	–	–	–	–	–	–
30	X-Ray	35.6	2.3	2.8	5.1	2.8	4.5	7.3	3.4	1.1	4.5	–	.6	.6	2.3	5.7	7.9	2.8	3.4	6.2	2.8	1.1	3.9
33	Pulmonary Treatment	1.7	–	–	–	–	1.1	1.1	.6	–	.6	–	–	–	–	–	–	–	–	–	–	–	–
34	Lab	13.0	1.7	1.7	3.4	1.7	1.1	2.8	1.1	2.3	3.4	.6	1.7	2.3	–	1.1	1.1	–	–	–	–	–	–
37	Major Surgery	1.7	–	1.1	1.1	–	.6	.6	–	–	–	–	–	–	–	–	–	–	–	–	–	–	–
39	Physical Therapy	.6	–	–	–	–	.6	.6	–	–	–	–	–	–	–	–	–	–	–	–	–	–	–
	Other	13.6	2.3	2.3	4.5	1.7	3.9	5.7	–	–	–	–	–	–	1.7	1.7	3.4	–	–	–	–	–	–
	Total	100.0	7.9	10.2	18.1	9.6	16.3	26.0	6.8	5.7	12.4	1.7	5.1	6.8	6.2	10.7	16.9	4.5	6.8	11.3	4.5	3.9	11.8

Figure 19-17. Distribution of Services by Day and Time Expressed as Percentage of Total Services

	Acute Illness			Injury			Chronic Illness			Initial Assessment			Routine and Preventive			Non-Physcian			Total		
Appointment Status	CT 308	CT 309	Tot	CT 308	CT 309	Tot	CT 308	CT 309	Tot	CT 308	CT 309	Tot	CT 308	CT 309	Tot	CT 308	CT 309	Tot	CT 308	CT 309	Tot
Appointment	—	—	—	—	—	—	4.0	9.3	13.3	1.3	4.0	5.3	8.0	1.3	9.3	6.6	10.7	17.3	20.0	25.3	45.3
Telephone	4.0	9.3	13.3	—	1.3	1.3	—	—	—	—	—	—	—	—	—	2.7	—	2.7	6.6	10.7	17.3
Direct Referral	—	—	—	—	—	—	1.3	1.3	2.7	—	—	—	—	—	—	5.3	8.0	13.3	6.6	9.3	16.0
Walk-in Emergency	9.3	10.7	20.0	10.7	16.0	26.6	—	—	—	—	—	—	—	—	—	—	—	—	20.0	26.6	46.6
Walk-in Non-emergency	1.3	2.7	4.0	2.7	1.3	4.0	—	—	—	—	—	—	—	—	—	—	—	—	4.0	4.0	8.0
Total	14.7	22.7	37.3	13.3	18.6	32.0	5.3	10.7	16.0	1.3	4.0	5.3	8.0	1.3	9.3	14.7	18.6	33.3	57.2	76.0	133.3

Figure 19-18. Derivation and Status of Encounters by Type Expressed as Rates per 100 Patients

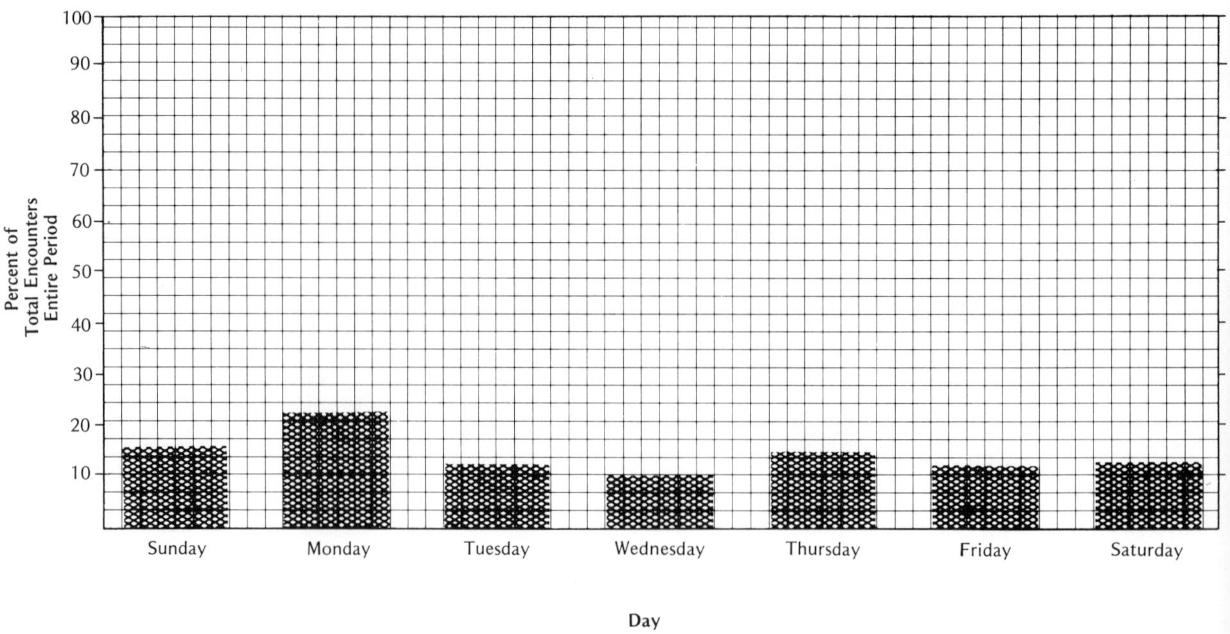

Figure 19-19. Distribution of Encounters by Day

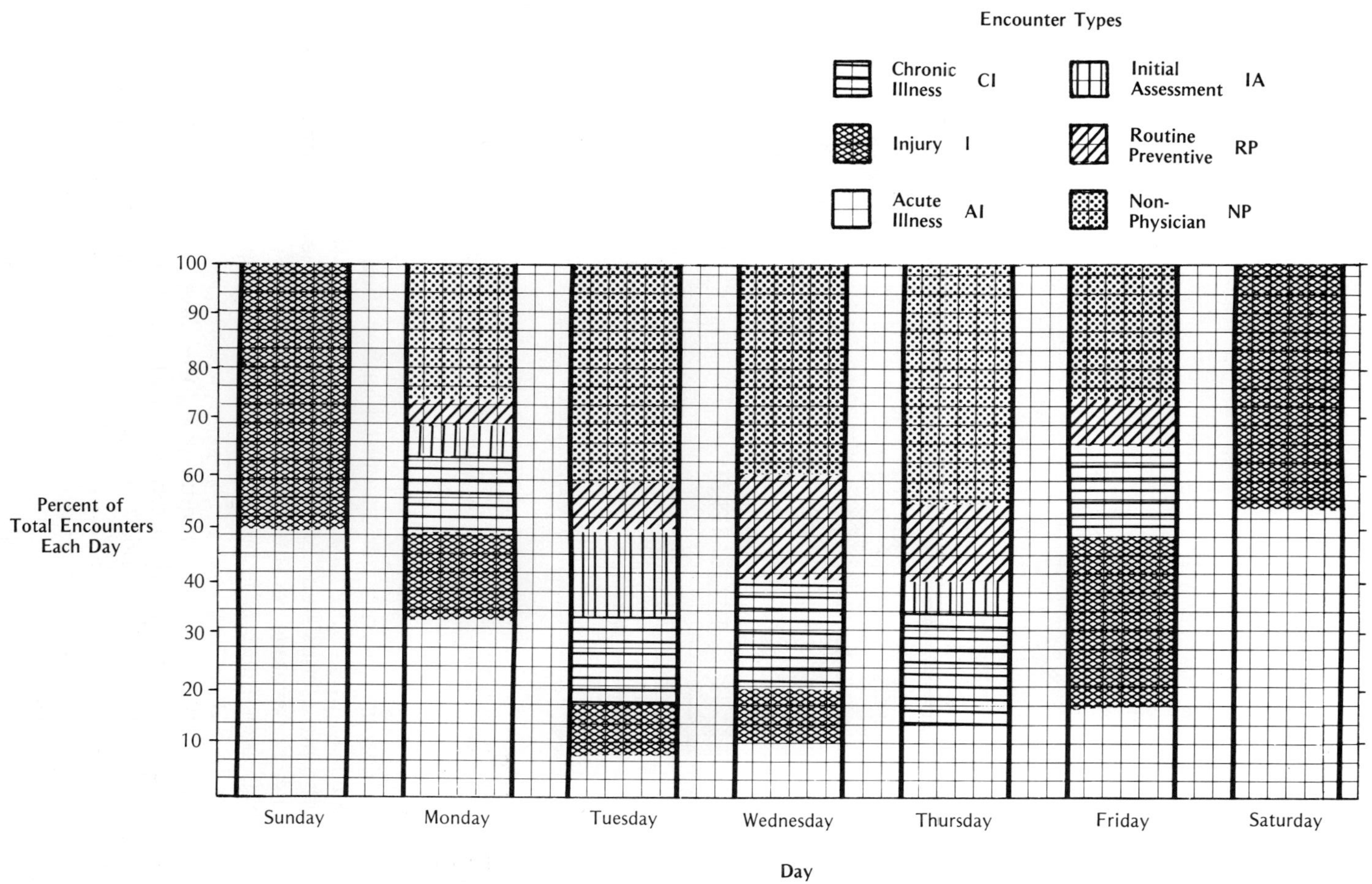

Figure 19-20. Encounter Type Mix by Day

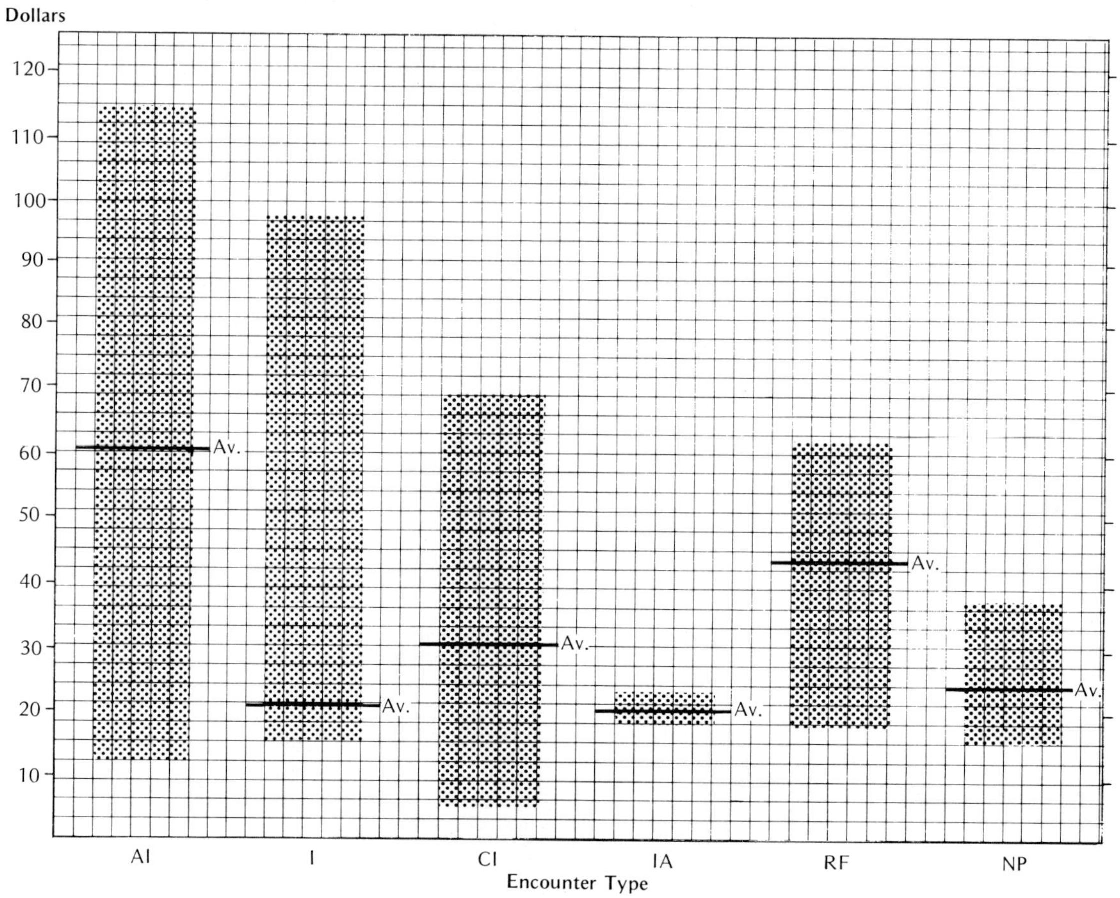

Figure 19-21. Revenue Per Encounter by Type, Range, and Average

lighting the *average* revenue per encounter rather than some "closing" figure. A format such as this immediately conveys the information that the encounter type with the most consistent price is an initial assessment encounter (IA) and that although the average revenue per injury encounter (I) is about the same as for an initial assessment it is far more variable, ranging from a high of about $97 to a low of $15.

Up to this point, ways of communicating the data from a particular reporting period have been discussed. Often, it is useful to combine in a single display data from more than one period. The bar chart shown in figure 19-22 parallels the distribution of dispositions from report P4 with the distribution from the comparable period during the previous year and provides comparisons between the two time periods.

For a more complete picture of some particular aspect of the program's performance, a number of reporting period outputs can be plotted in a time series. As an example, the total revenue associated with each of the major payment sources taken from report A1 can be plotted on the same time scale with comparable outputs from prior periods in figure 19-23. Carrying this approach

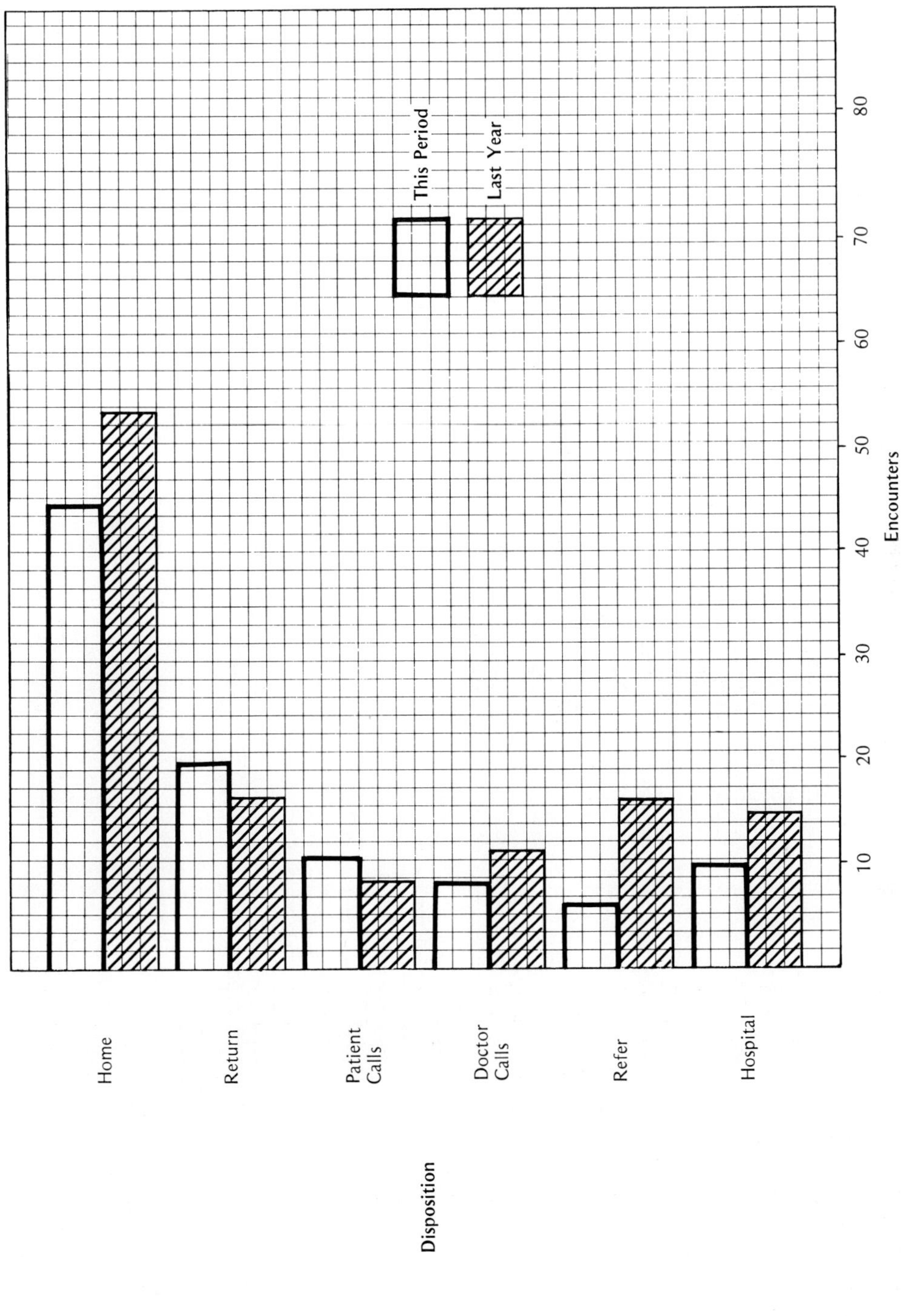

Figure 19-22. Distribution of Dispositions—This Period vs. Comparable Period Last Year

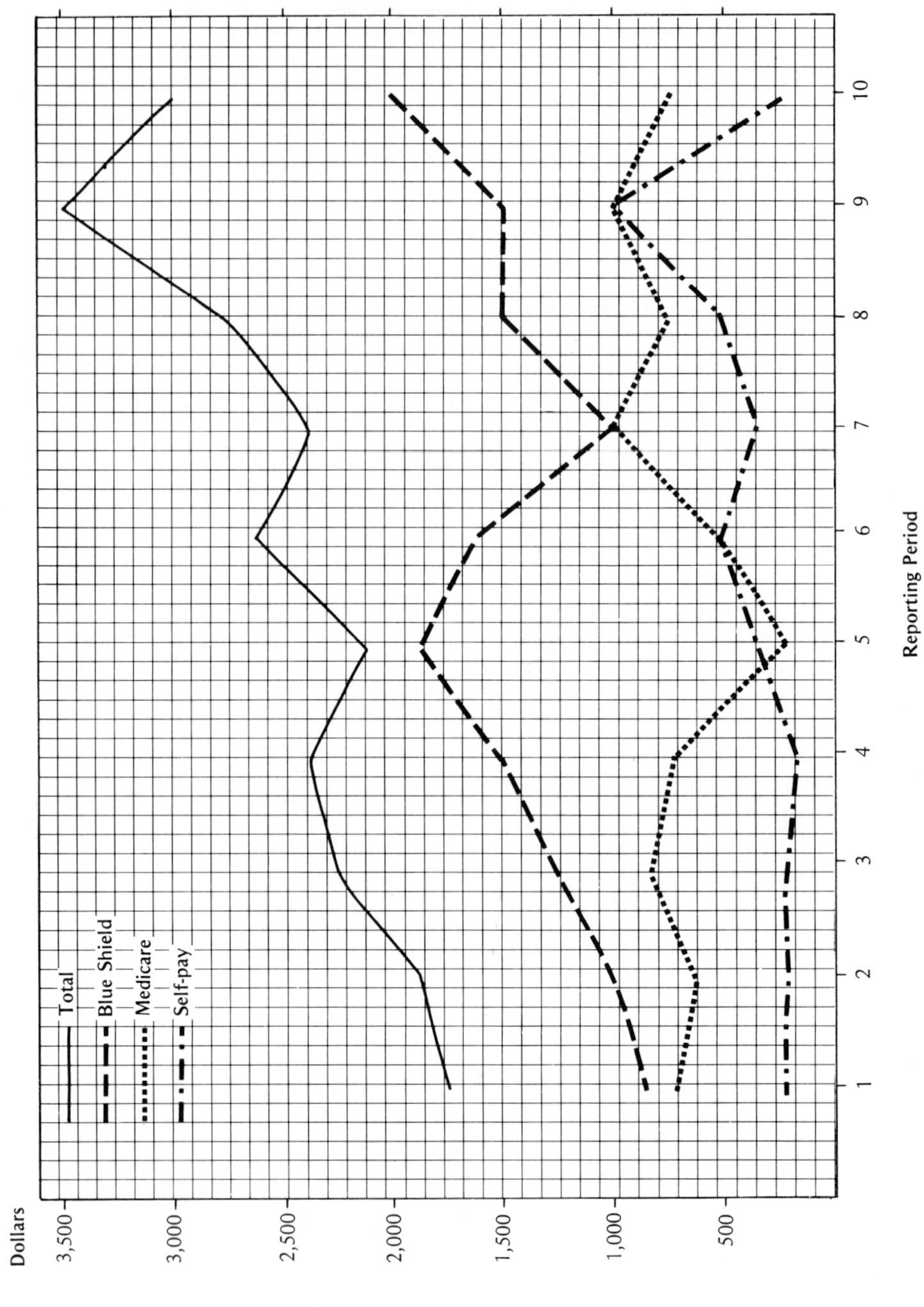

Figure 19-23. Revenue per Period Total and by Payment Source (Periods 1-10)

a step further, in figure 19-24 the same data are displayed cumulatively. Assuming each period to be a month, a sense of the "year to date" performance of the program is achieved, both in terms of total revenue generated and the relative contribution of each of the payment sources. Indeed, by highlighting the composition of the cumulative total through the use of distinctively shaded areas, the proportion of total revenue derived from each source is illustrated without explicitly stating the percentages involved.

Variance Reports. In an attempt to highlight the deviations of actual performance from planned or forecast performance, some form of variance reporting can be used. Figure 19-25 is a graphic display of actual financial data compared against a monthly plan.

The dotted lines roughly paralleling the forecast plots are the variance limits. Actual performance, indicated by the light solid lines, which is outside the maximum acceptable variance limits signals the group to take steps to compensate for the divergence. In the early months, variance limits are more liberal than those used once the program is beginning to stabilize. Initial divergence from plans is to be expected while operational snags and bottlenecks are being smoothed out. This form of variance analysis enables planners to judge whether actual performance is acceptable in relation to the budget. In the event basic changes are made in the program, cash flow projections must be adjusted accordingly.

Exception Reports. The foregoing formats typically are used to present data on a routine basis; however, certain data may need to be reported only when they are of special interest. Presenting data in this way is called "exception reporting." As figure 19-26 suggests, a report generated on an exception basis presupposes certain assumptions as to what constitutes an exceptional situation. In other words, there must be an established range of nonexceptional performance for each variable or data element reported. Only when performance is outside of the established range is it presented on the exception report. In this way the amount of information that is available to decisions makers is minimized and yet the issues of critical importance are not overlooked. Of course, all of the back-up data would be available for review at any time.

External Reporting. Outputs generated in response to external agency and third party payor requirements typically will be cast in formats dictated by these agencies and payors. Attempts should be made, however, to persuade external data recipients to accept data in the same formats as those used for internal purposes. An example of this would be the superbill concept described earlier in the discussion of charging and claims processing systems (Chapter 15). Another possibility worth exploring is the transmission of claims data in card or magnetic tape form directly to the payors, thereby eliminating an additional transformation step.

SPECIFYING INPUTS

Knowing the range of desired outputs, the next step in the process of system design is the determination of what these outputs call for in terms of input

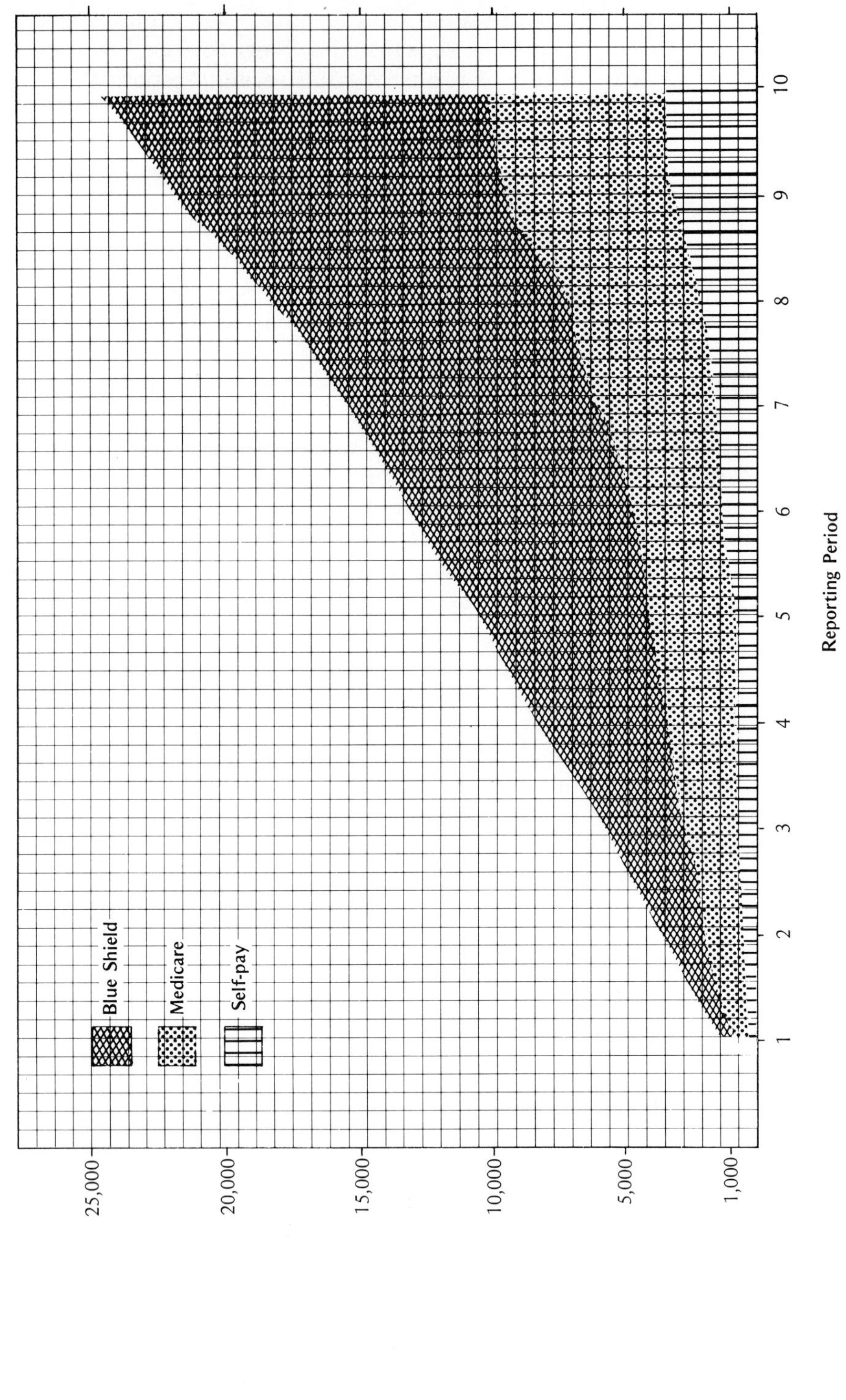

Figure 19-24. Cumulative Revenue By Payment Source (Periods 1-10)

MONITORING DISBURSEMENTS

MONITORING OPERATING RECEIPTS

MONITORING NET OPERATING CASH FLOWS

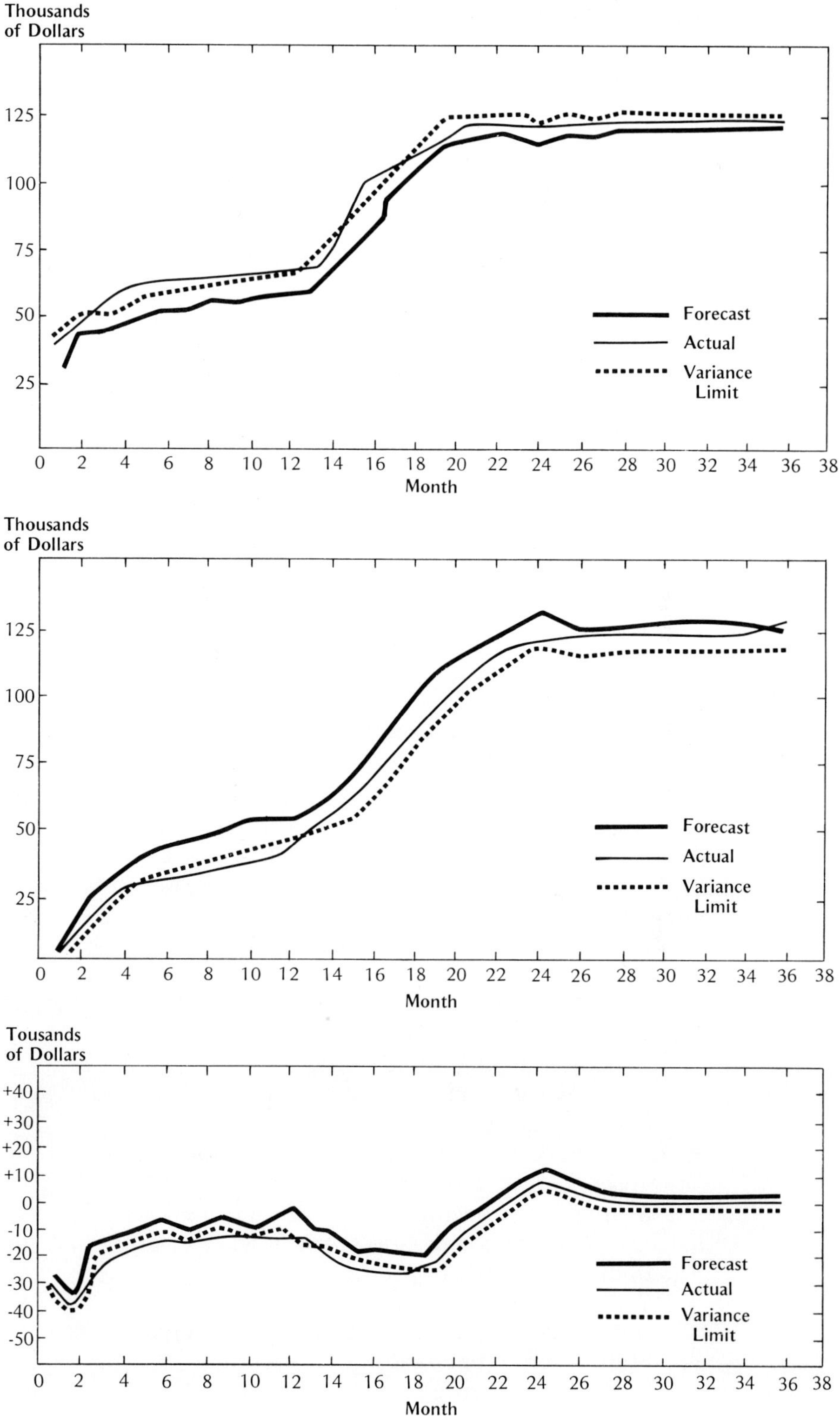

Figure 19-25. Examples of Variance Displays

		Report Reference	Does Performance Meet Standard?	If NO, Present Supporting Data
1.	The number of patients seen is more than 50 and less than 100.	A1	Yes [X] No [ ]	
2.	The number of encounters with any one provider is no less than 20% and no more than 40% of total Center encounters.	A1	Yes [ ] No [X]	Smith = 15%
3.	The number of encounters on any one day of the week is no less than 10% and no more than 25% of total Center encounters.	R1	Yes [X] No [ ]	
4.	No more than 20% of total Center encounters occur within a given two hour period.	R1	Yes [X] No [ ]	
5.	The number of x-rays per patient does not exceed 1.5 on average.	P2	Yes [ ] No [X]	X-rays per Patient = 1.6

Figure 19-26. Example of Exception Report

data. One way to approach this task is to develop a matrix listing the outputs along one axis and inputs along the other. Using the sample system described above as a model, the matrix shown in figure 19-27 can be developed. Below is displayed a listing of the sixteen output reports and tabulations and the data required as inputs to produce them.

A. Data related to *who* the patient is
 1. patient identification:
  name, history number, social security number, contract number
 2. patient demographic characteristics:
  age and sex
 3. census tract

B. Data related to *what* happens to the patient
 4. services rendered
 5. ancillary procedures:
  lab tests and X-rays
 6. drugs prescribed
 7. disposition

C. Data related to *how much* service is rendered
 8. duration of encounter
 9. charges incurred

D. Data related to *why* the encounter took place
 10. encounter type
 11. diagnosis

OUTPUTS	INPUTS															
	Who			What				How Much		Why		How			When	
Tabulations	Patient ID	Patient Demog.	Census Tract	Services	Ancillary Procedures	Prescrip-tions	Disposition	Duration	Revenue	Encounter Type	Diagnosis	Provider	Appt. Status	Payor	Day (Date)	Time
T1 Chronological Encounter Summary	x								x			x		x	x	
T2 Current Caseload Summary	x									x		x			x	
Administrative																
A1 Revenue Distribution by Payment Source									x			x		x		
A2 Revenue Distribution by Encounter Type									x	x		x				
A3 Revenue Distribution by Service				x					x			x				
A4 Age and Sex Profile of Caseload		x										x				
A5 Derivation of Caseload by Age and Sex		x	x									x				
Resource Management																
R1 Duration of Encounter Types by Day								x		x					x	
R2 Duration of Encounter Types by Time								x		x						x
R3 Distribution of Services by Day and Time				x											x	x
R4 Derivation and Status of Encounters by Type		x								x			x			
R5 Status of Encounters by Day and Time													x		x	x
Patient Management																
P1 Distribution of Services by Major Diagnosis				x						x	x					
P2 Distribution of Ancillary Procedures by Encounter Type					x					x						
P3 Drugs Prescribed by Diagnosis						x					x					
P4 Distribution of Disposition by Diagnosis							x				x					

Figure 19-27. Example of Input/Output Matrix

E. Data related to *how* the encounter took place
   12. the provider name and type
   13. appointment status
   14. payor:
       Blue Shield, Medicare, Medicaid, commercial, and self-pay

F. Data related to *when* the encounter took place
   15. day or date
   16. time

A. Patient

1. Patient Identification:
   a. name; b. number unique to that patient
2. Residence (include zip code)
3. Date of Birth
4. Sex
5. Expected Source of Payment (one or more):
   a. self; b. private insurance; c. government; d. no charge

B. Provider

6. Provider Identification:
   a. name; b. unique number
7. Professional Address
8. Profession:
   a. physician; b. specialist; c. dentist; d. nurse; e. other
9. Date of Encounter
10. Place:
    a. office; b. clinic; c. hospital outpatient department; d. emergency;
    e. home f. other

C. Encounter

11. Reason for Encounter (principal problem in patient's words)
12. Findings Information (pertinent to diagnosis):
    a. history; b. physical examination; c. lab tests
13. Diagnosis/Problem (provider's current assessment, principle problem first)
14. Service and Procedures (performed during encounter, before next encounter):
    a. diagnostic; b. therapeutic; c. preventive
15. Itemized Charges (all charges made during encounter and prior to next encounter)
16. Disposition:
    a. none; b. return; c. P.R.N.; d. telephone follow-up;
    e. referral to other provider; f. return to referring provider;
    g. hospital admission; h. other

Source: Jane Murnaghan, ed., *Report of the Proceedings of the Conference on Ambulatory Medical Records* (Chicago: U.S. National Committee on Vital and Health Statistics, 1972).

Figure 19-28. Uniform Minimum Basic Data Set for Ambulatory Care Records

Input Ducuments and Mechanisms

At the beginning of this chapter it was noted that an overall statistical analysis system incorporates data from a variety of other operating systems, such as patient registration, accounting, charge and claims processing, medical records, etc. Indeed, every effort should be made to utilize data already being generated for other purposes to satisfy the input requirements of the statistical analysis system. In some cases, particular data items, although available from other sources, may not be compatible with the system's needs. These items may not be generated with the appropriate frequency or defined at the required level of specificity, or they may be stored in a form not easily or economically converted for use in the system. Thus, it may be necessary to create a second data source. Actually, the redundance of a parallel data collection process can in certain cases prove beneficial. For example, it may provide a check on the accuracy of the data or may ensure against data loss.

In its report on the *Uniform Minimum Basic Data Set* the National Committee on Vital and Health Statistics suggests an array of source document types that would be appropriate in the ambulatory care setting for producing the minimum data set.[6] Figure 19-28 presents the recommended minimum data set and figure 19-29 relates these data elements to four types of source documents:

1. Provider record
2. Patient record
3. Billing record
4. Encounter record

Data Item	Provider Record	Patient Record	Encounter Record	Billing Record
Provider name	X		X	X
Provider identification number	X		X	X
Provider address	X			
Patient name		X	X	X
Patient identification number		X	X	X
Patient residence address		X		X
Patient date of birth		X		
Patient sex		X		
Principal source of payment		X		
Date of encounter		X		
Place of encounter			X	
Reason for encounter			X	
Findings			X	
Diagnoses			X	
Services and procedures			X	
Charges				X
Disposition			X	

Source: Jane Murnaghan, ed., "Record Format Study," *Report of the Proceedings of the Conference on Ambulatory Medical Records* (Chicago: U.S. National Committee on Vital and Health Statistics, 1972).

Figure 19-29. Suggested Record Format for Uniform Minimum Basic Data Set

Generally speaking, one-time and periodically updated input sources, such as patient registration and history forms and provider background data forms, pose few problems. Typically, the creation of these documents tends to occur either so infrequently or so independently of the medical care delivery process that elaborate procedures are unnecessary. (In Appendix 19A a sampling of such documents used in a variety of group practice settings is provided.) The collection of input data that can be produced only in the course of medical care *encounters* between the patient and the program is a far more complicated process. An important issue in this area is the amount of time that must be devoted to the clerical task of generating the encounter-based data—particularly by physician and nursing personnel. These professionals already are under a great deal of pressure to satisfy a multitude of clerical requirements generated by third party payors, administrators, health officials, researchers, etc. Many of these clerical chores appear to have little, if any, immediate medical benefit to the patient. How can needed encounter data be derived without totally alienating the providers of health care? And more importantly, how can health care providers be encouraged to want to generate these data accurately and in a timely fashion? It is clear that the system output is only as good as its input and that the control of that input is in the hands of the physician and his colleagues. They must be motivated to do a good job.

Simply to point out the medical benefits inherent in better performance analysis is not enough. There ought to be some realization of the benefits that result from the data-gathering effort itself. It must not complicate the physician's life by increasing the paper overload. Rather, data gathering should be incorporated into daily routine. When possible, data gathering actually should simplify the physician's work while at the same time producing the encounter-based data. This combination of features—clinical benefits and paperwork simplification—is likely to be the most persuasive argument for gaining the physician's cooperation in the timely and accurate recording of encounter data.

Another potential problem which should not be overlooked prior to introducing the physician to the encounter data collection process is the issue of style of practice. While most physicians recognize the legitimate interest shown by third party reimbursers in the medical services provided to their beneficiaries and also recognize the interests that senior medical staff, administrators, and, indeed, they themselves have in utilization review, there is likely to be a strong proprietary sense—even within a group setting—in maintaining individual styles of practice. Care must be taken, therefore, to involve the medical staff in every step of the development process so that data collection instruments do not impose upon then an alien style of practice. It is necessary, therefore, to distinguish between those data elements which can be encoded on the collection instrument and those which should be left to the physician himself. The very presence of prerecorded items to be checked off on a form implies a preconception of acceptable procedural alternatives—a preconception which the physician himself may not share. By the same token and in the interest of saving time, one cannot in every case ask for open-ended responses. From a practical point of view, this also would not be conducive to the data comparability necessary for analytical purposes and actually would impose such a burden of interpretation on the physician that he might not respond at all. A balance must be struck between structure and flexibility in the design of the data collection instruments, and the physicians themselves must be involved in the design process.

With these considerations in mind, the group should undertake the task of designing an encounter form and data collection procedure. One way to start is to review a variety of encounter forms already in use in ambulatory health programs around the country (see Appendix 19A). Although adequate in content, most of these forms tend to be deficient in the effectiveness with which they can be integrated into a provider's ongoing activities. In many cases, they do not simplify the physician's paperwork, but rather add to it.

A possibility for simplifying paperwork lies in developing an *integrated encounter form* that combines several documents in a single package, thereby reducing the number of parallel recording tasks. As an example of what can be done in this regard, consider the package illustrated in figure 19-30.[7] This encounter form package (8½ by 11 inches in size) consists of a set of shingled pages of progressively longer length and of different colors. Selected sections of a given page could be reproduced on successive pages through the use of specially treated paper. The pages are in the order of their sequence in the package:

1. X-ray Order
2. Laboratory Order
3. Patient's Copy
4. Cashier's Copy
5. Physician's Copy
6. Business Office Copy
7. Claims Form

Paperwork is simplified by combining in one package not only an encounter form but also a medical record, patient's bill, and ancillary service requisition. The physician and nurse would thus be relieved of a number of repetitive clerical tasks, while at the same time encouraged to complete the encounter form accurately. The inputs to this form are simultaneously inputs to the physician's own medical record and to the patient's bill—which in a fee-for-service situation may be the basis of the physician's compensation. The need to demonstrate tangible clinical benefit is addressed in two important ways. First, the physician's medical record is an integral part of the system. Secondly, the data bank of encounter forms provides the physician with a reservoir of historical information on his patients which can be assessed in a wide variety of ways to help him in their treatment.

The problem of balancing structure and flexibility is handled by precoding only those elements of the encounter form that do not impinge on the physician's professional judgment. Diagnosis, for example, is left completely to the physician to express in his own terms. Moreover, the medical record component of the package contains a special section to allow him to write his own notes in whatever manner and however completely he desires. The package also contains another important feature—the capacity to serve as a claims form for purposes of third party reimbursement. On the reverse side of the Business Office Copy can be included all of the language unique to Blue Shield, Medi-

X-ray Order

X-RAY ORDER

PATIENT'S NAME	SOCIAL SECURITY NO.	HISTORY NO.	DATE	Sequence

PATIENT'S ADDRESS	BIRTH DATE	AGE	SEX	Enc. Type	Appt. Status	DAY	TIME

CITY OR TOWN	STATE	ZIP CODE	Census Tract	TELEPHONE NO.	PROVIDER NO.

BILLING NAME	Payer	CONTRACT NO.	Payer	CONTRACT NO.

BILLING ADDRESS	SUBSCRIBER'S NAME

CITY OR TOWN	STATE	ZIP CODE	SUBSCRIBER'S ADDRESS	CITY	STATE	ZIP

X-RAYS ORDERED					
CHEST	GI	UPPER EXT.		EXPLANATION	
IVP	GALL BLADDER	LOWER EXT.			
BE	MAMMO-GRAPHY			PHYSICIAN'S SIGNATURE	

Laboratory Order

LABORATORY ORDER

PATIENT'S NAME	SOCIAL SECURITY NO.	HISTORY NO.	DATE	Sequence

PLEASE ATTACH RESULTS OF LAB TESTS HERE

LAB TESTS ORDERED					
URINAL-YSIS	URIC ACID	PAP		EXPLANATION	
CBC	BUN	SMA			
GLUCOSE	CHOLES-TEROL			PHYSICIAN'S SIGNATURE	

Figure 19-30. Integrated Encounter Form

Patient's Copy

PLEASE RETURN TO BUSINESS OFFICE BEFORE LEAVING — PATIENT'S COPY

PATIENT'S NAME	SOCIAL SECURITY NO.	HISTORY NO.	DATE	Sequence
PATIENT'S ADDRESS	BIRTH DATE / AGE / SEX / Enc. Type / Appt. Status		DAY / TIME	
CITY OR TOWN / STATE / ZIP CODE	Census Tract	TELEPHONE NO.	PROVIDER NO.	
BILLING NAME	Payer / CONTRACT NO.		Payer / CONTRACT NO.	
BILLING ADDRESS	SUBSCRIBER'S NAME			
CITY OR TOWN / STATE / ZIP CODE	SUBSCRIBER'S ADDRESS / CITY / STATE / ZIP			

PLEASE SAVE THIS STATEMENT FOR REIMBURSEMENT UNDER MAJOR MEDICAL INSURANCE.
ACCOUNTS ARE PAYABLE IN FULL WITHIN THIRTY DAYS.

SERVICES RENDERED

SERVICE	FEE	SERVICE	FEE	SERVICE	FEE	SERVICE	FEE	SERVICE	FEE	Last Pay. Date
Office Visit		Minor Surgery		Laboratory		Dispensary Visits				/ /
Consultation		Injection		Home Lab Call		Utilization Fee				Last Paid Amt.
Insurance Examination		Dressing		Abstract		Welfare				Previous Balance
Home Visit		Sigmoidoscopy		Major Surgery		State Medicaid				
Hospital Visit		Allergy		Assisting Surgeon		Prepaid				Charges this Visit
EKG		History and Physical		Physical Therapy						Total Charges
Dr. Service in Acc. Room		X-ray		Traction Set						
Use of Acc. Room		X-ray Call Back		Audiogram						Credits
Suturing		Pediatrics		Anesthesia						Balance
Cast Application		Pulmonary Treatment		Total Units						

DISPOSITION Home ☐ Return ☐ Patient Calls ☐ Doctor Calls ☐ Refer ☐ Dr. Name — Hosp. ☐ Hospital Name

Figure 19-30. (Cont.)

care, and Medicaid claims forms that apply in a particular jurisdiction. Data common to all these forms already are accounted for elsewhere in the package. Assuming that these third parties would be willing to accept a data tape instead of individual hard copy claims forms (the encounter form itself would still be available on an ad hoc basis for purposes of auditing patient and physician signatures and determines the validity of certain data items), the value of the package to the group practice would be increased significantly.

This integrated encounter form is an example of a package which captures all of the data elements presented earlier in figure 19-27 and should be capable of generating at minimum all of the internal management reports in the sample

Cashier's Copy

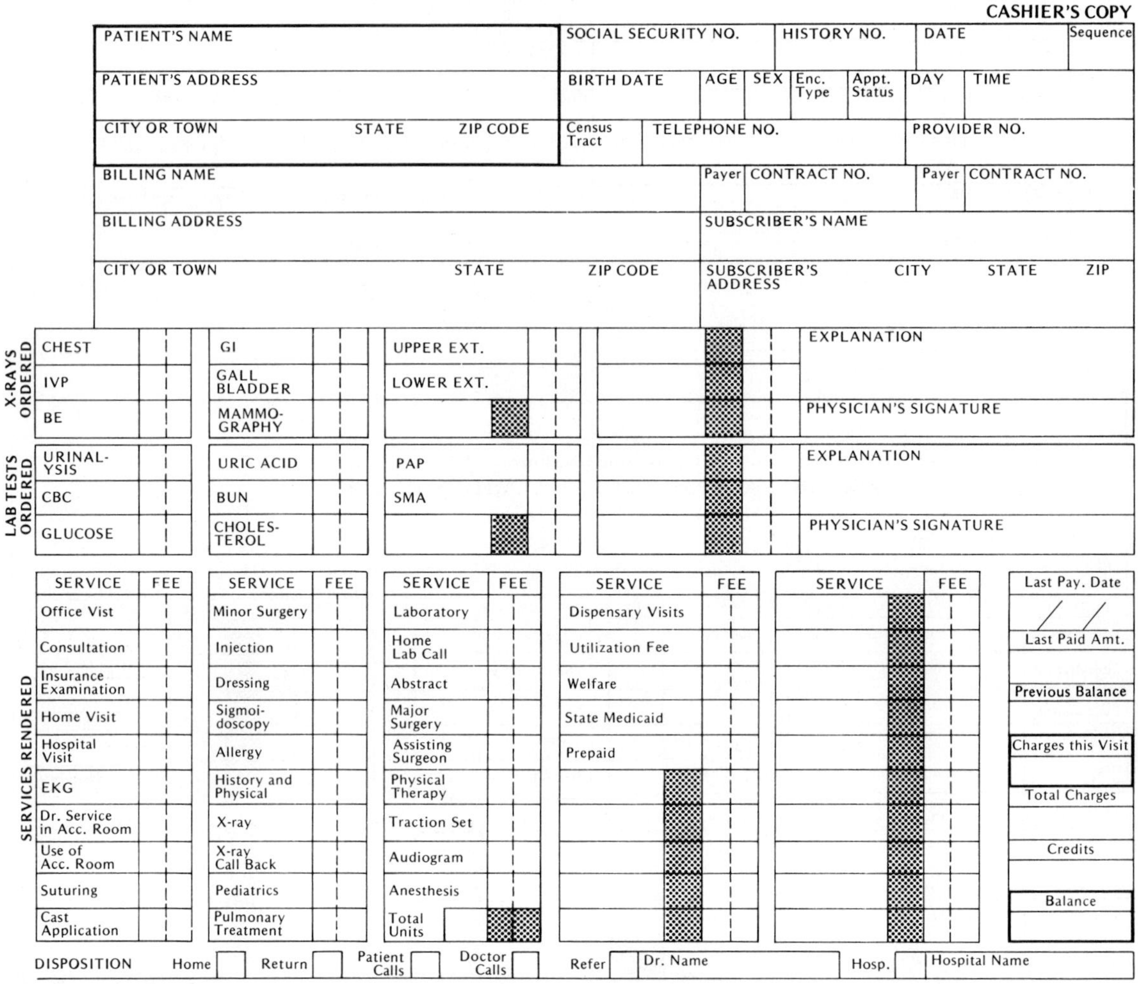
CASHIER'S COPY

PATIENT'S NAME | SOCIAL SECURITY NO. | HISTORY NO. | DATE | Sequence

PATIENT'S ADDRESS | BIRTH DATE | AGE | SEX | Enc. Type | Appt. Status | DAY | TIME

CITY OR TOWN | STATE | ZIP CODE | Census Tract | TELEPHONE NO. | PROVIDER NO.

BILLING NAME | Payer | CONTRACT NO. | Payer | CONTRACT NO.

BILLING ADDRESS | SUBSCRIBER'S NAME

CITY OR TOWN | STATE | ZIP CODE | SUBSCRIBER'S ADDRESS | CITY | STATE | ZIP

X-RAYS ORDERED: CHEST | IVP | BE | GI | GALL BLADDER | MAMMO-GRAPHY | UPPER EXT. | LOWER EXT. | EXPLANATION | PHYSICIAN'S SIGNATURE

LAB TESTS ORDERED: URINAL-YSIS | CBC | GLUCOSE | URIC ACID | BUN | CHOLES-TEROL | PAP | SMA | EXPLANATION | PHYSICIAN'S SIGNATURE

SERVICES RENDERED

SERVICE	FEE	SERVICE	FEE	SERVICE	FEE	SERVICE	FEE	SERVICE	FEE	
Office Vist		Minor Surgery		Laboratory		Dispensary Visits				Last Pay. Date
Consultation		Injection		Home Lab Call		Utilization Fee				Last Paid Amt.
Insurance Examination		Dressing		Abstract		Welfare				Previous Balance
Home Visit		Sigmoi-doscopy		Major Surgery		State Medicaid				
Hospital Visit		Allergy		Assisting Surgeon		Prepaid				Charges this Visit
EKG		History and Physical		Physical Therapy						Total Charges
Dr. Service in Acc. Room		X-ray		Traction Set						
Use of Acc. Room		X-ray Call Back		Audiogram						Credits
Suturing		Pediatrics		Anesthesis						
Cast Application		Pulmonary Treatment		Total Units						Balance

DISPOSITION | Home | Return | Patient Calls | Doctor Calls | Refer | Dr. Name | Hosp. | Hospital Name

Figure 19–30. (Cont.)

set. It also meets most of the Minimum Data Set requirements. Assuming additional linkages between these encounter data and other data from patient, provider, and accounting records, the potential for responding to a broad range of data requests can be greatly enhanced.

Collection Procedures

The manner in which data are entered into the system often is viewed as a trivial consideration compared to the kinds of fundamental systems design issues already described. Yet, from the perspective of the staff who must work on a day-to-day basis with the input documents, this aspect of the system can be either a source of constant irritation or a useful exercise. Basically, the problem is one of weighing the needs of the system for accuracy of recording and

Physician's Copy

PATIENT'S NAME			SOCIAL SECURITY NO.	HISTORY NO.	DATE	Sequence
PATIENT'S ADDRESS			BIRTH DATE / AGE / SEX / Enc. Type / Appt. Status		DAY	TIME
CITY OR TOWN	STATE	ZIP CODE	Census Tract	TELEPHONE NO.	PROVIDER NO.	

BILLING NAME			Payer	CONTRACT NO.	Payer	CONTRACT NO.
BILLING ADDRESS			SUBSCRIBER'S NAME			
CITY OR TOWN	STATE	ZIP CODE	SUBSCRIBER'S ADDRESS	CITY	STATE	ZIP

X-RAYS ORDERED

CHEST	GI	UPPER EXT.		EXPLANATION
IVP	GALL BLADDER	LOWER EXT.		
BE	MAMMO-GRAPHY			PHYSICIAN'S SIGNATURE

LAB TESTS ORDERED

URINAL-YSIS	URIC ACID	PAP		EXPLANATION
CBC	BUN	SMA		
GLUCOSE	CHOLES-TEROL			PHYSICIAN'S SIGNATURE

SERVICES RENDERED

SERVICE	FEE	SERVICE	FEE	SERVICE	FEE	SERVICE	FEE	SERVICE	FEE	
Office Visit		Minor Surgery		Laboratory		Dispensary Visits				Last Pay. Date
Consultation		Injection		Home Lab Call		Utilization Fee				Last Paid Amt.
Insurance Examination		Dressing		Abstract		Welfare				Previous Balance
Home Visit		Sigmoi-doscopy		Major Surgery		State Medicaid				
Hospital Visit		Allergy		Assisting Surgeon		Prepaid				Charges this Visit
EKG		History and Physical		Physical Therapy						Total Charges
Dr. Service in Acc. Room		X-ray		Traction Set						Credits
Use of Acc. Room		X-ray Call Back		Audiogram						
Suturing		Pediatrics		Anesthesia						Balance
Cast Application		Pulmonary Treatment		Total Units						

DISPOSITION Home ☐ Return ☐ Patient Calls ☐ Doctor Calls ☐ Refer ☐ Dr. Name Hosp. ☐ Hospital Name

	Acute	Chronic
PRIMARY DIAGNOSIS		
SECONDARY DIAGNOSIS		

DRUGS PRESCRIBED

NOTES

MEDICARE
Do you accept assignment of this patient's bill?
Yes ☐ No ☐

BLUESHIELD
Do you accept this patient under the full payment provision?
Yes ☐ No ☐

REASON FOR NON-ACCEPTANCE

Duration of Visit			
Under 15 min.	15-30 min.	30-60 min.	Over one hour

1 2 3 4 5 6 7 8 9

PHYSICIAN'S SIGNATURE (The undersigned certifies that services were personally rendered by him or under his supervision.)

M.D.

SIGNATURE

PHYSICIAN'S COPY

Figure 19-30. (Cont.)

Business Office Copy

PATIENT'S NAME	SOCIAL SECURITY NO.	HISTORY NO.	DATE	Sequence
PATIENT'S ADDRESS	BIRTH DATE / AGE / SEX / Enc. Type / Appt. Status	DAY	TIME a.m. p.m.	
CITY OR TOWN / STATE / ZIP CODE	Census Tract	TELEPHONE NO.	PROVIDER NO.	
BILLING NAME	Payer	CONTRACT NO.		
BILLING ADDRESS	Payer	CONTRACT NO.		
CITY OR TOWN / STATE / ZIP CODE	SUBSCRIBER'S NAME			

X-RAYS ORDERED

Chest	61	GI	64	Upper Ext.	67			EXPLANATION
IVP	62	Gall Bladder	65	Lower Ext.	68			
BE	63	Mammography	66					PHYSICIAN'S NAME

LAB TESTS ORDERED

Urinalysis	01	Uric Acid	04	PAP	07			EXPLANATION
CBC	02	BUN	05	SMA	08			
Glucose	03	Cholesterol	06	Serology	09			PHYSICIAN'S NAME

SERVICES RENDERED

SERVICE		FEE	SERVICE		FEE	SERVICE		FEE	SERVICE		FEE	SERVICE	FEE	
Office Visit	14		Minor Surgery	24		Laboratory	34		Dispensary visits	43				Last Pay. Date / /
Consultation	15		Injection	25		Home Lab Call	35		Utilization Fee	44				Last Paid Amt.
Ins. Exam	16		Dressing	26		Abstract	36		Welfare	45				Previous Balance
Home Visit	17		Sigmoidoscopy	27		Major Surgery	37		State Medicaid	46				Charges this Visit
Hospital Visit	18		Allergy	28		Assisting Surgeon	38		Prepaid	47				
EKG	19		History & Physical	29		Physical Therapy	39							Total Charges
Dr. Serv. in Acc. Rm.	20		X-ray	30		Traction Set	40							
Use of Acc. Rm.	21		X-ray Call Back	31		Audiogram	41							Credits
Suturing	22		Pediatrics	32		Anesthesia	42							
Cast Appl.	23		Pulmon. Treat.	33		Total Units								Balance

DISPOSITION Home 1 Ret. 2 Pat. Calls 3 Dr. Calls 4 Ref. 5 Dr. Name Hosp. 6 Hospital Name

	Acute	Chronic	Primary Diagnosis
PRIMARY DIAGNOSIS			M 1 2
SECONDARY DIAGNOSIS			Secondary Diagnosis
DRUGS PRESCRIBED			BS 1 2
			Drugs
NOTES			Duration of Visit
			1 2 3 4

1 2 3 4 5 6 7 8 9

PHYSICIAN'S SIGNATURE (The undersigned certifies that services were personally rendered by him or under his supervision.)

M.D.

SIGNATURE

BUSINESS OFFICE COPY

Figure 19-30. (Cont.)

Common Claims Form
Reverse of Business Office Copy

PATIENT INFORMATION

BLUE SHIELD: Answer the following questions with a check mark and/or explanation in the appropriate space:

a) IS THIS A JOB CONNECTED INJURY? Yes ________ No ________

b) IF AN ACCIDENT, WHERE DID IT OCCUR? Work ______ Home ___ Highway ___ Other ______

c) IF YOU HAVE OTHER COVERAGE: Policy No. ________ Name of Company ________________

If you are enrolled under Plan A, Plan B or the Federal Employee Low Option Plan, participating physicians *are not required* to accept the Blue Shield payment as full settlement *unless all of the following requirements are met.* (Medical and maternity cases, except caesarian delivery and anesthesia, are not covered under the full payment provision.)

A. PLAN A/FEP LOW OPTION ▶ INDIVIDUAL INCOME UNDER $2,800; FAMILY INCOME UNDER $4,000

PLAN B ▶ INDIVIDUAL INCOME UNDER $4,000; FAMILY INCOME UNDER $6,000

▶ Limits include all income before deductions—please check your Plan Income Category in the box below.

B. YOU HAVE NO OTHER SURGICAL-MEDICAL HEALTH INSURANCE COVERAGE.

C. YOU DID NOT OCCUPY A PRIVATE ROOM—UNLESS IT WAS MEDICALLY NECESSARY.

TYPE OF MEMBERSHIP: PLAN A/FEP LOW OPTION ▶ INDIVIDUAL ________ FAMILY ________ PLAN B ▶ INDIVIDUAL ________ FAMILY ________

INCOME: UNDER $2,800 ________ $2,800—$4,000 ________ $4,000—$6,000 ________ OVER $6,000 ________

I HAVE READ THE ABOVE REQUIREMENTS AND I AM___ AM NOT___ ENTITLED TO THE FULL PAYMENT PROVISION.

NOTE: *If you are enrolled under the Blue Shield "100" Plan or the Federal High Option Plan,* participating physicians will accept the Blue Shield payment as full settlement of these charges regardless of income, unless there is a deductible amount which you must pay.	Signature of Subscriber or Applicant	Date Signed

MEDICARE NOTICE: ANYONE WHO MISREPRESENTS OR FALSIFIES ESSENTIAL INFORMATION REQUESTED BY THIS FORM MAY UPON CONVICTION BE SUBJECT TO FINE OR IMPRISONMENT UNDER FEDERAL LAW.

Describe the illness or injury for which you received treatment:	Was your illness or injury connected with your employment? ☐Yes ☐No

If you have other health insurance or if your state Medical Assistance Agency will pay part of your medical expenses and you want information about this claim released to the insurance company or state agency upon its request, give the following information:

Insuring Organization or State Agency Name and Address	Policy or Medical Assistance Number

I authorize any holder of medical or other information about me to release to the Social Security Administration or its intermediaries or carriers any information needed for this or a related Medicare claim. I permit a copy of this Authorization to be used in place of the original, and request payment of medical insurance benefits either to myself or to the party who accepts assignment.	Signature of Patient	Date Signed
PUBLIC ASSISTANCE I certify these services to be just, correct, and complete as rendered and received this date. This bill has not been previously paid.	Signature of Patient or Agent	Date Signed
AUTHORIZATION FOR OPERATIVE PROCEDURES I hereby give permission for the staff of the Medical Associates of Bristol County, Inc. to perform the necessary operative procedures which they deem advisable in the treament of: Patient: ________	Signature of Parent or Guardian	Date Signed

PHYSICIAN INFORMATION

Please describe your services in sufficient detail to enable Blue Shield to apply the appropriate allowance:

SPECIAL INFORMATION REQUESTED ◀

- DIAGNOSIS —If the cause is traumatic, specify the date of injury.
- MEDICAL —If your fee is for consultation, enter the name of the referring physician.
- " —Give the date of any surgery performed during this admission.
- SURGERY —Include the size and location of any lesion, burn, laceration, etc.
- RADIOLOGY —X-ray: Report films taken and findings—Therapy: Report the type and number of treatments.
- LABORATORY —If laboratory profile, specify name and charge as well as your charge for collection and handling.

0 1 2 3 4 5 6 7 8 9 10 11 12 CM

(If you are reporting a skin lesion please indicate the size of the lesion in centimeters.)

Figure 19-30. (Cont.)

for economical operation, on the one hand, and the needs of the people recording the data on the other. One problem alluded to in the description of an integrated encounter form package is that the need of the physician to retain control over his style of practice should not be arbitrarily constrained by the methodology for entering data into the medical record. Every detail of the data entry phase of system design should be examined from this perspective—arrangement of items on the form, precoding of entries, multiple choice check-off boxes, etc. Whether the data need to be entered on a so-called real-time basis will determine the appropriateness of entry techniques other than manually produced forms. In most cases, and particularly in group practices of less than ten physicians, batch processing of data will be adequate and probably desirable.

Flow Charts and Instruction Manuals. Often, it is extremely useful to develop flow charts showing the sequence of activities involved in the processing of each input document into the system. Flow charts need not be very sophisticated, but at minimum they should specify:

1. Initiator of each document (if not by name then by job title)
2. Individual responsible for each entry
3. Decision process determining sequential movements of the document and its copies
4. Disposition of each copy.

In the course of developing such flow charts, one can identify potential problems or bottlenecks ahead of time and can correct them before they create difficulties during actual program operations. Much internal dissension can be avoided in this manner. In addition to the flow charts themselves, instruction manuals usually will be necessary for professional and clerical personnel handling these documents. All terms and entries should be defined and decision rules for recording data should be spelled out. For example, when should an encounter be designated an *emergency*? If there is more than one third party responsible for payment of a patient's bill, how should *primary payment source* be identified?

Ensuring Accuracy. Not every piece of data entered into the system will require that a high degree of care be taken to ensure its accuracy. For example, the patient identification number (a number unique to each patient, possibly the social security number) is one piece of data that should receive careful attention. The accurate recording of this number and the extent to which it is used to link multiple records of the same patient together as a unit record, both within the group practice and the hospital, can be very important. The accuracy of other data may be of less concern.

All data inputs should be reviewed in terms of how entry errors could affect decisions based on derived reports. For those items calling for a high degree of accuracy, the use of preprinted entries, rubber stamps, and patient identification cards should be considered. In the discussion of registration systems

(Chapter 12) it was noted that identification cards can be initiated on the spot during registration or at the same time as the patient's medical history is initiated. Such cards can help to ensure that the identification number is always recorded correctly. There are other ways to approach the problem of ensuring accuracy. Staff training programs can be devised for clerical, administrative, and medical personnel. Edit check procedures can be designed which specifically target particular items after they have been recorded. Provision then can be made for their correction, should this be necessary.

Data Preservation. The preservation of certain source documents may be critical, especially if subsequent use of data from these documents is subject to electronic processing. Patient signatures authorizing medical procedures and physician signatures attesting to the accuracy of medical information are notable examples of data elements that need to be preserved in their original form. Appropriate steps should be built into the data collection procedure to account for the movement and storage of such documents.

Data Confidentiality. Earlier, the subject of data confidentiality was discussed more specifically in relation to medical record information. The following discussion treats the issue of responsibility in a broader sense. The possibility for misuse of sensitive medical, financial, and other data related to the patient or his physician should be considered at every juncture of system design, and safeguards should be introduced to minimize potential misuse. In this regard, consideration should be given to:

1. Eliminating or disguising patient or physician identification on certain output reports
2. Restricting distribution of documents and accounting for all copies
3. Physical safeguarding of particularly sensitive files, including the use of protection systems
4. Controlling the handling and transmittal of data.

This last effort can be rendered more difficult or can be simplified greatly when data are being processed electronically. Handling and transmitting can be more difficult when there is no tangible document involved; it may be harder to track the movement of the data. On the other hand, through appropriate use of codes that limit to particular individuals access to all or to parts of records in computer files, there actually can be greater assurance that confidentiality is being protected.

Phase-in Possibilities. In order to allow the problems that inevitably arise in data collection systems to be worked out, thought might be given to phasing in components of the system over a period of time, thus allowing personnel to become reasonably familiar with one component before another is introduced. Once the system is functioning, a number of ways to improve it will become obvious. If all components are implemented simultaneously, however, the cost of revised forms and procedures may increase substantially.

MAKING THE SYSTEM WORK

In the final analysis, how will the physician, administrative, and clerical staffs know if the statistical analysis system is an effective one? Howerton has offered these measures of system effectiveness:[8]

1. *Convenience* to the user (location of facilities, formalities required to obtain service, media, or input)
2. *Ease of translation* from request to system language
3. *Cycle time*—time required for information to flow through the system (backlog, response time for retrieval, etc.)
4. *Recall*—completeness with which the file has been searched and appropriate matches have been made
5. *Relevance*—degree to which a single item is related to the initial request.

It might be added that cost also is an important measure of effectiveness. Attaining a uniformly high degree of convenience, ease of translation, cycle time, recall, and relevance for all system uses is an expensive proposition. The approach suggested causes the group to set priorities based initially on the mission priorities and modified when necessary by external forces and internal logistical considerations. Even with this more tailored approach, the overall system costs may be deemed excessive given its uses. If this is the case, one should try to distinguish between what the system is capable of doing for the group practice and how it actually is being used. Until a meaningful effort has been made to close the gap between these two system states, it would be unfortunate if the cost-benefit decision were made in the direction of reducing the system's capabilities. It would certainly be important to ascertain if there were ways in which its full potential could be realized.

This effort may involve major internal education, but much of that effort should have been built into the process of system design. As it has been described, a considerable amount of physician and other staff involvement is essential to that process; nevertheless, the educational job never ceases. Moreover, it works in both directions; not only must the system's users—the decisionmakers—be aided in their understanding of how to get the most out of it, but also their comments and suggestions regarding the system in operation represent the most important source of feedback to management for improving the system's usefulness. Put simply, the usefulness of a statistical analysis system is a function of how effective its outputs are in improving the group's performance. The gap between an understanding of the causes of poor performance and the translation of that understanding into corrective action can be wide. There are, however, several ways to bridge it—to relate the analysis system to a control system.

Control Through Monitoring

A useful, but often ignored, tool for controlling organizational performance is the pressure imposed by the existence of the statistical analysis system itself. The various measures of performance that are monitored on a continuing basis and for which data are routinely collected can act as signals to the program staff—medical and administrative—that certain aspects of performance are viewed as important. The reasons these signals are not always as clear as they might be are that, first, there may be insufficient staff commitment to the performance measures used and, secondly, there may be insufficient visibility of these measures in use. Unless others in addition to management are involved in selecting performance measures, there is not likely to be a commitment to corrective action should these measures reveal a need for it. By the same token, early involvement in the selection of performance measures cannot generate ongoing commitment. This sense of commitment must be constantly reinforced by making the application of these measures highly visible to the staff throughout the program. Performance data that are not even disseminated to those in decision-making positions obviously have no impact.

Control Through Incentives

The possibilities for control implicit in the performance monitoring process are augmented by tying incentives to the performance measures. There are, of course, positive and negative incentives or rewards and penalties. The most powerful incentive is the possibility of improving the health status of the individual patient, but it would be unrealistic to ignore the fact that members of any organization are to some degree motivated by other factors as well, and of these the most powerful are not necessarily monetary. Rewards other than financial ones can act as strong inducements toward improved performance. These rewards can range from commendation by one's professional peers to expressions of gratitude from patients. There are financial incentives as well, but as long as they are tied to performance that is ultimately in the best interest of the patient, they fulfill a proper role. Indeed, the whole concept of risk-sharing within a prepaid program of health care builds in part upon the positive use of financial incentives. (The reader's attention is called to Chapter 9, where the issue of physician compensation is discussed in greater detail.) There is no magic about the way such incentives work. There may be as much danger of fostering inadequate utilization of the program's services in a prepaid setting as there is danger of promoting unnecessary utilization in the fee-for-service setting. There must in each case be forces at work within the organization to counteract these tendencies. Creating a strong peer review capability can be very important in this regard.

Control Through Explicit Action

Up to this point the discussion has centered on implicit mechanisms for correcting program performance. Clearly, there will be times when performance measures reveal the existence of specific problems that must be resolved explicitly: the physicians are spending too much time on clerical chores; waiting times are inordinately long during peak load periods. In cases such as these, nothing less than clear corrective action may suffice. One cannot rely simply on the dissemination of the data or the evolutionary effects of incentives. Rather, decisions must be made to cope with the problems at hand: hire more administrative staff to handle the clerical chores; revise the hours of operation to encourage utilization during off-peak periods. Generally speaking, it is through the continuous application of such explicit modifications that the overall program is maintained at the levels of performance originally intended.

System Impact on Planning

Program planning (as described in Chapter 4) is by nature an open-ended activity. Outputs from the statistical analysis system can validate or reveal the need to revise assumptions used in planning. Projected utilization rates may be off; certain costs may have been budgeted too low. Any number of external circumstances may have changed in such a way as to alter the validity of the existing plan—ranging from epidemics to the emergence of a competing health facility. Internal circumstances may also change. The group practice may evolve into new forms. Fee-for-service may give way to prepayment; the facility may expand its capacity, or new facilities may be added.

The group practice must be prepared to reassess not only assumptions as to demand, capacity, and cash flow, but basic program priorities and missions as well. In other words, it must be prepared to cycle back into the strategic as well as the program planning process. Of course, at this time the group will have a history of its own—a history replete with mistakes from which to learn and achievements to inspire continued success in meeting the health care needs of the community.

Appendix 19A

A Sampling of Patient Record Documents

ASSURANCE OF CONFIDENTIALITY – All information which would permit identification of an individual, a practice, or an establishment will be held confidential, will be used only by persons engaged in and for the purposes of the survey and will not be disclosed or released to other persons or used for any other purpose.

1 DATE OF VISIT

__ __ __
Mo / Da / Yr

NATIONAL AMBULATORY MEDICAL CARE SURVEY

PATIENT RECORD

2 DATE OF BIRTH

__ __ __
Mo / Da / Yr

3 SEX

1 ☐ Female
2 ☐ Male

4 COLOR OR RACE

1 ☐ White
2 ☐ Negro/Black
3 ☐ Other
4 ☐ Unknown

5 PATIENT'S PRINCIPAL PROBLEM(S), COMPLAINT(S) OR SYMPTOM(S) THIS VISIT *(In Patient's own words)*

____

6 SERIOUSNESS OF PROBLEM IN ITEM 5 *(Check one)*

1 ☐ Very Serious
2 ☐ Serious
3 ☐ Slightly Serious
4 ☐ Not Serious

7 HAVE YOU EVER SEEN THIS PATIENT BEFORE

1 ☐ Yes 2 ☐ No

If yes, for the problem indicated in Item 5

1 ☐ Yes 2 ☐ No

8 MAJOR REASON(S) FOR THIS VISIT *(Check all major reasons)*

01 ☐ Acute Problem
02 ☐ Acute Problem Follow-up
03 ☐ Chronic Problem, Routine
04 ☐ Chronic Problem, Flare-up
05 ☐ Postoperative Care
06 ☐ Prenatal Care
07 ☐ Postnatal Care
08 ☐ Well Adult/Child Exam
09 ☐ Family Planning
10 ☐ Counseling/Advice
11 ☐ Immunization
12 ☐ Referred by Another Physician/Agency
13 ☐ Administrative Purpose
14 ☐ Other *(Specify)* ________________

9 PHYSICIAN'S PRINCIPAL DIAGNOSIS THIS VISIT

a. Diagnoses Associated With Item 5 Entry

____

b. Other Significant Current Diagnoses *(In Order of Importance)*

____

10 TREATMENT/SERVICES ORDERED OR PROVIDED THIS VISIT *(Check all that apply)*

01 ☐ None Ordered/Provided
02 ☐ Prescription Drug
03 ☐ Non-Prescription Drug
04 ☐ Injection/Immunization
05 ☐ History/Physical Exam
06 ☐ Lab Procedure/Test
07 ☐ X-rays
08 ☐ Office Surgical Treatment *(Specify)* ________________
09 ☐ Psychotherapy/Therapeutic Listening
10 ☐ Medical Counseling/Advice
11 ☐ Other *(Specify)* ________________

11 DISPOSITION <u>THIS</u> VISIT *(Check all that apply)*

1 ☐ No Follow-up Planned
2 ☐ Return at Specified Time
3 ☐ Return if Needed, p.r.n.
4 ☐ Telephone Follow-up Planned
5 ☐ Referred to Another Physician/Agency
6 ☐ Admit to Hospital
7 ☐ Returned to Referring Physician
8 ☐ Other *(Specify)* ________________

12 DURATION OF <u>THIS</u> VISIT *(Time actually spent with Physician)*

________ Minutes

Source: Jane H. Murnaghan, ed., "Ambulatory Medical Care Data," *Medical Care*, 2, No. 2 (1973 Supplement), 199.

NAME OF PLAN ______________________________
(Code to identify specific center if Plan has multiple centers)

(1)

Patient Name ________________
ID Number ________________
Family Number ________________
Sex ________ Date of Birth ________
Method of Payment ________________

(2) DATE OF ENCOUNTER ________________

(3) CLASS (Encircle Code No.)
1 Enrolled 2 Registered 3 Fee-for-Service

(4) SITE OF ENCOUNTER (Encircle Code No.)
1 Center 2 Home 3 Hospital Inpatient
4 Hospital OPD 5 Other ________________
Specify

(5) APPOINTMENT STATUS (Encircle Code No.)
1 Appointment (this encounter) 2 Walk-in

(6) PROVIDER ______________________________ (Code No. of Type of Provider)

(7) PURPOSE OF THIS ENCOUNTER (Encircle Code No.)

Illness Care	Non-Illness Care	
1 Illness	3 Pre/Post Natal	6 Well Baby/Child Health Review
2 Injury	4 Initial Health Assessment	7 Immunization
	5 Adult Health Review	8 Other ________ Specify

(8) LABORATORY TESTS AND PROCEDURES ORDERED (Encircle all that apply)

1 Hematology	4 Microbiology	7 Serology
2 Urinalysis	5 Blood Bank	8 EKG
3 Chemistry	6 Tissue Studies	9 Special Procedures ________ Specify

(9) X-RAY EXAMINATIONS ORDERED (Encircle all that apply)

1 Chest	4 Spine and Pelvis	6 Special Radiologic Procedures ________ Specify
2 Abdomen	5 Extremities	7 Other ________ Specify
3 Head and Neck		

(10) DIAGNOSIS/PROBLEM (at this encounter)
1 Diagnosis ________________ (write in) 2 Problem ________________ (write in)

(11) DISPOSITION (Encircle all that apply)

1 No follow-up necessary
2 Return appointment scheduled
3 Follow-up visit by provider:
________ Specify (home, hospital, nursing home, etc.)
4 Telephone to/from patient
5 Referred to hospital for admission
6 Referred to hospital for out-patient care
7 Consultation/referral outside plan's facilities
8 Consultation/referral inside plan's facilities
9 Other ________________
Specify

(12) ______________________ ______________________
Signature of Provider I.D. Number (Individual Staff I.D. No.)

Source: Jane H. Murnaghan, ed., "Ambulatory Medical Care Data," *Medical Care,* 2, No. 2 (1973 Supplement), 156.

OUTPATIENT DATA FORM

HOSPITAL CODE | PATIENT'S MEDICAL RECORD NO. | CONTROL NO.

PATIENT'S LAST NAME | INITIAL

STREET NO. | N/S-E/W | STREET NAME | AV/ST | ZIP CODE

AGE — 00 - UNDER 1 YEAR; NB - NEW BORN; 01 - 99

SEX & RACE — 1 - M; 2 - F; 3 - WM; 4 - WF; 5 - BM; 6 - BF; 7 - OM; 8 - OF

MARITAL STATUS — 1 - SINGLE; 2 - MARRIED; 3 - WIDOWED; 4 - DIV. OR SEPARATED

TRANSPORT — 1 - PRIVATE CAR; 2 - BUS; 3 - TAXI; 4 - AMBUL.; 5 - POLICE CAR; 6 - RESCUE SQUAD

MO. DAY YR. ADM. DATE

HOUR ADM. — 01 - 24

FIRST CLINIC (See Guide)

REFERRAL SOURCE (See Guide)

DIAGNOSES: LIST PRINCIPAL DIAGNOSIS FIRST

A

B

C

D

E

F

G

FOR ALL NEW PATIENTS COMPLETE ITEMS ABOVE

RESERVE ITEMS BELOW FOR LATER FOLLOW-UP

MO. DAY YR. LAST DATE ACTIVE

DISCH. STATUS — 1 - DISCHARGED; 2 - PRN. RETURN; 3 - FAILED APPT.; 4 - RET. TO PVT. DR.; 5 - ADM. TO HOSPITAL; 6 - REF. ELSEWHERE; 7 - STILL ACTIVE; 8 - DIED

PAY STATUS — 1 - SELF-PAY; 2 - BLUE CROSS; 3 - COMMERCIAL; 4 - MEDICARE; 5 - OTHER GOVT.; 6 - WORK COMP.; 7 - FREE; 8-9 - OPTIONS

PREGNANCY OUTCOME — 1 - LIVE BIRTH; 2 - STILL BIRTH; 3 - ABORTED; 4 - NOT YET TERM

ATTENDING PHYSICIAN

NO. CLINICS ATTENDED

TOTAL NO. CLINIC VISITS

MODEL CITIES — 1 - YES; 2 - NO

CODED BY

CODING GUIDE

CLINIC CODES

01. Allergy	18. Hemodialysis	35. Planned Parenthood
02. Amputee	19. Inhalation Therapy	36. Plastic Surgery
03. Audiology	20. Internal Medicine	37. Poison Control
04. Cardiology	21. Metabolic	38. Post Partum
05. Catheterization	22. Minor Surgery	39. Proctology
06. Chest	23. Neurology	40. Psychiatry
07. Chiropody	24. Neurosurgery	41. Pulmonary Function
08. Dental	25. Nutrition	42. Renal
09. Diabetic	26. Obstetrics	43. Special Development
10. Diathermic	27. Occupational Therapy	44. Speech
11. E. N. T.	28. Orthopedic	45. Spinal Punctures
12. Eye	29. Otology	46. Surgery
13. General Medical	30. Outpatient Emergency	47. Urology
14. Genetics	31. Pacemaker	48. X-Ray & Lab
15. G. I.	32. Paracentesis	
16. Gynecology	33. Pediatrics	
17. Hematology	34. Physical Therapy	

50. Specialty Clinic — Unspecified

REFERRAL SOURCE

1. Self referral — general care
2. Self referral — specialty care
3. Referred by other medical institution for general care
4. Referred by other medical institution for specialty care
5. Referred by M.D. for general care
6. Referred by M.D. for specialty care
7. Referred by M.D. for consultation or tests
8. Decision by emergency vehicle driver
9. Referred for follow-up of in-pt. care
0. Other

Source: Jane H. Murnaghan, ed., "Ambulatory Medical Care Data," *Medical Care,* 2, No. 2 (1973 Supplement), 180.

1. Family Identification Number __ __ __ __

2. Plan Code __ __ __: 3. Medicare [A] [B] (Check) 4. Title XIX Cat. [1] [2] [3] (Check)

5. Registration (Effective Date) __ __ __

6. Census Tract Number __ __ __ 7. Income Source __ 8. Income Amount __ __

9. Social Security Number __ __ __ __ __ __ __ __ __

10. Medicare Number __ __ __ __ __ __ __ __ __ __ __ __ __

11. Present Address ______________________
Number Street City State Zip Phone

12. In Case of Emergency Contact ______________________

____
Number Street City State Zip Phone

13. Education of Head of Family (Enter Last Grade Completed) ____________

14. Type of Residence (Check) [1] House [2] Apartment [3] Public Housing [4] Other

15. Tenancy Status (Check) [1] Own [2] Rent [3] Other

16. (Optional) Head of Family - Racial Ethnic Profile (Check) [1] White [2] Black [3] Spanish Speaking [4] Other

17.

Individual Computer Number	Last Name, First Name, Initial	Medicaid Suffix	Sex	Birthdate	Family No. Prefix
	Head of Household 1				
	2				
	3				
	4				
	5				
	6				
	7				
	8				
	9				
	10				
	11				
	12				
	13				

Interviewed By ______________________ Date ____________

NHC-1002-A-5M-5/71 **BUSINESS OFFICE COPY**

Source: Jane H. Murnaghan, ed., "Ambulatory Medical Care Data," *Medical Care*, 2, No. 2 (1973 Supplement), 57.

HIST. #

091806

NAME

1st CARE SOURCE ____________

SEX DOB INS PL FAMILY# DATE

PROBLEM LIST STATUS

Add Del Fam

DIAGNOSIS (PROBLEMS THIS VISIT)

I _ O O O _ I ____________

II _ O O O _ II ____________

III _ O O O _ III ____________

DRUG REACTION (DRU) ____________

RELATED TO: EMPLOYMENT 1 O

PREGNANCY 1 O IF SO, APPROXIMATE DATE PREGNANCY COMMENCED ____________

APPOINTMENT STATUS

- O 1 Scheduled in Advance
- O 2 Walk-in
- O 3 Scheduled Today
- O 4 No Show

PLACE

- O 1 Office (normal day hrs.)
- O 8 Office (normal evening hrs.)
- O 2 Hospital
- O 3 Home
- O 4 Home (night)
- O 5 Home (weekend)
- O 6 Office (night)
- O 7 Office (weekend)
- O 9 Other

DURATION OF CONTACT

1st Care Source

- O 1 1-15 Mins.
- O 2 16-30 Mins.
- O 3 31-45 Mins.
- O 4 45 + Mins.

2nd Care Source ____________ (Enter care source number)

- O 1 1-15 Mins.
- O 2 16-30 Mins.
- O 3 31-45 Mins.
- O 4 45 + Mins.

PURPOSE CATEGORIES

- O A Illness-initial visit
- O B Illness-follow-up
- O C Injury-initial visit
- O D Injury-follow-up
- O E Pre-natal
- O F Post-natal
- O G Consultation (Referral from other physician)
- O H Well Baby
- O J Initial Health Assessment
- O K Health review
- O L Immunization only
- O M Injection only
- O N Pharmacy/Lab/X-ray only
- O R Post-Operative Follow-up
- O T Family Planning
- O W Routine Gyn Check

SPECIAL PROCEDURES

Ear, Nose and Throat

- O 201 Ear Myringotomy
- O 202 Irrigation-Ear Canal
- O 210 Nose-Polypectomy
- O 211 -Excision of other lesions
- O 212 -Control of Epistaxis
- O 213 Oral-Excision Biopsy
- O 214 Sinus Irrigation

Ophthalmology

- O 215 Complete Refraction Exam
- O 216 Ophthalmologic Follow-Up Exam
- O 217 Prescription Check

Psychiatry

- O 301 Initial Evaluation

Continuing Psychotherapy

- O 302 a Family Therapy
- O 303 b Single
- O 304 c Group
- O 305 d Pharmaco Therapy
- O 306 e Couple

Orthopedic

- O 501 Injection
- O 502 Long Arm Cast
- O 503 Short Arm Cast
- O 504 Long Leg Cast
- O 505 Short Leg Cast
- O 506 Cylinder Cast
- O 507 Aspiration
- O 508 Follow-up

Surgery

- O 550 Minor Surgery-Excision
- O 551 Minor Surgery-Suture
- O 552 Minor Surgery-Incision and drainage
- O 553 Minor Surgery-Removal of foreign body
- O 554 Vasectomy

General

- O 401 Audiometry Sweep Check
- O 402 Audiometry Threshold Check
- O 403 Allergy Testing
- O 405 Psychometric Testing
- O 406 Vision Screening
- O 407 Tuberculin Testing
- O 411 EKG
- O 412 Tonometry
- O 413 Pulmonary Function Study

Other ____________

____

DISPOSITION

- O 10 No Specific Disposition
- O 11 Follow-up visit within __ mos.
- O 21 Telephone to/from patient if necessary
- O 26 Arrange Hospital Admission (elec)
- O 27 Arrange Hospital Admission (emer)

Consultation Referral Outside Plan

41 ____________ ☐☐☐
(Clinic or Physician)

Consultation/Referral Inside Plan

- O 50 Dentist
- O 51 Surgeon
- O 52 Ophthalmologist
- O 53 Optometrist
- O 54 Psychiatrist
- O 55 Psychologist
- O 56 ENT
- O 57 OB-GYN
- O 58 Pediatrician
- O 59 Internist
- O 60 Radiologist
- O 61 Speech and Hearing
- O 62 Health Associate
- O 63 Social Service
- O 64 Mental Health Couns.
- O 65 PHN
- O 66 Neurologist
- O 67 Orthopedic Surgeon
- O 68 Allergist
- O 69 Dermatologist
- O 70 Urologist

(Reverse side of this encounter form is shown on the following page.)

LABORATORY (LABR.)

SEROLOGY

- 4510 R.P.R.
- 4515 VDRL
- 4535 Heterophile Titer
- 4560 ASTO
- 4550 R. A. Test
- 4600 Febrile Agglutinations
- 4564 C-Reactive Protein

URINALYSIS & PARASITOLOGY

- 5200 Routine U.A. (all of the below)
- 5204 Specific Gravity
- 5203 Ph
- 5205 Sugar and Albumin
- 5207 Protein
- 5230 Ketone Bodies
- 5210 Microscopic

Qualitative Screening Test

PKU

- 5300 Bence-Jones Protein
- 5234 Bilirubin
- 5236 Cystine
- 5240 Urobilinogen
- 5242 Porphobilinogen

Quantitative Test

- 5555 Protein (24-hr. urine)
- 5510 Glucose (24-hr. urine)
- 9380 PSP
- 9310 Urea Clearance
- 9300 Creatinine Clearance
- 6460 Occult Blood
- 7800 Ova & Parasite Stool
- 7800 Ova & Parasite Urine
- 7800 Pin Worm Prep

HEMATOLOGY

- 3057 C.B.C.
- 3060 R.B.C.
- 3085 W.B.C.
- 3050 Hemoglobin
- 3055 Hematocrit
- 3090 Differential
- 3075 Sedimentation Rate
- 3080 Platelets Count
- 3070 Reticulocyte Count
- 3250 Exam. Smear for Platelets
- 3200 Eosinophil Count
- 6051 Sperm Count
- 3200 Nasal Smear for Eosinophils
- 3330 Prothrombin Time
- 3550 Hemoglobin Electrophoresis
- 5010 Spinal Fluid Cell Count (CSF)
- 3205 Sickle Cell Prep

Misc. ______

BACTERIOLOGY & MYCOLOGY

- 7150 Throat
- 7140 Nasopharyngeal
- 7152 Sputum Culture
- 7120 Urine Culture
- 7220 Stool Culture
- 7110 Spinal Fluid Culture
- 7200 Vaginal Culture
- 7100 Blood Culture

Wet Prep ______
TBC ______
Fungi ______
Miscellaneous ______

CHEMISTRY

- 5020 Glucose - CSF
- 9000 - Glucose Tol.
- 0150 - AC
- 0155 - PC
- 0180 CO_2
- 0175 C1 - CSF Other ______
- 0165 NA - Other ______
- 0170 K - Other ______
- 0160 Blood Urea Nitrogen
- 0100 6 Channel - All of above
- 0360 Triglycerides
- 0195 Calcium
- 0200 Phosphorus
- 0340 Uric Acid - Body Fluid ______
- 0210 Total Protein Serum ______ Other ______
- 0215 Albumin
- 1700 T4 (by column)
- 0225 Bilirubin
- 0245 SGOT
- 0235 Alkaline Phosphatase
- 0350 Cholesterol
- 0250 SGPT
- 0255 LDH
- 0240 Acid Phosphatase
- 0110 SMA 12-60 Survey
- 1502 Carotene
- 0315 Creatinine
- 0400 B. S. P.
- 0230 Thymol Turbidity
- 1375 Serum Acetone
- 1000 Serum Iron
- 1005 Iron Binding Capacity
- 1701 T3
- 1710 Thyroxine Binding Globulin
- 0205 Magnesium
- 1830 17 Keto
- 1733 17 OHC
- 5880 VMA

Misc. 1 ______
2 ______
3 ______
4 ______
5 ______

CYTOLOGY

- 9875 Huhner Test
- 9850 Cervical

Biopsy ______ (Source)

- 9713 Endometrical Biopsy

VIROLOGY

- 4650 Rubella
- 4651 Influenza
- 4692 PPLO

Other (1) ______
(2) ______
(3) ______

TOXICOLOGY

Specify ______

BLOOD BANK

- 4020 Grouping & Rh and Antibody Screening
- 4070 Coombs Test
- 4170 Rh Titers
- 4165 Isoagglutinin Titer

MISCELLANEOUS

- 9851 Pregnancy Test

X-RAY (RAD.)

RT	LT	BIL	
			HEAD AND NECK
		010	Facial Bones
020	021	022	Mandible
		025	Mastoids
		030	Nasal Bones
035	036	037	Optic Foramen
		040	Orbits
		045	Paranasal Sinuses
		055	Sella Turcica
		060	Skull series, Comp.
		062	Skull series, Ltd. or pediatric
		064	Skull, single film
		080	Tempero mandibular joints
		085	Temporal Bones
		090	Zygomatic Arches
			CHEST
		101	Chest (PA and Lat.)
		103	Chest (AP)
		107	Chest, Cardiac Ser. w/fluoroscopy
		119	Chest, Single film
130	131	132	Ribs
			ABDOMEN
		201	Abdomen (supine & erect)
		207	Abdomen, single film
		210	Barium Enema
		215	Barium Enema (Air contrast)
		240	Esophagus Study
		245	Esophagus Study, Acid barium
		250	Gallbladder, scout film
		280	Small Bowel Series
		284	Upper G.I. Series
		288	Upper G.I. & Small Bowel Series
			GENITOURINARY
		301	Cystogram
		350	Pyelogram, hypertensive
		353	Pyelogram, intravenous
		356	Pyelogram, intravenous drip
			SPINE AND PELVIS
		401	Cervical Spine
410	411	412	Hip
		420	Lumbar Spine
		430	Lumboscaral Spine
		440	Pelvis
		450	Sacriliac Joints
		460	Sacrum and Coccyx
		480	Spine, single film
		490	Thoracic Spine
			EXTREMITIES
512	513	514	Ankle
521	522	523	Clavicle
525	526	527	Elbow
530	531	532	Femur
540	541	542	Foot
551	552	553	Hand
559	560	561	Humerus
562	563	564	Knee
569	570	571	Radius and Ulna
575	576	577	Shoulder
578	579	580	Tibia and Fibula
585	586	587	Wrist
			SPECIAL
		972	Bone Age Survey
		974	Bone Survey metastatic
		918	Hysterosalpingogram
		980	Joint Survey
		942	Pelvimetry
			OTHER

MEDICATION (RXX)

RX #	NDC	QTY.	UNIT	REFILL OK	REFILL YES

Source: Jane H. Murnaghan, ed., "Ambulatory Medical Care Data," *Medical Care,* 2, No. 2 (1973 Supplement), 58-59.

OUT PATIENT VISIT DATA

DEPARTMENT OF BUSINESS SERVICES – YALE-NEW HAVEN HOSPITAL

CARD 5 MUST BE COMPLETED WHENEVER PATIENT HAS A CLINIC VISIT

CARD	COL.		MONTH	DAY	YEAR
ALL CARDS	1-6	VISIT DATE			
	7-12	ACCOUNT NO. (NOT UNIT NO.) →			
2 GUARANTOR	15-38	NAME LAST, FIRST, M.I. FIRST NAME NOT BEFORE COL. 23 →			
	79-80	CARD CODE 9 1			
	15-38	NAME MR. MRS. MISS FIRST M.I. LAST			
	39-58	STREET			
	59-78	CITY, STATE			
	79-80	CARD CODE 9 2			

3 PATIENT DATA

	COL.
BIRTH DATE (MONTH DAY YEAR)	15-21
RESIDENCE CODE	22-24
RELIGION: 1 CATHOLIC 2 JEWISH 3 PROTESTANT 4 OTHER	25
M.O. REFERRAL: 1 PRIVATE M.D. 2 E.S. 3 SELF 5 YALE PRIVATE CLINIC 6 AGENCY 8 OTHER	26
RACE: N – NEGRO W – WHITE O OTHER	27
SEX: M MALE F FEMALE	28
MARITAL STATUS: S SINGLE D DIVORCED P SEPARATED M MARRIED W WIDOWED	29
FAMILY INCOME – ALL SOURCES: 0 Less than $1000; 1 1000 – 1999; 2 2000 – 2999; 4 4000 – 4999; 5 5000 – 5999; 6 6000 – 6999; 7 7000 – 7999; 9 9000 and Over	30
MEDICAL INSURANCE HELD: 0 NONE; 1 BLUE CROSS AND CMS; 2 BLUE CROSS ONLY; 3 CMS ONLY; 4 COMMERCIAL INSURANCE ONLY; 5 BLUE CROSS AND COMMERCIAL INSURANCE; 6 OTHER	31
PRIME SOURCE OF MEDICAL CARE: 1 OSTEOPATH; 2 CHIROPRACTOR; 3 PRIVATE PHYSICIAN; 4 YNH EMERGENCY SERVICE; 5 YNH CLINIC; 6 OTHER – PLEASE STATE; 7 NONE	32
OCCUPATION OF HOUSEHOLD HEAD: 1 PROFESSIONAL AND TECHNICAL; 2 MANAGER, OFFICIAL, PROPRIETOR (NON FARM); 3 CLERICAL AND KINDRED; 4 SALES; 5 CRAFTSMAN, FOREMAN, KINDRED; 6 OPERATIVES, KINDRED; 7 PRIVATE HOUSEHOLD WORKER; 8 SERVICE WORKER (NOT PRIVATE HOUSE); 9 LABORER	33

CARD 3 – CONTINUED	COL.
EMPLOYMENT STATUS – HOUSEHOLD HEAD: 1 EMPLOYED (On Vacation, On Strike, Laid Off, Temporary); 2 LOOKING FOR WORK; 3 KEEPING HOUSE; 4 GOING TO SCHOOL; 5 DISABLED; 6 OTHER – PLEASE STATE	34
YEARS AT PRESENT ADDRESS	35-36
YEARS IN PRESENT TOWN	37-38
CARD CODE	79-80 9-3

CARD 4 – METHOD OF PAYMENT

BILL PLAN NO. 1	CODE: PUNCH FOR ALL VISITS PUNCH ZEROS IF BLANK (15 17 19 21 23 25)
	ASSIGNED UNASSIGNED: PUNCH ALPHAS AS CIRCLED OR WRITTEN (27-42)
BILL PLAN NO. 2	CODE: PUNCH ONLY IF CODED (43 45 47 49 51 53)
	ASSIGNED UNASSIGNED: PUNCH ALPHAS AS CIRCLED OR WRITTEN (55-70)

CARD CODE COL. 79-80 9 4

CARD 5 – CLINIC FEE CHARGE CODE 15-9

9

CARD CODE 9 5 79-80

Source: M. Harvey Brenner and E. R. Weinerman, "An Ambulatory Data System," *American Journal of Public Health,* 59, No. 7 (July 1969), 1, 156.

PHYSICIAN'S ENCOUNTER FORM 1 0 1 | 4 1

1 2 3 CENTER NO. | 4 5 FORM NO.

DATE: MONTH (16) DAY (17 18) YEAR (19)

Patient's Name

Last ___ (6 7)

First ___ (8)

I.D. No. ___ (9 10 11 12 13 14 15)

PROVIDER NO. ___ (20 21 22) SERVICE LOCATION ___ (23)

1. TYPE OF ENCOUNTER: Check only one, the primary nature of care provided during the encounter.

24
- 1 ○ EPISODIC CARE (INCLUDING EMERGENCY CARE)
- 2 ○ INITIAL HEALTH ASSESSMENT (NEW PATIENT)
- 3 ○ LONG-TERM HEALTH CARE MANAGEMENT
- 4 ○ ROUTINE AND PREVENTIVE CARE

2. SERVICES RENDERED DURING ENCOUNTER: Check as many as are appropriate, but only one (or none) of the first three.

25
- 1 ○ COMPREHENSIVE PHYSICAL EXAM (NEW PATIENT OR RE-EXAMINATION)
- 2 ○ EXAMINATION/EVALUATION (NEW CONDITION OR SPECIALTY EXAM)
- 3 ○ FOLLOW-UP CARE (INCLUDING CONTINUATION OF AN EXAM)

- 26 ○ IMMUNIZATION(S)
- 27 ○ MEDICATION (INCLUDING INJECTIONS)
- 28 ○ DIAGNOSTIC TEST(S)

OTHER SERVICES: (SPECIFY & CODE)

29 ☐ ___

30 ☐ ___

3. LENGTH OF ENCOUNTER: Check only one.

31
1 ○ BRIEF 2 ○ ROUTINE 3 ○ PROLONGED

4. DIAGNOSIS:

A. List (in order of priority) only those conditions dealt with during *this encounter.*

B. If a *Physical Exam* is in process but not completed, check *Deferred.* Upon completion, list the conditions found on the form for the encounter completing the exam.

C. *Initial Health Assessment* should be checked as the Type of Encounter for each encounter of a new patient's work-up.

(i) PRIMARY (CHECK BELOW OR SPECIFY) ___

32.33 ___ Dx CODE ☐☐ (32 33)

00 ○ DEFERRED

○ NONE. IF NONE, CHECK ONE:
- 01 ○ PRENATAL CARE
- 03 ○ POSTPARTUM CARE
- 05 ○ WELL-CHILD CARE
- 07 ○ WELL-ADULT CARE
- 08 ○ FAMILY PLANNING
- 09 ○ OTHER

(ii) SECONDARY ___ Dx CODE ☐☐ (34 35)

(iii) ___ Dx CODE ☐☐ (36 37)

(iv) ___ Dx CODE ☐☐ (38 39)

(v) ___ Dx CODE ☐☐ (40 41)

5. RETURN APPOINTMENT(S) REQUIRED?

42	WHEN	WHICH PROVIDER
1 ○ YES	(i)	
	(ii)	
	(iii)	

Source: *Ambulatory Health Care Information System: Overall System Description.* U. S. DHEW Publication No. (HSM)72-6202, (Cambridge, Massachusetts: Bio Dynamics, 1972), p. B-4.

DENTAL ENCOUNTER FORM

Center No. Form No.

1. Patient's Name ____________________

I.D. No. ☐☐☐☐☐-☐☐

Date: Month ☐☐ Day ☐☐ Year ☐☐ Provider No. ☐☐☐ Service Location: ☐

General Instructions: Check circles. Enter numbers or letters in boxes.

1. TYPE OF ENCOUNTER: Check only one, the primary nature of care provided during the encounter.

○ Initial Dental Assessment/Treatment Series
○ Episodic Care (including emergency care)
○ Subsequent Dental Assessment/Treatment Series (Periodic Recall Series)
○ Consultation

2. SERVICES RENDERED DURING ENCOUNTER: Check as many as are appropriate, but only one in Section 2. A.

2.A. Continuity

○ Dental Examination or Evaluation
○ Follow-up Care

2.B. Diagnostic Services

○ Charting

Radiography: Enter the number of films of each type

☐ Posterior Bitewing
☐ Panoramic films
☐ Periapical
☐ Other (Specify: ____________)

The films entered above represent

A ○ Less than full mouth survey OR B ○ Full mouth survey OR
☐ More than full mouth survey—enter number of films in excess of those needed for a full mouth survey

○ Other diagnostic aids (Check and specify: ____________)

2.C. Preventive Services

Check preventive services performed:
A ○ Prophylaxis (Routine/Preventive)
B ○ Topical Fluoride Application
C ○ Structured Dental Health Education (not informal remarks)
○ Other Preventive Service (Check and specify: ____________)

2.D. Therapeutic Services

2.D.1. Restorations

Amalgams—enter number of fillings

Deciduous Teeth		Permanent Teeth	
☐ 1 Surface	☐ 2 Surfaces	☐ 1 Surface	☐ 2 Surfaces
☐ 3 or more Surfaces		☐ 3 or more Surfaces	

☐ Number of cement bases used
☐ Number of Sedative/Emergency Fillings

Silicates and Resins—enter number of surfaces

☐ Deciduous Teeth
☐ Permanent Teeth

Pulp Treatment—enter number of teeth

Deciduous Teeth		Permanent Teeth
☐ Pulpcapping	☐ Pulpotomy	☐ Pulpcapping
☐ Pulpotomy		☐ Pulpectomy

Endodontics	One Tooth	Two Teeth	Three or more Teeth
Root Canal In Process	○		
Completed 1 Root Canal	○	○	○
2 Root Canals	○	○	○
3 or more Root Canals	○	○	○
Apicoectomy	○	○	○

○ Other Restorative Work—Check and specify: ____________

2.D.2. *Oral Surgery—enter number of teeth in appropriate box.*

Extractions—

Deciduous Teeth		Permanent Teeth	
☐ Routine	☐ Surgical	☐ Routine	☐ Surgical

○ Other oral surgery—check and specify:

2.D.3. *Prosthetics*

Removable Prosthetics (enter letter codes from Coding List)
Note: Each encounter involving removable prosthetics should result in at least one entry left of the double line and at least one entry right of the double line.

○ Case in Process (check) ‖ ☐ Constructed ☐ Relined
☐ Delivery ‖ ☐ Repaired ☐ Adjusted

Fixed Prosthetics
Note: Each encounter involving fixed prosthetics should result in at least one entry above the double line **and** at least one entry below the line.

○ Case in Process
Delivered Number of:
☐ Abutments ☐ Pontics

Crowns ○ Constructed ○ Repaired

Type (from Coding List)	Number
☐	☐
☐	☐

○ Other Prosthetic Work—Check and Specify: ____________

2.D.4. *Periodontics (Check all appropriate circles)*

○ Scaling and Curettage
○ Polishing (Periodontal Prophylaxis)
○ Occlusal Adjustment
○ Gingivectomy
○ Vincent's Treatment
○ Other—Specify: ____________

2.D.5. *Orthodontics. Check and Specify.*

○ Active ____________
○ Interceptive/Preventive ____________

2.D.6. *Anesthesia. If Anesthetic used, check appropriate circle (only one).*

○ Local Anesthetic Only
○ General Anesthetic Only
○ Both Local and General Anesthetics

2.D.7. *Medication.*

Record all medication **except** that administered by the dentist topically or locally in the mouth. Check medication given:
A ○ Fluoride Tablets
B ○ Antibiotics
C ○ Other medication: Specify: ____________

3. RETURN APPOINTMENTS INDICATED. Check; complete table if necessary.

○ Not until next dental assessment—recall periodic checkup
○ For Initial Dental Assessment (as a result of Episodic Encounter)
○ Return indicated for reason other than 1 and 2 above

When?	Which Provider?	Why?

4. Check if "Care Completed"

Note: If this encounter is the result of an Initial Assessment or Periodic Checkup, the circle should only be checked by, or under authority of, the dentist performing the Initial Assessment or Periodic Checkup. See instruction sheet for details.

○

Source: *Ambulatory Health Care Information System: Overall System Description.* U.S. DHEW Publication No. (HSM)72-6202, (Cambridge, Massachusetts: Bio Dynamics, 1972), p. B-6.

OTHER PROFESSIONAL'S ENCOUNTER FORM

1	0	1	–	6
1	2	3		4

Center No. Form No.

1. Patient's Name ______________________

I.D. No. [ ][ ][ ][ ][ ]–[ ][ ] (5 6 7 8 9 10 11)

Date: Month [ ] (12) Day [ ][ ] (13 14) Year [ ] (15)

Provider No. [ ][ ][ ] (16 17 18)

Service Location [ ] (19)

1. TYPE OF ENCOUNTER: Check only one, the primary nature of care provided during the encounter.

20-
1 ○ Episodic Care (including emergency care)
3 ○ Initial Assessment/Evaluation (new patient)
2 ○ Long-Term Care Management
4 ○ Routine and Preventive Care

2. SERVICES RENDERED DURING ENCOUNTER: Check as many as are appropriate.

21- 1 ○ Examination/Evaluation/General Care
22- 1 ○ Sensory Testing (speech, vision, hearing)
23- 1 ○ Medication (including injections)
24- 1 ○ Psychometric Testing
25- 1 ○ Immunization(s)
26- 1 ○ Other Diagnostic Testing (including dental X-rays)
27- 1 ○ Therapy (speech, physical, occupational, psychological)
28- 1 ○ Counseling/Education/Training (including diet and nutrition)
29- 1 ○ Special Treatment (dressing change, prophylaxis, etc.)
○ Other (specify) ______________________

Service Code [ ][ ] (30 31)

3. LENGTH OF ENCOUNTER: Check only one.

32-
1 ○ Brief
2 ○ Routine
3 ○ Prolonged

4. RETURN APPOINTMENT(S) REQUIRED?

33-
1 ○ Yes

	When	Which Provider
(i)		
(ii)		
(iii)		

Source: *Ambulatory Health Care Information System: Overall System Description.* U.S. DHEW Publication No. (HSM)72-6202, (Cambridge, Massachusetts: Bio Dynamics, 1972), p. B-7.

HOME VISIT FORM

1	0	1	8	1
1	2	3	4	5

CENTER NO. FORM NO.

Patient's Name

Last ___ 6 7

First ___ 8

I.D. No. [ ][ ][ ][ ][ ]-[ ][ ] 9 10 11 12 13 14 15

DATE: MONTH [ ][ ] DAY [ ][ ] YEAR [ ][ ] 16 17 18 19

PROVIDER NO. [ ][ ][ ] 20 21 22

1. VISIT REQUESTED BY: Check only one.

23
1 ○ PATIENT 2 ○ PHYSICIAN 3 ○ FHC 4 ○ PHN 5 ○ OTHER CENTER STAFF MEMBER 6 ○ OTHER (SPECIFY) ______

2. SERVICES RENDERED DURING ENCOUNTER: Check as many as are appropriate.

24 ○ MEDICAL CARE	30 ○ HYGIENE
25 ○ POSTPARTUM/PRENATAL CARE	31 ○ SOCIAL SERVICE
26 ○ WELL-CHILD CARE	32 ○ EDUCATION/TRAINING
27 ○ INJECTION(S)	33 ○ NURSING CARE
28 ○ MEDICATION CHECK	34 ○ OTHER (SPECIFY) ______
29 ○ DIET AND NUTRITION	______ SERVICE CODE [ ][ ] 35 36

3. FOLLOW UP CARE REQUIRED: (Check and note if applicable)

37	DATE	PLACE	PROVIDER	REASON
1 ○ YES	(i)			
	(ii)			
	(iii)			

Source: *Ambulatory Health Care Information System: Overall System Description.* U.S. DHEW Publication No. (HSM)72-6202, (Cambridge, Massachusetts: Bio Dynamics, 1972), p. B-8.

SPECIALIST – CONSULTANT REFERRAL ENCOUNTER

1 0 1 9 1
1 2 3 4 5

Patient's Name

Last ___ (6 7)

First ___ (8)

I.D. No. ___ (9 10 11 12 13 14 15)

DATE: MONTH (16) DAY (17 18) YEAR (19)

REFERRED BY: ______________________
NAME

PROVIDER NO. ___ (20 21 22)

1. REASON FOR REFERRAL: Check only one.

23

DIRECT HEALTH CARE SERVICES	INDIRECT HEALTH SERVICES
1 O HOSPITALIZATION	5 O FOOD STAMPS
2 O CONSULTATION	6 O EMPLOYMENT
3 O MANAGEMENT/TREATMENT	7 O WELFARE
4 O DIAGNOSTIC PROCEDURE(S) (EXCEPT X-RAY AND LABORATORY WORK – USE SEPARATE FORMS)	8 O MEDICAID/MEDICARE REG.
	9 O SOCIAL SERVICE
	0 O OTHER (SPECIFY)

2. INSTRUCTIONS: To be completed by referrer.

24

a. SPECIALTY: Check only one.

1 O DENTISTRY	3 O OBSTETRICS	5 O OPHTHALMOLOGY
2 O SURGERY	4 O UROLOGY	6 O OTHER (SPECIFY)

b. NOTES: ______________________

3. REFERRAL REPORT: Referree, please use this form for submitting your report to the Medical Records Department of the Center.

(Continue on back if more space is needed.)

____

HOSPITALIZATION CASES: TOTAL NUMBER OF INPATIENT DAYS (e.g., six is 06) ___ (25 26)

27 SERVICE DISCHARGED FROM: (Check only one)

1 O MEDICINE	3 O SURGERY
2 O OBSTETRICS	4 O GYNECOLOGY
5 O OTHER (SPECIFY) ______	

OBSTETRICAL CASES: Number of Live Births ___ 28

Number of Still Births ___ 29

______ Signature ______ Date

4. REFERRAL STATUS: To be completed by Medical Records Department after 30 days, hospital discharge, or initial referral appointment, as appropriate.

Check only one.

30

1 O REFERRAL COMPLETED (IF HOSPITALIZATION, PROVIDE INFORMATION ABOVE)
2 O REFERRAL REQUIRES RE-VISITS
3 O PATIENT DID NOT FOLLOW THROUGH (INITIATE NEW REFERRAL, IF APPROPRIATE)
4 O OTHER (SPECIFY) ______

Source: *Ambulatory Health Care Information System: Overall System Description.* U. S. DHEW Publication No. (HSM)72-6202, (Cambridge, Massachusetts: Bio Dynamics, 1972), p. B-10.

PATIENT'S NAME ____________________

PHYSICIAN'S ENCOUNTER [2 0 2] [4]

IDENT. NO. [| | | |]-[|]

DATE Month [|] Day [|] Year [|]

NAME OF PROVIDER ____________________ NO. [| |] SERVICE LOCATION [ ]

	I. TYPE OF ENCOUNTER *(Check One)*	III.	SERVICES RENDERED DURING ENCOUNTER *(Check One or None of First Three)*	IV.	PRIMARY DIAGNOSIS *(Check Below or Specify)*	V.	SECONDARY DIAGNOSIS
	EPISODIC CARE (INCL. EMERGENCY CARE)		COMPLETE PHYSICAL EXAM (NEW PATIENT OR RE-EXAM)	Code		Code	
	INITIAL HEALTH ASSESSMENT (NEW PATIENT)		EXAMINATION EVALUATION (NEW CONDITION OR SPECIALTY EXAM)			Code	
	LONG-TERM HEALTH CARE MANAGEMENT		FOLLOW-UP CARE *(Incl. continuation of exam.)*		DEFERRED *(Always check if initial Health Assessment incomplete)*	Code	
	ROUTINE AND PREVENTIVE CARE	ALSO CHECK OR SPECIFY AS APPROPRIATE:		NO DISEASE-- *(Check one box below)*		Code	
II.	LENGTH OF ENCOUNTER *(Check one)*		IMMUNIZATION(S)		PRENATAL CARE		RETURN APPOINTMENT REQUIRED? *(Check if "Yes")*
	BRIEF		MEDICATIONS (INCL. INJECTIONS) (EXCLUDE ALLERGY CARE)		POSTPARTUM CARE	When?	With Whom?
	PROLONGED		DIAGNOSTIC TEST(S) (EXCLUDE EKG, REFRACTION OF EYES)		WELL CHILD CARE		
	ROUTINE	Serv. Code	OTHER SERVICES *(Specify)*		WELL ADULT CARE		
					FAMILY PLANNING		LAB WORK—Complete if ordered. 1 = Center 2 = Non-center
					OTHER		Was this a Consultation? *(Check if "Yes")*

Source: *Ambulatory Health Care Information System: Overall System Description.* U. S. DHEW Publication No. (HSM)72-6202, (Cambridge, Massachusetts: Bio Dynamics, 1972) p. B-2.

Patient's Name

Last 6 7

First 8

I.D. No. 9 10 11 12 13 14 15

CENTER NO. | 1 | 0 | 2 | (1 2 3)

FORM NO. | N | 1 | (4 5)

DATE			PHYSICIAN'S NUMBER	SERVICE LOCATION
MONTH	DAY	YEAR		
16	17 18	19	20 21 22	23 24

1. **APPOINTMENT STATUS:** Check one. → 25 1 ○ Appointment 2 ○ Walk-In 3 ○ Direct Referral 4 ○ Other

2. **TYPE OF ENCOUNTER:** Check one. → 26 1 ○ EPISODIC CARE (Including emer. care) 2 ○ LONG-TERM HEALTH CARE MANAGEMENT 3 ○ INITIAL HEALTH ASSESSMENT (new patient) 4 ○ ROUTINE & PREVENTIVE CARE

3. **GENERAL SERVICE RENDERED:** Check one. → 27 1 ○ COMPREHENSIVE PHYSICAL EXAM. (New patient or re-examination) 2 ○ EXAMINATION/EVALUATION (New condition or specialty exam.) 3 ○ FOLLOW-UP CARE (Including continuation of an exam.)

4. **SPECIFIC SERVICE(S) RENDERED:** Check as many as are appropriate. →
   - 28 ○ IMMUNIZATION(S)
   - 29 ○ MEDICATIONS (Including injections - exclude allergy care)
   - 30 ○ DIAGNOSTIC TESTS (i.e., Tire., Pulmonary, PKU-EKG, Refraction of Eyes)
   - CODE 31 32 OTHER SERVICES - (specify and enter code)

5. **LENGTH OF ENCOUNTER:** Check one. → 33 1 ○ Routine 2 ○ Brief 3 ○ Prolonged

6. **DIAGNOSIS:** Check one circle in the box below.

34 - 35

01 ○ DEFERRED

If a disease condition is suspected but not diagnosed at the time of the encounter, check deferred. Also check deferred if a physical exam (including initial health assessment) is in process but not completed. Upon completion of the examination, check the primary condition found for that encounter.

NONE

If no diagnosis, check one of the following circles:

- 02 ○ –PRENATAL CARE
- 03 ○ –POSTPARTUM CARE
- 04 ○ –WELL CHILD CARE
- 05 ○ –WELL ADULT CARE
- 06 ○ –FAMILY PLANNING
- 07 ○ –OTHER

If Diagnosis, check or code **one** of the following:

10 ○ –ALCOHOLISM	18 ○ –HEARING PROBLEMS	26 ○ –OBESITY
11 ○ –ALLERGIC DISORDERS	19 ○ –HEART DISEASES	27 ○ –REFRACTIVE ERRORS
12 ○ –ANEMIA INCLUDING SICKLE CELL	20 ○ –HYPERTENSION	28 ○ –SKIN DISORDERS
13 ○ –ARTHRITIS AND RHEUMATISM	21 ○ –INFLUENZA AND PNEUMONIA	29 ○ –STOMACH ULCERS
14 ○ –ASTHMA	22 ○ –INJURY/ACCIDENT	30 ○ –STREPTOCOCCAL SORE THROAT
15 ○ –COLDS	23 ○ –LEAD POISONING	31 ○ –TEETH AND SUPPORT STRUCTURE DISORDERS
16 ○ –DIABETES	24 ○ –MALIGNANT NEOPLASMS	32 ○ –TUBERCULOSIS
17 ○ –DRUG DEPENDENCE	25 ○ –MENTAL DISORDERS	33 ○ –VENEREAL DISEASES

IF DIAGNOSIS OTHER THAN ABOVE, ENTER CODE HERE (SEE NHSP CODE SHEET) 34 35

7. **SELECTED ITEMS OF SERVICE AT THE CENTER:** Check circles for as many items as are applicable.

A. X-RAYS (ordered)	B. LABORATORY TESTS (ordered)	C. CONTRACEPTIVES	D. PRESCRIPTIONS (issued)
36 ○ –CHEST	42 ○ –HEMATOLOGY	48 ○ –ORAL PILL Rx ISSUED	51 ○ –PRESCRIPTION PHARMACEUTICAL (excluding oral contraceptive Rx)
37 ○ –BARIUM SWALLOW, UPPER G.I., SM. BOWEL SERIES	43 ○ –URINALYSIS	49 ○ –I.U.D. FITTED	
38 ○ –GALL BLADDER	44 ○ –BAC. & PARA.	50 ○ –ALL OTHER	
39 ○ –BARIUM ENEMA	45 ○ –SEROLOGY		52 ○ –Non-Prescription Pharmaceutical
40 ○ –I.V. PYELOGRAM	46 ○ –PAP SMEAR		
41 ○ –OTHER X-RAYS	47 ○ –OTHER LAB TESTS		

8. **EXTERNAL REFERRALS REQUESTED:** Check as many as are applicable.

DIRECT HEALTH SERVICE		INDIRECT HEALTH SERVICE	
53 ○ –HOSPITALIZATION	57 ○ –DENTAL MANAGEMENT	61 ○ –FOOD STAMPS	65 ○ –VOCATIONAL REHABILITATION
54 ○ –MEDICAL CONSULTATION	58 ○ –X-RAY PROCEDURES	62 ○ –EMPLOYMENT	66 ○ –SOCIAL SERVICE
55 ○ –MEDICAL MANAGEMENT	59 ○ –LABORATORY TESTS	63 ○ –WELFARE	67 ○ –HOUSING
56 ○ –DENTAL CONSULTATION	60 ○ –OTHER	64 ○ –MEDICAID/MEDICARE REGISTRATION	68 ○ –OTHER

9. **OTHER PROVIDER:** Enter other provider number only if physician does not see patient during encounter. → PROVIDER NO. 78 79 80

Source: *Ambulatory Health Care Information System: Overall System Description.* U. S. DHEW Publication No. (HSM)72-6202, (Cambridge, Massachusetts: Bio Dynamics, 1972), p. B-3.

PATIENT'S NAME ____________________

CENTER NO. 6 0 1 (1 2 3) FORM NO. N (4)

PATIENT'S IDENTIFICATION NUMBER (5 6 7 8 9 10 11)

DATE: MONTH (12)	DAY (13 14)	YEAR (15)	PHYSICIAN'S NUMBER (16 17 18)	SERVICE LOCATION (19 20)

1. APPOINTMENT STATUS Check one. 21 1 O Appointment 2 O Walk-in 3 O Direct Referral 4 O Other
2. TYPE OF ENCOUNTER: Check only one, the primary nature of care provided during the encounter.
   22 1 O EPISODIC CARE (Including emer. care) 2 O LONG-TERM HEALTH CARE MANAGEMENT 3 O INITIAL HEALTH ASSESSMENT (new patient) 4 O ROUTINE AND PREVENTIVE CARE
3. SERVICES RENDERED DURING ENCOUNTER: Check only one (or none) of these 3 circles.
   23 1 O COMPREHENSIVE PHYSICAL EXAM (New Patient or re-examination) 2 O EXAMINATION/EVALUATION (New condition or specialty exam) 3 O FOLLOW-UP CARE (Including continuation of an exam)

   Check as many as are appropriate below:
   - 24 O IMMUNIZATION(S)
   - 25 O MEDICATIONS (Including injections—exclude allergy care)
   - 26 O DIAGNOSTIC TESTS (i.e., Tire.,Pulmonary, PKU—but exclude EKG EKG, Refraction of Eyes)

   OTHER SERVICES – (specify and intercode): ____________ CODE (27) ____________ CODE (28)
4. LENGTH OF ENCOUNTER: Check only one. 29 1 O Brief 2 O Routine 3 O Prolonged
5. DIAGNOSES: A. List (in order of priority) only those conditions dealt with during *this encounter.*
   B. If a *Physical Exam* is in progress but not completed, check *Deferred.* Upon completion, list the conditions found on the form for the encounter completing the exam.
   C. *Initial Health Assessment* should be checked as the Type of Encounter for each encounter of a new patient's work-up.

I. PRIMARY ____________________ ICDA CODE

Specify or Check Below

- 30-33 XXOO O DEFERRED
- O NONE — CHECK ONE →
- 30-33 XXO1 O PRENATAL CARE
- XXO3 O POSTPARTUM CARE
- XXO5 O WELL CHILD CARE
- 30-33 XXO7 O WELL ADULT CARE
- XXO8 O FAMILY PLANNING
- XXO9 O OTHER

ICDA CODE

II. SECONDARY ____________________ (34 35 36 37)

III. ____________________ (38 39 40 41)

IV. ____________________ (42 43 44 45)

6. SELECTED ITEMS OF SERVICE AT THE CENTER: Check circles for as many items as are applicable.

A. X-RAYS (ordered)	B. LABORATORY TESTS (ordered)	C. CONTRACEPTIVES	D. PRESCRIPTIONS (issued)
46 O –CHEST	52 O –HEMATOLOGY	58 O –ORAL PILL Rx ISSUED	61 O –PRESCRIPTION PHARMACEUTICAL (excluding oral contraceptive Rx)
47 O –BARIUM SWALLOW, UPPER G.I., SM. BOWEL SERIES	53 O –URINALYSIS	59 O –I.U.D. FITTED	62 O –EYE GLASSES
48 O –GALL BLADDER	54 O –BAC. & PARA.	60 O –ALL OTHER	
49 O –BARIUM ENEMA	55 O –SEROLOGY		
50 O –I.V. PYELOGRAM	56 O –PAP SMEAR		
51 O –OTHER X-RAYS	57 O –OTHER LAB TESTS		

7. EXTERNAL REFERRALS REQUESTED: Check as many as are applicable.

DIRECT HEALTH SERVICE		INDIRECT HEALTH SERVICE	
63 O –HOSPITALIZATION	67 O –DENTAL MANAGEMENT	71 O –FOOD STAMPS	75 O –VOCATIONAL REHABILITATION
64 O –MEDICAL CONSULTATION	68 O –X-RAY PROCEDURES	72 O –EMPLOYMENT	76 O –SOCIAL SERVICE
65 O –MEDICAL MANAGEMENT	69 O –LABORATORY TESTS	73 O –WELFARE	77 O –OTHER
66 O –DENTAL CONSULTATION	70 O –OTHER	74 O –MEDICAID/MEDICARE REGISTRATION	

8. OTHER PROVIDER: Enter other provider number only if physician does not see patient during encounter. → PROVIDER NO. (78 79 80)

Source: *Ambulatory Health Care Information System: Overall System Description.* U. S. DHEW Publication No. (HSM)72-6202, (Cambridge, Massachusetts: Bio Dynamics, 1972), p. B-5.

Family Registration Form
Name of Comprehensive Health Center
(City, State)

1	2	3	4
Center No.			Form No. [1]

FAMILY REGISTRATION FORM
Page 1 of 2

FAMILY IDENTIFICATION NUMBER: → 5 6 7 8 9

REGISTRATION DATE: (Month - Day - Year) → 10 11 12 13

1. NAME OF HEAD OF FAMILY: 14 15 16 17 18 19 20 21 22 23 24 25 26 27 28 29 30 31 32 33 34 35
Last (one blank space) First — M.I.

2. DATE OF BIRTH OF HEAD OF FAMILY: (month - day - year) → 36 37 38 39 40

3. SEX OF HEAD OF FAMILY: 1 = Male 2 = Female → 41

4. PRESENT ADDRESS ________ PHONE ________

CHANGE OF ADDRESS: ________ PHONE ________

LENGTH OF RESIDENCE AT PRESENT ADDRESS: (years - months) → 42 43 44 45

LENGTH OF RESIDENCE IN NEIGHBORHOOD: (years - months) → 46 47 48 49

5. NUMBER OF ROOMS IN HOME: → 50
Enter tne number of rooms. (Use 9 for nine or more rooms)

6. CENSUS TRACT NUMBER: → 51 52

In Target Area: 1 = Yes 2 = No → 53

7. LIST ALL FAMILY MEMBERS (If surname differs from that of head, indicate)
AND ASSIGN A NUMBER TO EACH MEMBER:

NAME, AGE, SEX	Relation to Head	Family member number	Date member registered
1. Head:	X	01	
2. Spouse:	X	02	
3.			
4.			
5.			
6.			
7.			
8.			
9.			
10.			

8. TOTAL NUMBER OF FAMILY MEMBERS (as listed above): → 54 55

9. TOTAL NUMBER OF OTHER INDIVIDUALS IN HOUSEHOLD: → 56 57

10. ACCESS TO CENTER: → 58
1 = Walk 2 = Bus 3 = Private Auto 4 = Taxi 5 = Center Provided
Average Time Required (Minutes) → 59 60

(Reverse side of this family registration form is shown on the following page.)

Family Registration Form
Name of Comprehensive Health Center
(City, State)

FAMILY REGISTRATION FORM – page 2 of 2 FAMILY IDENTIFICATION NUMBER ______________

11. SPECIAL REQUIREMENTS: 1 = Yes 2 = No

Physical Assistance Required (Name of Family Member______________) → [ ] 61

Other (specify) → [ ] 62

12. PRIMARY REFERRAL SOURCE: → [ ] 63

1 = Self	6 = Private M.D. or Dentist
2 = Neighbor, Relative	7 = School
3 = Community Health Program Staff	8 = Hospital
4 = Community Action Agency	9 = Other (specify): ______________
5 = Health, Welfare, or Social Agency	

13. FAMILY INCOME CODE: → [ ][ ] 64 65

14. FAMILY RECEIVING WELFARE PAYMENTS: 1 = Yes 2 = No → [ ] 66

15. CERTIFICATION:

I certify that the above information is correct to the best of my knowledge.

____
Signature of Head (or Spouse)

16. PERIODIC RE-CENSUS AND RECERTIFICATION OF REGISTRANTS:

End of Period	Signature of Head (or Spouse)	Date
1.	______________	________
2.	______________	________
3.	______________	________
4.	______________	________
5.	______________	________

17. TEAM NUMBER OF FAMILY TEAM ASSIGNED: → [ ][ ] 67 68

Source: *Ambulatory Health Care Information System: Overall System Description.* U. S. DHEW Publication No. (HSM)72-6202, (Cambridge, Massachusetts: Bio Dynamics, 1972), pp. 2-6 and 2-7.

Individual Registration Form

Name of Comprehensive Health Center

(City, State)

[ ][ ][ ]-[2] — 1 2 3 Center No. — 4 Form No.

INDIVIDUAL REGISTRATION FORM
page 1 of 2

PATIENT'S IDENTIFICATION NUMBER: → 5 6 7 8 9 Family No. — 10 11 Family Member No.

REGISTRATION DATE: (Month – Day – Year) → 12 — 13

1. PATIENT'S NAME: 14 15 16 17 18 19 20 21 22 23 24 25 26 27 28 29 30 31 32 33 — 34 M.I.
   Last (one blank space) First

2. SEX: 1 = Male 2 = Female → 35

3. DATE OF BIRTH: (month – day – year) → 36 37 38 39 40

4. MARITAL STATUS: → 41
   1 = Never Married 2 = Now Married 3 = Divorced 4 = Widowed 5 = Separated

5. RACE: → 42
   1 = Black 2 = White 3 = Oriental 4 = American Indian 5 = Other

6. ETHNIC GROUP: → 43
   1 = Puerto Rican 2 = Mexican American 3 = Other Spanish Speaking 4 = Other

7. EMPLOYMENT STATUS: (Select the one which most closely describes the individual's current major activity) → 44
   1 = Going to School or Pre-School
   2 = Keeping House
   3 = Working, Full-Time (35 hrs. or more)
   4 = Working, Part-Time
   5 = Unemployed (but not disabled or retired)
   6 = Disabled
   7 = Retired

   USUAL OCCUPATION: __________

   EMPLOYER OR SCHOOL: __________

   LENGTH OF TIME EMPLOYED: __________

8. EDUCATION: Presently Enrolled in School: 1 = Yes 2 = No → 45
   Highest Grade Completed: → 46 47
   Any Special Class? (If yes, specify) __________

9. LENGTH OF TIME SINCE LAST ENCOUNTER WITH MEDICAL DOCTOR: → 48
   0 = never
   1 = less than 6 months
   2 = 6 months to 11 months
   3 = 1 year to 2 years
   4 = more than 2 years to 5 years
   5 = more than 5 years

10. NUMBER OF ENCOUNTERS WITH A MEDICAL DOCTOR DURING THE PAST YEAR: (Enter the number of encounters. Use 0 for none and 9 for nine or more). Exclude hospital encounters with medical doctors. → 49

(Reverse side of this individual registration form is shown in the following page.)

Individual Registration Form

Name of Comprehensive Health Center

(City, State)

INDIVIDUAL REGISTRATION FORM – page 2 of 2 PATIENT'S IDENTIFICATION NUMBER ______________

11. MEDICAL PAYMENT STATUS:

Status Code	Payment Source(s)	Coverage		Remarks	Check (✓) the Primary Payment Source
		Yes	No		
1.	Medicare, Part B				
2.	Title XIX				
3.	Public Assistance				
4.	Private Insurance				
5.	Cash Payment				
6.	None—PHS Pays Cost				
7.	Other (specify)				

	Status Code (from above)	Coverage No.													
Primary Payment Source	50	51	52	53	54	55	56	57	58	59	60	61	62	63	64
Other Payment Source (if any)	65	66	67	68	69	70	71	72	73	74	75	76	77	78	79

12. AUTHORIZATION FOR MEDICAL CARE:

(Each center will use the appropriate legal wording for its state)

DATE______________ 19 ____

______________ AUTHORIZED SIGNATURE

WITNESSED BY:

______________ INTERVIEWER

______________ RELATIONSHIP TO PATIENT

13. PERSON TO BE CONTACTED IN CASE OF EMERGENCY:

Name ______________ Phone ______________

Address ______________

14. PHYSICIAN NUMBER OF PHYSICIAN ASSIGNED: ——→ | | | |

Source: *Ambulatory Health Care Information System: Overall System Description.* U. S. DHEW Publication No. (HSM)72-6202, (Cambridge, Massachusetts: Bio Dynamics, 1972), pp. 2-9 and 2-10.

Health Services Encounter Form

NAME OF COMPREHENSIVE HEALTH CENTER
(City, State)

CENTER NO. (1 2 3) FORM NO. Y 1 (4 5)

PATIENT'S NAME
LAST (6 7)
FIRST (8)
I.D. NO. (9 10 11 12 13 14 15)

2. DATE: MONTH (16) DAY (17 18) YEAR (19)

3. SITE OF ENCOUNTER: (20)
1 = CENTER 2 = HOME 3 = HOSPITAL 4 = OTHER (specify) ______

4. APPOINTMENT STATUS: (21)
1 = APPOINTMENT 2 = WALK-IN 3 = DIRECT REFERRAL 4 = OTHER (specify) ______ 5 = MISSED APPOINTMENT

5. HEALTH CARE PROVIDER: (22 23)

01 = PHYSICIAN–GENERAL
06 = PHYSICIAN–ADULT
11 = PHYSICIAN–CHILD
16 = OBSTETRICIAN/GYNECOLOGIST
21 = PSYCHIATRIST
24 = OTHER PHYSICIAN SPECIALIST
30 = DENTIST–GENERAL
33 = DENTIST–SPECIALIST
41 = PSYCHOLOGIST
44 = OPTOMETRIST
46 = PODIATRIST
48 = OTHER INDEPENDENT PROFESSIONAL PROVIDER
56 = NURSE
66 = DENTAL HYGIENIST
68 = SOCIAL WORKER
74 = OTHER PROFESSIONAL AND FORMALLY TRAINED TECHNICAL PROVIDER
81 = HEALTH AIDE
86 = FAMILY HEALTH WORKER
91 = OTHER NON-PROFESSIONAL PROVIDER

PROVIDER I.D. (see instructions) (24)

6. TYPE OF ENCOUNTER: (25 26)

Medical Care
01 = EPISODIC (INCLUDING EMERGENCY)
02 = INITIAL HEALTH ASSESSMENT IN PROCESS
03 = INITIAL HEALTH ASSESSMENT COMPLETED

Preventive Care
04 = PRENATAL
05 = POSTPARTUM
06 = WELL-BABY
07 = IMMUNIZATIONS ONLY
08 = OTHER PREVENTIVE CARE (specify) ______
09 = MENTAL HEALTH CARE
10 = FAMILY PLANNING
11 = LONG-TERM CARE MANAGEMENT
12 = OTHER MEDICAL CARE (specify) ______

Dental Care
21 = INITIAL ASSESSMENT
22 = PREVENTIVE
23 = RESTORATIVE
24 = OTHER DENTAL CARE (specify) ______

Social Service
31 = INITIAL SOCIAL ASSESSMENT
32 = FOLLOW-UP SOCIAL SERVICE
33 = OTHER SOCIAL SERVICE CARE (specify) ______

40 = ALL OTHER CARE (specify) ______

7. SELECTED ITEMS OF SERVICE AT THE CENTER: **Check circles for as many items as are applicable and enter numbers as appropriate for items 46 and 47.**

A. X-RAYS (ordered)	B. LABORATORY TESTS (ordered)	C. CONTRACEPTIVES	D. DENTISTRY	E. PRESCRIPTIONS (issued)
27 ○ CHEST	33 ○ HEMATOLOGY	41 ○ ORAL PILL Rx ISSUED	44 ○ DENTAL X-RAYS	49 ○ PRESCRIPTION PHARMACEUTICAL (excluding oral contraceptive Rx)
28 ○ BARIUM SWALLOW, UPPER G.I., SM. BOWEL SERIES	34 ○ BLOOD CHEMISTRY	42 ○ I.U.D. FITTED	45 ○ PROPHYLAXES	50 ○ NON-PRESCRIPTION PHARMACEUTICAL
29 ○ GALL BLADDER	35 ○ URINALYSIS	43 ○ ALL OTHER	46 □ EXTR. (NO. TEETH)	
30 ○ BARIUM ENEMA	36 ○ BAC. & PARA.		47 □ FILLINGS (NO. SURF.)	
31 ○ I.V. PYELOGRAM	37 ○ SEROLOGY		48 ○ DENTAL CASE COMPLETED	
32 ○ OTHER X-RAYS	38 ○ PAP SMEAR			
	39 ○ EKG			
	40 ○ OTHER LAB TESTS			

8. EXTERNAL REFERRALS REQUESTED: **Check as many as are applicable.**

A. DIRECT HEALTH SERVICE		B. INDIRECT HEALTH SERVICE	
51 ○ HOSPITALIZATION	55 ○ DENTAL MANAGEMENT	59 ○ FOOD STAMPS	63 ○ VOCATIONAL REHABILITATION
52 ○ MEDICAL CONSULTATION	56 ○ X-RAY PROCEDURES	60 ○ EMPLOYMENT	64 ○ SOCIAL SERVICE
53 ○ MEDICAL MANAGEMENT	57 ○ LABORATORY TEST	61 ○ WELFARE	65 ○ OTHER
54 ○ DENTAL CONSULTATION	58 ○ OTHER	62 ○ MEDICAID/MEDICARE REGISTRATION	

SPECIAL STUDIES (see instructions)
STUDY NO. (66 67)
STUDY DATA (68 69 60 71)

Source: *Ambulatory Health Care Information System: Overall System Description.* U. S. DHEW Publication No. (HSM)72-6202, (Cambridge, Massachusetts: Bio Dynamics, 1972), p. 2-12.

Part IV

Facility Design, Construction, and Financing

Chapter 20

Long-Range Planning

THE MASTER PLAN

Health care agencies increasingly are advocating that adequate planning be instigated to respond not only to future governmental regulations, community growth, facility expansion, and changes in zoning, but also to many social, economic, and political needs. For medical groups that have been in existence for some time and wish to improve inadequate quarters as well as for the group that wishes to build a new facility, the importance of a comprehensive master plan cannot be overestimated. A master plan embodies the synthesis of various goals and objectives within a specified concrete approach to the anticipation of change. In the context of a building program the goal of any such plan is to provide a site and physical plant which will adequately serve both present and future demands, while at the same time remaining flexible in the face of rapid change. Fluctuations in interest rates and building codes as well as rising construction costs can contribute to problems in projections for future growth. Deciding upon how to save money on construction costs may be replaced by a reexamination of whether a new facility is necessary and what servcies are to be provided. A master plan serves the function of simplifying decision-making by providing a narrative of projected activities and conceptual plans. It usually is very general and reflects a number of basic influences such as the medical community and the patient community as well as typical requirements for medical space, ancillaries, other general support areas, and parking.

Some group practice administrators claim that they do only what is immediately necessary and obvious in terms of planning. Indeed, with a field that is changing as rapidly as that of medicine, a prediction of future needs may be difficult. The development of a master plan and a method for its continuous evaluation and updating throughout a group's existence may be the activity most important to a medical group's viability. The more flexible yet thorough a master plan, the more likelihood that the group will be able to anticipate changes brought about by expanded services and increased staff. In fact, the plan itself may stimulate innovation and produce changes.

Reasons for Master Planning

The advantages of a master plan make it a virtual necessity for every group. Social and technological change within the health care field can be accommodated more effectively by groups who have planned for staged development of their medical programs and facilities. A successfully master planned facility precludes the need for extensive programs to identify and evaluate potential alternatives in future remodeling and expansion. The initial design of a group practice facility, therefore, should incorporate a reasonable plan for future expansion, which includes allocation of space as well as provision for the expansion of mechanical, electrical, and plumbing systems.

Allowing for the purchase of sufficient land is a major purpose of the master plan. Future expansion within an existing center may take place either horizontally or vertically. A commonly held opinion is that horizontal expansion is easier and less costly, but this is not always true. The alternatives must be carefully weighed, considering future operating costs as well as initial capital outlay. It is obvious that horizontal expansion requires additional land, and even if expansion does take place in a vertical direction, with no more land taken up by the building itself, parking facilities must be expanded. A multilevel parking facility is one alternative to grade level parking but can be very expensive; therefore, the cost of a parking structure must be considered in light of the corresponding cost of land. While bearing in mind that a parking structure is expensive, it may be the only feasible option under conditions such as extremely high land cost or unavailability of adjacent land. It is probably more advantageous to locate on a site larger than the group thinks necessary and to consider selling any excess land in the future; land adjacent to a successful center may later become very expensive to acquire and, conversely, very profitable to sell.

A master plan for long-range expansion constitutes insurance for the future. Ideally, each successive building program is an intermediate step toward an ultimate goal, involving minimal interruption to the medical practice. It may cost very little to provide for expansion potential during initial construction. One existing clinic spent $1,200 to install the caissons for future horizontal expansion. These caissons are now buried, but they will lower greatly the cost of any future expansion. It is presently estimated that it would cost $2,500 just to bring in the equipment for this operation. The $1,200 expense to accommodate future expansion constituted a very small amount in a building program that had an overall budget of $350,000. Projecting the medical needs and practices of the future can be based on forecasting changes in the community. If the area or the characteristics of the population change, revisions in plans for both the medical services and the business operations of the group practice may be necessary. Those individuals involved in master planning should consider such possibilities and may even be instrumental in determining future medical practices. Long-range plans perhaps should include the expanded use of computers, the introduction of surgicenters which are acceptable for third party payment, and increased cooperation and coordination with local hospitals and other health facilities.

Of increasing concern to health care planners in the future will be the part played by federal and state governments in the delivery of medical services. Whether this involvement is found in the development of programs such as health maintenance organizations or in the peripheral field of finance, master planning may be especially important to meet the government's requirements. Many states already have considered legislation dealing with the certification of need for health care facilities. Simply stated, this means that the granting of state licenses or governmental reimbursement may be dependent upon an evaluation of the need for a particular facility in light of other existing facilities. Without an adequate master plan, the inability to predict these needs may make future expansion difficult if not impossible.

Components of the Master Plan

When long-range plans are formulated one of the first factors to be considered is the length of time covered by the master plan. Variables which influence the choice of time segments generally are the type and size of the community in which the practice is located and the projected growth patterns of the area. A forecast of community growth may be obtained from the Chamber of Commerce, from the local government, or from utility companies who have completed studies to facilitate their own future planning. One clinic, located in a suburb of Chicago, has expanded in just ten years from six physicians in a two-story building to thirty-eight physicians in a four-story building. During the past year alone, the group has hired nine new physicians. Plans for a four-story addition to house still another twenty-five to thirty physicians are now in the initial stage and scheduled for completion during the next year. Another clinic, located in rural Kentucky, was founded in 1953 by five physicians. It now has fifty-eight physicians. The clinic has a long-range planning committee that studies short-range needs and helps to direct current recruiting activities. The committee can project to three years and then to five years; they even "dream" to ten years. Obviously, in rural Kentucky a ten-year "dream" may be adequate, while in metropolitan Chicago a ten-year detailed plan may be necessary.

While it is often difficult to predict how much expansion may be needed, an educated estimate based on reasonable projections is probably the best place to start. A group might look at its history as a source for such projections. Present programs and facilities should be evaluated and justifications presented for projected changes in services. Planning should progress with a concern for compatibility between new systems and existing ones and for operational efficiency of these combined systems. In addition, master plan assumptions need to be reevaluated continually. Communicating with comprehensive health care planners could contribute to this endeavor. Few groups feel that they have really overplanned. The majority will probably agree that, somewhere in the past, they have in fact grossly underplanned.

Once the time limit covered by the plan has been ascertained, a number of strategic decisions related to the projection of future demands for services can be made. Professional help is available from medical consultants and architectural firms, particularly those with experience in medical group facilities, who may have procedures or questionnaires designed to aid in the development of a master plan. Change in demand is affected by the composition of the existing medical community as well as by the characteristics of the community as a whole. Long-range planning for a medical group located in a small community without a hospital, medical school, medical library, or specialist consultation services poses a set of problems different from long-range planning for a group with access to these facilities. It should be determined by the group whether the community is overstaffed by physicians or whether there is a need for additional physicians. The feasibility of sharing facilities and services with other institutions should be evaluated, as should the possibility of mergers and affiliations. The composition of the community from which the patients will come also is important to the development of the master plan and can be estimated by considering the following trends: What is the patient load in relation to the total population? What is the prospect or direction of population growth? Is the age average of the community population increasing, decreasing, or remaining constant? Is the community an industrial, a residential, or an agricultural area? How many physicians should be in the group initially and how many physicians may be in the group ultimately? What are the factors determining the addition of a new physician and what are the space requirements?

Prior to developing space allocation programs and architectural feasibility studies, the group needs to review and agree upon the basic concepts of the practice of medicine within the group setting. It may be unwise for physicians to engage in a building program before they have had a chance to develop their practices and thereby estimate just what their future needs might be. After forecasting the growth of the community, physicians must decide if they will set a limit on the growth of the group, or if they will accept new physicians to meet the expanding needs of the community. Such planning can be facilitated by initiating a monthly analysis of each physician's patient load which will indicate not only which physicians are able to accept new patients and which are not, but also which departments need additional staff so that new patients can be accepted. Within its area of influence, which generally increases with success, the group must decide how many medical specialties it will support. In this respect, it should be remembered that if one doctor is brought into the group in a specialty not previously covered, the group can plan to add eventually at least one more doctor in that same specialty. The addition of one doctor per year for ten years by an average-sized group represents substantial growth. The formulation of a growth policy emerging from decisions made early in the life of the practice is important to future generations of the group. Members also must consider the terms of physician withdrawal from the group; that is, both the conditions under which a physician may choose to leave and the conditions under which a physician may be asked to leave. If physicians leave during a building program, any plans previously made may have to be reformulated.

Should the group later decide to modify its growth policy it may find that expanding or remodeling an existing building can be an expensive endeavor if the original design plan did not incorporate a master plan for expansion. The original building should be designed to accommodate the current staff plus a reasonable staff addition. The inclusion of a basement, large storage spaces, or facilities that can be rented until expansion of the group is necessary, can provide a means for future expansion. Another alternative is to incorporate shell space or undeveloped space in the initial building design and construction. Later, when the group practice has grown and added more physicians, suites can be designed and built to fill the undeveloped space. Some building industries specialize in the production of efficiently designed modular units. These units can be assembled into facilities that fit the group's present needs with the provision that additional units can be incorporated should future space requirements make expansion necessary. A building adequately planned for expansion may be more marketable and more adaptable for other uses. The impact that construction may have on the operation of the facility must also be considered. In a facility that is planned for expansion, the clinic should be able to operate effectively during the expansion process.

In order for the building to serve its proper function, it must be designed to meet the needs of the individual patients, the physicians, and the clinic personnel. For this reason, physicians also must determine just how group-oriented they are. For the purpose of discussion, consider three hypothetical classifications for groups. The first group is highly individualistic. The space set aside for each physician is highly personalized, specially designed, and self-contained. Generally, patients of this group have a preference for a particular physician. While this type of medical practice often is thought of as individualistic, the physicians do share common ancillaries and business office management in a group practice setting. The second category for physician groups involves a unified team-type approach to medical practice. These physicians practice in a multiphysician medical corridor or suite, and share personnel, common waiting areas, and examination/consultation rooms. They may use private offices or have their offices in an examination/consultation room. Patients often are considered to be the patients of the group rather than of a single physician. Again, these physicians share common ancillaries and management. The third category of physician group is the mechanized, almost futuristic medical practice which is highly organized, automated, and computerized, in order to serve a large number of patients. Compared to the first two types of practice, this group type may be relatively impersonal. Nevertheless, it represents a potentially efficient means of providing a large number of patients with quality medicine at a minimum cost. It may well be that no one of these classifications is really superior, yet these three alternatives should illustrate that physicians considering forming a group must fully contemplate their philosophy of group practice. They must attempt to develop a medical practice within a physical setting that will permit rational growth, utilize modern technology, increase efficiency and accuracy, and allow for the desired individuality of both patients and medical staff.

The designing or redesigning of facilities should be preceded by planning or analyzing the practice itself: patient flow, utilization of personnel, and effective management of the physicians' time, activities, and tasks. In order for the clinic to react to unscheduled patients on an emergency or short-notice basis, it may be necessary to provide space for physicians who will have something less than a full practice. The requirements of all operating systems, such as the medical records system and the appointments system (see Part III), should be analyzed and documented prior to engaging an architect or design team. The professional then will be able to suggest ways in which a building can be designed to accommodate these systems. A logistical analysis describing how all supplies are received, processed, distributed, used, collected, and disposed of will also influence the final design. By studying the traffic patterns of nonambulatory patients, outpatients, emergency patients, visitors, doctors, nurses, technicians, and staff, the designer can plan the most efficient means of routing both people and paper throughout the building. A systems analysis of the process by which registration, appointments, and billing and insurance collections are accomplished also may be productive.

In general programming, architects assign space in terms of requirements per group physician; therefore, plans for number of physicians and types of specialities to be included are important in determining gross square footage estimates, which usually vary from 1,000 to 1,200 square feet per physician for an operational plan of one shift per day. Of this 1,000 to 1,200 square feet, examination room space may constitute only one-quarter or less; the gross footage figure includes the examination/consultation rooms, as well as physician offices, business offices, waiting rooms, corridors, expandable mechanical space, electrical equipment room space, stairways and elevators in multistory buildings, pharmacies, labs, X-ray rooms, physicians' and employees' lounges, exterior walls and interior partitions—everything necessary for a group practice facility. Single-speciality space and special support areas in multispecialty groups usually are programmed and planned for very special functions. These areas may be more efficient in terms of square foot space utilization than many areas of multispecialty group practice facilities, in which space must be planned for flexibility and typical rooms must be adaptable to the needs of different specialists. Regardless of group type, however, increasing use of paramedical personnel, the introduction of sophisticated equipment, the additional requirements for administrative personnel, and more pleasant working and patient areas have resulted in a general increase in the total space requirements for a medical group practice.

As a part of the master plan a feasibility study should be conducted which will evaluate the various options available to a group. Such a study includes a statement of the advantages and disadvantages of remodeling, expanding, renting or leasing facilities, or constructing a new facility. Also inherent in the general feasibility of the project are the financial commitments necessary to complete and maintain the planned facility, and the ownership options which the group should consider.

Evaluation of Present Building or Space

The various needs of the group and the preliminary program which evolves from discussion of these needs may determine conclusively what the expansion program should contain. If not, variables such as building costs, financing, and utilization of property may become determining factors. A newly formed group either may buy or rent an existing building, construct a new one, or rent space within a building. An existing group must look at the facilities that it now uses and the financial arrangements that are in effect. This is as true of an already existing group occupying a building as it is of a physician who presently is in private practice, owns a facility, and is considering group practice. The space may be owned, leased, rented month-to-month, or occupied under some other arrangement. If the existing building has not been master planned for expansion, it may be that a group has no choice but to acquire a new facility. The group must consider when it will be free to relocate, whether the present building can be sold if the group decides to build elsewhere, and the value of the property in relation to funds required for a new facility. The present land and building may be a better investment than purchasing another site.

Local real estate firms usually can supply an analysis of the buyers' market value of an existing building. There are, however, serious financial implications involved in selling a single-purpose medical building. Remodeling a former clinic for another use is often extremely costly when compared to the potential dollar return. Nonmedical persons seeking space for their profession may find it more economical to buy or rent a general office building. It may be difficult, therefore, to sell the building profitably. Zoning restrictions at the present site also must be considered. A group that is leasing or renting should determine whether an option can be obtained to buy the property or whether arrangements can be made with the present owner to construct a building without restrictions. The cost of new construction versus a new addition should be weighed carefully.

Alternatives to New Construction

An alternative that may be of particular interest to new groups is that of renting medical office space, and an already existing group may consider renting space as a means of developing a satellite facility. The site should be selected with the greatest possible care, and studies should be conducted to determine population densities, proximity of other medical buildings, means of transportation, traffic flow and congestion, and adequacy of parking. Since there may be other physicians in the building, an analysis of their specialties and services also should be conducted. One major problem involved in renting space is that the group's desire to expand may be thwarted by conditions entirely beyond its control. For example, other physicians in the building may not be willing to relinquish space for the expansion of a competing medical group. Even if an entire building is rented by a single group, it might be difficult to require that the building landlord expand the facilities for the sole purpose of meeting a particular group's needs. Ownership, therefore, carries with it the prerogative of control in adapting the existing quarters to projected needs. On the other hand, renting space for the new group practice removes the elements of risk and loss which can result from a potentially ill-conceived investment in an owned facility.

Another factor to be studied is whether an existing building can be sufficiently remodeled at a cost as reasonable or more reasonable than the cost of a new building. Personnel salaries will continue to represent a large portion of group practice overhead. Inefficient or poorly designed space may have to be staffed too heavily to be financially feasible over the long term. In addition, due to the constraints of construction-code restrictions currently in effect, remodeling can present some unique problems. Present building codes and requirements may be difficult to adhere to in a building constructed under earlier and now outdated codes and requirements. In addition, extensive remodeling may cost more per square foot than new building space because new facilities and equipment often require different spatial arrangements. Remodeling also may be greatly disruptive to the operation of the clinic.

Thus, if expansion is not considered during the master planning period, it may become extremely difficult to expand a facility without extensive and costly remodeling which may in turn produce inefficiency in operation. Some limited expansion may take place internally in space originally used for storage, or medical space that was rented out to physicians not associated with the group. If expansion does take place, care should be taken that any addition is compatible with the existing structure. For example, one existing group contemplating expansion kept a record of the name of the brick yard that had manufactured brick previously used in the facility's construction. They knew the mixture by number and procured samples to ensure that an addition to the building would match exactly the original portion of the structure. Care also should be taken that drawings for any addition be as detailed as were those for the original building. These aspects of the project can be coordinated with the architect in charge.

Finally, under some circumstances, building a new facility will emerge as the only alternative. A group may have a good building which is at maximum utilization and was not master planned for future expansion. Adjacent property may be very high in price. If alternate and adequately sized sites are available, a new building designed to meet the particular and special needs of a specific group may be more efficient not only in cost, but also in the utilization of personnel within the facility. It is important to consider the relative cost of a new building in comparison with other available options. Remodeling may be expensive because new facilities must be constructed while old facilities are removed. Renting available medical space may appear inexpensive initially, but the overall costs during the entire life-cycle of the group also must be considered.

Disadvantages to New Construction

There are some inherent problems in any building program, especially in a new building program. Problems of cost overruns, time delays, etc., can affect adversely both the physicians personally and their practice of medicine. While in a new or larger building, operating costs may increase, maintenance costs may be considerably less; however, unless the capacity of the existing staff is increased or the staff itself increases, earnings may decrease. In addition, an appreciable cost increase may have an adverse effect on the group's recruiting capabilities. These problems may be viewed differently by various members of the group. Younger physicians, with their entire careers ahead of them, may not look negatively upon high initial costs; however, older members of the group may not want to involve themselves in a building program.

The clinic administrator may become deeply involved in the building program, but he must coordinate this activity with his other administrative functions. The same is true of all other personnel, unless they have been delegated the responsibility to concern themselves primarily with the building program while others substitute for them and assume operational responsibilities. In order for patients to adjust adequately to a potential change in the group practice operation, they should be made aware of any new building program. This should be done even if it is a new building on a new site, because patients will consider the new facility to be "their" clinic. Advance notice assumes even greater importance if the program is the expansion or remodeling of an existing facility, because inconvenience to the patient may result.

Advantages to New Construction

While there are many disadvantages to a building program, there are many, often overriding, advantages in the construction of a new facility. A new facility designed to meet specific needs of the group will be much more effective in providing medical services because the gross area of a totally new facility, while usually smaller, is inherently more efficient than the expanded and remodeled building. Because most facilities are constructed to accommodate more capabilities with increased efficiency, it is only natural that a new facility should be expected to serve a greater number of patients. In general, the construction of a new facility will result in an increase in the group's patient load capacity. This may be due either to the potential for greater productivity of the present staff, or to the addition of physicians and staff personnel in the new facility. Personnel can receive a great deal of personal satisfaction and psychological motivation from working in a new facility, particularly if they have shared in some of the original design decisions.

The construction of a new facility may increase the operating costs of a group, but the long-term financial outcome should reflect a savings. A facility that is owned by the physicians and rented back by the group is usually less expensive than one rented from a third party. This procedure allows the savings of ownership to flow back to the group rather than to a landlord. The investment opportunities inherent in the ownership of a new medical facility also should be considered. A medical group in Minnesota, having established a separate corporation for building ownership, is renting space from the corporate organization for $7 per square foot. The cost of this rental space includes the taxes, utilities, and maintenance of the building. The same medical group also is renting space for a satellite clinic at a minimum rate that is now $9 per square foot on the commercial market. It can be assumed that this $9 rate will increase in keeping with the entire rental market of the area. While it is also true that the $7 rate may rise in the future, it will not rise as quickly as commercial market rates. In addition, there are tax advantages involved in ownership, whether by a partnership or corporation.

A new building also will have an effect on the group's ability to recruit new members. An aesthetically attractive building may appear very impressive to a physician contemplating membership in the group. A potential group member also may be attracted by the investment opportunities offered by ownership of a new building. If situated in relation to the entire medical community, the facility should better serve the overall medical needs of the area. As more patients are served, the health of the entire community can be upgraded. The group should consider the public relations impact of an attractive new building. An effectively designed building may offer the group an opportunity to give its patients more private, personal, and individualized attention. At the dedication ceremonies for a new clinic in the state of Washington, the local mayor reported that improvements initiated by the group resulted in a general "sprucing up" of the area, including the installation of curbs and gutters. He said that the city felt the clinic to be a great asset. One of the physicians of the group commented that the attractiveness of the medical clinic can make a patient feel good even before medical treatment is administered.

Finally, a group of physicians may consider a new building after observing colleagues from the medical community in new facilities. The excitement and interest generated by a new building program may be psychologically rewarding. Because a successful building program depends upon the eventual satisfaction of the owners, the ideas, attitudes, and feelings of all physicians involved should be considered.

THE FEASIBILITY STUDY

After the group has made a preliminary decision to embark upon a building program, it may be expedient to conduct a feasibility study to consider the many alternatives open to it. It should be emphasized that a feasibility study is not the same as a master plan. The master plan is a *solution* adopted by the group to meet its particular needs. It involves a great deal of future planning. A feasibility study is a *study of alternatives* that may lead to a solution for a specific building program. A feasibility study may consider the many options that were master planned into an existing structure years earlier and will take into account building and zoning codes currently in effect.

Reasons for a Feasibility Study

Depending upon the particular needs of a group, it is possible that a detailed feasibility study may be unnecessary. The conditions under which a feasibility study may not be needed fall into three categories:

1. A new group which *must* have a new facility
2. An existing group which finds that, for a number of reasons, expansion on the existing site is obviously impossible or impractical
3. An existing group which has either a facility already master planned for expansion, or a facility with obvious and reasonable expansion potential.

Although the preceding conditions may make a detailed feasibility study unwarranted, groups which must consider a new site may wish to consider some of the available options. A typical situation in which an architectural feasibility study may be in order is as follows:

1. A well-established, balanced, twenty-physician, multispecialty group is presently housed in a good building which is being utilized to its full capacity.

The facility was not master planned for future growth and has no inherent expansion potential.

2. Adjacent property is available but is expensive and may or may not satisfy the expansion requirements; however, alternate sites of adequate size are available.
3. The short-term goals and objectives of the group include balanced addition of twelve physicians in specific specialties and appropriate expansion of the support facilities. This addition will increase the size of the group to thirty-two physicians in the next six years. It is possible to develop a program of space requirements for the first construction phase, whether it is an addition and remodeling of the existing facility or an entirely new building project.
4. The long-range goals and objectives are such that the group must continue to grow in response to the needs of the community. The maximum size of the group is anticipated at approximately seventy-five physicians in balanced composition of medical and surgical specialties and subspecialties. Most of the present physicians feel that they themselves will not see the group grow to such a size and several question whether in fact it should. It is agreed, however, that the master plan should not limit the expansion to less than seventy-five.

More than one type of feasibility study may be necessary prior to making the decision to begin a specific building program. Based on a demographic and statistical analysis of the needs of the patients served, it must be determined whether the goals and objectives of the group are feasible. The following questions need to be considered: Can the goals and objectives be achieved architecturally by expanding the existing facility or must a totally new base be initiated? Which alternative is more feasible economically? Finally, in light of the anticipated income of the group, and based on the cost estimates developed in the architectural feasibility study, is the proposed project financially feasible?

One major advantage of a feasibility study is that it offers the opportunity to predict and possibly reduce costs of a building program. With several options available, the group should be able to establish both which option will offer the lowest initial costs and which options may result in lower life-cycle costs. In addition, the group may find that in order to be eligible for government approval or government financing, a feasibility study of the alternatives is required.

The architectural feasibility study is, in part, a graphic representation in schematic form of the short- and long-range program. The study should include various alternatives for each site under consideration as well as alternatives for remodeling and expanding an old facility. For each site alternative, preliminary cost estimates, including figures for land acquisition, new construction, demolition, required parking, architects' fees, and financing costs, usually are developed. These systematic plans describe total areas with basic circulation, and relationships of the immediate and ultimate additions. Inpatient facilities are included if they constitute a part of the program. Proposed locations and basic layouts of new areas and remodeled existing areas for phase one construction often are indicated in some detail, while areas to be developed for future construction may be detailed to indicate appropriate structure, functional relationships, internal traffic, and record flow. The architectural feasibility study may be accepted as the basis from which to begin the schematic design phase and standard architectural services. In some cases, with only minor modification, the study may be approved as the final schematic design. Also included may be a buyers' market value of the existing building, which can be obtained through a local real estate firm. A commentary on the advantages and disadvantages of each solution is often a part of the study report.

Early in the project, the group must evaluate the options for financing the project. Alternatives include arranging a new lease, refinancing the present loan, or arranging personal loans rather than mortgaging the property. A financial feasibility study of some degree usually is required by a lending institution, but physicians themselves will want to know how the cost of a building program may affect their incomes. For these reasons the following questions need to be asked: Will the rates on the money needed be cheaper on mortage rather than on personal loans? In addition to interest rates, what will be the other costs of borrowing money? The group will want to project operating costs for heating, cooling, utilities, staff, and taxes. It will be important to ascertain whether increased efficiency and anticipated higher patient loads can be expected to offset increased costs. For a sophisticated financial study, a group should engage the appropriate financial specialists.

It should be remembered that while in the past, medical groups customarily have owned their own buildings, certain difficulties may arise if, for example, the medical partnership itself owns its facilities. As the group expands and takes on new personnel, it usually does not want to limit its selection of new doctors to those able to invest a large share in the assets. Conversely, when a physician is leaving the group, his departure should not be tied to liquidating his share of the assets. It is not unusual, therefore, to divorce the organization established to practice medicine from the organization established to own and administer the physical assets. The most common forms of ownership for physical assets are: partnership arrangements, condominiums, incorporation where nonpractitioners may be included as members of the corporation, formation of a holding company, and in some cases, divesting of ownership in a nonprofit foundation. Another alternative is the possibility that a hospital may build a group facility adjacent to or within the hospital and include no unusual concessions to the physicians or vice versa. On the other hand, physicians may lease only the land from the hospital while owning the building themselves.

Developing the Feasibility Study

Although professional help is available for the development of feasibility studies, some groups may not want or need such help. A detailed feasibility study may be unnecessary, for example, when a parcel of land is available in an obviously prime area at a very reasonable cost. In most instances, a well-established group can assemble, through its own statistics, a record of patient residency and population trends.

If it is decided that detailed feasibility studies are necessary, professional assistance is available from architectural and engineering firms, design/build firms, and consultants. It should be emphasized that these professionals should be sought by the group as early as possible in the building program. Early involvement of the architect in the planning process is most valuable, since his plan/design-oriented contribution should influence the critical process of early decision-making.

The costs for developing feasibility studies vary, depending upon the complexity and scope of a project. Fees are negotiable and can be determined only after a discussion with the building committee concerning the group's goals and objectives. Some architect/engineer firms are able to provide the group with feasibility studies and economic analyses, assistance in site definition and requirements, preliminary schematic drawings, and a guaranteed price for what is considered to be a minimal cost. The feasibility study may be included as part of the overall contract. A preliminary agreement which covers this early phase of the project is simply a method of assuring the firm that it will be reimbursed for a portion of its cost if the project does not proceed. While the services of these firms are approximately the same, the main difference lies in the fee that is charged and the time of payment. Some firms may ask for a lump sum fee governed by the size of the project. Such a fee may cover the feasibility study and several subsequent steps leading to the signing of a contract for design development. Other firms may ask for a graduated fee, charging the client for each step. Still others may not charge a fee for the feasibility study since they prefer to allow both themselves and their clients the freedom to terminate the project if it is unsatisfactory to either party. It should be pointed out, however, that most firms will not begin a project until the owners are sincere about building, have completed their own preliminary studies, and have arrived at preliminary decisions.

The following chapter will outline the areas in which these early decisions must be made and will describe the organization structure necessary for a building program.

Chapter 21

Organizational Structure

DECISION-MAKING

The future productivity of any medical practice will be influenced heavily by the physical environment in which the physicians work. Whether remodeled or new, owned or leased, physician offices can be convenient, efficient, and pleasant or may be a source of continual irritation to the individuals occupying them. Decisions concerning facility planning, therefore, are extremely critical. Many groups will find it necessary to rely on a variety of advisors for assistance with decisions concerning the building or remodeling of a medical facility; however, advice should be sought only from those who are experts in their fields. Accepting the advice of an accountant on the practicality of a suite layout or the advice of an architect on the wording of buy/sell agreements in a partnership could have serious consequences. Five general areas into which decisions relating to a building program will fall are listed below, along with the suggestions for a choice of advisor(s) in each category.

1. *Ownership Entity*
   Group Administrator
   Practice Consultant
   Attorney
   Accountant
   Investment Counselor
2. *Design*
   Architect
   Contractor
   Financial Consultant
   Attorney

3. *Site*
   Real Estate Agent
   Contractor
   Architect
   Attorney
   Accountant

4. *Construction*
   Architect
   Contractor
   Attorney

5. *Finance*
   Attorney
   Accountant
   Financial Consultant

Making a decision in one area will have an effect on subsequent phases of the project. An obvious example is site selection. If the site selected is inadequate in size, expansion of the building must be vertical or involve multiple sites. Most decisions have similar ramifications requiring evaluation before a conclusion is reached. In the example above, the architect might be able to answer various questions. He may not be aware, however, that increased cost involved in providing vertical expansion capability probably will add little or nothing to the present economic value of the building, but may increase the equity requirement, although perhaps not the loan amount. This could result in a cash requirement in excess of that agreeable to the group of physicians. Vertical expansion, in this particular case, becomes unacceptable, thus making the site unacceptable.

The Decision-makers

The primary decision-makers probably will be all the members of the group; however, the task also might be assigned to a committee representing the total group; a corporate or partnership entity composed of all, part, or none of the physicians; or possibly a hospital board. For the purposes of this chapter, it will be assumed that a total group of physicians, in one form or another, is the primary decision-maker. Some decisions, of course, will be beyond the control of the medical group. For example, it may be decided by the group that all of the site not used for the actual building be devoted to parking, thereby increasing the number of patient parking stalls while reducing initial landscaping costs and the on-going cost of maintaining landscaped areas. The city or the governmental jurisdiction under which the project falls may insist, however, that a minimum of 2 percent of the total site area be devoted to green belt or landscaped areas. The group also may decide that a minimum of seven cars per physician will provide adequate parking for patients, staff, and physician convenience; however, the Air Pollution Control Board or Environmental Protection Agency may grant permission to park only five cars per physician on the site. In either case, the decision is beyond the owner's control. In fact, often in many substantive areas governmental agencies will be at least a strong influence, if not the actual decision-makers.

If a group requires financing, an additional decision-maker will be the lender or source of funds for the project. Although the money market is a competitive area and there are periods when it is a borrower's market, the lender still makes the final decision concerning who will borrow what amount, on what terms, and under what conditions. For example, the borrower may feel that the real estate together with his corporate signature constitute adequate security, but the lender may decide that the personal signatures of each member of the group also are required. A variety of other individuals may be included in the decision-making category even if the building is to be owned by the group physicians. For example, a hospital acting through a land lease or through contracts with those physicians who usually provide service to the hospital, such as radiologists or pathologists, may strongly influence decisions.

The Decisions

Decisions are comparable to building blocks, with early decisions influencing all subsequent action. To change an initial basic decision at a later date can mean that all work completed in the interim has to be modified accordingly, or possibly redone completely. In addition, every project is based on a predetermined time table. A delayed decision resulting in a substantially altered time table can be just as destructive and costly, if not more so, than a decision altered at a later date. The most expedient approach is to determine initially the actions that will result from various decisions to be made, thereby indicating what information is pertinent and requisite to making the decision. As an example, if the group is contemplating beginning with a one- or two-story building and expanding as much as three stories later, and if the site the group desires to purchase contains a height restriction of forty-eight feet (adequate for four stories), the decision to purchase the land should not necessarily be delayed until a variance is obtained for a five-story building, which may take as long as two or three months. Considering not only the cost of preparing the necessary applications but also the possibility of an increase in construction costs, acquiring a change in the zoning need not be a prerequisite for the group's decision to buy the site. On the other hand, it would be just as foolish to purchase a site for which zoning restrictions were in doubt. These examples should illustrate the prudence of determing what information is *necessary* to arrive at a purchase/non-purchase decision for a particular site. Peripheral information which only serves to delay and confuse the decision-making process should be set aside.

Other decisions will be made on a more subjective basis. For example, one such decision might involve the selection of a method for financing the project. The group must decide which of the many terms and conditions contained in a mortgage commitment are vital to the decision process and which are simply desirable or supplemental. It may decide that the maximum annual constant (the figure by which the loan amount is multiplied to determine the monthly payments for interest and principal) cannot exceed 10.49, which would be equal to a 9½ percent loan over twenty-five years. The commitment, however, may be for 9¾ percent for thirty years (a 10.31 constant). According to the original decision, this arrangement would be acceptable because the group had decided previously that the constant would be the criterion, not the specific rate or loan period. In the financing area, other possible examples would include loan period versus amortization period, fees or points versus interest rate, and limited liability versus joint and several liability.

In essence, the decision-making process should be characterized by compromise in dealing with the issues. Decisions should be neither unduly delayed nor hastily made on the basis of inadequate information. Early in the planning process the medical group must identify the key issues to be considered, specify when such decisions should be made and delegate the appropriate responsibility to certain individuals. A chart illustrating the organizational authority of the individuals who are to participate in the building program may be helpful. It is advisable in many cases to specify that a consultant or advisor is to use his best judgment, with his decision being subject to the group's veto if it is totally unacceptable. Decisions concerning the structural system to be employed or the choice of specific structural materials should be left to those individuals conversant with the design and cost of the project. The same is true for many of the technical sections of contracts and leases. This does not imply that the group should remain unaware of the processes and potential results, but if it has selected and is paying for professional help, it should attempt to maximize the benefits.

Convenience and interest may influence the delegation of authority. If, in a ten-physician group, it is stipulated that all decisions are to be approved by the total group, months of unnecessary delay may be added to the project. In addition, individuals having little or no interest in or knowledge about the actual development of the project will make few constructive contributions to the validity of decisions. Without question, there are certain decisions which the group as a whole should be given the opportunity to review and possibly to veto. Major decisions concerning financial liability, overall building functions, and site selection should be the concern of at least the total building committee, and perhaps even the entire medical group. The involvement of the total group in making routine decisions, however, is better kept to a minimum. In any case, to ensure quality decisions the group should encourage the participation of those with past experience and/or the greatest interest in the project. Routine decisions often can be left to the committee chairman, and will occur most commonly during the construction phase. Usually, these types of decision will not affect the quality or cost of the project, but will be requested by the contractor on a day-to-day basis in order to prevent unnecessary delays and to promote orderly, uninterrupted progress. Some routine decisions also will be required during the design stage.

Assuming the size of the group is such that a building committee is formed, some consideration should be given to the additional effort and time spent by committee members on behalf of the group's interest. Those involved either are contributing extra time in addition to their practice hours or are being forced to reduce their practice hours and, consequently, their income, for the benefit of the group. In this case, some form of compensatory adjustment is justified. If, however, other members of the group serve on committees involving the organization of the group or some other aspect of group practice, reasonable equality of effort already may have been achieved. Often, the building committee is a composite of those active in the group's management or leadership and those who simply would not be happy if they were not involved; therefore, no specific compensation may be required. Of course, if the group has truly competent advisors and consultants, the actual time requirement imposed on the physician should not be excessive.

Among the group's first design and construction decisions will be those concerning the financial feasibility of the project. Interim and long-term financing will be discussed in the following chapter.

Chapter 22

Financial Considerations

OWNERSHIP OPTIONS

In order to initiate any building program, a group must establish itself as a borrowing entity so that it may obtain adequate financing. While it is common for a single individual to own a building, from a lender's standpoint this type of ownership is the least desirable because there is no continuity of responsibility if something should happen to the owner, especially during the construction phase. Although facility ownership has been covered in detail in Chapter 7, ownership as it relates to facility financing requires additional consideration at this point.

Traditionally, the investors who own the building are the physicians who also occupy the office space. This arrangement is convenient because it precludes landlord/tenant conflicts over such items as rent, maintenance, and parking space. The investors should be financially responsible individuals with similar practice, economic, and retirement goals. Such commonality of interests helps to maximize the chances of a smooth relationship among the owners.

In a mutual ownership, the doctors forming the group will invest funds either equally or in accordance with mutually acceptable agreements. In cases of unequal investment, it usually is advisable to establish a plan whereby small investors can increase their investment gradually until all owners are on an equal basis. One form of mutual ownership is the general partnership agreement, in which all partners are equally responsible and one partner can bind all others. This type of ownership, however, is less popular and is seldom used for a number of reasons. In a general partnership, each and every partner is jointly and severally liable for repayment of the loan. If one or more of the partners have a substantial net worth, their personal advisors may not permit them to sign jointly and severally on the loan. Those partners having a smaller net worth will have substantially less to lose in the event that there is a default. Under any ownership plan, it is important to negotiate this potential problem with a lender who will often agree to limit the liability of each partner to his prorated share of ownership in the entity, to his share multiplied by some factor, or to a negotiated dollar maximum.

The limited partnership represents a different type of ownership arrangement in which two or three individuals, or possibly a corporation, act as general partners and are responsible for all acts of the partnership. Other individuals may be limited partners and may purchase an interest in the project, but have no voice in the management or operation of the building. The funds from the sale of partnership interests are used as initial capital, with general partners financially responsible for the project, and limited partners responsible only to the extent of their original contributions. In this type of ownership, the partnership usually is composed of physicians who are tenants of the building.

The limited business partnership offers a means of minimizing the liability exposure of the individual partners since the liability of each partner is limited to the amount of his investment. By definition, however, such a partnership requires at least one general partner, who usually is subject to the claims of the creditors, while the limited partners may be exposed only to the extent of their investment. The problem, then, becomes one of identifying a person or entity willing to assume this responsibility. If the physicians are unwilling to be associated in a general business partnership and there are no physicians willing to assume the unlimited liability of the general partner, it may be wise to engage a "professional" general partner, such as a builder or developer in the community, or an institution, perhaps a bank, which is willing to assume financial risk for sufficient incentive, which may be a promotional interest in the partnership. Such an arrangement is an ownership agreement whereby the general partner invests no funds, but assumes liability to the creditors. If the general partner is a contractor, an added incentive may be the contract for the construction of the facility. Unless the general partner is financially strong, however, the lending institution still may require guarantees from the limited partners.

Corporate structure is yet another form of ownership. In this case, a corporation is formed to own both the building and its equipment, and physicians then lease facilities and equipment from the corporation. When the corporation is formed, funds accruing from the stock issued can be used as initial capital to start the project. Officers are elected and given the authority to conduct the business of the corporation as well as to construct and operate the clinic. The formation of the corporation can be structured to accommodate the particular needs and desires of the individuals involved. In the foreseeable future, it is entirely possible that all group practices may be required to be licensed by the state in which they operate. If such licensing becomes obligatory and if, for this purpose, the definition of such a group includes all physican affiliations which have achieved corporate status, the medical group may wish to reevaluate its decision to incorporate.

The question often arises as to whether it is better for the building to be owned by a partnership or by a corporation. Most lawyers advocate corporate ownership. From a tax standpoint, however, a partnership arrangement may be more advantageous during the first few years of a project's existence. Most medical buildings are heavily mortgaged due to financing arrangements and correspondingly heavy interest payments. The interest plus depreciation on the building will produce a sizable tax loss during the building's early years. These tax losses are more likely to benefit individual owners rather than a corporation. If the building is owned by a partnership, such tax losses can be passed along to the individual partners and used to offset ordinary income. Usually, however, this tax write-off cannot be taken by a corporation. While a partnership has more liability exposure than a corporation, this exposure often can be covered by insurance. When the building begins to produce a taxable income, the group may wish to consider a change to corporate ownership.

LAND PURCHASE

The first financial commitment made by a group contemplating a new building is the purchase of land. If care is not exercised in the selection and purchase of land, permanent financing for a building project may be impossible. The loan will be much more attractive to the lending institution if the medical facility is well-located in relation to the community and other medical facilities, is easily accessible, and has ample parking space. If surveys are conducted before land is purchased, the previous owner may assume full or partial payment for the services. It is advisable that control of land be secured before construction begins and that the group have enough working capital to realize the completion of certain building phases. In order to obtain permanent financing commitments for construction of the facility, it usually is necessary to establish some legal relationship between the owners of the proposed facility and the owners of the land upon which the facility will be constructed. Depending upon the specific situation, this relationship may be established through option to purchase, long-term leases, or outright purchase.

A purchase option is a contract giving an intended purchaser time in which to decide whether or not to effect that purchase. In order for the option to be legally enforceable, it must contain all of the terms and conditions for purchase of the land. The option, however, does not entitle the buyer to any rights of ownership of the land. Often the seller is unwilling to grant a purchase option because, in effect, the land is being removed from the market during the option period; however, a seller may be convinced of the prospect for success of the project and this conviction, together with payment to him for the privilege of obtaining the option, often will enable the buyer to obtain a three-, six-, nine-, or even twelve-month option. The seller may be willing to credit any monies paid for the option against the purchase price of the land at such time as the option is exercised. If the group should find at a later time that it does not wish to exercise the option, it then has forfeited these payments.

An alternative to the purchase option approach is a conditional contract through which land is procured under contract to a straw party with a provision that the straw party have the right to assign his rights under the contract to whomever he chooses. By this method, when the time arrives to exercise the option, the contract is simply assigned to the physicians or to a corporation, and purchase is made by the physicians. Whether the contract is an option to purchase or a conditional contract, it should state a number of conditions. These conditions may reflect the reasons for not purchasing the land immediately, such as availability of proper zoning, results of any soil boring test, and the obtaining of permanent financing. The length of the option period should be sufficient to allow for arrangement of all permanent financing as well as for arrangement of a short-term construction loan, which may provide the money for purchase of the land.

If the project's financial structure and requirements are such that the group cannot afford to restrict money in land, a facility may be constructed upon leased land. A long-term lease has the further advantage of permitting rental payments to be tax deductible as an ongoing expense during periods of time when the facility will be generating income. Furthermore, a lessor may be willing to grant a lease/option which would provide for a later purchase of the land at a presently negotiated price. The lease/option arrangement also presents a possible advantage for the seller because he may avoid a substantial tax burden resulting from the sale of the property. For example, an older person may own property that was acquired many years before. In the hands of the seller, the property is likely to have a low cost basis; if the land was acquired for $10,000 and it is now worth $50,000, the cost basis remains at $10,000. Upon sale of the land, the difference between the cost and the sale price is taxable as a gain. A capital gains tax, however, would not be the only result of the sale. Whatever amount of the proceeds remaining in the estate of the seller at his death also would be taxable.

As more and more medical communities cluster around hospital facilities, it is probable that medical building construction will be hospital linked and will involve larger structures. A common problem arising from this situation is whether the medical building should be owned and operated by the physicians or by the hospital. Both parties may want to be the landlord and both have a good case. Hospitals are obligated to guarantee that assets owned by them are properly utilized and prudently disposed of. A community hospital which loses permanent control of part of its land to a group of physicians could be open to considerable criticism. On the other hand, physicians often feel threatened by the prospect of a hospital in the role of landlord because they fear interference in their practices by the hospital administration. Traditionally, most physicians have preferred to develop and manage their own facility. A fairly simple solution to this dilemma is a long-term lease arrangement in which land is leased from the hospital to the group of physicians who then own, construct, and manage their own building. As landlord, the group physicians avoid any interference with their practices by the hospital and are able to control the conditions under which they lease office space. On the other hand, the long-range disposition and use of the property remains under the control of the hospital. In addition, the hospital is spared the necessity of spending considerable funds which may be needed for other purposes and both parties gain advantages inherent in a hospital-based group practice. In negotiating such an arrangement, there need be no unusual concessions made by the hospital to the physicians, such as leasing the land below the usual rental rate. The physicians, in turn, should not be expected to give up any of their ancillaries, such as laboratory and X-ray, even if the hospital views these services as competitive. If both parties deal in good faith, a long-term lease of this type can make possible a hospital-based medical practice while safeguarding the legitimate interests of both the physicians and the hospital. During negotiation of such a lease arrangement, there are many details that should be covered, including terms of the lease, rental rate, conditions under which the building is to be managed and can be sold, provisions for any services by the hospital to the physicians, liaison between building management and hospital administrations, local economic conditions, land availability, and various relationships between hospital and medical staff.

An alternative arrangement consists of a profit sharing or pension plan's loaning money to the purchasing entity for purchase of land, construction of a building, and possibly purchase of equipment. Determining that a fair rate of interest is charged and that there is adequate security for the loan is extremely important. The term "adequate security" means submitting something of value in addition to and to support the promise to pay. This security is pledged to the lending plan trust in such a way that it may be sold, foreclosed upon, or otherwise disposed of in the event of default in repayment of the loan. The anticipated value and liquidity of the security is such that, should the loan not be repaid, no loss of principal or interest will result. Adequate security may consist of mortgages or liens on the property or accommodation endorsements from those capable of meeting the amount of the loan. Interest payments made by the borrowers are deductible expenses for income tax purposes and the interest income received by the plan trust is not taxable.

Finally, an outstanding opportunity may be available to individuals who are interested in acquiring the land and have a substantial interest in a profit sharing/pension plan. While income received by the profit sharing/pension plan may be taxable as unrelated business income, the tax rate may be substantially lower than that paid by those wishing to use the land. If the profit sharing or pension plan group then purchases the land upon which the facility is to be built and rents it to the physicians, the rental payments made for the use of the land can be deductible expenses to the physicians. The terms of such an arrangement, however, must be made reasonable, and the rental payments must reflect a fair rental for the use of the land. The 1974 pension reform act does raise some questions concerning whether a qualified retirement plan may own such facilities. It would be advisable, therefore, not only to obtain written opinions from respected real estate appraisers and brokers as to the fair rental value of the land, but also to secure legal advice from an attorney familiar with the recent pension reform act.

PREREQUISITES TO FINANCING

Although extensive negotiations with a specific lender will not occur until construction costs have been determined and the architect has formulated his plans, the group should begin to seek available funds early in the development process. Loan terms and loan availability may be determined in great part by local conditions. It is probably best, therefore, to negotiate with local lenders or with those who are fully aware of local conditions.

Of prime importance in evaluating a loan application is the ability of the borrowers to pay off the loan. The lender will be interested in whether the borrowers is a partnership or corporation, and may require signed financial statements from the borrowers, as well as a short biography of each of the borrowers, or each member of the group or corporation. These precautions are taken so that in case of default of payment the actual liability of the borrowers can be determined. In connection with this evaluation, there should be a projection of estimated rental income and operating expenses of the building. Many lenders prefer a current financial statement audited and prepared by a competent accountant or auditing firm, and often it is helpful to have a statement which compares the previous year with the current year. A lender can and usually will obtain credit reports. The financial condition of a limited partnership is somewhat difficult to document because the partnership itself usually is organized and formed for the sole purpose of that particular project and probably will have limited assets. Since the partnership has no history, it is to the lender's advantage to determine the credibility of those individuals who are involved. It also is helpful to obtain a financial statement of the limited partners even though they have no liability. This evaluation gives credibility to the project and facilitates a more favorable analysis of the ownership. Corporate ownership of a group facility is similar to that of a limited partnership, if formed primarily for the particular project, and it presents the same problems as the limited partnership in the analysis of information relevant to financial responsibility.

In addition to financial statements, a long-term lender usually will require a profit and loss statement. A new project, which cannot be documented, will necessitate a profit or loss projection which a lender will analyze carefully to ascertain if it is realistic compared with other groups and to determine if there is sufficient net income to pay the debt service (interest, amortization, and taxes) of the loan.

It is unwise for a group to start an ambitious building program without sufficient operating capital. Although physicians are considered good financial risks, they should realize that there is still some limit to their borrowing capacity. It is important that the building be backed by sufficient funds, and even more important that the group's income be large enough to enable the paying back of loans needed both during construction and during operation. Land should be secured before construction begins and the group should have enough working capital to finance the primary building phases. The lender will be interested in the economic feasibility of the project, and must be assured that there are sufficient funds to complete construction. This assurance is particularly necessary for the short-term lender who makes a construction loan. A short-term lender will want to guarantee the completion of the project either through a bond or title company disbursement, either of which assures the construction company of completion free of any lien. The construction lender also will want to be sure that the group will satisfy all of the terms of the long-term loan since it is the long-term lender who will pay off the construction loan.

In addition to evaluating the financial capabilities of the borrowers, the lender also may require some other pertinent information concerning the project. While working drawings may not be necessary in the early negotiations, the lender will need preliminary site plans and floorplans. Because all negotiations will revolve around the cost of the project, a preliminary cost estimate should be made. In evaluating the site, the lender will want to know what land will be encumbered, its zoning, its cost, its current value, and the condition of its title. The lender probably would find useful a demographic survey of the community in which the facility is to be built. In addition, if there will be other tenants in the building, signed leases or intent to lease forms will be required.

A lender will want to be assured of both the professional and financial capabilities of the contractor and the architect, both of whom should be asked to submit a validated financial report. A completion and performance bond also may be necessary, and while there may be resistance to this requirement, the owner, as well as the lender, needs assurance that the building will be completed according to plan.

Cost Estimates

Because the financial commitment will be made long before construction is completed and actual costs are known, it is important that the cost estimates be as accurate as possible. Building costs are seldom stable and generally tend to increase. These increases can be highly volatile and financial estimates should allow for the impact of cost escalation both in the short- and the long-term period. It is important, therefore, to take into account the lapse of time between the making of the estimate and the actual construction. Several types of long-term cost estimates should be brought up to date periodically if they are to provide an accurate picture of what the costs actually will be. First, the cost of the building must be projected. Secondly, the group should estimate the income from the building, the expenses incurred, and the cash flow. Finally, the group should consider both the capital needed for the project and the rent to be charged.

It is extremely important that the cost estimate of the building be as accurate as possible because this estimate will influence all subsequent projections. Depending on the area, construction costs may range from $25 to $40 or even $50 per square foot. Although construction costs may be inflating rapidly, the group should be able to secure a square foot estimate from either a local banker, architect, or contracting firm. The group must be certain that it has all the available cost information, and that it distinguishes between initial costs and life-cycle costs. In the long run, a building inexpensively constructed may become very expensive to operate due to high maintenance and utility costs. The use of quality materials and insulation can reduce unnecessarily high utility costs, and good equipment can mean lower operation and maintenance costs. If the structure is adequately master planned, substantial life-cycle savings can be realized by including expansion capabilities in the original structure. If the group uses the services of a design/build firm, it may benefit greatly through the use of the firm's manufacturing, bulk buying, and time saving capability. Finally, some cost savings can be realized by simply obtaining the permission of adjoining landowners to use portions of their land during construction. Costs such as these should be considered in a life-cycle analysis or energy use evaluation.

In evaluating the cost of the building, it must be determined whether the tenants or the owners will pay for tenant improvements, such as basic provisions for the covering of floors, walls, and ceiling, and the installation of plumbing and partitions, etc. These considerations will have a crucial bearing on the total cost estimate. One way to approach the problem is to state in the lease the extent to which owners will furnish tenant improvements. Work which exceeds these limits is paid for by the tenants. In addition to actual building costs, the group should consider cost of the land and site improvements such as parking, sidewalks, exterior lighting, and landscaping. Service fees for the architect, lawyer, and professional manager, as well as for the financing, engineering, and appraisal also should be included. Fees paid for building permits and other related licenses, construction loan interest, and insurance are a part of the overall cost of the building as well.

As will be discussed in detail in Chapter 24, architects' or engineers' fees usually are negotiable. The architect's fee can be paid either in a lump sum, or as a percent fee contract in which the architect receives a percentage of the overall construction costs. A percent fee usually ranges from 7 percent to 10 percent. Understandably, owners may become concerned that an architect who will receive a percentage of the construction costs may be tempted to escalate these costs as high as possible to increase his overall fee. Conversely, the architect, as a professional, actually may try to provide the most efficient design possible for the least amount of money. In a percent fee contract, the harder the architect works, the lower his fee is going to be. This dichotomy suggests that other contractual arrangements might be preferred. When the scope of the project is fully understood before work begins, negotiating a lump sum fee is a practical approach.

The total fee, whether percent fee or lump sum contract, when analyzed in terms of total project cost is a relatively minor portion of the overall life cycle analysis. A reputable and experienced architectural firm will be well worth the fee; nevertheless, it is important that fees be negotiated carefully. Furthermore, a considerable amount of time may be saved by using a design/build firm. The fee for these firms, as well as for major architectural firms, will depend upon the amount of work done. If the firm is retained to handle the project from the master plan through construction, fees obviously will be higher than if the firm is involved only in design and construction.

Construction costs based on early estimates may not be the same as actual construction costs. Time delays, therefore, represent a cost that must be considered. Whether they are intentional, caused by the group waiting for lower interest rates, or whether they are the result of unforeseen strikes or material shortages, these delays will affect adversely the costs of the project. These additional costs are more noticeable in terms of both construction inflation and the payment of interest on borrowed money.

The mortgage loan usually is obtained on the basis of the estimated, not the actual costs. When a project the size of a medical building is under consideration, any substantial excess of actual cost over estimated cost can place a severe additional burden on the investors. In order to protect the group against such contingencies, some consulting firms routinely will include an additional fee for cost overruns. In evaluating architectural and contracting firms, one quality that should not be overlooked is the firm's ability to estimate costs. The firm's previous record can be evaluated by comparing actual costs for projects with the firm's initial cost estimates. Early involvement of the contractor in the project is another method for ensuring accurate cost estimates. With his knowledge of costs and construction methods, the contractor should be able to offer valuable design input. While his contribution may not radically affect major design decisions, the contractor may be in a position to point out less expensive or higher quality alternative solutions. Cost analysis should be an ongoing process conducted by the architect, contractor, construction manager, or possibly by a combination of these individuals.

In estimating the rental income of the facility, the group should consider the total square footage available and an appropriate rental rate per square foot. This rental rate may vary depending upon location of the space and its intended use. After considering a percentage of estimated vacancy, an estimated gross income can be established. Taxes, insurance, utilities, and maintenance, as well as services such as management, legal, administrative, and accounting, will contribute to the operating expenses of the facility. The group also must consider payments on interim and long-term loan, including both principal and interest. The tables presented in figures 22-1, 22-2, and 22-3 should be helpful in making some of these estimates. Estimated vacancy rates and estimated mortgages are based on percentages which will depend on local conditions. Information on these percentages should be available from local real estate firms and lending institutions. Assuming that the building owners are paying for air conditioning, heat, water, and interior upkeep, in addition to the usual owner-assumed responsibility for management, such as insurance and taxes, estimated operating expenses should fall between 30 percent and 35 percent of the estimated gross income. This 30 percent to 35 percent rule will not necessarily apply during times when the building is only partially rented.

If the primary aim of the group for its facility is investment value, it should receive a yield which at least equals what might be expected from a completely passive investment in which the group is not involved as a developer. In fact, the yield should be even larger because of the larger risk involved in general real estate development. A common way of expressing investment yield is in terms of the ratio of cash flow to money invested. Eight percent to 10 percent of the capital investment should be expected. This figure, however, does not represent the total yield. A medical building offers considerable tax shelter for taxable income and provides additional yield in the form of tax benefits. Assuming that the market value of the building remains stable or increases, the equity the investors theoretically gain through payment of the mortgage principal may further increase this yield. Real estate investments are currently available in which the investor is not required to participate as developer, and which carry total yield of 15 percent to 20 percent and higher. The developers of a medical building, for whom return on their investment is a primary concern, should expect to receive a yield similar to this.

Loan Terms

In negotiating the financial arrangements for the building project, the borrowers should be familiar with some of the terms and conditions of a loan con-

Land	
Building (Including any tenant capital improvements)	
Site Improvements (Including parking, roadways, sidewalks, exterior lighting, landscaping, sewer and water connections, etc.)	
Service Fees:	
Architect	
Legal	
Professional Management	
Financing	
Engineering (Including soil testing, site and topographical surveys, etc.)	
Appraisal	
Building Permit and Related Licenses	
Construction Loan Interest	
Insurance and Interest (interim)	
Contingencies	
TOTAL ESTIMATED COST	

Source: *Physician's Management*, December 1971, p. 40.

Figure 22-1. Estimate of Cost

tract, such as the determination of the interest rate. It has been customary for the interest rate to remain constant during the entire term of a loan; however, some lenders are becoming increasingly concerned with the concept of a floating interest rate. This provision is much the same as that found in the cost of living increase provision of many commercial leases. The floating interest rate has an obvious disadvantage to the borrower because in considering cash flow or cash requirements for any given period of time during the operation of the facility, he cannot be assured of the amount of his monthly payment.

Estimated Rental Income

Floor or Facility	Rentable Sq. Ft.	Rental per Sq. Ft.	Gross Income
Totals			

Estimated Vacancy Loss (%)

ESTIMATED GROSS INCOME

Estimated Operating Expenses

Taxes (real estate, personal property, payroll)
Insurance (land and building)
Electricity
Salaries (maintenance)
Water
Snow Removal
Service Contracts
Scavenger Service
Management
Legal, Administrative and Accounting
Repairs and Replacements
Maintenance Supplies

Total

ESTIMATED OPERATING NET INCOME

Acquisition Costs
Mortgage Principal (average)
Interest (average)
ESTIMATED ANNUAL SURPLUS (before federal taxes)

Estimate of Federal Tax
Estimated Operating Net Income
Interest
Depreciation

Taxable Income
Tax

ESTIMATED NET ANNUAL SURPLUS

Source: *Physician's Management*, December 1971, p. 41.

Figure 22-2. Estimate of Income, Expense, and Cash Flow

Fees or charges by the loan broker or the lending institution for making the loan are called "loan points"; a point is equal to 1 percent of the loan. These fees are subject to negotiation and usually involve a one-time charge covering the cost of the paper work and the loan broker's fee. In a short-term loan, one loan point is not the same as 1 percent interest. It is the same, however, if the

Capital Requirement		
1. Total project cost (from estimate of cost sheet)		$ ______
2. Less: Any portion of land not allocable to project	______	
Any portion of site improvements not allocable to project	______	______
3. ESTIMATED NET PROJECT COST		______
4. Estimated mortgage obtainable (% of net project cost)		______
5. Balance (Line 3–Line 4)		______
6. Land and site improvements not allocable to project		______
7. ESTIMATED CAPITAL REQUIRED (Line 5 + Line 6)		______

Rental Rate Requirement	
1. Total estimated operating expenses (From estimate of income, expense and cash flow sheet)	______
2. Depreciation (@ 2% of total depreciation basis of building)	______
3. Investment yield (% of total net project cost)	______
4. Total Lines 1, 2, and 3	______
5. Adjustment for estimated vacancy loss (% of line 4)	______
6. Estimated gross rental income requirement (Line 4 + Line 5)	______
7. Rental rate (annual per square foot—line 6 ÷ net rentable square foot in building)	______

Source: *Physician's Management*, December 1971, p. 41.

Figure 22-3. Estimate of Capital and Rental Rate Requirements

full amount of the loan is outstanding for one year and is paid off at the end of that year. A construction loan is neither paid out all at one time nor paid only during the construction. For example, on a $1,000,000 construction loan, it may be that the average outstanding is only approximately $500,000. In this case, a point on the $1,000,000 ($10,000) would be the same as 2 percent interest on the outstanding $500,000. On the other hand, if the construction loan runs a term of eighteen to twenty months, the loan point on yield might be less than 1 percent.

There usually are several conditions included in the loan contract regarding payment of the loan. One of these conditions, the "lock-in," is becoming more and more popular with most lenders because it prohibits the borrower from paying off the loan during a certain period without the payment of some penalty or the renegotiation of loan terms. In the medical facility construction field, these lock-in periods usually range from five to ten years. In addition to being unable to refinance at a more advantageous rate, other problems, resulting from failure to prepare for the future, may arise during a lock-in period. If the loan has a lock-in period the group is dependent upon the existing lender for obtaining additional funds for expansion of the facility. It is very difficult to circumvent this problem, but if the group is reasonably able to foresee the future expansion needs of the facility, it can, at the same time the loan for the present facility is negotiated, include some agreement with the lender for the eventuality of financing future expansion. This is not a fully satisfactory solution because most lenders are unwilling to commit themselves to a future loan with an interest factor based on the present rate. A more manageable, although equally difficult approach, would be to master plan the facility. When financing the original structure, any portion of the land required for known future development can be left unencumbered by the lender. Should the lender be unwilling to lend upon favorable terms, this arrangement will allow a subsequent lender to become involved in financing the expansion; however, because the expanded portion of the facility may not be a self-contained unit, a new lender might be unwilling to loan upon a structure which, in itself, cannot be operated as a separate facility and cannot be considered as such in the event of default.

Most lenders include a provision in the loan agreement which stipulates that upon the sale or transfer of a property, the loan may be accelerated at the lender's option, thus making the total loan immediately due and payable. Typically, the physicians who combine to form a group practice are the initial borrowers in connection with the construction of the facility. Subsequently, two or three new physicians may be added to the group. These new physicians may be permitted to invest in the facility, thereby changing the composition and identity of the original borrowing group. This action could be considered a "sale or transfer" according to the acceleration provision of the loan agreement and could require an immediate repayment of the loan. Acceleration is a distinct possibility if the current interest rate is appreciably greater than the rate on the existing loan. This acceleration may be avoided, however, by requiring the lender to exclude from his definition of a "sale or transfer" a sale of ownership interest to physicians who subsequently become members of the group, or to others at the discretion of the owners. Avoiding acceleration of the loan is important because money markets may change. Additional expense to the group may include a higher interest rate, higher loan points, and the costs of a "new" loan to replace the accelerated loan. While these acceleration and assumption provisions usually are negotiable, the group should safeguard against a very poor bargaining position in the future by negotiating wisely at the beginning of the project.

Any prepayment penalties included in the loan contract also should be considered. If a group makes payments on the principal which are in addition to the regular payments as stipulated in the note, a prepayment penalty may be levied. A prepayment penalty is an extra charge required under the provisions of the loan. Prepayment penalties generally are a problem when the owners wish to distribute the cash value of equity which has resulted from an increase in the value of the facility. The terms of a prepayment penalty can sometimes be negotiated with the lenders. A typical prepayment penalty will give the lender six months additional interest on the amount of prepayment. Many lenders, however, will permit from 10 percent to 25 percent of the original loan to be prepaid in any year without a penalty. They also may reduce the amount of the penalty once the loan has been in existence for several years.

If possible, the group should avoid arrangements through which the lender exacts a share of the property or other income as a condition of making the loan. Securing a loan without such lender involvement usually is possible under current market conditions. In the past, lenders were not satisfied with a maximum return of 10 percent to 12 percent per year. Most states now have usury statutes which legally limit the maximum interest which may be charged on a loan. When money is scarce, there is a tendency for lenders to attempt to obtain more than interest as a return on the loan advanced by them. In this way the lenders, in effect, charge from 12 percent to 18 percent and more per year on property leased back to the borrowers. If such an arrangement must be made, the borrowers should negotiate an option to buy the facility back from the lender at some future date. Another arrangement to be considered is that of "balloon payments." It is becoming common practice to write, for example, a twenty year loan which has an amortization schedule based on twenty-five years. Any unpaid balance on the loan at expiration of the twenty year period is made in one lump sum, commonly called a "balloon payment."

LONG-TERM FINANCING

With increasing specialization in the medical field, various lenders may offer exclusively either take-out loans or construction loans. The take-out loan is the final loan made once the structure is completed and often is referred to as the permanent financing. It is this loan that runs from ten to thirty years in duration and incorporates some or all of the loan provisions previously discussed. The construction loan, on the other hand, is an interim loan, usually made by banks during the construction period and only for the purpose of financing construction. As a general rule, banks are unwilling to commit their funds for long-term real estate loans, and they fill the gap prior to completion of the facility by providing short-term construction financing. The construction lender, however, wants to be assured that the borrower is able to pay off the construction loan once the building is completed. Consequently, it is best to obtain the take-out loan first and then go to the construction lender with a firm commitment letter from a take-out lender. Each of the lenders charges points and interest, and may have acceleration and assumption provisions as well as prepayment penalties. These provisions, however, are much more important in connection with the take-out loan which may encumber the property for as long as thirty years.

In obtaining a construction loan, it is important to be certain that the loan runs for a period sufficient to ensure completion of the structure. The group must be prepared for such unforeseen circumstances as labor strikes, shortages of materials, and unfavorable weather, so that no time gap occurs between the termination of the construction loan and the commencement of the take-out loan. The two lenders should cooperate in coordinating their documentation in order that lost time, legal fees, and undue conflict do not result from lenders' disputes.

There are a variety of sources from which long-term financing can be obtained. The first of these is a mortgage banker who will know the loan market and will have an established relationship with various lenders, such as insurance companies. It is recommended that the group ask its commercial banker to supply a list of three or four reputable mortgage bankers in the community. The commercial banker can indicate to the group which insurance companies are represented by the mortgage bankers and what loans they recently have placed in the community. The mortgage banker usually can be depended upon to accommodate the group. Often, he can provide an approximation of the terms he expects to obtain, and he will charge the group a fee, usually 1 percent of the loan amount, for obtaining the permanent commitment. Assuming he places the loan with one of the companies he represents, in addition to this fee he will continue to receive income from servicing the loan. The mortgage banker accounts for the payments to the insurance company and sees that the property is properly insured, thereby protecting the interests of both the lender and the mortgagee as well. He also may make an annual inspection of the property, and will ensure that the group pays its taxes. If the loan is not made locally, he represents the lender and receives a fee for doing so.

The reputation of the mortgage banker must be thoroughly evaluated. It is possible that he may make promises he is unable to fulfill. For example, he might lead the group to believe that he could obtain a loan at a certain percent and later report that the best available loan is 2 percent higher; or, wanting more loan points, he may try to extend a shorter time period for payment than previously agreed upon. Thus, one of the main reasons for suggesting that the group ask the advice of its commercial banker is that he will be more aware of the reputation of local mortgage bankers. The market is fairly homogeneous and all bankers know, within a certain range, what the rates should be.

If the members of a group agree to consult a mortgage banker, they will be asked to sign a letter giving the banker the exclusive right to find a loan for the group. Mortgage bankers sometimes ask for six months to find such a loan, and these arrangements could be unacceptable to most groups. In most cases, sixty days should be sufficient and a quality mortgage banker should have a preliminary indication from one of his lenders in thirty to forty-five days, at which time he must submit a plan to that lender. A thorough evaluation of the group's plan, however, and approval by the lender may involve some time. Assuming the mortgage banker has obtained a commitment from the lender, he usually will return to the group with a commitment letter. Some mortgage bankers also will add their own commitment. The group then is able to go to the construction lender to show him how the loan will be paid. Since the construction lender will evaluate this commitment, it is important that the commitment be issued by a financially responsible lender who has the ability to fund the project when the building is completed.

It also is possible for the group to deal directly with the primary lender without using the mortgage banker as a liaison and long-term representative. These institutions may be life insurance companies, whose actuaries can forecast how much money the company will have to pay in claims for the next forty years.

They know how much money will be incoming and by coordinating cash inflows with cash outflows they can make long-term loan commitments. In addition, many large insurance firms have their own mortgage originator officers who deal directly with the borrower and may not use mortgage bankers as their representatives.

The group should not overlook the possibility of going to a local savings and loan institution or a local savings bank. It may be that some of the physicians in the group serve on the boards of these institutions. Many savings and loan institutions are restricted in the amounts they can loan; only a certain percentage of their assets can be used for loans on such specialties as medical group facilities. They are, however, permitted to make this type of loan if their existing portfolio is not already at the top of the percentage limitation. Savings banks usually are under no such limitation. If members of the group have a good relationship with the local commercial bank, it may be possible for them to secure a relatively short-term loan from that institution. These loans may run from fifteen to twenty years, or they may involve ten-year loans with a twenty-year amortization, thereby necessitating a balloon payment at the end of the ten-year period. Most commercial banks, however, are not long-term lenders on major projects and do not actively seek this type of long-term financing.

If the group building the facility is large enough, it may be able to self-finance the facility. Such self-financing may mean that each investor will go to his own bank and borrow his percentage of the total money needed for the financing of the facility. When the facility is operating in a positive cash flow position, the group can operate from a stronger negotiating position to secure longer term financing which will then provide the cash proceeds to pay back the individual loans of the owner group. A group should keep in mind that, generally, lenders have considered medical facilities to be single purpose structures and, therefore, a substantial number of lenders have been reluctant to grant loans on them. With a facility already built and operating profitably, such reluctance should be overcome and a group may be able to negotiate a larger loan with a lower interest rate and more favorable loan provisions.

In an effort to stimulate interest in the formation of new group practices, the Federal Housing Administration and the Department of Housing and Urban Development, authorized by Title XI of the National Housing Act, administers the Group Practice Mortgage Loan Guarantee Program which represents a government guarantee to mortgagors of group practice facilities. Loans of up to 90 percent of the building project, including only capital expenses of land, building, and equipment, are offered. There are, however, a number of disadvantages to Title XI funding. The real estate transaction must be conducted by a nonprofit corporation established for that purpose; and the land, building, and equipment then are leased to the medical group. The depreciation accrues to the corporation rather than to the physician-owners. This type of loan is restricted to urban and suburban groups of over five physicians and rural groups of three or more physicians. In addition, a number of charges amounting to a surcharge of approximately 8 percent are levied against the total project. The completed facility can be sold or refinanced at the end of twenty-five years, however, providing group members with an opportunity for a potentially large capital gain or for an investment in other ventures. The safety provided by the government guarantee of the loan is an incentive for lenders to give lower interest rates. The group must be able to show, however, that it can become a viable financial entity. Another loan source is the sale of state-approved industrial bonds. Many states have passed laws allowing the sale of tax exempt bonds up to $5,000,000 per project. They represent an excellent means of low-cost financing for health facilities. Universities, charitable organizations, and union and corporate pension funds have a great deal of money to lend and generally constitute additional low-cost financial sources. If other possibilities for financial assistance have been exhausted, the Small Business Administration also will lend money to an organized group of physicians regardless of whether the group functions as a profit or nonprofit organization.

A final source for the long-term financing may be the firm that gives the construction loan. Certain lenders will provide a construction loan which converts to long-term financing at the completion of construction. Obvious advantages to this type of loan include lower points and other related fees, as well as substantial savings in such areas as title reports, legal fees, and escrow charges. If the lender is committed to long-term financing, he obviously has confidence in the project and may want to make the construction loan because typically it is a higher yielding loan for lenders.

Of greatest concern to the borrowers will be the cost of the loan. The range of interest rates is fairly broad and depends upon a great many factors. For example, many insurance companies are much more reluctant to lend money in small towns than they are in metropolitan areas; publicity of a foreclosure would be much more adverse in a small town than in a large community. Another aspect affecting the cost of the loan is the time when it is made. Some borrowers may want to wait to secure a loan, hoping that interest rates will eventually decrease. Waiting may have been a reasonable approach several years ago, but it is unlikely that interest rates will drop appreciably in the foreseeable future. Even if rates were to drop slightly during the course of a year, inflated construction costs might significantly outweigh the decrease. For example, if a group needs a $1,000,000 loan for its building and the current interest rate for twenty-five years is 9 percent, the loan, including principal and interest, would be $100,800 per year. It also is reasonable to assume that construction costs may rise at least 10 percent during the next year. A one year delay, therefore, could mean that the group would have to borrow, $1,100,000, and at 9 percent interest it would be paying $110,880 per year. Were interest rates to drop a full 1 percent, the group could arrange a $1,100,000 loan for twenty-five years at 8 percent; however, it would then be paying $101,970 per year, which is slightly higher than payment would have been on the 9 percent loan obtained one year earlier. In fact, a group would have to secure a 7 7/8 percent interest rate (a payment of $100,870 a year) in order to equal the payments on the 9 percent loan which had been available the previous year. Due to rising construction costs, the longer a group waits for lower interest rates, the greater the reduction in interest rates must be in order for the group not to lose money as a result of inflation. In addition, while waiting for lower rates, the physicians may not have an adequate facility in which to practice as they had planned.

Returning briefly to the mortgage banker alternative, it may be noted that he will charge at least one loan point for structuring the loan agreement. An insurance company may commit itself to giving the group $1,000,000 for permanent financing in twelve to eighteen months, but it may ask for as much as two points ($20,000) which will be refunded when the loan is closed. A group should not hesitate about paying a refundable fee to any reputable and responsible financial institution. By withholding this fee, the insurance company then obligates itself to have the funds available to the group. If upon completion of the project interest rates have gone down, the group may decide to negotiate a better loan elsewhere. The insurance company is willing to take this chance; if the group arranges a loan elsewhere, the insurance company will retain the $20,000.

Insurance companies also protect themselves by including in the loan contract a buy/sell agreement, which is sometimes called a triparty agreement. In this agreement among the construction lender, the long-term lender, and the group, the construction lender agrees to sell the note to the insurance company and the insurance company agrees to buy that note only if the borrower has satisfied all terms of the commitment. The borrower is then asked to agree not to do anything to prevent the consummation of this arrangement. If the group enters into such an agreement, even if it has paid a refundable fee, it loses all control and any legal right to take advantage of lower rates that may be available upon completion of the project.

THE CONSTRUCTION LOAN

When the group has obtained a commitment for permanent financing, it should approach a lender for a construction loan. Since the construction lender must be assured of repayment upon completion of the facility, the permanent financing commitment is a necessary prerequisite. The construction loan is used to pay an expense incurred in building on the property, including the acquisition of the site, any interest due during the construction period, and, of course, the payment to the general contractor. This money is not paid in one lump sum but is disbursed as construction progresses.

The group's own commercial bank probably is the best and least expensive source for a construction loan. Most commercial banks approve this type of loan since its duration usually is only twelve to twenty months. Banks are in the business of making short-term loans and are not in the long-term market; however, some banks do not make construction loans as a matter of policy because they are not staffed adequately to administer the loan and protect their interests. Real estate investment trusts usually are anxious to offer short-term construction loans, but may charge more than local banks. The long-term lender may want to offer the permanent financing and make the construction loan as well.

When the group is negotiating with its commercial bank, any favorable financial information that can be presented to the commercial banker will have a bearing on the interest rate finally charged. A construction loan at a commercial bank usually will cost at least 1½ percent over the prime interest rate, adjusted as the prime rate moves higher or lower; real estate investment trusts usually will charge 3 percent to 4 percent over the prime rate. In order to qualify for the lowest rates possible, therefore, it is important that the group maintain a good relationship with its bank and then search for the most favorable rate. The construction lender also may want to charge points for the loan. In comparing one loan arrangement with another, a group must evaluate thoroughly all conditions of the loan in order to determine which is the least expensive arrangement. In addition to interest rates, additional costs, such as legal fees, travel for inspection, builder's risk insurance, and title insurance, must be considered as well. Some lenders will insist that their own architect inspect the progress of the building. This inspection is made at the borrower's expense and takes place before payment is made.

Among the major concerns of the construction lender are that the borrower satisfy all conditions of the permanent financing commitment, and that the facility be completed within a certain time period, within the cost estimates, and in accordance with the plans and specifications. If these conditions are not met, the permanent commitment may not be operative and the construction lender will, in effect, be left with the permanent loan. The lender, therefore, must be assured that there are sufficient funds to complete construction. For example, if the construction loan is for $1,000,000 and the final cost is $1,200,000, the construction lender will want to be sure that the medical group has sufficient funds to complete construction. If the project is 90 percent completed and the group fails to secure the additional $200,000, the construction lender will have no choice but to complete the project at his own expense. Only upon satisfactory completion of the project will the construction lender be paid by the long-term lender. Because it is the completed project which he is paying for, any and all changes should be approved by the permanent lender. If the project is not completed in accordance with the plans and specifications as well as within the agreed upon time, the permanent lender has no further commitment. The short-term lender, therefore, must be reasonably satisfied that the project will be completed within the allotted time.

In order to guarantee the completion of the project according to specifications and predetermined costs, it is possible to obtain payment and performance bonds which guarantee completion of the project for the contract amount, free from liens for material, men, or equipment. There are several forms of payment and performance bonds which should be reviewed by the group's attorney. An alternative to the use of payment and performance bonds is the use of a construction escrow service at a rate sufficient to cover its costs. The service usually charges from 1 to 1½ percent of the total contract price and guarantees that the group will have a project that is fully paid for at the end of the contract.

The permanent financing arrangements become effective when the Notice of Completion is signed. When the Notice of Completion is filed, the final payment to the contractor, including any retainage, must be made. Before signing this notice, therefore, the medical group should be certain that the project is totally completed. When the permanent financing begins, there will be an additional expense to the group. During the construction period only interest on the construction loan is paid. Upon completion of the project, however, it will be necessary to pay the principal on the long-term loan as well as the interest.

Site selection, location, and planning can have various financial implications which will be discussed in the following chapter. In addition, the method chosen for the design of the facility also will affect financing. This relationship is discussed fully in Chapter 24.

Chapter 23

Site Selection

LOCATION

Of obvious importance in any building program is the site on which construction takes place. A site must be evaluated not only for its immediate environment and aesthetic qualities, but also its adequacy in serving the group's needs. In Chapter 4 location is discussed from the perspective of group mission and the planning of a practice. In this chapter the group's location will be considered in relation to facility planning. While the location of a medical clinic is important, there are those who argue that it is not of primary importance in predicting if a patient will avail himself of the group's services. When seeking a qualified physician, a patient probably would be willing to go to any area in which the group practice is located. For this reason, paying a premium for location may not be a necessity but, nonetheless, a thorough evaluation of location is important.

There are two population entities to which the medical group must relate, the medical community and the patient community as a whole. These communities are of interest to a planner not only in relation to site selection but also in relation to the provision of information required by the lending institution. Locating near a hospital provides convenience primarily to the physicians but also to the patients, particularly if the group sends a majority of its patients to one hospital. The most useful and convenient facility would be one close enough to the hospital so that the physicians can walk to it from their offices, thus eliminating time consumed in driving and parking. In certain communities, a hospital might build a group practice facility adjacent to it or may renovate space within the hospital. If the group physicians send their patients to several hospitals, the ideal location for the clinic would be a site centrally located among the hospitals served. It also is advisable to evaluate the potential construction site in relation to the physicians' homes.

In assessing the possibilities of various locations, it is important to consider the patient community. The site must be analyzed not only in terms of patient locations, but also with respect to the particular neighborhood and its probable future. The site should be easily accessible and have ample parking spaces. Location in a shopping center, however, is often undesirable. It is preferable that a medical facility preserve its identity, which easily may be lost amidst a multitude of unrelated shops and a sea of automobiles. The facility's visibility and its proximity to well-traveled thoroughfares and public transportation are additional considerations.

MASTER PLANNING OF THE SITE

While attempting to locate the ideal site, the group should be giving thought to master planning as discussed in Chapter 20. Group members should be concerned with the potential for growth, the number of physicians to be included, and the medical specialties which should be covered. When master planning the site, there are a few simple guidelines to be considered. Experience shows that the floor area of an efficiently designed building planned for a group practice of twenty physicians will cover approximately 25,000 square feet. While it is possible that the original building may house many fewer physicians, if it is anticipated that the group will expand to twenty, ground for the expanded building should be considered at the outset. Space for one physician is estimated to encompass from 1,000 to 1,200 square feet. Parking area requires at least 300 square feet per car and the group should plan to allow for six to ten spaces per physician; therefore, a one-story building housing twenty physicians requires approximately 25,000 square feet of floor area for the building plus at least 36,000 square feet for parking. This results in a total of 61,000 square feet, which is roughly one and one-half acres. Added to this area should be another 50 percent for open space and landscaping, resulting in a total of two and one-quarter acres. If yet another 50 percent is added for future contingencies, such as parking, the minimum sized site for a potential twenty-physician group would be approximately three and one-half acres. Regardless of the characteristics of health care systems in the future, adequate space in the present can result in efficient and cost effective construction and expansion. In fact, success in coping with the future may depend upon having an adequately-sized site.

Site Adequacies

In evaluating a site, it must be ascertained whether the site meets both the group's present and future needs. The facility should be accessible to pedestrians, automobiles, and public transportation, and have available necessary utilities. An investigation of the site property may reveal that it is properly zoned but, in fact, that it may be necessary to go before an environmental impact review board to secure permission for the type of building the group wishes to construct. Because the group purchases a site with the intent of building and adding stories in the future does not guarantee that utilities and zoning will support the addition. The sewer configuration, for example, may not be able to support a multistory facility.

Having the land thoroughly evaluated by an engineer provides the group with information which not only will be valuable in the construction of the facility but also may be required by the financing institution. It is advisable not only to appraise utilities, but also to conduct soil tests and surveys of the terrain upon which the building is to be located. A site that is steep or has a great deal of rock and other impediments would require costly grading. Building on wet, boggy land would require piling and reinforcement to sustain the building and thus greatly increase building costs. A civil engineer should be able to assess the problems associated with drainage, grading, and subsoil conditions, such as high water tables, unstable soil, and uncompacted landfill. A competent engineer also should be able to provide estimates of the cost necessary to correct certain deficiencies of the site. It even may be expedient to make acquisition of the land dependent upon the results of soil boring tests. Additionally, clearing a site of trees could prove more costly than demolishing an existing building to construct another. A decision relating directly to the future expansion of the group and the results of engineering tests is whether or not to include a basement in the facility. Some soil conditions, such as the location of the water table, may make basement facilities impossible; however, if the site does permit the construction of a basement, such areas often represent space far less expensive to construct than those facilities which are above ground, and only can be excavated feasibly at the time the building is constructed.

Land Titles and Deeds

When a site has been tentatively selected, the group's attorney should check the title policy of the site to ascertain whether there are any provisions which would affect the proposed building. This information can be secured by a preliminary title report from a title company. Items of record which are identified as conditions, covenants, and restrictions recorded in specific books on specific pages at the tax recorder's office are listed in the report. Should there be impediments or encumbrances, the title report will place the group on notice. It may be valuable to obtain copies of the actual title in order to ensure that there is nothing to prohibit the group from building the type of structure or from using the property in the manner which they desire.

A lender may require that the group obtain an American Land Title Association policy which differs from a standard policy obtained for the purchase of a home. While a standard policy insures almost anything, it sets forth only what is of record and does not insure access to the property. In other words, the property can be insured, but it could be landlocked in such a way as to be inaccessible or it could have other defects not identified in a standard policy. An ALTA policy shows accessibility and identifies, after a visual inspection has been made of the property, any items which are determined to be detrimental including easements, encroachments, and leases. The inspection indicates whether work already started on the property could possibly contribute to a mechanic's lien, or if there were items that would have prior rights ahead of a buyer or lender. If work has been started, the group can still provide a lender with the desired type of protection by obtaining an indemnity agreement from the title company. This agreement is a bond that is given to the title company stating that any mechanic's lien will be paid by the owner or contractor and that the title company will not be held responsible. In turn, the title company then provides the lender with the type of policy needed for a prior lien.

In determining the condition of the title, the group should examine the deed for any restrictions placed upon the property, since such deed restrictions may supercede any provisions of the local zoning ordinances. For example, a city may permit commercial construction on a particular site as far as zoning is concerned but the land deed of the site may not. In this case, restrictions of the deed would govern the use of the property.

Landscaping and Parking

Landscaping on the group's new property generally must conform to the community's master plan which may indicate what types of trees and shrubs may be used and what views must be maintained. Group members also should determine whether the land can support the type landscaping they desire.

When planning for parking facilities, it is important to give a great deal of thought to the possibility of future expansion and it is therefore important that sufficient land be available. On the other hand, obtaining information concerning the future mass transit routes also is important. If there are no provisions for parking on the premises an assessment of the facilities available for parking must be made. A group may be able to negotiate parking privileges on adjacent or nearby parking lots or facilities for patients and staff. It is unsatisfactory, however, to rely completely upon on-street parking to provide the necessary spaces. Because of the expense involved in building multilevel parking structures, groups who have done so find that they must charge their patients for parking. These additional considerations should remind the group again of the implications of purchasing sufficient land before the site is developed.

Utilities

Engineers, employed by local governments having jurisdiction over possible city sites, can supply information concerning the availability of utility and sewer connections as well as utility company regulations for such constructions. Information necessary to determine the location and availability of sewer, gas, water, and electric lines can be provided. Such information could have an important effect on construction costs, if, for example, a building should require new storm or sanitary sewers. City or county engineers also should be questioned concerning regulations governing the building of roads or drives within the site or regulations on any contemplated changes to adjacent streets. If a piece of land is acceptable except for the location of easements, it may be possible to have some of the easements changed. This problem should be discussed with the city engineers or local utility companies.

Zoning Considerations

It is important that the particular site which the group chooses be properly zoned. The best land, as far as price is concerned, often is not zoned for the use the group intends. Property for a medical facility usually is considered a high use area and often carries a top price. If the group can secure the proper zoning, good agricultural or nonurban land in suburban areas often is suitable. If the land is not zoned properly already, purchase should be made contingent upon obtaining the required zoning. Securing permission to build on a site that is not properly zoned usually is accomplished by forming a team consisting of the group's attorney, architect, and some member of the group to negotiate with the proper zoning authorities.

If the site is improperly zoned, the group may incur difficulties and elect not to buy the site. The group should first determine, however, the chances of having the site rezoned, obtaining a variance, or securing permission for a planned unit development. Rezoning a plot of land can be a very difficult and time consuming process. In many respects, it is a political process requiring sensitive negotiation. It may be necessary to conduct public hearings or to initiate a public relations effort to build community support for the group's project. It may even be worthwhile to meet with the city councilperson from the area so that the group can present a favorable interpretation of its project. If the land cannot be rezoned, a conditional use variance is another possibility. A variance is not a zoning change but an exception to a zoning ordinance. Such special use permits, however, can result in future difficulties when selling the facility. While the group may have been given permission to build a medical facility on a particular site, permission for some other use of the site may not be possible when and if the group should decide to sell the facility.

A final alternative is that of a planned unit development. This alternative is a relatively new concept and may not be a possibility in all communities. In approving a planned unit development, the local government may decide that although the facility is in violation of local zoning laws and other local ordinances, the overall impact of the project is such that it may be of great value to the community. It is the group's responsibility, however, to prove that the proposed facility, though in violation of local regulations, will be better than a facility that could be developed under the current regulations.

Once a facility site is secured, the group is ready to consider various construction approaches. In the next chapter, the activities involved in new construction—architectural and engineering design, pricing and/or bidding the design, acquisition of financing, and construction and its management—will be discussed in terms of alternative approaches which include the traditional, the design/build, and the turnkey.

Chapter 24

The Planning and Construction Process

THE TRADITIONAL APPROACH: THE DESIGN-BID-BUILD PROCESS

Design-bid-build describes the framework of action within which a building traditionally has been produced. As the name implies, there are three basic and distinct elements in the sequence. The design process, which is carried out by an architect working in conjunction with the medical group to establish firmly the entire scope of the project, culminates in the contract documents—the drawings and specifications which represent the technical development of the design. These contract documents are used during the second phase of the process, the bid period. Contractors obtain prints of the documents from the architect, establish the cost of construction, and submit their bids in the form of sealed proposals to the architect and/or the medical group. After the contractors' proposals have been evaluated, the contractor(s) selected is notified, and the third and final step in the process begins, the actual construction of the building. Within the second phase of the process, it may be anticipated that a lending institution will be involved to some degree. In addition, contract negotiation may take the place of actual bidding.

The advantages of the design-bid-build process emanate from its logical, step-by-step nature, starting with rudimentary preliminary sketches and ending with owner occupancy. The process permits maximum control for both the group and the architect, as well as careful review, analysis, and approval at the various check points occurring in the overall process. Once the bids are received or contract negotiations completed, the medical group knows what the construction cost of the building will be, and, subject to the vagaries of weather and strikes, when the building can be occupied.

Essentially, there are three disadvantages to the system. Traditionally, the design-bid-build method is a linear process; each step must be completed before the next step can be taken. Often, three years may elapse between the hiring of an architect and the actual occupancy of the new building. The second most common concern of any client is the potential variance between the estimate made by the architect and the lowest bid actually submitted by the contractor. Admittedly, it is difficult to estimate the cost of a building that will be bid by contractors a year later, and it can be a traumatic experience for all concerned—the group, the architect, and the contractor—when the low bid substantially exceeds the estimate; however, if cooperation and understanding prevail, adjustments can be made and a satisfactory building project can remain a very real possibility. A third potential problem is the adversary relationship which may develop between architect and contractor during the construction phase of the project. The group and the architect have as their goal maximizing the space to be constructed at a minimum cost commensurate with good design. The contractor has as his goal minimizing his risk and maximizing his profit. The variance of these goals occasionally can cause conflicts; consequently, it may be necessary to seek mutually satisfactory compromises. By incorporating a number of alternatives within traditional processes, however, some of these limitations can be overcome.

Fast Tracking

Fast tracking is considered by many to represent a unique design and construction method; however, the fast tracking concept easily can be employed within the traditional design-bid-build sequence. In addition, it often is included in turnkey methods, which will be discussed later in this chapter. The fast track method was developed to reduce the overall elapsed time in the design-delivery process (see figure 24-1). While the fast track system almost certainly would be employed in an emergency situation, such as the rebuilding of a structure damaged due to fire, it was not developed initially as an answer to catastrophic occurrences. Rather, it emerged as a method for producing a building more rapidly. In an inflating economy, shortening the overall elapsed time for completion of the project by six months can mean a 6 percent reduction in the total cost. Furthermore, interim financing required during the construction period, which usually is carried at a much higher rate than is long-term financing, is necessary for a shorter period when fast tracking is used, thus resulting in a lower cost.

The early phases of the fast tracking process are almost identical with those of the design-bid-build sequence. The primary difference is that the contract documents are not totally completed before contractors are invited to bid on the project. Rather, the contract documents are broken down into a series of bid packages based on the usual construction procedure. For example, a bid package may be produced for the preliminary site work, excavation, footings, and foundations. This bid package would be awarded to the successful low bidder and the work would be started even though the remaining contract documents had not been completed. Structural steel might be bid as a separate package on a tonnage basis, even though the actual steel members had not yet been designed by the structural engineers. Thus, inflationary costs are avoided

PROCESSES

Fast tracking phases the design and construction of a facility so that the owner may obtain earlier use of the building. The time needed to design and construct the structure is compressed by overlapping activities that are normally performed in sequence. This process places a premium on comprehensive initial planning and requires a high degree of coordination between owner, architect/engineer, and constructor.

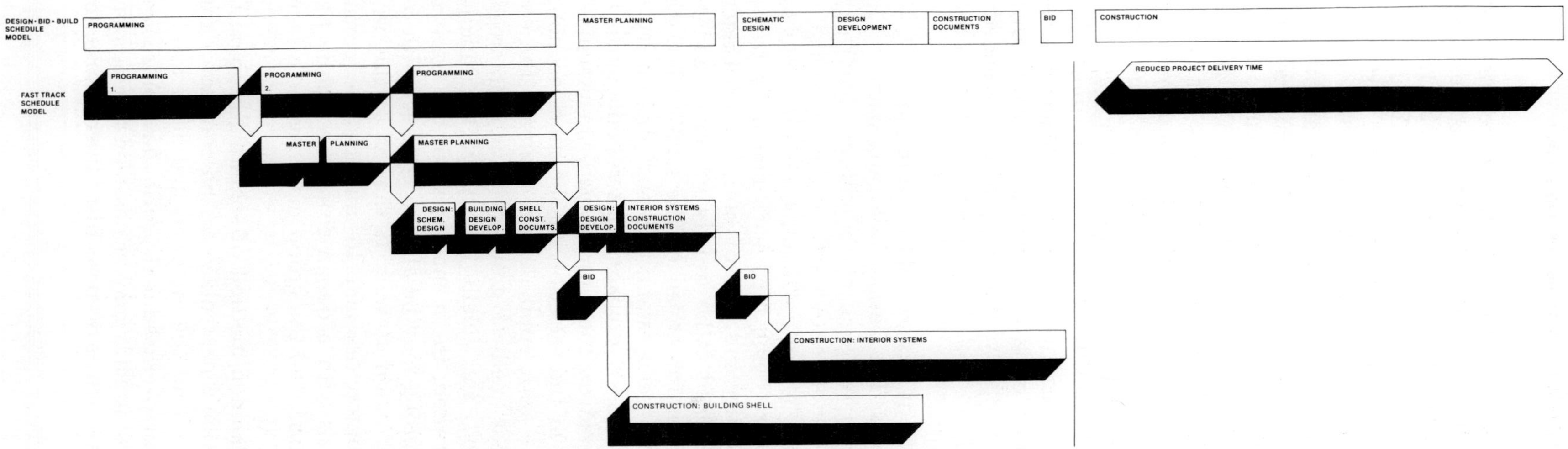

Figure 24-1. Comparison of Design-Bid-Build Sequence and Fast Tracking

and delivery at a time when the steel is required is assured. Equipment systems having long lead delivery schedules also are determined and ordered as early as possible, again to assure their timely arrival at the site. As few as one-half dozen or as many as thirty to forty separate bid packages can be part of the fast track process. Obviously, a system of this nature requires considerable organization and control if it is to succeed, and above all requires firm and timely decision-making on the part of the medical group and architect.

There are essentially two disadvantages involved in fast tracking. Required changes in the design can be difficult and expensive to implement after construction has started. Hence, both the group and the architect must be convinced that the scope of the project has been established firmly and has been agreed upon, and that the approved preliminary documents are an accurate representation of the group's needs. The second major problem concerns the final cost of the construction. Obviously, with many bid packages involved, determining the final cost is not possible until the last bid package has been executed; therefore, the system demands a very close estimation of probable construction costs to avoid cost overruns toward the end of the construction phase. This disadvantage may be compounded by the fact that no single prime contractor is responsible for coordination of the entire project.

Concurrent Design and Construction Contracts: The Design/Build Approach

Although the legal considerations involved in design and construction will be treated more extensively in the next chapter, a discussion of a few specific contracts is important here. Concurrent but separate design and construction contracts are being used with increasing frequency in an attempt to give the group practice the best of both worlds. Under these arrangements, the architect is retained as he usually would be and assumes the same duties and responsibilities for design of the facility; however, as soon as the scope of the project has been established and preliminary drawings and outline specifications have been prepared, interested contractors are invited to submit proposals based on these *preliminary* documents. The contractors then assist the architect in the selection of the most economical construction systems commensurate with good design; estimate the construction cost of the project; provide the medical group with a guaranteed maximum construction cost, if required; and finally, construct the building. When the design/build approach is used, the management of the construction project is less of a problem; the group may be able to contract with *one* firm not only for design, but for construction as well. It then is to the benefit of this firm to engage reputable contractors and to manage the construction efficiently. When the group deals with a design firm, the architect's responsibility may end at the design phase, and the group may have to hire a construction management firm as well.

One common method of soliciting proposals from contractors on this basis is to provide a percentage to the contractor for overhead and profit based on the final cost of the materials and labor involved in the construction. The percentage for overhead and profit that contractors require does vary, and selection of a contractor may be based on this factor alone. Since it is not uncommon to find as much as 80 percent of the construction completed by subcontractors on a competitive bid basis, rather than by the selected prime contractor, the element of competitive bidding is not reduced substantially through this method. When a contractor is involved early in the design process, he is available as an independent consultant to the architect and group and can assist in the determination of building systems and in the estimation of probable construction costs. Additionally, he becomes more intimately involved in and knowledgeable about the functional and aesthetic goals of both the group and the architect. Finally, the potential for conflicts is certainly minimized, if not eliminated. Members of the design and delivery team—medical group, architect, and contractor—essentially have a common goal and can work in a more cooperative framework to achieve that goal. The major requirement for the success of this method is compatibility and professional respect between architect and contractor. An adversary relationship during the construction phase can be damaging enough, but an adversary relationship during the design phase can be chaotic.

The Turnkey Approach

Another alternative approach to the design-bid-build process involves the turnkey option. Using this method, the group contracts with the firm for all services *including the arranging of financing.* The turnkey approach enables a group to deal with only one firm, and for a guaranteed price to move from the inception of the project to the turning of the key in the door.

During the initial stages of the turnkey approach, a medical facility planning specialist and the medical group usually establish ground rules for the building project. Objectives are discussed, target dates established, budgets reviewed, and the approximate quantity of space required is determined. The group will be asked to list services needed to complete the project, to choose the architectural style for the project, and to discuss many other facts that may affect the project or that are important to the physician group. This period allows for free discussion and exchange of ideas. As the project begins to take shape, the turnkey firm assumes the responsibility for testing various components for compatibility and for determining if the entire concept is economically feasible before any significant amount of time and money is spent or any major commitments are made. The group will be asked to sign a preliminary contract authorizing the turnkey firm to conduct engineering studies, cost analyses, feasibility studies, and functional programming studies for use in formulating the design of the facility. These tasks will be performed during various phases of the project by specialists assembled as a team who will remain with the group's project from the beginning of the development program through completion and delivery of the facility. Each team member is responsible for and contributes his expertise to a particular phase or function of the project in a coordinated effort with other team members.

The next step is the choice of a site. If the group has not acquired a satisfactory site, the turnkey specialist can analyze all appropriate sites according to the physicians' present operational needs and according to size requirements for accommodating expansion. Zoning requirements and economic considerations of the project also contribute to the analysis. At this point, the architectural member of the project team begins his work. He will sketch some conceptual drawings which, together with the preliminary specifications and a project estimate, enable other team specialists to seek sources for financing the project. Assuming favorable responses are generated in relation to rate and term appropriate for the estimated project cost, the team will proceed with the development of more detailed drawings, definitive specifications, and a detailed cost analysis for the project. As soon as plans, specifications, and cost analyses are developed to the extent that they can be used for financial documentation, the entire project is reviewed with the medical group to ensure that all goals and objectives as originally established are being met. The financial program is then prepared for submission by the group to *selected* lenders for both long-term and construction financing. With a firm financial commitment assumed, plans and specifications complete, a fixed price determined and agreed upon, and a building permit granted, construction contracts can be initiated and a completion date can be established. During the construction period, in addition to periodic inspections and approvals by both the local building department and the financing institution, formal inspections are arranged with the group, culminating in a final inspection and acceptance of the completed facility. At appropriate stages throughout this operation, various team specialists will resolve problems associated with zoning, environmental impact statements, special use permits, lease negotiations, changes the group may wish to make, and other items required for orderly progress and completion.

Often, the turnkey approach has been criticized because it may eliminate the competitive bidding used in more traditional approaches for the selection of a construction firm. Due to their obligation to perform at a guaranteed price, most turnkey firms remain informed on costs and prices pertinent to the project. When the design-bid-build sequence is approached more traditionally, as considered earlier in this chapter, it is possible that by the time plans and specifications are sufficiently complete for bidding, decisions already have been made that may result in the building's costing more than the group's budget will allow. Another alleged disadvantage of the turnkey method is the possibility of the contractor's not being adequately supervised by the project architect. When an independent contractor is employed, however, the probability of infrequent inspection by the architect or project representative may be less, but an adversary relationship between contractor and architect may develop as a result of overly restrictive supervision.

Regardless of the group's specific approach to its construction project, the process involved remains basically the same: design-bid-build. The important consideration is that there are different approaches to this process which can produce varying products and results. At one end of the continuum is the traditional design approach in which the group hires an architect to design a facility. Construction and construction management usually are not included in the arrangement. At the other end of the continuum is the turnkey approach in which the group contracts with one firm for a total package of services, including the arranging of financing. While formal bidding may not occur in this method, agreement must be reached on costs and prices. In the middle of the continuum is the design/build approach. Using this alternative, the group contracts with one firm for both design and construction. The design/build firm supervises any necessary bidding and manages construction; however, it does not arrange financing. The descriptions of the three approaches considered in this chapter are of ideal types; variations of each exist. Groups contemplating the construction of new facilities would be well-advised to examine buildings constructed from these various approaches before making any final decisions.

GUIDELINES FOR SELECTING A DESIGN, DESIGN/BUILD, OR TURNKEY FIRM

At the inception of the facility program, the group is presented with the problem of identifying qualified design, design/build, or turnkey firms. Most physicians and group practice administrators know of other groups who recently have been involved in a construction program or are now engaged in one. Meeting with these individuals provides an excellent means for determining which firms are most competent in facility design. Other business associates who have been involved in building programs also are good resources for identifying qualified firms. State and national conventions offer an opportunity to discuss potential firms with members of other groups, and exhibitors at such conventions may suggest additional possibilities. Finally, many state architectural societies maintain offices and often are capable of providing names which a group may wish to consider. In selecting professionals for the project, it is important to understand why an architect rather than an engineer should be selected for *primary* design responsibility. Most states have legal statutes requiring that a registered architect be responsible for the design of buildings that serve the public, or when health and safety must be considered. Each group, however, should review the laws in effect in its community, as there are some exceptions, and regulations do vary among states. It should be emphasized that, in general, an architect may have a broader range of experience in building design than an engineer. Most architectural schools require students to take some courses in structural, mechanical, and electrical engineering in addition to their architectural design classes. This exposure gives them the potential for an awareness of the many problems inherent in the total design process. Architects are not registered immediately upon graduation from an accredited architectural school. They must have three years of practice under a registered architect before they are eligible to take the architectural registration examination.

After compiling a list of firms, it is advisable for the group to send a letter to each firm describing the group's present status and what the anticipated construction program will be. Any other pertinent details of interest and importance to the firms also should be included. The group should ask for a letter in return that will indicate each enterprise's emphasis and capabilities. A brochure describing the firm and including descriptions of recent work it has accomplished can be helpful. In describing its past experience with medical groups, the firm should indicate names of clients and other knowledgeable people whom the medical group could contact for more information on past projects. The original group of firms under consideration may be quite extensive, perhaps a dozen or more. After the written information has been received, however, it is suggested that the list of those eligible be narrowed to from three to five possibilities. Two methods of selecting the firm are through interviews and direct selection or by competition.

The competition procedure for selection generally is reserved for large buildings and projects. The American Institute of Architects (AIA) has a published guide of standard practices used in conducting architectural competitions and architects are obligated by ethical codes to conform to these practices. One disadvantage of this procedure for the selection of an architect for a group practice facility is that the architect is selected by an AIA jury based on the design of a building submitted in the competition. The winning design may or may not be an accurate representation of the owner's practical and aesthetic goals. When using the interview method, however, the building committee generally conducts sessions of approximately one hour each. During this time, each firm's representative discusses his background and his firm's capabilities and presents his credentials by showing his previous building designs. The list of candidates then may be limited to the two or three considered to be the most suitable for the project. At this time, a detailed review of buildings designed, and perhaps built, by each firm, together with references from the owners of these buildings, is made. Field research of the buildings should be a major influence in the selection process. An interview with the physicians and administrators, as well as with the maintenance staff, can be very helpful in providing information about the durability and the functional and mechanical design of the building.

Professional Qualifications and Experience

The firm's experience, particularly in the design of medical facilities, is of considerable importance; however, this aspect may be given too much emphasis by the prospective owner. Health care facilities are specialized and often costly because of complex mechanical requirements and unique layout and design. Previous medical building experience, therefore, can be a definite advantage; a firm that specializes in medical facilities spends a great deal of time in keeping abreast of current developments in medical facility design. Still, a design firm that has not had past experience with such facilities should not necessarily be eliminated from further consideration. A skillful architect approaching a new building type will begin with current research and may design a fresh and innovative building. Members of the group should be prepared, however, to spend a considerable amount of time relaying information to him to ensure that some of the details involved in functional design are brought to his attention. If the group cannot spend this kind of time with an inexperienced architect, a further alternative exists; it may be possible to locate a firm that has had a great deal of experience in designing medical facilities whose architects may be willing to act as design consultants on the project. In this case, the inexperienced architect could be briefed by the consulting firm rather than by members of the medical group.

The group should be assured that the firms under consideration are financially responsible. Such information is not only valuable to a group but also may be required by the lending institution financing the project. The group must be assured that the firm chosen is solvent and will remain in business over the course of the project. The group may wish to secure a financial statement from the firm's banks as well as a financial report through a reputable organization offering such a service; the firm, in turn, may seek similar information from and about the medical group.

The location of the firm can present a problem and should be considered during the selection process. Close proximity of the design offices to the facility site would be ideal. If the group is negotiating with a design/build firm, an understanding of the architect's responsibilities will reveal the necessity for his developing a close rapport with the group and the importance of his being available to inspect the project during construction. Should a nonlocal firm be chosen, problems relating to the architect's accessibility can be solved through communication by telephone or letter. It also may be possible to hire a local firm to inspect the construction on a consultation basis. If the firm whose location is miles away from the project has had varied experiences in working in states other than its own, and if problems inherent in being in a place other than where the building is being constructed can be overcome, the firm's address should not be a deterring factor. If a local firm meets all the necessary criteria for selection, however, engaging it would be preferable.

The size of the firm and its methods of operation, both internally and with clients, should be evaluated. It should not be so large as to preclude the group's talking with the principal architect at any time. On the other hand, if the firm is small it may not be able to design and perhaps manage a building project within reasonable time constraints. For example, the sequence of procedures within a design/build firm usually involves design, working drawings, bid supervision, and construction inspection. For a substantial project, large design/build and turnkey firms make a practice of utilizing specialists for each phase of the project, usually with a "project architect" guiding the progress, especially during the design of the basic floor plan and style. Smaller design firms may utilize only one architect who may or may not be the principal being interviewed. In any event, the project architect should be evaluated along with the principal during the interview periods. If several specialists will be working on the project, the group should obtain information concerning each member's professional qualifications and work experience. The firm also should present a schedule for organizing these members into a team. Once the group has established that the firm has the desired background, the group should seek assurance at the outset that they will meet with individuals within the firm who will be in daily responsible control of the project.

Time Schedules and Budget

While the size of a firm may not be of major importance, the internal organization should be of concern to the group. During the early planning of the project, the group probably will adopt a time schedule, including a date at which it expects the project to be completed and a time for occupying the new facility. The architect and/or other firm members may be helpful in developing such a schedule. It is essential that the firm be able to finish the project within a reasonable amount of time, even if it becomes involved in other projects. Past projects completed by members of the firm should be helpful in assessing their ability to work within allocated time constraints.

The firm, regardless of its size, must be capable of proceeding with the project as soon as the group is ready to begin and should be willing to satisfy the group's time schedule by completing contract documents in order that a bidding and construction schedule can be met. An analysis of the management and organization of the firms under consideration also may be useful. Communication is extremely important and the group should satisfy itself that the firm has a management system that will keep the group informed of the progress of the work and provide it with the information it needs. From inception to completion, the average construction project can take as long as three years. The group should realize that it is becoming involved in a temporary partnership with a firm which may last for this length of time. To ensure continuity, it is a good practice to insist that at least two individuals be in responsible control of the project as far as the firm is concerned, thereby resolving problems of absences due to vacation, illness, or perhaps even death.

In order to meet the budget for design and construction, it is wise to hire a firm that is cost-conscious. It should be determined what prospective firms know about cost estimates. In discussing past projects, the architect should be asked for information on costs per square foot and on additive costs to basic bid figures. Cost figures can be updated by applying the historic inflation index to the quoted costs. If change orders to the original bid figure are more than 5 percent, the extra cost indicates poor planning in the design phase or inadequate working drawings from the architect's office. The firm should be willing to do a life-cycle analysis and should be willing to submit such analyses from previous projects. If a small design firm is engaged for a large portion of the work, it will be necessary to hire engineering consultants, including civil, structural, mechanical, electrical, and acoustical engineers. Landscape architects, interior designers, communications consultants, and others are retained at an additional fee and at the owner's option. When evaluating the quality and compatibility of the design team, consultants certainly should be included and should be evaluated under the same basic guidelines used to evaluate architects.

When negotiating a contract with a particular firm, it is important to have a thorough discussion and agreement on what the firm's fee will be. For example, architects generally work under one of two basic contract types. The first of these is a percent fee based on overall construction costs. This fee usually will range somewhere between 7 percent and 10 percent, depending upon certain conditions and the complexity of the project. A basic conflict of interest, however, may exist under such a contract arrangement. The owner usually is concerned that since the firm will receive a percentage of the construction costs, it could be to its advantage to project these costs as high as possible. On the other hand, it is hoped that the members of the firm are professionals and are doing their best to provide the group with the most efficient design possible. A negotiated fixed fee is the other most popular contract arrangement. Under such a contract, however, a full knowledge of the scope of the project is required before the architect arrives. Such a fee approach is generally more applicable to remodeling projects and partial architectural services. When employing an architect on a consulting or part-time basis, it is not unusual to pay on an hourly basis. This fee is most commonly used when nonlocal architects design a facility and a local architect is responsible for inspection during construction.

THE DESIGN PHASE

The first order of business after an architect has been hired should be a thorough *review of the contract provisions* of the owner-architect agreement. A contract is a rather formal document and often requires further interpretation. Obviously, caution must be exercised so that basic provisions are not violated. The American Institute of Architects' Document B-141 represents a typical agreement between owner and architect and includes a number of options to reflect individual circumstances (see Appendix 24A). For example, Article 1.1.14 (page 651) under the "Administration of the Construction Contract" begins with the stipulation that the architect shall make periodic visits to the site. This is an excellent example of the need for further interpretation. A clear understanding of the contract is important so that both owner and architect understand the authority and responsibility that each has accepted. As indicated in Chapter 21, the organizational structure representing the group can serve as an important adjunct in delineating appropriate authority and responsibility during the construction process.

As in any profession, architects and engineers have a jargon all their own and it can be a barrier to clear communication with those outside the field. It is understandable that the group could evidence some confusion when an architect initiates a conversation about a STC rating for a particular wall or when an engineer suggests the use of a variable volume system for the ventilation of a building. It is incumbent upon both the architect and the engineer to recognize that the communication barrier exists and to work diligently to eliminate it. For example, as an additional means of reinforcing and elaborating vocal agreements, the architect/engineer should initiate memoranda or letters describing his interpretation of all oral communications.

Article 1.1.1 of AIA Document B-141 (see Appendix 24A, page 651) indicates that in order to *ascertain the requirements of the project*, the architect will review a program furnished by the owner, and will confirm the requirements with the owner. Some groups have sufficient in-house expertise to develop a detailed program, but in most cases the architect must play a major role in the task. An architect experienced in medical facility design should be able to incorporate the ideas of group members into a workable plan and should have an idea of what is best for a particular group in terms of design, materials, and costs. It is his professional responsibility to tell members of the group when and why he feels that their ideas may be impractical or unfeasible. The final design should be a workable combination of the design envisioned by the architect and the expectations of the group. It is important that the architect organize and coordinate all planning sessions, as they may involve a variety of interested parties, including not only the architect and the group, but also bankers, lawyers, and the nonmedical personnel of the group.

A well-conceived program usually contains three basic parts: the immediate needs, the long-term goals, and a master plan describing how immediate needs and long-term goals will be accomplished. Immediate needs include the physician's requirements which will be provided for in the construction program. They should be thought out carefully and, in addition to delineating space needs and relationships, they should include the requirements for equipment that the group intends to use in those spaces. A statement about the quality of the space to be provided, along with a statement about the administrative and operational goals of the medical group, also is necessary. For example, if a nurse is assigned permanently to a particular physician, the space requirements for both individuals should be integrated closely. Similarly, a central appointment system versus a departmental appointment system is an administrative and operational decision that can have significant ramifications in terms of space allocation and space relationships.

Long-term goals require far less specificity than do immediate needs. This lack of required detail, however, in no way diminishes the importance of a definition of long-term goals if orderly expansion is to be achieved in the future. As discussed in Chapter 20, long-term goals should do much more than vaguely delineate future horizontal and/or vertical expansion. Medical groups usually expand at the rate of one or two physicians at a time. How these added physicians will be accommodated and at what point expanded space will be required are issues that must be considered in long-range planning. The plan also should include methods for the orderly expansion of departments which would be difficult and expensive to relocate, should the overall size of the group increase. Finally, some decision should be made as to the maximum size that the center can achieve based on the amount of land owned and the current codes and zoning ordinances of the community. The immediate needs and the long-term goals culminate in a facility master plan.

The design process, begun with a definition of the group's immediate needs, long-term goals, and the development of the master plan, proceeds with the *schematic design phase.* This phase begins with a graphic delineation of the department requirements of the group without regard to interior or room development of specific departments. The locations of individual departments are established commensurate with required interdepartmental relationships, as they may or may not exist. If the building is to be a multistoried structure, departmental relationships must be worked out on a floor-by-floor basis to achieve a square footage balance for the entire structure. Traffic patterns for both patients and staff must be determined along with consideration for the distribution of materials, both incoming and outgoing. After these basic criteria have been established, the design is carried forward with the development of space for individual departments as well as for ancillary and support facilities, in keeping with the group's needs and philosophy of operation, administration, and management.

Design of the exterior of the building usually is initiated along with the planning of various floors. Presumably one of the criteria for selecting a particular architect is his design philosophy. Exterior elevations of the building, three-dimensional preliminary sketches, perhaps a rough model, will help to illustrate his philosophy in relation to the proposed building. Too often, forming medical practices assume one of two roles as they review the proposed exterior appearance of their building. Individuals in the first category say little, ask few questions, and generally allow the architect to determine the building's appearance. Some architects actually may prefer this arrangement. The second type of client has some preconceived ideas of how the building should appear and continually asks for additional ideas. Neither of these two extremes is the more desirable. Rather, the architect should be given an opportunity to develop a total design concept that embodies the group's needs and philosophies and, as stated earlier, shows concern for the patients. Most architects are very articulate in describing their proposed solution and their reasons for it. Members of the group should ask questions about the design to be certain they understand that the proposed solution does indeed embody their documented needs.

As the schematic design nears completion, the first opportunity arises to make a preliminary judgment about the projected cost of the facility. In this early phase of the work, the estimate usually is made on a square footage basis by calculating the gross square feet of the total facility and multiplying by the cost per square foot, using current construction costs. Since the building is at least six months to one year away from actual construction, an inflationary factor should be added to this per square foot cost. In addition, a minimum contingency of 5 percent should be included as a hedge against future changes in the design. It is not at all unusual to find that gross square footage may increase as building plans develop and group requirements become better defined and understood. Modification in the design is an inevitable and ongoing process during this phase of the work. This is the time for testing ideas and for a mental tour of the building to visualize how medical staff, paramedical staff, and support personnel will function in terms of efficiency of operation. After the schematic design has been completed to the mutual satisfaction of group and architect, an in-depth review is called for. The program written earlier should now be compared to the actual schematic design in terms of both immediate needs and long-term goals. In addition to a careful review of architectural considerations, preliminary studies for mechanical and electrical systems should be reviewed with equal care. Because the architect will rely on the medical group's approval of these preliminary design documents, a careful review is necessary to avoid major changes at a later date. This review also should include an examination of the code and zoning ordinances along with a report by the architect concerning various regulatory agencies from which ultimate approval must be obtained. Usually, formal review and approval by these regulatory agencies will not be obtained at this time. As a general rule, however, such agencies are more than willing to make a preliminary review of the documents and comment on their compliance with codes and zoning ordinances.

The next step, *design development*, involves refinement of earlier schematic design documents plus overall detailed development of the design approved earlier. It is perhaps the most critical stage in terms of the functional requirements of the building as they relate to equipment locations and mechanical and electrical systems. For a typical examination room, the type of room most often repeated in a clinic setting and usually similarly equipped for the majority of the medical staff, provisions must be made for a heating, ventilating, and air conditioning system, as well as for plumbing, electrical lighting, electrical power, and communication systems. In special cases, a compressed air system and a gas and/or oxygen system may be required within this relatively small area. The terminating points of each system in the form of a valve, a grille, a switch, or an outlet are critical to successful and efficient use of space. Space must also be allocated both for built-in equipment and movable furniture. A design which can be used repeatedly for all exam rooms as well as a unique room design must be developed carefully during this phase to ensure that space is used functionally. Simple things are easy to overlook—such as the direction in which the door swings open into an examination room. If swung properly, the examination table is protected from casual observers in the corridor. It is very difficult to motivate medical and paramedical staff to become involved deeply in this kind of detail, and yet it is very important that they do so. The requirements of specific work areas, such as storage requirements and the arrangement of shelving and drawer space, are best obtained from those who are intimately involved with the use of the space on a daily basis. The specialty requirements in ENT, ophthalmology, and radiology departments, as well as in the laboratory, further complicate various system requirements and require intensive review with both staff and technicians if a satisfactory design is to be obtained.

The interfacing and establishment of all basic systems will be accomplished during this phase. While members of the group may not have a keen interest in structural systems being developed for the building, they should receive an in-depth review of medical and electrical systems being contemplated. The group should seek a detailed explanation of the capacity of such systems—how they function, their energy efficiency, and their regular maintenance requirements. Temperature control probably is the simplest example of a mechanical system which should be reviewed in this manner. The group should inquire if broad temperature control zones are being established with a single thermostat controlling the temperatures for a number of spaces, or if each room in the building will have its own thermostat. While a thermostat in each room might be considered ideal, it obviously increases the construction cost of the project. Final decisions in regard to sophistication of control and use of materials must be made in light of initial costs, operating costs, and maintenance costs. A common term for an equation expressing this relationship is life-cycle analysis. Decisions such as these must be made by the medical group based on advice from and consultation with the architect. It is well to remember that while the construction cost constitutes a one-time only expense, operating and maintenance costs remain a part of the annual operating budget.

At the end of the design development phase, sufficient information should be available to permit an estimation of the probable construction cost of the facility based on quantity purchase of materials and equipment, and potential inflationary trends. When the design development phase is completed and submitted to the owner for final review and approval, it should include an outline specification of materials to be used, actual samples of these materials when appropriate, and catalog descriptions of the more important items of equipment, the fixtures, and the furniture to be included in the basic contract. A second courtesy review of these documents by the appropriate regulatory agency also would be advisable.

Usually, the total design has been established at the completion of the design development phase. Very often it is one of the most difficult concepts for an owner to understand from a two-dimensional drawing. A three-dimensional colored rendering of the exterior of the building as well as of the more important interior spaces will help the group understand the appearance of the new building. Whether or not this work is included in the basic contract or stipulated as an additional service on the part of the architect, medical groups should avail themselves of the opportunity for a clearer understanding of the building's architecture.

THE BID PHASE

Contract documents are developed for use in the bid period and in the actual construction. These documents consist of drawings and specifications produced and submitted to the contractors for bidding purposes. Questions usually arise during this bid phase, and to ensure that everyone has access to the same information, addenda are issued periodically to clarify questions raised by the contractors. Generally, such addenda are revisions in the drawings or specifications originally produced. Change orders, which will be discussed in more detail later, constitute another element of the construction documents. When the contract documents are approximately 75 percent complete, the final estimate of the probable construction cost which was made at the end of the design development phase is rechecked against the contract documents. With the contract documents completed, a formal review is held with the governing regulatory agencies and a written approval of the documents is obtained from those agencies. Subject to any omission which may have been identified, initial approval may carry the qualification of full approval to be based on an actual inspection of the completed building and does not relieve the architect from the responsibility of code and zoning compliance. The completion of the review by regulatory agencies, and the final review and approval of the construction documents by the group, set the stage for the bid period. If a design/build or turnkey firm has been retained, the group's involvement in this phase may be diminished considerably, especially when compared to its involvement in the schematic design and design development phases. This is not to suggest that meetings and conversations will not be necessary, but if the previous phases have been completed correctly, the vast majority of the decisions required of the group already have been made.

Primarily, there are two basic ways to engage a contractor—by single contract or split contract. The single contract provides for the submission of a single dollar amount for the total construction of the project by one prime contractor. All other contractors involved in the construction process are considered to be subcontractors to the prime contractor. In addition to his duties as general contractor, the prime contractor also is responsible for the overall coordination and completion of the work. On the other hand, split contracts specify more than one prime contractor and usually include a general, a mechanical, and an electrical contractor. When multiple contracts are used, all other contractors are considered subordinate to these three, and often there is no single point of responsibility. The general contractor, however, may be responsible for overall coordination of the work.

There are several ways to determine the contractor's fee: through open or closed bidding, negotiated contract, or partial facility ownership. If contractors are requested to submit bids under an open invitation method, any contractor who meets the qualifications established in the specifications may bid. A common example is a project funded by state or federal governments who require that an open invitation be issued to all interested, qualified contractors. Bids are opened in alphabetical order and read aloud in an open meeting which any interested individual is permitted to attend. In the closed invitation method, selected prime contractors are invited to bid and the project is not advertised in local news media. Bids are opened in a closed session with the architect and the owner's legal counsel in attendance. Depending upon the financing of the building project, the lender also may be involved.

The major advantage of going through a competitive bidding process is that the group can be relatively sure that the price it is paying is the best price available at that time. Bids, however, will not tell the group if its building is designed economically or if it is designed to take advantage of a certain contractor's specific talents and abilities. If a building costs 20 percent to 30 percent more than the amount budgeted, it will be of little value to the group to know they have received the lowest bid. Thus, if a competitive bid process is used, there will be no means of evaluating the cost implications of the architect's proposal until the design phase has been completed. Also, competitive bidding is more time consuming than other processes, and usually requires 30 days after the architect has completed the working drawings for bids to be prepared. In addition, the competitive bid process prohibits beginning any construction work until after the working drawings, bidding procedures, and signing of the contract have been completed. There also is the danger that if the lowest bidder has bid the project too low, he may shortchange the group in order to make what he considers to be a reasonable profit.

The second most popular type of contract is the negotiated contract, based on either a fixed fee or a cost-plus basis. Under a negotiated contract, the contractor will build the project at cost and then ask for either a fixed fee or a percentage of the total costs to cover overhead and profit. A major advantage of a negotiated contract is that selection can be made on the basis of the contractor's qualifications and his ability to work with the group. This type of contract eliminates the temptation to select a contractor with the lowest bid who may lack qualifications and may be difficult to work with. The contract guarantees the contractor his profit, which in itself may make for a more pleasant working relationship. Another major advantage to a negotiated contract is that the construction phase can begin before all of the working drawings are completed. For example, it may be possible to pour the foundation before roof materials are even chosen. A negotiated contract eliminates the time consuming bidding process and also permits the contractor to make constructive contributions during the design phase. The major disadvantage to a negotiated contract is that the contractor has no incentive to keep costs down. If a cost plus percent contract is used, the contractor will realize a larger profit if building costs are higher. One means of keeping costs low is to establish a maximum fixed price very early in the project. An arrangement then can be made whereby any savings under the fixed price will be split between the owner, contractor, and the architect. In this latter case it is wise for the group to keep a record of all resources consumed.

A third means of paying the contractor is by permitting him to have a partial ownership in the completed building. This arrangement is most commonly used when a project, such as an apartment or office building, has a rental income. Depending upon how the group has been organized, it may be possible for the contractor to realize his profits based on a percentage of the group's income. Such an arrangement may be particularly helpful if the group, as a limited partnership, has found it necessary to have a contractor or developer act as a general partner for the group.

Identifying Qualified Contractors for the Bid Phase

Design/build and turnkey firms usually have established relationships with certain contractors and need not carry out lengthy investigations. If the group must identify qualified contractors for the bid phase or if a design/build or turnkey firm is handling an out-of-town project, some guidelines may be necessary. An architect should be helpful to the group in identifying qualified contractors, and if the architect will be involved in construction management, securing his advice ensures some measure of compatibility between the contractor and the architect in the project. Bankers also may be helpful in providing lists of qualified contractors and will know contractors who have a record of successfully completed projects. In addition, local insurance agents and bonding companies will be able to recommend qualified contractors. A final source of information may be the local branch of the Associated General Contractors, which is the only national organization of general contractors representing all types of construction. This organization acts as a leading spokesman for the construction industry and was created to represent the industry in working with public officials and labor unions. While membership is voluntary, a contractor must have been engaged in the business of general contracting for two or more years prior to making application, and he must possess the essential attributes of skill, integrity, and responsibility. The AGC is comprised of over 8,500 members from 134 chapters and branches through the country.

Professional Qualifications and Experience

Perhaps the most important point to consider when selecting a contractor(s) is whether or not he has had experience with medical facilities. Correcting the mistakes of an inexperienced contractor can be both costly and time consuming. The experienced contractor, on the other hand, is able to discover and solve problems before construction begins. He will be aware of the most frequent trouble areas and will check them thoroughly as a matter of course. The competency and experience of the general contractor should be investigated just as carefully as that of the architect. How well a building is constructed from any architect's plans depends entirely upon the ability and integrity of the general contractor. Only contractors whose records reflect cooperation and who take pride in their workmanship should be considered. Many general contractors regularly check on a job year after year to make sure there are no problems with the completed project. Hopefully, any necessary adjustments and repairs are not additionally assessed. If a local contractor is hired, he will, of necessity, regard the present project in light of his future reputation. Most contractors will try to maintain good public relations with their clients.

Because a contractor must be able to control costs, his knowledge in this area is essential. His past performance should be evaluated in order to determine the relationship between actual costs and contract bids. If a contractor is not able to finish a building for the contract price, there always is the chance that he may be financially unable to complete the project or may attempt shortcuts, sacrificing quality for profit. Contractors also must be evaluated in terms of their ability to adhere to time schedules. The group assumes that the completion date will be met, and permanent financing may be dependent upon the facility being completed in the allotted time. The financial reliability of each of the contractors under consideration should be documented. It is almost certain that the group's financial lending institution will require such information. Contractors should have substantial bank balances with very few indications of past liens, defaults, or unpaid bills. This financial assessment can be accomplished by securing a formal financial report or comparable rating on the contracting firm, or by contacting bankers and asking them to appraise candidly the contractor's financial reliability. In exercising his financial responsibilities, the responsible contractor will not depend upon income from one contract to pay for another.

In evaluating the contractor's financial capabilities, it should be ascertained if he is bondable. Should a contractor become bankrupt during the construction project, a payment and performance bond will ensure that construction is finished and that materials and labor are paid for. Such bonds, however, cannot guarantee quality workmanship or job progress schedules, and a group may elect not to purchase them since they do constitute an additional expense. Bonds usually account for about three-quarters of 1 percent of the total contract but may be in excess of that amount depending upon the qualifications of the contractor. A bond may constitute a reasonable risk, however, if contractors are highly qualified, financially sound, and capable of being bonded.

One of the best means of evaluating potential contractors is to visit projects they have completed and to question owners of recently completed projects to discover if there has been any dissatisfaction. These clients should be asked if the contractor has been willing to return to make repairs and if there has been any charge for such repairs. The owners and the architects of previously completed projects can supply information about the ease of working with the contractor and whether he followed all plans and instructions carefully. The current construction schedule of each of the contractors under consideration must be evaluated and the contractors' willingness to devote time to the group's project must be ascertained. A contractor's location in relation to the site of the construction project is important. A local contractor may be desirable strictly from a public relations point of view; local workers may prefer to work with local contractors, and if the contractor is from outside the community, there may be delays due to worker shortages. Union or non-union requirements also must be determined. In some communities, all work must be done by union employees, even to the extent of unloading materials from trucks. If out-of-town contractors are selected, they may not be aware of such conditions and may later find it necessary to hire union employees. It should not be assumed, however, that contractors who use only union employees necessarily will charge a higher fee. Finally, the superintendents chosen to work on the job should be rated. Careful attention must be given to their qualifications, and it should be learned whether the general contractor would be willing to use the particular superintendents the group or its representative may request.

After interviewing and determining the qualifications of a variety of contractors, four or five qualified and competent contractors may be selected to bid on the project or to begin contract negotiations with the group or its representative. By having several contractors to choose from, the possibility of collusion among those bidding on the project is minimized. After the bids have been submitted, and if only contractors who are fully qualified for the project have been selected, it is reasonable that the contractor finally chosen will be the one who submits the lowest bid. If the low bid is over the building's budget, the architect should be willing to make changes in the design. The standard American Institute of Architects' contract provides for this responsibility if specifically requested by the owner. A group is, of course, free to choose any contractor, but if the bid method is used the group should have good reasons for not selecting the lowest bidder. In order to avoid any adverse feelings, if some criterion other than lowest bid is to be used in selecting the contractor, this criterion should be made clear to every contractor who is bidding the project.

If a bid bond is made part of the specifications, the contractor must submit a bond with his bid, usually in an amount of 5 percent of the construction contract. If the contract is awarded to him, a bid bond obligates the contractor to the bid he has submitted, usually for a period of thirty days, and ensures that he will proceed in good faith with the signing of the construction contract. This bid bond can be forfeited if it can be proven that the contractor has defaulted substantially.

Substitutions may be requested and approved during the bidding period, with specifications written so that the contractor has the opportunity to select from two or three previously qualified manufacturers of a particular piece of equipment. When a contractor requests approval of a manufacturer or supplier who has not been approved previously and whose name does not appear in the specifications, the request must be reviewed to determine whether it is acceptable based on the quality earlier established. If it is found acceptable, an addendum is sent to all contractors, notifying them that another manufacturer or supplier has been approved. All of this activity should take place during the bidding period and no requests for substitutions should be considered after bids are submitted.

THE CONSTRUCTION PHASE

The first order of business after a contractor has been selected and the construction contract has been signed is a preconstruction meeting of the medical group or its building committee with the contractor and his field superintendent as well as with the group's representative—an architect or a project representative, if the group has been working with a design/build or turnkey firm, or possibly a construction management firm representative. While the contractor should be thoroughly familiar with the drawings and specifications, a general review of these documents may be helpful and further clarification should be made as required. The contractor should present affidavits of the insurance stipulated in the specifications, along with a payment and performance bond if needed. All required forms should be reviewed at this time with special attention given to the contractor's request for payment, change orders, lien waivers, etc. A discussion of the procedures to be followed by each member of the team will contribute to common understanding and will help to minimize future problems. The responsibility and authority of each individual should be stated clearly and lines of communication firmly established. If confusion is to be avoided during the construction process, these lines of communication must be adhered to without exception. Assuming that there will be periodic site visits rather than full-time project representation, a preliminary schedule for such visits by the group's representative should be recorded, although it should be recognized that unscheduled visits also may be required as the construction progresses. If the project is relatively large, it may be highly desirable to employ a full-time representative who will be the official interpreter of the contract's conditions and the judge of the resulting performance. In actions under this status, it is incumbent upon such a representative to side neither with the owner nor with the contractor. He must use his authority under the contract to enforce its faithful performance by both parties. If the group is not dealing with a design/build firm, it may enlist the services of a professional construction manager; or, if construction management was not included in the original design/build contract but is deemed advisable later, it can be implemented under the Additional Services Article of the AIA contract (see Appendix 24A). When the architect acts as construction manager and thereby moves from owner's agent to impartial arbitrator between owner and contractor, the transition often is misunderstood by owners. While in this capacity it is the architect's responsibility to make periodic visits for inspection and review, the contractor has the prime responsibility of proper performance under the contract. The frequency of the inspection visits will have to be negotiated to the satisfaction of all parties involved, giving due consideration to costs and the availability of local inspections. The manager's right to reject work is provided for in order to enable him to meet his obligation to the owner, and is not intended to extend to the areas of safety precautions in connection with the work. It also is not his right to determine the adequacy of construction means, methods, techniques, sequences, or procedures.

The contractor has a variety of responsibilities, depending upon when he joins the group and the extent of the building project. If a design/build or turnkey approach is used, the contractor may have joined the group at the beginning of the project. It is not only wise to have the architect with the group during the early planning phases, but also valuable to have a contractor available for help with decisions during the early design phase. The contractor's most valuable contribution can involve construction methods and related construction costs. How well a building is constructed from any architect's plans depends entirely upon the ability and integrity of the general contractor. The contractor must stay abreast of the latest developments in the construction industry, particularly if he considers himself especially qualified in any one type of building project.

During the construction of a new building, the general contractor has two basic responsibilities. First, he must carry out the plans and specifications as stated in the building contract. Secondly, he must comply with the city, state, and federal laws and regulations. He also must furnish the labor, materials, and equipment for the building, as well as employ and supervise responsible subcontractors, and he should pay all permits, licenses, and taxes. In addition, it is the contractor's responsibility to provide protection on the job, both for the workers and the building itself. The contractor may be held liable for any injuries to the public during the construction phase, and the medical group should see to it that all of these provisions are included in the contract.

Many contractors keep daily logs, noting any trouble encountered from the weather, labor problems, or other situations they may consider beyond their control. These logs may provide the contractor with evidence that allows for extensions in time and for the avoidance of penalties. Since the contractor's log may or may not be accurate, it is suggested that the medical group or its representative also keep a record of the project's progress, carefully noting those events which later may lead to negotiations for time extensions.

The contractor usually submits a monthly request for materials stored on the site, materials used, and labor expended during the previous month. The group's representative should arrange to visit the site near the end of the month to discuss with the field superintendent the amount of work in place and the materials stored on the site, so that all parties concerned are satisfied that the contractor's request for payment is an accurate representation of the work and so that he receives the money due him. Change orders, sometimes called field modification orders, can be a general irritant; however, if all individuals bound by the contract recognize that situations will occur that could not be foreseen and if the construction contingency is funded in anticipation of these situations, the irritation of change orders can be reduced substantially.

The contractor should be partially responsible for solving various problems during the construction phase. While certain problems may not be attributable to him, he should seek the solution with the help of the owners, the architect, and/or the construction manager. The contractor also must understand and approve the construction manager's responsibility to inspect the project. While an honest contractor will not deliberately construct a facility below specifications, he should be aware of the possibility of mistakes inadvertently made by workers. If defects are suspected in the construction, it is the manager's right, on behalf of the owner, to have any work he may think defective uncovered. If work is in fact defective, it is the contractor's responsibility to make corrections at his own expense. Uncovering and redoing work which was done properly, however, becomes the owner's financial responsibility. The group's representative develops the so-called punch-list immediately prior to final review and approval of the completed construction. The list enumerates remaining items to be completed before final approval can be gained, and is turned over to the contractor as he completes the work. At the end of the construction, it is the responsibility of the contractor or the owner to file a notice of completion. If, after thirty days, no liens have been filed on the project, the portion stipulated by the contract to be retained is paid. At this time, the project should be totally completed. It behooves the owner to check the project thoroughly before paying out the retainage fee. After it has been paid, there is no financial incentive for the contractor to continue work on the project.

It is the contractor's responsibility to pay for all labor and materials. If the parties who have supplied labor and materials are not paid by the contractor, it is possible for them to file a lien against the project which will prevent the owner from occupying the building until the unpaid parties have been reimbused. The owner must be certain that all such payments have been made before the general contractor is reimbursed. There are a number of ways to ensure that the owner receives a finished project unencumbered by liens. A very common method is withholding payment to the contractor pending certification by the architect that the payment is in order. The lien laws of most states, however, leave the owner who does not take the necessary steps for his protection completely vulnerable to paying for a job twice. In most cases, the contractor must be able to produce a lien waiver or some other form of proof that materials have been paid for. The contractor may complain that he cannot possibly procure a lien waiver from a certain supplier. If this should happen, it is best for the group to make a check jointly payable to both the contractor and the supplier. The group then will have fulfilled its responsibility of paying for the work, and any conflicts between the contractor and the supplier must be settled between them.

Once again, emphasis should be placed on the importance of the communication process during the construction phase. A failure on the part of the contractor to ask questions and to clarify what ultimate results are expected too often has created large problems from what could have been minor difficulties. Lack of communication only contributes to the development of an adversary relationship. The means, methods, and techniques that a contractor chooses to use to achieve the desired results are his prerogatives and will vary among contractors. As long as the system used complies with the contract documents and contributes to the efficient completion of the work in terms of time constraints, these responsibilities should be left where they properly belong, with the contractor.

Appendix 24A

AIA Standard Form of Agreement Between Owner and Architect

THE AMERICAN INSTITUTE OF ARCHITECTS

AIA Document B141

Standard Form of Agreement Between Owner and Architect

THIS DOCUMENT HAS IMPORTANT LEGAL CONSEQUENCES; CONSULTATION WITH AN ATTORNEY IS ENCOURAGED WITH RESPECT TO ITS COMPLETION OR MODIFICATION

AGREEMENT

made this day of in the year of Nineteen Hundred and

BETWEEN the Owner:

and the Architect:

For the following Project:
(Include detailed description of Project location and scope)

The Owner and the Architect agree as set forth below.

MULTIPLE OF DIRECT PERSONNEL EXPENSE

I. THE ARCHITECT shall provide professional services for the Project in accordance with the Terms and Conditions of this Agreement.

II. THE OWNER shall compensate the Architect, in accordance with the Terms and Conditions of this Agreement.

A. *FOR BASIC AND ADDITIONAL SERVICES,* as described in Paragraphs 1.1 and 1.3, compensation shall be computed on the basis of a MULTIPLE OF DIRECT PERSONNEL EXPENSE, as follows:

Principals' time at the fixed rate of dollars ($) per hour.
For the purposes of this Agreement, the Principals are:

Employees' time (other than Principals) at a multiple of
( ) times the employees' Direct Personnel Expense as defined in Article 4.

Services of professional consultants at a multiple of
( ) times the amount billed to the Architect for such services.

B. *AN INITIAL PAYMENT OF*
dollars ($)
shall be made upon the execution of this Agreement and credited to the Owner's account.

C. *FOR REIMBURSABLE EXPENSES,* amounts expended as defined in Article 5, including computer time for professional services.

III. THE OWNER AND ARCHITECT agree in accordance with the Terms and Conditions of this Agreement that:

A. *IF SCOPE* of the Project is changed materially, compensation shall be subject to renegotiation.

B. *IF THE SERVICES* covered by this Agreement have not been completed within
( ) months of the date hereof, the amounts of compensation, rates and multiples set forth in Paragraph II shall be subject to renegotiation.

PROFESSIONAL FEE PLUS EXPENSES

I. THE ARCHITECT shall provide professional services for the Project in accordance with the Terms and Conditions of this Agreement.

II. THE OWNER shall compensate the Architect, in accordance with the Terms and Conditions of this Agreement.

A. *FOR BASIC SERVICES,* as described in Paragraph 1.1, Basic Compensation shall be computed on the basis of a PROFESSIONAL FEE PLUS EXPENSES, as follows:

(1) a Professional Fee of
dollars ($)

plus (2) expenses computed as follows:

Principals' time at the fixed rate of dollars ($) per hour.
For the purposes of this Agreement, the Principals are:

Employees' time (other than Principals) at a multiple of
( ) times the employees' Direct Personnel Expenses as defined in Article 4.

Services of professional consultants at a multiple of
( ) times the amount billed to the Architect for such services.

B. *FOR ADDITIONAL SERVICES,* as described in Paragraph 1.3, compensation computed as follows:

1. Principals' time at the fixed rate of dollars ($) per hour.
For the purpose of this Agreement, the Principals are:

2. Employees' time (other than Principals) at a multiple of
( ) times the employees' Direct Personnel Expense as defined in Article 4.

3. Services of professional consultants at a multiple of
( ) times the amount billed to the Architect for such services.

C. *AN INITIAL PAYMENT* of dollars ($)
shall be made upon the execution of this Agreement and credited to the Owner's account.

D. *FOR REIMBURSABLE EXPENSES,* amounts expended as defined in Article 5.

III. THE OWNER AND ARCHITECT agree in accordance with the Terms and Conditions of this Agreement that:

A. *IF SCOPE* of the Project is changed materially, compensation shall be subject to renegotiation.

B. *IF THE SERVICES* covered by this Agreement have not been completed within
( ) months of the date hereof, the amounts of compensation, rates and multiples set forth in Paragraph II shall be subject to renegotiation.

PERCENTAGE OF CONSTRUCTION COST

I. THE ARCHITECT shall provide professional services for the Project in accordance with the Terms and Conditions of this Agreement.

II. THE OWNER shall compensate the Architect, in accordance with the Terms and Conditions of this Agreement.

A. *FOR BASIC SERVICES,* as described in Paragraph 1.1, Basic Compensation shall be computed on the basis of one of the following PERCENTAGES OF CONSTRUCTION COST, as defined in Article 3, for portions of the Project to be awarded under

A Single Stipulated Sum Construction Contract

percent (%)

Separate Stipulated Sum Construction Contracts

percent (%)

A Single Cost Plus Fee Construction Contract

percent (%)

Separate Cost Plus Fee Construction Contracts

percent (%)

B. *FOR ADDITIONAL SERVICES,* as described in Paragraph 1.3, compensation computed as follows:

1. Principals' time at the fixed rate of dollars ($) per hour.
For the purpose of this Agreement, the Principals are:

2. Employees' time (other than Principals) at a multiple of
( ) times the employees' Direct Personnel Expense as defined in Article 4.

3. Services of Professional consultants at a multiple of
( ) times the amount billed to the Architect for such services.

C. *AN INITIAL PAYMENT* of

dollars ($)

shall be made upon the execution of this Agreement and credited to the Owner's account.

D. *FOR REIMBURSABLE EXPENSES,* amounts expended as defined in Article 5.

III. THE OWNER AND ARCHITECT agree in accordance with the Terms and Conditions of this Agreement that:

A. *IF SCOPE* of the Project is changed materially, compensation shall be subject to renegotiation.

B. *IF THE SERVICES* covered by this Agreement have not been completed within
( ) months of the date hereof, the amounts of compensation, rates and multiples set forth in Paragraph II shall be subject to renegotiation.

FIXED FEE

I. THE ARCHITECT shall provide professional services for the Project in accordance with the Terms and Conditions of this Agreement.

II. THE OWNER shall compensate the Architect, in accordance with the Terms and Conditions of this Agreement.

A. *FOR BASIC SERVICES,* as described in Paragraph 1.1, Basic Compensation shall be computed on the basis of a FIXED FEE
dollars ($).

B. *FOR ADDITIONAL SERVICES,* as described in Paragraph 1.3, compensation computed as follows:

1. Principals' time at the fixed rate of dollars ($) per hour.
For the purpose of this Agreement, the Principals are:

2. Employees' time (other than Principals) at a multiple of
( ) times the employees' Direct Personnel Expense as defined in Article 4.

3. Services of professional consultants at a multiple of
( ) times the amount billed to the Architect for such services.

C. *AN INITIAL PAYMENT* of
dollars ($)
shall be made upon the execution of this Agreement and credited to the Owner's account.

D. *FOR REIMBURSABLE EXPENSES,* amounts expended as defined in Article 5.

III. THE OWNER AND ARCHITECT agree in accordance with the Terms and Conditions of this Agreement that:

A. *IF SCOPE* of the Project is changed materially, compensation shall be the subject to renegotiation.

B. *IF THE SERVICES* covered by this Agreement have not been completed within
( ) months of the date hereof, the amounts of compensation, rates and multiples set forth in Paragraph II shall be subject to renegotiation.

TERMS AND CONDITIONS OF AGREEMENT BETWEEN OWNER AND ARCHITECT

ARTICLE 1

ARCHITECT'S SERVICES

1.1 BASIC SERVICES

The Architect's Basic Services consist of the five phases described below and include normal structural, mechanical and electrical engineering services and any other services included in Article 14 as Basic Services.

SCHEMATIC DESIGN PHASE

1.1.1 The Architect shall review the program furnished by the Owner to ascertain the requirements of the Project and shall confirm such requirements to the Owner.

1.1.2 Based on the mutually agreed upon program, the Architect shall prepare Schematic Design Studies consisting of drawings and other documents illustrating the scale and relationship of Project components for approval by the Owner.

1.1.3 The Architect shall submit to the Owner a Statement of Probable Construction Cost based on current area, volume or other unit costs.

DESIGN DEVELOPMENT PHASE

1.1.4 The Architect shall prepare from the approved Schematic Design Studies, for approval by the Owner, the Design Development Documents consisting of drawings and other documents to fix and describe the size and character of the entire Project as to structural, mechanical and electrical systems, materials and such other essentials as may be appropriate.

1.1.5 The Architect shall submit to the Owner a further Statement of Probable Construction Cost.

CONSTRUCTION DOCUMENTS PHASE

1.1.6 The Architect shall prepare from the approved Design Development Documents, for approval by the Owner, Drawings and Specifications setting forth in detail the requirements for the construction of the entire Project including the necessary bidding information, and shall assist in the preparation of bidding forms, the Conditions of the Contract, and the form of Agreement between the Owner and the Contractor.

1.1.7 The Architect shall advise the Owner of any adjustments to previous Statements of Probable Construction Cost indicated by changes in requirements or general market conditions.

1.1.8 The Architect shall assist the Owner in filing the required documents for the approval of governmental authorities having jurisdiction over the Project.

BIDDING OR NEGOTIATION PHASE

1.1.9 The Architect, following the Owner's approval of the Construction Documents and of the latest Statement of Probable Construction Cost, shall assist the Owner in obtaining bids or negotiated proposals, and in awarding and preparing construction contracts.

CONSTRUCTION PHASE — ADMINISTRATION OF THE CONSTRUCTION CONTRACT

1.1.10 The Construction Phase will commence with the award of the Construction Contract and will terminate when the final Certificate for Payment is issued to the Owner.

1.1.11 The Architect shall provide Administration of the Construction Contract as set forth in AIA Document A201, General Conditions of the Contract for Construction, and the extent of his duties and responsibilities and the limitations of his authority as assigned thereunder shall not be modified without his written consent.

1.1.12 The Architect, as the representative of the Owner during the Construction Phase, shall advise and consult with the Owner and all of the Owner's instructions to the Contractor shall be issued through the Architect. The Architect shall have authority to act on behalf of the Owner to the extent provided in the General Conditions unless otherwise modified in writing.

1.1.13 The Architect shall at all times have access to the Work wherever it is in preparation or progress.

1.1.14 The Architect shall make periodic visits to the site to familiarize himself generally with the progress and quality of the Work and to determine in general if the Work is proceeding in accordance with the Contract Documents. On the basis of his on-site observations as an architect, he shall endeavor to guard the Owner against defects and deficiencies in the Work of the Contractor. The Architect shall not be required to make exhaustive or continuous on-site inspections to check the quality or quantity of the Work. The Architect shall not be responsible for construction means, methods, techniques, sequences or procedures, or for safety precautions and programs in connection with the Work, and he shall not be responsible for the Contractor's failure to carry out the Work in accordance with the Contract Documents.

1.1.15 Based on such observations at the site and on the Contractor's Applications for Payment, the Architect shall determine the amount owing to the Contractor and shall issue Certificates for Payment in such amounts. The issuance of a Certificate for Payment shall constitute a representation by the Architect to the Owner, based on the Architect's observations at the site as provided in Subparagraph 1.1.14 and the data comprising the Application for Payment, that the Work has progressed to the point indicated; that to the best of the Architect's knowledge, information and belief, the quality of the Work is in accordance with the Contract Documents (subject to an evaluation of the Work for conformance with the Contract Documents upon Substantial Completion, to the results of any subsequent tests required by the Contract

Documents, to minor deviations from the Contract Documents correctable prior to completion, and to any specific qualifications stated in the Certificate for Payment); and that the Contractor is entitled to payment in the amount certified. By issuing a Certificate for Payment, the Architect shall not be deemed to represent that he has made any examination to ascertain how and for what purpose the Contractor has used the moneys paid on account of the Contract Sum.

1.1.16 The Architect shall be, in the first instance, the interpreter of the requirements of the Contract Documents and the impartial judge of the performance thereunder by both the Owner and Contractor. The Architect shall make decisions on all claims of the Owner or Contractor relating to the execution and progress of the Work and on all other matters or questions related thereto. The Architect's decisions in matters relating to artistic effect shall be final if consistent with the intent of the Contract Documents.

1.1.17 The Architect shall have authority to reject Work which does not conform to the Contract Documents. Whenever, in his reasonable opinion, he considers it necessary or advisable to insure the proper implementation of the intent of the Contract Documents, he will have authority to require special inspection or testing of any Work in accordance with the provisions of the Contract Documents whether or not such Work be then fabricated, installed or completed.

1.1.18 The Architect shall review and approve shop drawings, samples, and other submissions of the Contractor only for conformance with the design concept of the Project and for compliance with the information given in the Contract Documents.

1.1.19 The Architect shall prepare Change Orders.

1.1.20 The Architect shall conduct inspections to determine the Dates of Substantial Completion and final completion, shall receive and review written guarantees and related documents assembled by the Contractor, and shall issue a final Certificate for Payment.

1.1.21 The Architect shall not be responsible for the acts or omissions of the Contractor, or any Subcontractors, or any of the Contractor's or Subcontractors' agents or employees, or any other persons performing any of the Work.

1.2 PROJECT REPRESENTATION BEYOND BASIC SERVICES

1.2.1 If more extensive representation at the site than is described under Subparagraphs 1.1.10 through 1.1.21 inclusive is required, and if the Owner and Architect agree, the Architect shall provide one or more Full-Time Project Representatives to assist the Architect.

1.2.2 Such Full-Time Project Representatives shall be selected, employed and directed by the Architect, and the Architect shall be compensated therefor as mutually agreed between the Owner and the Architect as set forth in an exhibit appended to this Agreement.

1.2.3 The duties, responsibilities and limitations of authority of such Full-Time Project Representatives shall be set forth in an exhibit appended to this Agreement.

1.2.4 Through the on-site observations by Full-Time Project Representatives of the Work in progress, the Architect shall endeavor to provide further protection for the Owner against defects in the Work, but the furnishing of such project representation shall not make the Architect responsible for construction means, methods, techniques, sequences or procedures, or for safety precautions and programs, or for the Contractor's failure to perform the Work in accordance with the Contract Documents.

1.3 ADDITIONAL SERVICES

The following Services shall be provided when authorized in writing by the Owner, and they shall be paid for by the Owner as hereinbefore provided.

1.3.1 Providing analyses of the Owner's needs, and programming the requirements of the Project.

1.3.2 Providing financial feasibility or other special studies.

1.3.3 Providing planning surveys, site evaluations, environmental studies or comparative studies of prospective sites.

1.3.4 Providing design services relative to future facilities, systems and equipment which are not intended to be constructed as part of the Project.

1.3.5 Providing services to investigate existing conditions or facilities or to make measured drawings thereof, or to verify the accuracy of drawings or other information furnished by the Owner.

1.3.6 Preparing documents for alternate bids or out-of-sequence services requested by the Owner.

1.3.7 Providing Detailed Estimates of Construction Cost or detailed quantity surveys or inventories of material, equipment and labor.

1.3.8 Providing interior design and other services required for or in connection with the selection of furniture and furnishings.

1.3.9 Providing services for planning tenant or rental spaces.

1.3.10 Making revisions in Drawings, Specifications or other documents when such revisions are inconsistent with written approvals or instructions previously given and are due to causes beyond the control of the Architect.

1.3.11 Preparing supporting data and other services in connection with Change Orders if the change in the Basic Compensation resulting from the adjusted Contract Sum is not commensurate with the services required of the Architect.

1.3.12 Making investigations involving detailed appraisals and valuations of existing facilities, and surveys or inventories required in connection with construction performed by the Owner.

1.3.13 Providing consultation concerning replacement of any Work damaged by fire or other cause during construction, and furnishing professional services of the type set forth in Paragraph 1.1 as may be required in connection with the replacement of such Work.

1.3.14 Providing professional services made necessary by the default of the Contractor or by major defects in the Work of the Contractor in the performance of the Construction Contract.

1.3.15 Preparing a set of reproducible record prints of drawings showing significant changes in the Work made during the construction process, based on marked-up prints, drawings and other data furnished by the Contractor to the Architect.

1.3.16 Providing extensive assistance in the utilization of any equipment or system such as initial start-up or testing, adjusting and balancing, preparation of operation and maintenance manuals, training personnel for operation and maintenance, and consultation during operation.

1.3.17 Providing services after issuance to the Owner of the final Certificate for Payment.

1.3.18 Preparing to serve or serving as an expert witness in connection with any public hearing, arbitration proceeding or legal proceeding.

1.3.19 Providing services of professional consultants for other than the normal structural, mechanical and electrical engineering services for the Project.

1.3.20 Providing any other services not otherwise included in this Agreement or not customarily furnished in accordance with generally accepted architectural practice.

ARTICLE 2

THE OWNER'S RESPONSIBILITIES

2.1 The Owner shall provide full information, including a complete program, regarding his requirements for the Project.

2.2 The Owner shall designate, when necessary, a representative authorized to act in his behalf with respect to the Project. The Owner shall examine documents submitted by the Architect and shall render decisions pertaining thereto promptly, to avoid unreasonable delay in the progress of the Architect's services.

2.3 The Owner shall furnish a certified land survey of the site giving, as applicable, grades and lines of streets, alleys, pavements and adjoining property; rights-of-way, restrictions, easements, encroachments, zoning, deed restrictions, boundaries and contours of the site; locations, dimensions and complete data pertaining to existing buildings, other improvements and trees; and full information concerning available service and utility lines both public and private, above and below grade, including inverts and depths.

2.4 The Owner shall furnish the services of a soils engineer or other consultant when such services are deemed necessary by the Architect, including reports, test borings, test pits, soil bearing values, percolation tests, air and water pollution tests, ground corrosion and resistivity tests and other necessary operations for determining subsoil, air and water conditions, with appropriate professional recommendations.

2.5 The Owner shall furnish structural, mechanical, chemical and other laboratory tests, inspections and reports as required by law or the Contract Documents.

2.6 The Owner shall furnish such legal, accounting, and insurance counseling services as may be necessary for the Project, and such auditing services as he may require to ascertain how or for what purposes the Contractor has used the moneys paid to him under the Construction Contract.

2.7 The services, information, surveys and reports required by Paragraphs 2.3 through 2.6 inclusive shall be furnished at the Owner's expense, and the Architect shall be entitled to rely upon the accuracy and completeness thereof.

2.8 If the Owner becomes aware of any fault or defect in the Project or non-conformance with the Contract Documents, he shall give prompt written notice thereof to the Architect.

2.9 The Owner shall furnish information required of him as expeditiously as necessary for the orderly progress of the Work.

ARTICLE 3

CONSTRUCTION COST

3.1 If the Construction Cost is to be used as the basis for determining the Architect's Compensation for Basic Services, it shall be the total cost or estimated cost to the Owner of all Work designed or specified by the Architect. The Construction Cost shall be determined as follows, with precedence in the order listed:

3.1.1 For completed construction, the cost of all such Work, including costs of managing construction;

3.1.2 For Work not constructed, (1) the lowest bona fide bid received from a qualified bidder for any or all of such Work, or (2) if the Work is not bid, the bona fide negotiated proposal submitted for any or all of such Work; or

3.1.3 For Work for which no such bid or proposal is received, (1) the latest Detailed Estimate of Construction Cost if one is available, or (2) the latest Statement of Probable Construction Cost.

3.2 Construction Cost does not include the compensation of the Architect and his consultants, the cost of the land, rights-of-way, or other costs which are the responsibility of the Owner as provided in Paragraphs 2.3 through 2.6 inclusive.

3.3 The cost of labor, materials and equipment furnished by the Owner for the Project shall be included in the Construction Cost at current market rates including a reasonable allowance for overhead and profit.

3.4 Statements of Probable Construction Cost and Detailed Cost Estimates prepared by the Architect represent his best judgment as a design professional familiar with the construction industry. It is recognized, however, that neither the Architect nor the Owner has any control over the cost of labor, materials or equipment, over the contractors' methods of determining bid prices, or over competitive bidding or market conditions. Accordingly, the

Architect cannot and does not guarantee that bids will not vary from any Statement of Probable Construction Cost or other cost estimate prepared by him.

3.5 When a fixed limit of Construction Cost is established as a condition of this Agreement, it shall be in writing signed by the parties and shall include a bidding contingency of ten percent unless another amount is agreed upon in writing. When such a fixed limit is established, the Architect shall be permitted to determine what materials, equipment, component systems and types of construction are to be included in the Contract Documents, and to make reasonable adjustments in the scope of the Project to bring it within the fixed limit. The architect may also include in the Contract Documents alternate bids to adjust the Construction Cost to the fixed limit.

3.5.1 If the Bidding or Negotiating Phase has not commenced within six months after the Architect submits the Construction Documents to the Owner, any fixed limit of Construction Cost established as a condition of this Agreement shall be adjusted to reflect any change in the general level of prices which may have occurred in the construction industry for the area in which the Project is located. The adjustment shall reflect changes between the date of submission of the Construction Documents to the Owner and the date on which proposals are sought.

3.5.2 When a fixed limit of Construction Cost, including the Bidding contingency (adjusted as provided in Subparagraph 3.5.1, if applicable), is established as a condition of this Agreement and is exceeded by the lowest bona fide bid or negotiated proposal, the Detailed Estimate of Construction Cost or the Statement of Probable Construction cost, the Owner shall (**1**) give written approval of an increase in such fixed limit, (**2**) authorize rebidding the Project within a reasonable time, or (**3**) cooperate in revising the Project scope and quality as required to reduce the Probable Construction Cost. In the case of (3) the Architect, without additional charge, shall modify the Drawings and Specifications as necessary to bring the Construction Cost within the fixed limit. The providing of such service shall be the limit of the Architect's responsibility in this regard, and having done so, the Architect shall be entitled to compensation in accordance with this Agreement.

ARTICLE 4

DIRECT PERSONNEL EXPENSE

Direct Personnel Expense is defined as the salaries of professional, technical and clerical employees engaged on the Project by the Architect, and the cost of their mandatory and customary benefits such as statutory employee benefits, insurance, sick leave, holidays, vacations, pensions and similar benefits.

ARTICLE 5

REIMBURSABLE EXPENSES

5.1 Reimbursable Expenses are in addition to the Compensation for Basic and Additional Services and include actual expenditures made by the Architect, his employees, or his professional consultants in the interest of the Project for the expenses listed in the following Subparagraphs:

5.1.1 Expense of transportation and living when traveling in connection with the Project; long distance calls and telegrams; and fees paid for securing approval of authorities having jurisdiction over the Project.

5.1.2 Expense of reproductions, postage and handling of Drawings and Specifications excluding duplicate sets at the completion of each Phase for the Owner's review and approval.

5.1.3 If authorized in advance by the Owner, expense of overtime work requiring higher than regular rates and expense of renderings or models for the Owner's use.

5.1.4 Expense of computer time for professional services when included in Paragraph II.

5.1.5 Expense of computer time when used in connection with Additional Services.

ARTICLE 6

PAYMENTS TO THE ARCHITECT

6.1 Payments on account of the Architect's Basic Services shall be made as follows:

6.1.1 An initial payment as set forth in Paragraph II is the minimum payment under this Agreement.

6.1.2 Subsequent payments for Basic Services shall be made monthly in proportion to services performed so that the compensation at the completion of each Phase, except when the compensation is on the basis of a Multiple of Direct Personnel Expense, shall equal the following percentages of the total Basic Compensation:

Schematic Design Phase	15%
Design Development Phase	35%
Construction Documents Phase ...	75%
Bidding or Negotiation Phase	80%
Construction Phase	100%

6.1.3 If the Contract Time initially established in the Construction Contract is exceeded by more than thirty days through no fault of the Architect, compensation for Basic Services performed by Principals, employees and professional consultants required to complete the Administration of the Construction Contract beyond the thirtieth day shall be computed as set forth in Paragraph II for Additional Services.

6.2 Payments for Additional Services of the Architect as defined in Paragraph 1.3, and for Reimbursable Expenses as defined in Article 5, shall be made monthly upon presentation of the Architect's statement of services rendered.

6.3 No deductions shall be made from the Architect's compensation on account of penalty, liquidated damages, or other sums withheld from payments to contractors.

6.4 If the Project is suspended for more than three months or abandoned in whole or in part, the Architect shall be paid his compensation for services performed prior to receipt of written notice from the Owner of such suspension or abandonment, together with Reimbursable Expenses then due and all termination expenses as defined in Paragraph 8.3 resulting from such suspension or abandonment. If the Project is resumed after being suspended for more than three months, the Architect's compensation shall be subject to renegotiation.

6.5 Payments due the Architect under this Agreement shall bear interest at the legal rate commencing sixty days after the date of billing.

ARTICLE 7

ARCHITECT'S ACCOUNTING RECORDS

Records of Reimbursable Expenses and expenses pertaining to Additional Services on the Project and for services performed on the basis of a Multiple of Direct Personnel Expense shall be kept on a generally recognized accounting basis and shall be available to the Owner or his authorized representative at mutually convenient times.

ARTICLE 8

TERMINATION OF AGREEMENT

8.1 This Agreement may be terminated by either party upon seven days' written notice should the other party fail substantially to perform in accordance with its terms through no fault of the party initiating the termination.

8.2 In the event of termination due to the fault of parties other than the Architect, the Architect shall be paid his compensation for services performed to termination date, including Reimbursable Expenses then due and all termination expenses.

8.3 Termination Expenses are defined as Reimbursable Expenses directly attributable to termination, plus an amount computed as a percentage of the total compensation earned to the time of termination, as follows:

20 percent if termination occurs during the Schematic Design Phase; or

10 percent if termination occurs during the Design Development Phase; or

5 percent if termination occurs during any subsequent phase.

ARTICLE 9

OWNERSHIP OF DOCUMENTS

Drawings and Specifications as instruments of service are and shall remain the property of the Architect whether the Project for which they are made is executed or not. They are not to be used by the Owner on other projects or extensions to this Project except by agreement in writing and with appropriate compensation to the Architect.

ARTICLE 10

SUCCESSORS AND ASSIGNS

The Owner and the Architect each binds himself, his partners, successors, assigns and legal representatives to the other party to this Agreement and to the partners, successors, assigns and legal representatives of such other party with respect to all covenants of this Agreement. Neither the Owner nor the Architect shall assign, sublet or transfer his interest in this Agreement without the written consent of the other.

ARTICLE 11

ARBITRATION

11.1 All claims, disputes and other matters in question between the parties to this Agreement, arising out of, or relating to this Agreement or the breach thereof, shall be decided by arbitration in accordance with the Construction Industry Arbitration Rules of the American Arbitration Association then obtaining unless the parties mutually agree otherwise. No arbitration, arising out of, or relating to this Agreement, shall include, by consolidation, joinder or in any other manner, any additional party not a party to this Agreement except by written consent containing a specific reference to this Agreement and signed by all the parties hereto. Any consent to arbitration involving an additional party or parties shall not constitute consent to arbitration of any dispute not described therein or with any party not named or described therein. This Agreement to arbitrate and any agreement to arbitrate with an additional party or parties duly consented to by the parties hereto shall be specifically enforceable under the prevailing arbitration law.

11.2 Notice of the demand for arbitration shall be filed in writing with the other party to this Agreement and with the American Arbitration Association. The demand shall be made within a reasonable time after the claim, dispute or other matter in question has arisen. In no event shall the demand for arbitration be made after the date when institution of legal or equitable proceedings based on such claim, dispute or other matter in question would be barred by the applicable statute of limitations.

11.3 The award rendered by the arbitrators shall be final, and judgment may be entered upon it in accordance with applicable law in any court having jurisdiction thereof.

ARTICLE 12

EXTENT OF AGREEMENT

This Agreement represents the entire and integrated agreement between the Owner and the Architect and supersedes all prior negotiations, representations or agreements, either written or oral. This Agreement may be amended only by written instrument signed by both Owner and Architect.

ARTICLE 13

GOVERNING LAW

Unless otherwise specified, this Agreement shall be governed by the law of the principal place of business of the Architect.

ARTICLE 14
OTHER CONDITIONS OR SERVICES

This Agreement executed the day and year first written above.

OWNER	ARCHITECT
______________________	______________________

Chapter 25

Legal Considerations

DOCUMENTS AND REGULATIONS

A group that is legally established has set down certain policies and may have retained a lawyer to solve its organizational problems. Because the group's attorney will be involved in any building project throughout its development, and because he will need to review and to negotiate a number of contracts with architects and contractors, he must have a thorough knowledge of real estate law and the relevant aspects of tax law. These contracts will become key and essential documents representing the constitution and framework within which disputes will be settled. There are numerous form contracts for the construction industry as represented by the American Institute of Architects and contractors' associations. Contracts coming from any particular segment of the industry are tailored for the benefit of that particular group and will not necessarily represent the best contract or contain the most appropriate language for the purposes of the physician group. It is best, therefore, to have a carefully tailored individual contract drawn up by a qualified, experienced attorney.

If the group is planning to build a new facility, it must enter into a real estate transaction in order to buy, lease, or option a piece of land. A legal document stating the price of the land and the method of payment should be drafted. When the land is owned by the group, the first thing to be documented is the hiring of an architect with whom the group must enter into some kind of binding agreement stating his duties and responsibilities as well as his fee. The architect will require a survey of the building site and a soil report. Completing these legal documents may involve a substantial expenditure, so care must be taken in selecting competent professionals.

Obtaining a building permit also must be arranged for. The following quote from the Los Angeles Building Code indicates some of the difficulties that can be encountered:

> No person shall erect, construct, alter, repair, demolish, remove or move any building or structure nor shall any person commence any sandblasting, liquid washing, compressed air cleaning or steam cleaning of exterior surfaces of any building unless he has obtained the permit hereafter from the Department of Building and Safety.

The building permit is a necessary document under the law. In evaluating the project for tax purposes, the first item examined by the assessor will be the building permit application. Before this permit can be issued, all departments having jurisdiction must issue their approvals. The zoning department will review the proposed building to ensure that it conforms to requirements such as building height, setback, and building area. The fire department will review the plans for exits, horizontal corridors and vertical stairs, standpipes, fire-hose cabinets, and extinguishers. In almost all communities the traffic department also will check the plans for the safety of vehicular egress and ingress to the property. In many communities the industrial waste department will want to know how solid waste is to be disposed of. They also will be concerned with the appropriate disposal of contaminated waste. The city planning department, by verifying the legal description of the land, will make sure that the group understands the extent of the property. The description of the plot, together with all restrictions, easements, and right-of-way limitations, may be confirmed by planning department maps. Some communities may require street improvements; information on the implementation of these improvements can be verified by the building department.

In some cities, architectural review boards are responsible for ensuring that the architecture of new buildings is compatible with the region. These boards also approve signs, exterior graphics, and parking requirements. Communities having a master landscape plan will insist that the group's landscaping conform to the community's plan. Environmental impact studies may be required to show the clinic's influence in a wide variety of areas. Such a study may include the clinic's relationship to recently enacted conservation acts.

A medical group wanting to include a pharmacy in its facilities must obtain approval from the appropriate pharmacy department. Some groups may be required to secure the approval of the Federal Aviation Administration if emergency heliport facilities are bieng considered. The state's industrial welfare department also may evaluate the plans. This department is concerned with employee requirements, such as lounges and lockers, X-ray protection, and elevator safety. Finally, if the group is adjacent to a freeway, it is necessary for the state highway department to check the plans, and at the insistence of some communities, local police departments will evaluate the plans for building security.

These various applications usually are completed by the group's architect. It should be remembered, however, that almost all of the forms require the owner's signature. The group depends upon its architect to establish a good working relationship with the building department, and must rely on his judgment for the interpretation of building codes and the selection of construction materials. Nonetheless, the forms should be reviewed by the group's attorney to ensure that they embody the intentions of the group and that they are consistent with other legal decisions.

THE CONSTRUCTION CONTRACT

There are a variety of ways in which a group can enter into a contract with a building contractor, including negotiated contracts during the design phase, bid contracts after the design phase, and either single contracts with a general contractor or multiple contracts with a variety of subcontractors. The decision on which type of contract to use may be influenced by time considerations, the labor market, and costs.

A contract between the group and the general contractor involves initiating several important construction documents. First, the contract states what work will be done and how payment will be made; second, there must be a complete set of working drawings to indicate what is going to be built, including specifications for such details as wall finishes and light fixtures. These drawings and specifications do not merely suggest how the work should be done, but rather indicate exactly what the contractor is to do. The plans indicate what the group is paying for—no more and no less. It is the architect's responsibility to see that the work is done according to these specifications. Thirdly, the construction documents usually include bulletins and instructions to bidders. It may be that during the bidding period a general contractor will suggest in his bid a less expensive, yet acceptable, alternative plan. If this change is considered worthwhile by the architects, they may incorporate into the contract an addendum which is sent to all bidding contractors, thus enabling everyone to work from the same plans. All drawings and specifications become part of the construction documents and all are legal documents. If, for some reason, there are court proceedings, these documents serve to substantiate the initial agreements.

The construction documents also include a statement of the time schedule the group expects the contractor to follow. Unless a time schedule is included in the contract, contractors may be inclined to follow a schedule best suited to their purposes. Some short-time delays can be anticipated, but lengthy delays can and should be avoided as they may affect arrangements both for permanent financing and for occupying the new quarters. An experienced architect can estimate the length of time necessary to complete the project, and should assist the group or its representatives in planning a time and progress schedule with the contractor and receive his assurance that he will maintain it; nevertheless, it is often necessary that built-in penalties for failure to abide by the time schedule be included in the contract.

If the contract, either bid or negotiated, is with a general contractor rather than several subcontractors, the group should discuss with him his choice of subcontractors. It is not unusual for subcontractors to go out of business during the course of a building project, and this is one of the main reasons for difficulty in maintaining time schedules. It is important, therefore, that each of the subcontractors be thoroughly investigated. If a group is able to select its own subcontractors, it should be free to insist upon the use of those subcontractors and may want to have them bonded separately from the general contractors. If the group discovers that the contractors or subcontractors it wants to use cannot obtain a bond, it should proceed with caution. The inability to bond a job has nothing to do with a man's capability or even his past record, but almost exclusively with how much financial backing he has to commit to the insurance company who will write the bond. The group should not necessarily infer, therefore, that the inability to receive a bond is any indication of lack of capacity to do a job, and should deal with the situation accordingly.

At the beginning of the construction phase, the group will want all necessary insurance coverages to be in effect. Even though the contractor's general liability policy purports to cover the group's exposure, the group also should maintain its own coverage on the job. In addition, there should be fire, vandalism, and general property damage coverage on the construction job. If there is vandalism on the site, it will be the owner's loss. The group, together with its insurance consultants, should review all insurance policies to be certain that the necessary coverage is in effect and is included in the contract. The group also must consider insurance necessary during the moving process. The limitational liability in intrastate and interstate tariffs is very low and does not bear any resemblance to the potential damage that can be inflicted on the group's equipment. For example, if the carrier moves an expensive X-ray machine and destroys it, the carrier may be willing to pay only thirty cents per pound for it. The group should be certain to insure the move and to obtain a separate agreement with the moving company concerning additional liability.

The construction contract should provide that the architect may reject work unsatisfactory to him and may order the builder to uncover work already done. If work is uncovered and defects are found, the cost of uncovering usually is borne by the contractor. If work is uncovered and found to have been properly completed, however, the cost of uncovering is borne by the owner. The owner also should preserve in the contract the right to stop the work at any point. If the group stops work for purposes of its own, it may be responsible for whatever damages the contractor might suffer. Nevertheless, the group should preserve this option in the contract; inability to stop the work at a certain point may cost the group significantly more than simply a damages payment to the contractor.

Even in the best planned and best designed projects, it will be necessary to make some changes which may affect time schedules and the building itself. The owner should be certain that the contract makes provision for such changes and that any changes anticipated are presented in writing. Also, any additions to the cost must be set forth at the time the changes are made. The group should not leave these decisions until the end of the project, because such problems do not become any easier to solve. Both the changes and the resultant costs must be neogitated on a day-to-day basis. If changes are necessary, all parties should negotiate what the additional cost is going to be. The change order should be priced, signed, and approved.

It is the owner's responsibility to pay for the job. There are a number of ways to protect the owner against liens and to ensure that the owner is receiving what has been paid for. Withholding payment to the contractor until the architect certifies that payment is in order is one very common procedure.

The architect will not certify any payment from the owner to the contractor until he has inspected and approved the work covered by the payment. At this time, he will be certain that all materials, labor, and other items delivered to the job site in connection with the work have been paid for. If the contractor does not pay for these services, the owner later may be held responsible.

The construction contract may provide for the owner to retain a certain portion of the total contract payment. It is unusual to make full payment to the contractor at the time all work is completed. Rather, it is customary to retain about 10 percent of all payments (retainage). If the contract stipulates that at a point when the construction is 20 percent completed the owner should make a payment for the work done to that point, this total cost less a 10 percent retainage would be paid. This money becomes part of the retainage deposit which will protect the owner and ensure completion of the job. Many owners move into substantially completed buildings with most of the fee paid, but there sometimes remain a number of things for the contractors to complete. Often, arranging for the contractor and his subcontractors to send men back to complete these small jobs is a problem; therefore, the owners should be sure to maintain suficient financial leverage with the contractor to be certain that at the completion of the job it is absolutely necessary for him to accommodate their needs.

REQUIREMENTS AND COMPLETION

As the building nears completion, two additional certificates must be secured. A Certificate of Occupancy is issued to the owner by the department of building and safety. Inspectors from this department only approve the building for occupancy, and do not certify that it is complete. The department is concerned with the protection and safety of people in the building, not with whether the walls have been painted or the air-conditioning works. Although the owner may have a Certificate of Occupancy, this means only that the building meets certain minimum standards for safe occupancy, and not necessarily that it is finished. At the end of construction, it is the responsibility of the owner or his agent to file a Notice of Completion which serves to alert all mechanics and suppliers of materials that if they have not been paid, they have thirty days in which to file a lien on the job. At the end of that time, if a lien has not been filed, suppliers have no further claim on the project. Generally, it behooves the owner to withhold signing of the Notice of Completion for a period of time, because once it has been signed, the owner must pay out the 10 percent retainage and thereby lose his financial leverage with the general contractor. It also should be remembered that, while the contractor will be anxious for final payment, the signing of the Notice of Completion will signal the end of the construction loan period and the beginning of long-term financing. The group must be certain that it is fully able to take over the obligation of long-term financing which will include the principal in addition to interest.

Architectural and engineering design considerations will be considered in the following chapter. Requirements for patient and physician needs, center staffing, ancillary services, and interfacing with the hospital are among the influences which will affect facility design.

❋ *Chapter 26*

Architectural and Engineering Design Considerations

SITE DESIGN

The design of group practice facilities is a total process; regardless of the particular approach chosen, all aspects of design are related closely to one another as well as to all the planning decisions discussed in Parts I and II and particularly in Part III. Usually, the same design considerations must be evaluated and understood thoroughly regardless of whether an established or newly forming group is contemplating constructing a new building, developing leased space, or expanding an existing facility. The specific design of the group practice building represents the culmination of the group's decisions regarding mission, strategic planning, systems development, and related design considerations. With each group physician requiring approximately 1,000–1,600 square feet of space (medical plus support) at construction costs in 1974 of approximately \$35 to \$45 per square foot, the design of the facility has major long- and short-term practice and economic implications.

Site design is an integral part of *total* facility design. For example, how patients and staff enter and exit the site from the public road system is as important as how they enter and exit the building from on-site dropoff and pickup points and parking areas. Generally, it is undesirable for vehicular traffic to enter or to exit the site at a point adjacent to public roadway intersections. The same rule applies to high traffic roadways unless pulloff and merge lanes are provided or unless adequate traffic control systems are in operation. As a group increases in size and its staff and patient load increase these concerns become more critical. Some groups may want to consider pulloff areas to provide a patient dropoff area away from main thoroughfares. Regardless of who pays for the area, the jurisdiction of the clinic concerning parking enforcement should be determined.

Patient parking areas should be designed to service main entrances and patient dropoff points. If subentrances must be used for special departments such as industrial medicine or pediatrics, they too should be served by main patient parking areas. Otherwise, special patient parking areas should be provided. In addition, the main patient entrance to the facility should be visible from the vehicular entrances, from the route of these entrances to the patient parking area, or from the patient parking area itself. Should the group elect to charge patients for parking, rates, accountability for parking time (time stamped tickets), the location of parking cashiering, the closing time of the lot and/or the cashiering closing time, the possibility of free parking at night and the use of control gates are important apsects of planning. Provision for staff parking areas should be related to staff entrances; however, parking areas used by employee staff might well be on more remote parts of the site. Where contiguous site restriction is a problem, off-street parking for employee staff located within reasonable walking distance of the clinic is a possible solution. Physicians' parking should be close to the appropriate entrances especially for those physicians who make frequent vehicular trips to hospitals, etc. Site design also can be influenced if the group chooses to have controlled parking for staff and physicians, such as token or magnetic entry into designated staff and physician parking areas. Although control access instruments usually require less space than does time stamped equipment, the electrical, treadle, and gate requirements remain the same. Figure 26-1 is a sample site plan which depicts possible patient, staff, and industrial/emergency entrances in relation to a site parking plan.

A sloped site often is used in site planning to artifically differentiate parking areas. For some patients it is much easier to walk increased distances on a level surface rather than up or down a slope. Likewise, it is easiest to walk parallel to rows of parked cars and not to traverse through the rows. In addition, stepping onto and off of curbs can be difficult and dangerous for some patients. Wheelchair ramps should be installed for all curbs in patient/pedestrian circulation routes and where steps occur.

Estimating the number of required staff and physician parking spaces usually is an easy task and is related to the resource projections discussed in Chapter 4. Estimating the required number of patient parking spaces, however, often can be difficult. Demand projections, services offered by the group, style of practice, etc. influence the length of time patients spend in the facility. Furthermore, the location of the facility site in relation to other business, particularly shopping and hospitals, may have a significant influence on the length of time a car remains in the facility lot. A general parking rule of thumb is six to ten parking spaces per physician, including physician, staff, and patient parking. As one further parking consideration, some clinics and local churches have found that arrangements allowing the church to use the clinic parking areas on Sundays and evenings and the clinic employees to use portions of the church parking area during usual clinic hours can be mutually advantageous.

A separate building area may be designated for deliveries to the clinic (general supplies, laboratory reagents, X-ray film, core, vending machine stock,

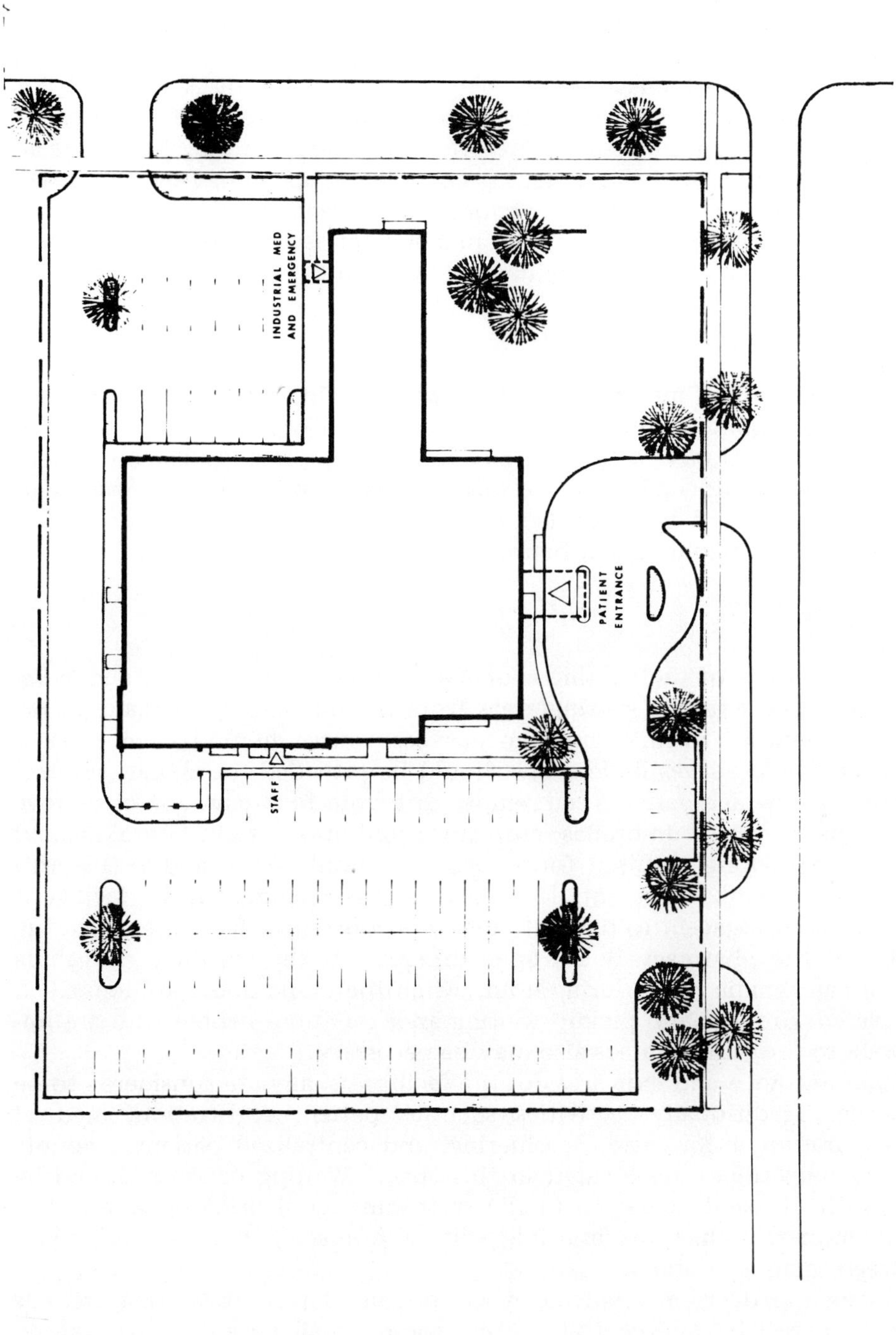

Figure 26-1. Sample Site Plan

etc.), especially as the clinic grows in size and in patient volume. To eliminate congestion, this area should be somewhat away from the busy on-site traffic pattern. It also may require visual shielding. Often, a receiving area relates well to outside mechanical equipment areas and their enclosures for maintenance, repairs, etc. In terms of image and public relations value, it is advantageous to present an attractive clinic frontage to major, off-site traffic routes. A special landscape design may soften the effect of a large parking lot and is an important facet of the total site design. Because landscape design services usually are not covered under a standard architectural agreement, the cost of design and of the actual landscaping should be planned for as a part of the total project budget and can vary significantly depending upon the group's interests.

BUILDING DESIGN AND FUNCTION

One basic philosophy of internal planning appears to dominate most successfully designed outpatient facilities and is appropriate to practices varying in size from the solo practitioner to the 100-physician group practice. The outpatient practice facility should include three basic types of space—public space and medical space separated by central control/administrative space. This philosophy is represented graphically in figure 26-2.

PUBLIC SPACE

Public space consists of the waiting rooms as well as their entrances and exits. Direct public access to the waiting areas from the main entry or main public circulation system is of prime importance; access routes should be well marked and obvious. Enclosed vestibule space should be provided for climate control and as a space in which patients can remove dirt from footwear, don or remove overcoats, open or close umbrellas, etc. Any prohibitions against smoking and stipulations concerning required footwear, etc., should be posted in this area to avoid possible embarrassment. If a pharmacy is included in the facility it should be located adjacent to the vestibule. It is convenient for patients leaving the facility if the pharmacy doors open directly off the vestibule. Vestibule doors then can remain open during hours when the clinic doors are locked. A small, covered, dropoff and pickup waiting area for those people who are unable to walk to the parking areas also may be necessary.

The main entrance and exit areas of the facility usually are considered to be prime space. Traditionally, activities such as patient registration, medical record preparation, information, cashiering, and centralized patient accounts (credit and collections) are located in this space. Waiting patients should be provided with efficient access to public restrooms, cool drinking water, and public telephones. If there are multiple waiting rooms, a public circulation system between them is desirable.

A fundamental decision involved in the design of patient waiting areas is whether there will be one central waiting room, small decentralized waiting rooms, or some combination of the two. Individuals who are proponents of one central waiting area (usually per floor) argue that:

1. One control desk with minimal duplication of support system and staff can serve many physicians.

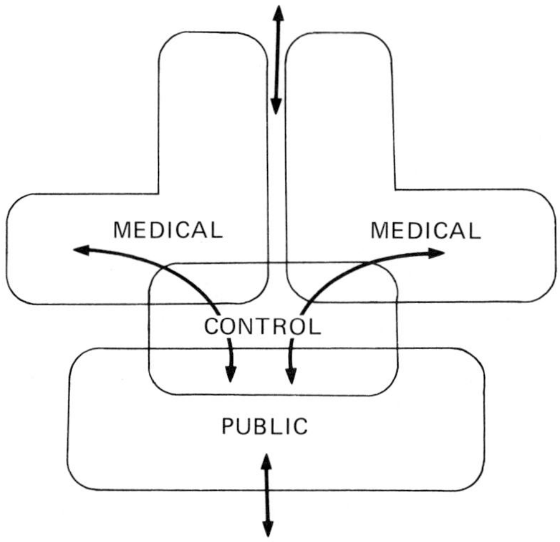

Figure 26-2. Three Basic Types of Space to Be Included in an Outpatient Facility

2. Small, subwaiting spaces can become individually overcrowded when a physician is behind schedule. In a central waiting room, however, this situation tends to average out.
3. A single waiting room can be subdivided into several waiting spaces through the technique of furniture arrangement, visual screens, planters, etc. The important functional consideration is that a single public space can serve several physicians through a single control point.
4. The central waiting area concept allows for greater potential flexibility in the planning of the medical space.

There are, however, three medical sections of the clinic which may have individual or subwaiting areas, including pediatrics, radiology (gowned patients), and emergency or industrial medicine. Supporters of decentralized waiting areas maintain that such areas provide more professional/medical control and are more individualized and personalized.

Whether centralized or decentralized, waiting area(s) should be within the visual command of the control function. Upon entering the area, the traffic flow should allow the patient to move directly to the receptionist. Controlling patients from a systems and design viewpoint also requires consideration. Many existing groups simply have the receptionist call out the patient's name as the physician is ready to see him. In large centralized waiting rooms where noise level may be high, the calling of patient names may be difficult and personally embarrassing. One alternative is to install a good quality paging system. If music is provided in waiting areas, the interface of a small amplifier and microphone with a feature to override the music is a very economical (approximately $100) and simple procedure. Several low volume speakers should be used in lieu of a few high volume speakers.

One final consideration in waiting room design is the potential for furniture arrangement. Furniture is usually arranged in waiting rooms to serve a specific purpose such as conversation and patient flow; to assume that the furniture will remain as arranged often is optimistic. One solution to the proper arrangement of furniture is to develop a diagram of the arrangement and fix responsibility for that continual arrangement on control personnel, maintenance personnel, or cleaning personnel.

CONTROL FUNCTION

The medical control station or desk (see figure 26–2, page 667) usually is located between the public space and the medical space and should be accessible from both these areas. The number and variety of functions that take place at the control desk will vary depending upon the size of the group and the manner in which particular specialties served by the desk operate. In a small, one-story facility all *medical* and *administrative* control functions may occur at or immediately adjacent to a single control desk. Such activities may include:

1. Patient reception and check-in
2. Both new and return *patient registration* and verification of recorded patient information
3. Insurance form activities
4. Credit interview (usually in adjacent office space)
5. Cashiering
6. Patient medical record preparation, control, and movement
7. Calling patients to the medical space
8. Telephone triage
9. Administrative and clerical work
10. Patient appointments.

In medium or large groups, some or most of these activities may be departmentalized, placed at separate administrative control desks, or completely removed from the control desk area. Those functions usually not removed from the main medical control desk are:

1. Patient reception and check-in for those sections served by the control desk, and often verification of registration information
2. Patient medical record control and movement
3. Calling patients to the medical space.

The control desk should be located adjacent to the medical record room or should be connected to it by a mechanical device designed for the transport of medical records and associated paperwork. If patient appointments are centralized at the control desk, the design and location of the desk will be influenced as will the mechanical requirements, such as conduit and counter openings for added telephones. Some form of sight and sound shield may be desirable at individual appointment and cashiering areas.

MEDICAL SPACE

The group's concept of medical practice should be built into the facility. It is unproductive to design a medical building that does not accommodate the group's mission(s) and objectives. The physician should have complete freedom to move about within the medical space without being seen by waiting patients, relatives, etc. Likewise, he should be able to enter and to leave the medical space and the building unobserved by waiting patients. Often, a great deal of medical activity occurs in or near the nursing stations (immunizations, routine tests, etc.) and in specialized rooms (measurement of aural and visual acuity, etc.). Lack of control in such areas easily can cause interruption of services and can violate the privacy reasonably due patients.

Examination Rooms

The style or manner of exam room utilization will influence room configuration. Exam rooms may be used only for examinations, with consultation rooms and offices provided separately or as combination examining rooms/offices. Examining rooms should be as close to the control complex as possible. Many architects feel that the optimum maximum walking distance from the control complex to the farthest examining room should not exceed ninety feet. Medical corridors radiating from the control complex with rooms on both sides have traditionally been an efficient and economical arrangement.

Medical space should be planned for internal growth, flexibility, and adaptability. To accomplish this goal, many architects contend that developing the largest reasonable number of functionally adaptable modular rooms along corridors of adequate width (approximately six feet) provides the greatest potential for accommodating the immediate and future needs of expanding groups. The same modular medical corridor that originally serves three family practice internists, two general surgeons, and one obstetrician can easily serve a seven-physician, or more, internal medicine section or a five- to six-physician obstetrics section. Suites specifically designed for two or three specialists will always remain two- or three-physician suites. In addition, a corridor serving six or seven physicians allows for efficient utilization of space as physicians rotate out of the clinic to hospital duties, vacations, etc. In small, specialized suites, however, such utilization becomes difficult.

The working cluster of rooms and the corridor or circulation system serving them should tie into the public space at the control desk. Medical corridors contain exam consultation rooms, exam rooms, offices, nurses' work rooms and stations, rooms designed for special use such as EKG, proctoscopy, minor surgery, X-ray and lab, plus other medically related functions. Usually, a ninety-foot medical corridor is sufficient for four to eight physicians, depending upon their specialties.

If the group decides to have each room specially designed, special suite arrangements must be made for each physician and activity within the group. Room size also is important. Unjustifiably oversized rooms are obviously wasteful, and undersized rooms are not only inflexible, less productive, and possibly inefficient, but also do not save construction costs proportionate to the reduction in area. Whether the exam room is 120 square feet or 80 square feet in area, it requires the same sink, door, and corner details. While lighting, heating, and cooling equipment costs may be reduced slightly, the basic components remain essentially the same. When a modular approach is used, however, the size and shape of a standard module can be established to satisfy the vast majority of such requirements. Different architects and groups have various opinions concerning the size of the optimum module.

Some feel that a space 9 × 13 feet in size is adequate. The 9 × 13 foot module and multiples of it can be designed to accommodate all of the activities usually found in a group practice facility. For example, a single 9 × 13 foot module can serve as a physician's office, an exam room, or a combination office/exam room. Figure 26–3 depicts a 9 × 13 foot module as an exam room, figure 26–4 as an office, and figure 26–5 as a dual purpose exam room and office. Space designed as multiples of the 9 × 13 foot module (18 × 13 foot module, 27 × 13 foot module, or 36 × 13 foot module) can accommodate specialized facilities for the ophthalmologist, otolaryngologist, radiologist, pathologist or pediatrician. In most instances, except for radiology and pathology, if specialized facilities are designed into areas which are multiples of the basic module, future conversion of these special facilities to standard sized modules is reasonably economical.

Visual and acoustical privacy are important requirements for any exam room. If the patient can hear conversation from the next room, he may be apprehensive and will be reticient to speak about his problems. Communicating doors, lightweight acoustical ceilings and untreated duct systems are common transmitters of sound. Building systems, including walls, ceilings, and doors, receive a rating—the Sound Transmission Class (STC)—according to their capacity to limit the transmission of sound. The higher the rating the more effective the sound barrier. Some architects contend that the minimum rating between exam room and consultation room should be in the STC forty to forty-four range. Others consider an STC of fifty to be common. Usually, it is not economically feasible to try to attain high sound attenuation through closed doors, ly feasible to try to attain high sound attenuation through closed doors, through the use of solid core doors. Because the corridor is not a conversation area, a weaker sound barrier is acceptable between the corridor and the room. Sound attenuation also can be improved by installing special weather stripping and drop bottoms on doors. This approach may be desirable on doors to rooms where psychiatric or hearing exams are conducted in which an STC rating of fifty-five to sixty may be required and also may help in areas such as cardiology where a physician's diagnosis is sensitive to corridor and other noise. An additional alternative in providing acoustical privacy in the exam rooms is the planned introduction of noise such as background music. Although initially expensive, when a central music system is employed, it may be appropriate to consider a volume control and even cut-off switches for each exam room. For example, although the cardiologist may not desire background music when performing a cardiac exam, he may wish to have music during consultation, dictation, etc.

Visual privacy can be achieved by draping windows adequately, by installing high window sills, by translucent glazing or omitting windows altogether, and to some degree, by screening the exam table from the opened door by having the door hinged in the direction opposite from usual installation. In addition, the exam table may be positioned at the left side of the room. By so doing, the foot or stirrup end of the table is angled away from the door, allowing placement of the dressing area behind the door and to the left so that persons entering the room must walk around an open door. Such an arrangement of the examination table usually is preferred by right-handed physicians because they usually prefer to examine the patient from the patient's right side.

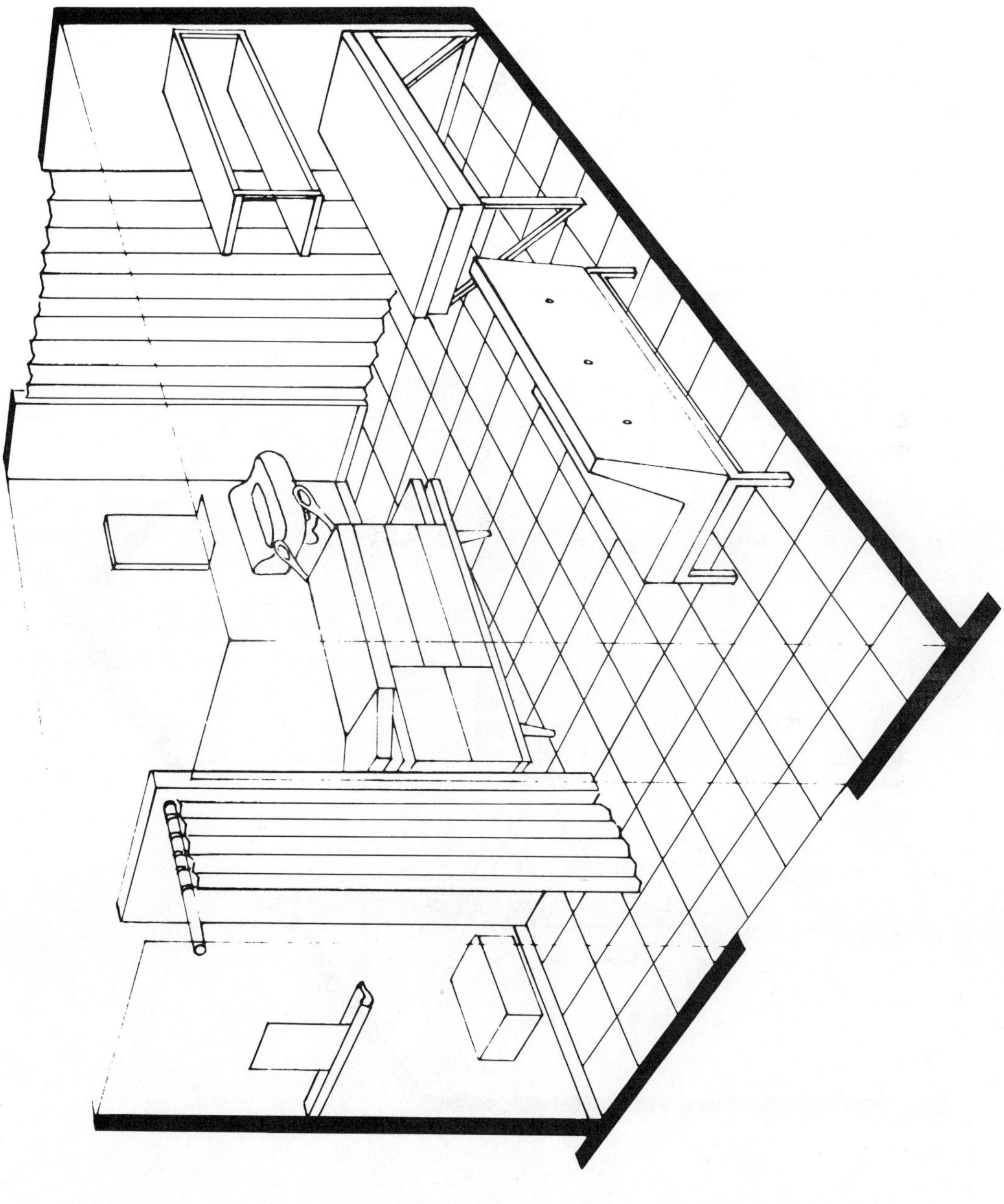

Figure 26-3. 9′ × 13′ Examination Room

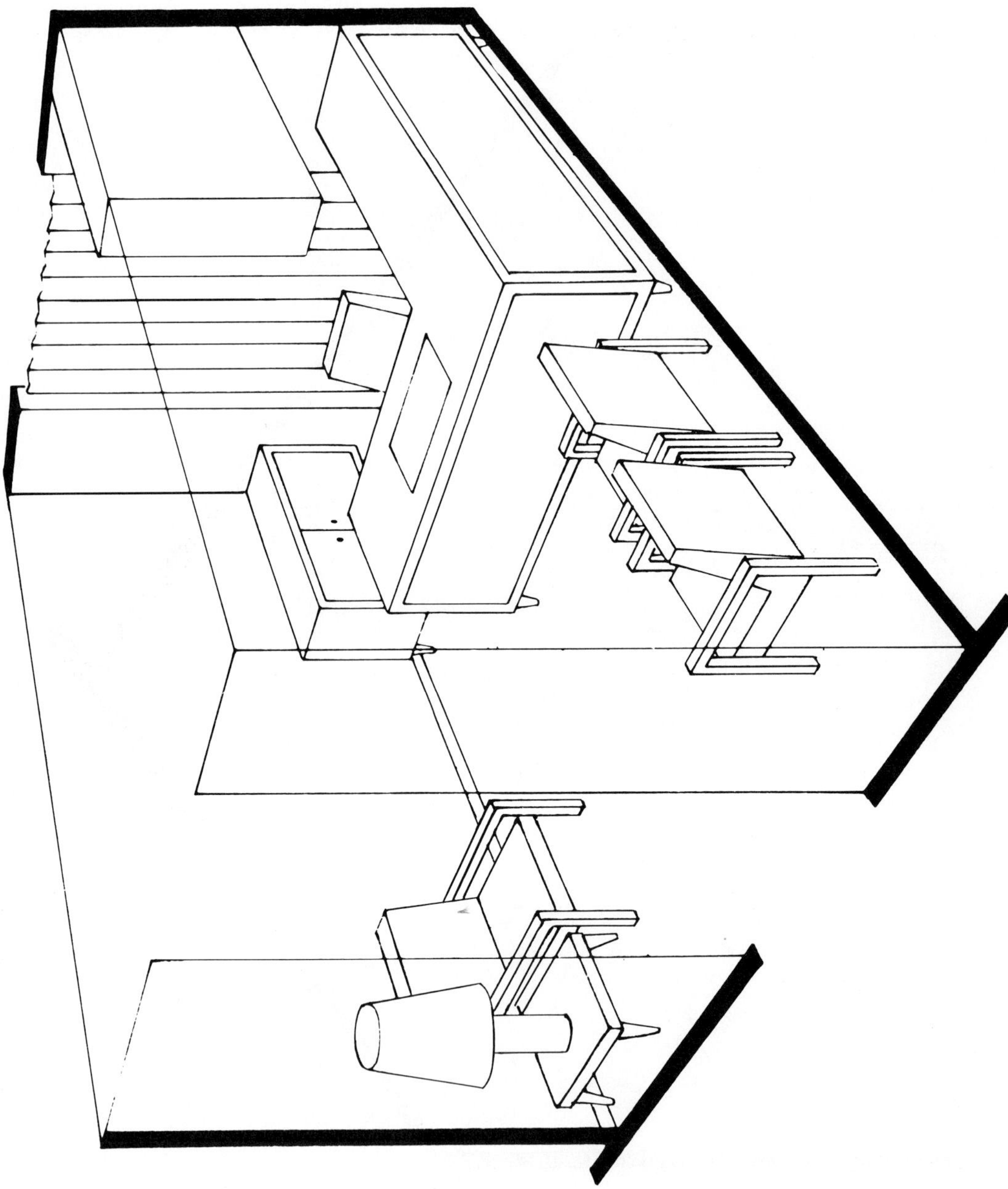

Figure 26-4. 9′ x 13′ Office

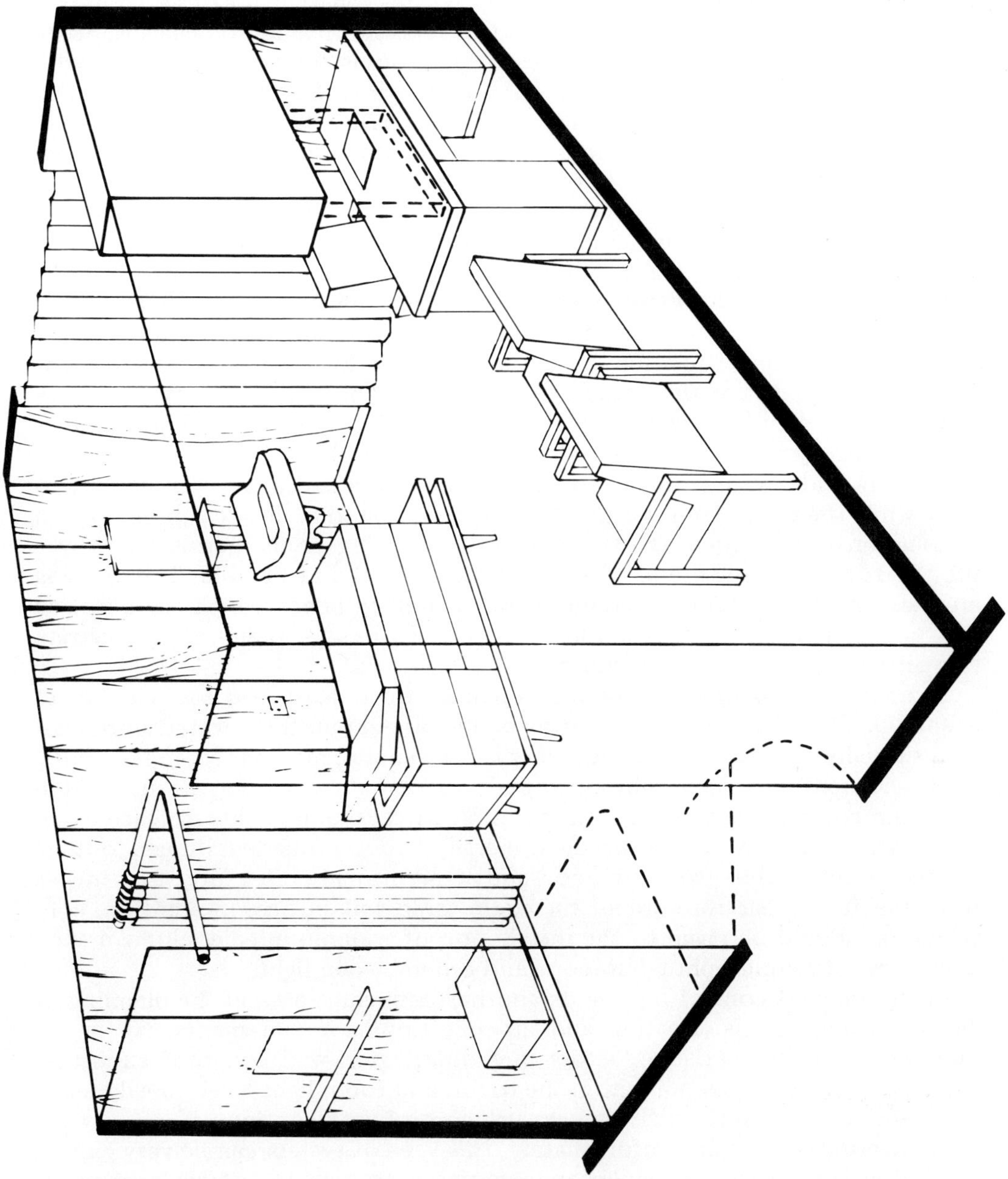

Figure 26-5. 9′ x 13′ Dual Purpose Room

Any electrical wires can be fed to the table at the point at which it comes closest to the wall, thereby avoiding the danger of exposed wires. An exam room for the left-handed physician is designed with the exam table at the right side of the room and with the dressing area behind and to the right of the door. Using a common wall for plumbing fixtures generally creates such mirror image rooms which are positioned for right- and left-handed physicians. Some physicians consider it a disadvantage to mix rooms for the left-handed with those for the right-handed. When all rooms are not identical, right-handed physicians may be forced to examine from the patient's left side. Although it may be economically advantageous to assemble plumbing and electrical outlets in a back-to-back configuration, the group will need to weigh such economies against its desire for rooms in which layouts are identical and interchangeable. Installing doors between examination rooms is generally discouraged by most group practice architects. Doors take up valuable wall space, cause acoustical problems, and further disturb room interchangeability. At a minimum, every exam facility should have a lavatory, an examination table and writing surface, a waste basket, one chair for the doctor and two for patients, an instrument stand, and a place for the patient to hang his clothes. When counter tops are installed, for stand up work the standard height is thirty-six inches while a height of thirty inches is acceptable for sit down work. A screened area for the patient to undress and dress also may be desirable and allows the patient to dress while the physician is writing his notes. If the group decides upon in-room dressing areas, a curtain suspended from the ceiling or the corner walls by a tubular rod or ceiling-mounted track is economical and flexible. The dressing area also might contain a wall-mounted or built-in bench which has a hinged seat and which can serve as a linen hamper. Figures 26–6 and 26–7 illustrate two different, typical room layouts.

Exam rooms require an illumination level of at least 100 foot-candles at exam table height (thirty to thirty-six inches). Four forty-watt fluorescent lamps usually will fulfill this requirement. If a general, modular room is decided upon and nonfluorescent lighting is used, a rheostat switch may be installed in the exam room to vary the illumination. Electrical requirements for each exam room also may be standardized. Generally, four grounded duplex outlets located twelve inches from the floor, and an additional outlet forty-four inches from the floor near the foot of the exam table will suffice. In addition, consideration should be given to the installation of wall-mounted equipment such as cautery, otoscope/ophthalmoscope and general exam light.

Environmental control represents another important area in the planning of medical exam rooms. Heating and air-conditioning requirements can be influenced by many variable factors including outer wall and roof exposure, weather, activity of people within the room, and room light level. Ideally, each room should have individual temperature control with continuous capacity for either heating or cooling. Unfortunately, this type of system can be very expensive. Alternative systems, which zone rooms according to typical occupancy and exposure are more economical, but not always as versatile. Environmental control in group medical corridors is particularly complex when compared to other medical facilities because the diversity of activity and procedures in rooms along a clinic corridor can vary from examining undressed patients to recording an EKG for a patient on a treadmill or ergometer. In hospitals, for

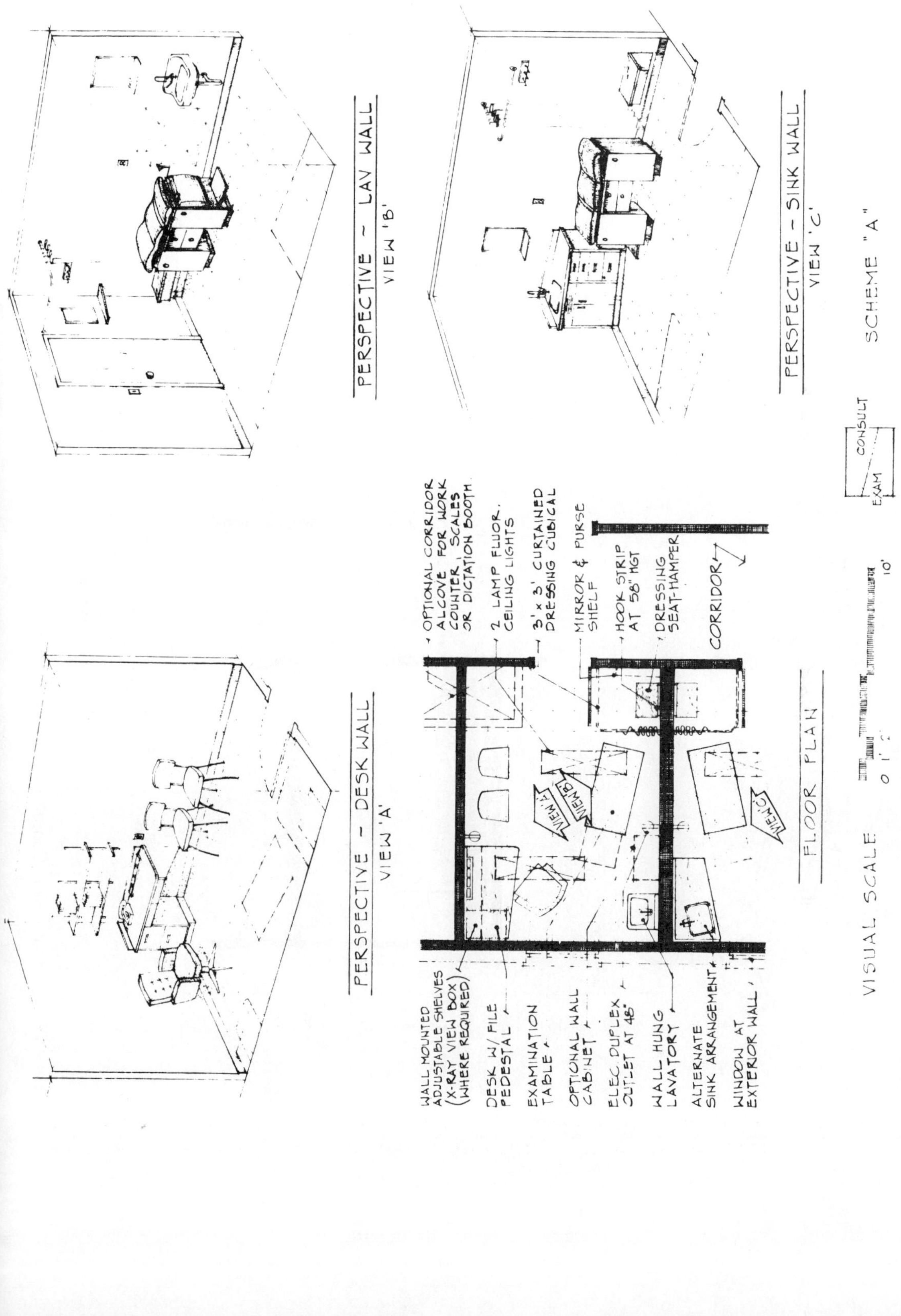

Figure 26-6. Clinic Exam-Consultation Room

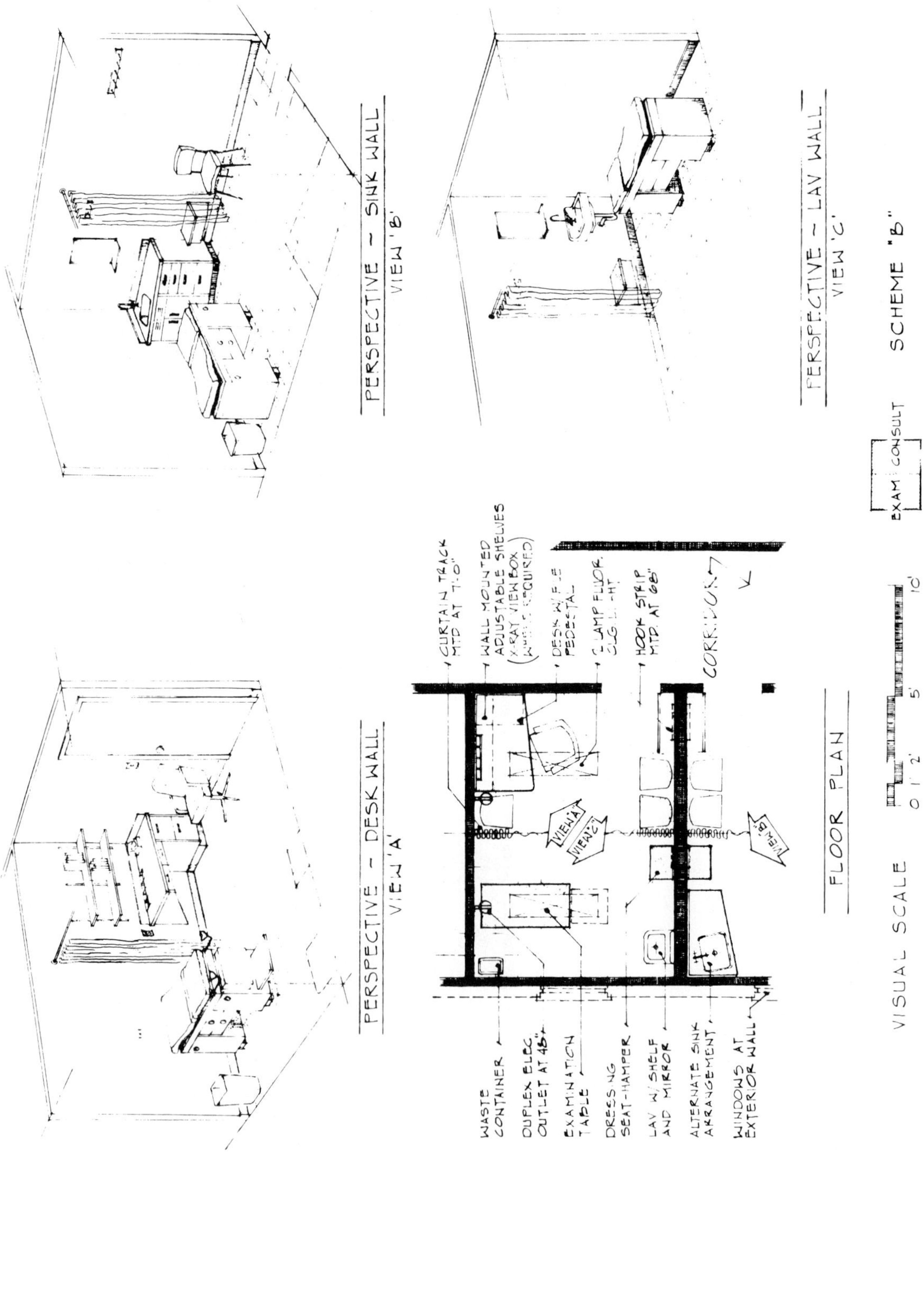

Figure 26-7. Clinic Exam-Consultation Room

example, similar activities usually occur over a larger area which may be more conducive to zone temperature ranges.

For either a tailored or a modular approach in the design of the medical corridor, consideration must be given to the placement of restroom facilities. From a purely economical and space allocation standpoint, restrooms in or directly accessible from each exam room are a prohibitively expensive convenience. Such facilities, however, must be easily available to urology and obstetrics patients. A sufficient number of restrooms also will be required to serve both staff and general patient needs.

After a specific room(s) design has been determined, the next major decision involves the number of specialized or modular rooms to be assigned each physician. Whether rooms are used for examination only, for consultation only, or for a dual purpose will influence this decision. The type of specialty, size of individual practices, and productivity are additional criteria that may be used to determine the number of rooms assigned and their specific locations. Among group practice architects, there is no universally accepted approach to the design of private office space for physicians. Many physicians do not require private offices as such, but rather employ the combination examination/consultation room concept with one such room assigned to each physician in which he can keep locked files and reference material. In some groups, this room is used by only one physician; in many groups, however, if a physician is not in the building, the room assigned to him may be used by other physicians as a combination consultation/examination room. In the event that group physicians choose to have offices apart from the examination rooms, it is possible to design the offices in standard modular size with plumbing and electrical services roughed in to allow for future conversion of the offices to combination rooms.

Within both individualized and modular approaches to the design of the medical corridor, the following specialists' rooms may require individual attention.

Allergy represents a potentially high volume practice in which traffic flow and adequate waiting space are important considerations. In order to determine reactions, most allergists will require observation of the patient for fifteen to thirty minutes following allergy procedures. The waiting room or a nearby room with a cot may be suitable for this period of observation.

Psychiatry does not represent a potentially high volume practice, but consideration should be given to whether a separate waiting area is required for psychiatric patients. Unless group therapy is a practice mode, the psychiatrist usually will need only one room with a residential living room environment. For group therapy, a 300 square foot area should be adequate. An exit which bypasses the main waiting area also may need to be planned for psychiatric patients.

Dermatology represents a potentially high volume practice. Because dermatologists usually receive and dispense large numbers of drug samples, an adequate-sized drug closet or cabinet may be required. In addition, the availability of natural light rather than artificial light may be necessary for making certain diagnoses. Other activities possibly associated with the dermatology area include X-ray therapy, ultraviolet therapy (requires aluminum foil walls), and electrolysis.

Obstetrics and Gynecology represent a potentially high volume practice. In the waiting room area, individual chairs with firm seats are more comfortable for pregnant women, than are low, overstuffed chairs. Because weight measurement and specimen collection are activities usually associated with each visit, accurate scales properly placed and an easily accessible restroom are important design factors. The location and placement of educational printed material and an area in which audiovisual media can be presented should be considered during the initial planning stages.

Ophthalmology requires special attention primarily because of the variety of practice methods currently employed. Traditionally, a distance of twenty feet between the patient and the refraction chart, plus the depth of the chair, produced a minimum depth requirement of 24 feet for refraction rooms. Through the use of projectors and mirrors, a shorter distance between chair and chart is now acceptable. In the specific design of the room and placement of the chair it is important to consider that the ophthalmologist have access to the patient from all sides. An electrically motorized chair as well as lights that can be dimmed may be necessary. Adjacent refraction rooms are diagrammed in figure 26-8.

Orthopedics represents a potentially high volume practice. Radiology, cast room requirements (storage and removals), injections, prosthesis, and physical therapy are functions usually associated with the practice. When radiology and physical therapy services are not included in the orthopedic suite, well-defined functional relationships and systems become necessary to accommodate the practice. The orthopedist often may require a six-foot exam table, placed against the wall, and six-foot corridors in order to observe patient gait and to accommodate patients on crutches, wheel chairs, etc.

Pediatrics is another specialty area which may require special design considerations. Pediatric exam rooms may be intentionally designed to be small to allow enough space for the patient, physician, and parent(s) but not for other family members. The design of pediatric waiting areas is highly controversial. The basic concern has been to avoid the spreading of contagious diseases among waiting children. Recently, however, a trend toward designing large waiting rooms with seating arranged to discourage social interaction between patients appears to be emerging as an acceptable approach. For patients who

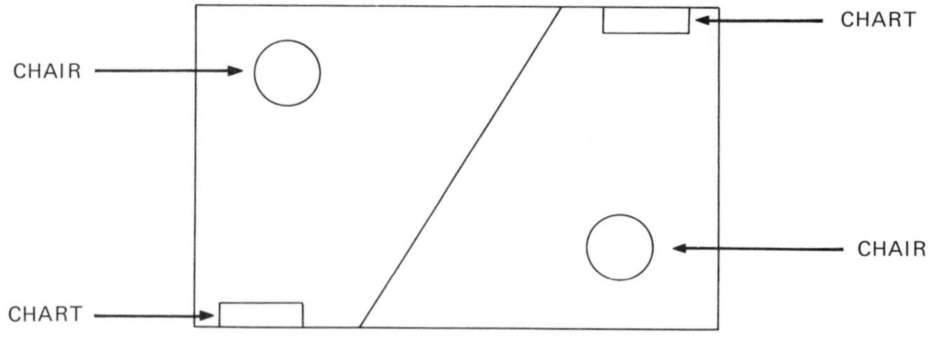

Figure 26-8. Adjacent Refraction Rooms

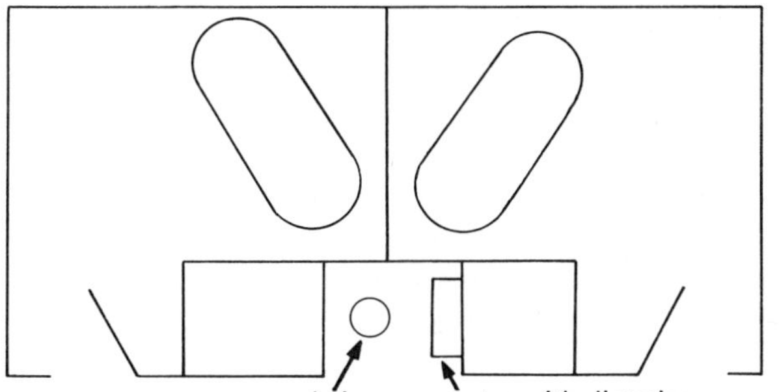

Figure 26-9. Dictation Booths

are identifiably contagious, however, waiting should be restricted to an isolated area.

After decisions have been made concerning examination and consultation rooms, attention should be directed toward arrangements for dictation. Dictation units may be installed in each exam room or dictation booths may be designed as part of the medical corridor. The system of medical dictation and the choice of centralization or decentralization of medical secretarial stations will influence this decision. If the group elects to include dictation booths in the medical corridor, one approach is the use of an alcove between two exam rooms, as shown in figure 26-9.

Nurses' Stations

Specific requirements for nurses' work areas in different specialties can vary somewhat. In a small facility with one or two medical corridors, one strategically located nurses' work area should suffice and can serve as a central nurses' supply area with wall and base cabinet storage units having ample countertop work area, a refrigerator, and a sink. The area also might serve as a small laboratory area with centrifuge and microscope. In addition, it often is desirable to locate a special nurses' triage exam room or injection room adjacent to the main nurses' work area. The area required for nursing stations will depend upon the duties of the nurses in the practice and the associated activities which must occur in the stations. In addition to housing supplies, other activities within the station might include:

1. Drug storage
2. Immunizations and reaction monitoring
3. Patient history
4. Patient height and weight
5. Routine laboratory procedures
6. Instrument sterilization
7. Telephone consultations

8. Appointments (decentralized)
9. Medical record administration, including progress notes, laboratory results posting, and radiology report inclusion.

It may be desirable to supplement the nurses' main work area with small (approximately five feet long and thirty inches deep) nurses' stations which are recessed in alcove fashion along the medical corridor. Nurses working out of these stations would have their primary base of operation directly adjacent to the rooms in which their physicians were working.

Architects generally agree that the *minimum* requirements for a nursing station are that it be a counter five feet in length and recessed in a corridor. In the typical group practice facility, nursing stations can be designed as alcoves, rooms, walk-through areas connecting medical corridors, or as a combination of these alternatives. The important consideration is that the functions of the nursing stations be detailed early in the planning process so that the design of the medical corridor can incorporate nursing activities.

Specialty Rooms

When modular specialty rooms are planned for activities such as minor surgery, proctoscopic exams, cast application and removal, pulmonary function and respiratory therapy, cystoscopic procedures, electrocardiograms, electroencephalograms, physical therapy, and multiphasic screening, it may be desirable to design such rooms as modules and a half—13 × 13 feet— or as multiple modules—18 × 13 feet, 27 × 13 feet, etc. This approach can provide additional space for storage and special equipment. A restroom adjacent to the *proctoscopy* room schould be accessible from both the proctoscopy room and the medical corridor. In addition, a built-in, water operated aspirator may be desired in the procto room. Floor drains often are desirable in *cystology* and *urology* exam rooms, and *proctology* rooms. In the cast room a plaster trap is required for the sink and a side drainboard is desirable on the surgeon's sinks in both *minor surgery* and *cast rooms*. Special electrical floor outlets also could be provided at the table location in both *minor surgery* and *proctology*. Specialty rooms are expensive and not always the most convenient when used for typical examinations; within smaller groups, therefore, one room may be established as a combination *minor surgery/cast room*. Many architects design the *cystoscopic* room with some of the features of an *X-ray room*, such as dark room, control area, and dressing area. In addition, a ceramic tile or terrazzo floor can be constructed with its base slanted to a floor drain.

Features of the *electrocardiogram area* are determined primarily by the type of EKGs to be performed, such as resting, phonocardiogram, echo cardiogram, masters two step, and treadmill or ergometer. In addition to specific procedural rooms, space for dressing, storage, tracing, cutting and mounting, and filing should be considered. If a dataphone is required to transmit EKGs to another location, planning for it should be considered as well as for the installation of a defibrillator, its storage, and its electrical requirements. Depending on the department's placement, shielding the room against radio frequency radiation may be important.

The types of minor surgical procedures to be performed in the facility will determine the design of the *minor surgical suite*. Generally, such rooms will require counters, a sink, and cabinets against one wall. An illumination level of 200 foot-candles at table height and an adjustable ceiling-mounted operating lamp also will be required. These fixtures are heavy and require special structural support frames. The design of the *multiphasic screening area* (automated or manual) will depend upon whether a carrel or station approach is used. When carrels are used, the patient is kept in one location with all the procedures of the screening performed at that location. When stations are used the patient moves from one station to the next to complete the screening. In terms of new construction operational efficiency and space economy, the carrel concept is preferred by many groups because one carrel requires only approximately 2400 square feet. Proponents of the carrel concept maintain that a four-booth unit can service 200 patients per day. Such activities usually include:

1. Medical history
2. Audio acuity
3. Visual acuity
4. Anthropometry (height and weight)
5. Pulmonary function
6. Tonometry (ocular tension)
7. Specimen collection (blood and urine)
8. Cardiovascular (EKG)
9. Mammography
10. Cytology
11. Physician consultation space.

Physical therapy represents another specialty area that will vary in design according to specific activities involved. In general, physical therapy can encompass therapeutic heat, diathermy, hydrotherapy, ultraviolet therapy, electrical stimulation, massage, and therapeutic exercise. If hydrotherapy is included, a floor drain usually should be provided. The typical therapy cubicle measures 5 × 8 feet with ceiling-mounted curtains, a therapy table (usually six feet), a clothes hook, and a chair or wall-mounted seat. The style of the group's practice can influence significantly the size of the physical therapy area. Therapeutic exercise equipment often requires structural ties to reinforced walls or ceiling structures.

The Walk-In or Immediate Care Section

Many groups are developing separate medical sections organized to satisfy their patients' requests for immediate care for nonappointment problems or minor emergencies, without disrupting the already tightly filled appointment schedules. Such a section may be described as an acute care area, an immediate care area, or a walk-in clinic. An area designed to serve these immediate care, minor emergency, and, possibly, related industrial medicine needs, also can serve as an after-hours clinic. The immediate care section, illustrated in figure 26-10, was designed so that it can be served by a separate mechanical system and can be closed off from the remainder of the clinic. The area contains its own public space—a patient entry, waiting room, and restrooms; a combination control desk/nurses' work room; a medical space made up of several combination examination-consultation rooms; a minor surgery-cast room; and a larger

Clinic Floor Plan

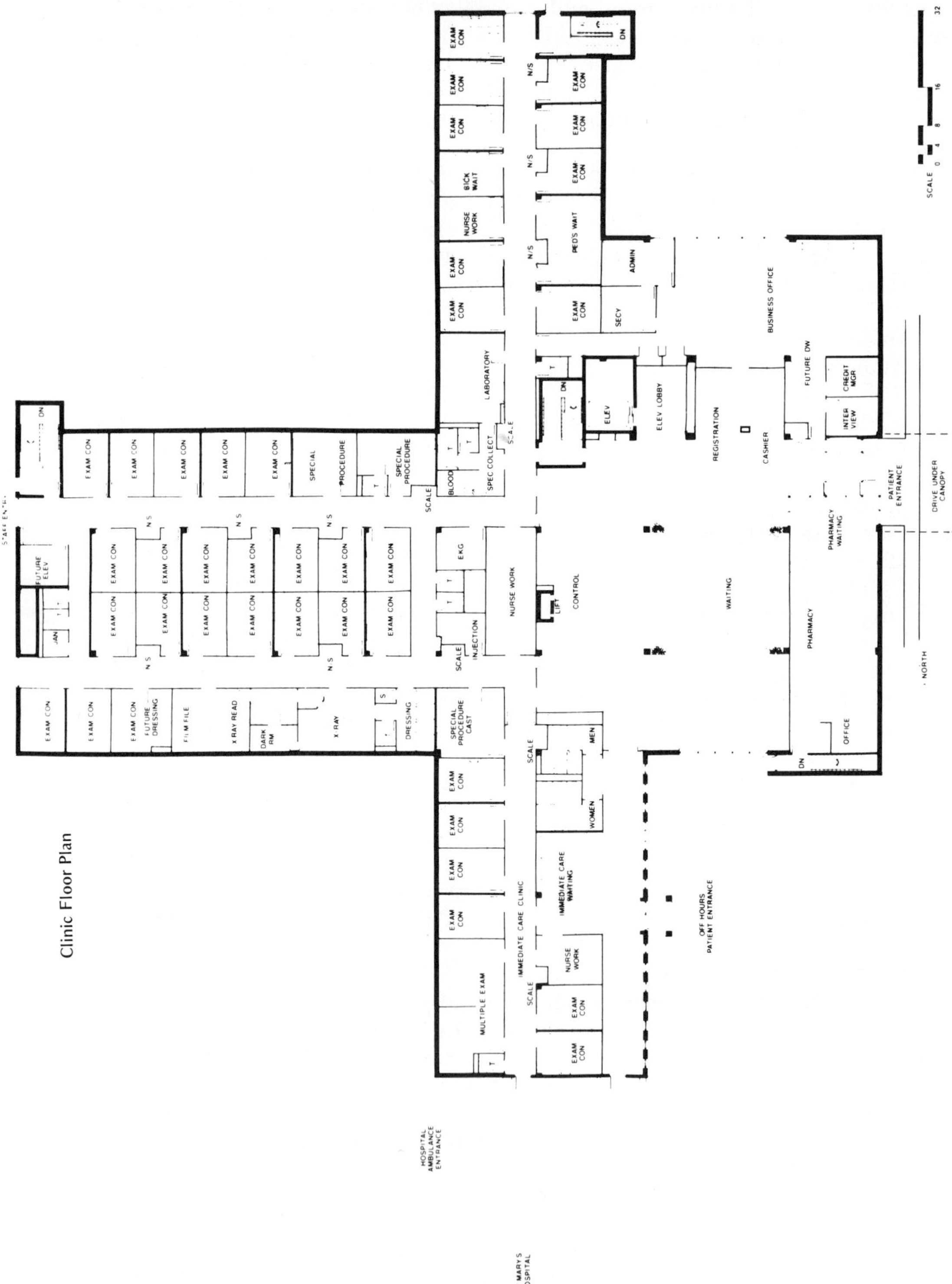

Figure 26-10. Immediate Care Section Designed to Be Served by Separate Mechanical System

general purpose module divided by curtains. After hours, medical personnel can have access to the remainder of the facility via the medical corridors. The special area may be used in lieu of a hospital emergency room by any of the group's physicians who wish to see a patient for a minor, acute need. If the facility is located adjacent to a hospital, patients can be transferred immediately to the hospital's emergency room if the need arises. During regular clinic hours, the special department is accessible through the main clinic entrance and lobby waiting room, except for those clinical emergency and industrial medicine patients who, because of their condition, must enter through the immediate care entrance.

Major Support Departments

Laboratory and radiology are the two largest medical support areas commonly housed within the medical group practice. Other than the mechanical equipment room, the *radiology* suite is probably the most expensive space in the facility in terms of building, remodeling, or relocating. The *laboratory* usually is second in cost to radiology. In terms of service operating expenses, Medical Group Management Association's 1975 *Cost Survey* (based on 1974 data) reveals that for the three- to ten-physician group, laboratory expenses account for 2.9 percent of gross revenue and radiology expenses for 1.5 percent. In comparison, the total expenses for all other medical and surgical supplies combined, including drugs, injectibles, laundry, linen, etc., total 3.3 percent of gross revenue. In a very small group, it often is difficult as well as undesirable to separate the laboratory and radiographic areas; it may be that one group of technicians can serve both departments. Furthermore, it is a convenience to a fairly large percentage of patients who must be seen in both departments on the same clinic visit if these departments are in close proximity. The experience of existing groups indicates that radiology usually grows faster than laboratory, and when these departments are located side-by-side, the expansion of one may cause the displacement of the other. Expansion can become extremely expensive when one of the departments must be relocated. With large groups, this problem often can be alleviated by placing the departments on different floors, perhaps directly over one another. Departmental growth then can be master planned into new adjacent space. When a multistory facility is being considered, the radiology department might well be located on the ground floor. Because of the weight and size of the equipment, and because of the weight of stored X-ray film, the floor structure must be carefully engineered. In addition, placement of doorways, elevators, and stairwells may not accommodate large, awkwardly shaped equipment.

The functions usually associated with the radiology department include patient dressing, waiting, radiographic control, processing, and film reading/reporting. One dressing room within the radiographic room can serve only one patient at a time, usually measures 4 × 5 feet, and generally is able to handle two patients per hour. Two to three dressing rooms should be adequate for each radiographic room. Providing lockers adjacent to the dressing area for storing patient clothing and valuables may increase the utilization of the dressing area and may lead to increased productivity of the radiographic rooms themselves. Because radiology patients usually are gowned while waiting, to prevent embarrassment, and if space permits, separate radiology waiting areas for men and women patients should be considered.

In most cases, one general purpose radiographic room should be sufficient to serve groups of from three to ten physicians. Most modern radiographic equipment operates most efficiently when structurally supported from above; a nine-foot ceiling is often the minimum required in a radiographic room. Depending upon specific equipment requirements, ceilings nine feet six inches or ten feet in height may be necessary. For the general radiology room, a minimum size of 13 × 15 feet (200 square feet) is required. Fluoroscopic rooms minimally require 15 × 16 feet. Because of the bulkiness of radiographic equipment, a minimum door size of thirty-six inches in width, and ranging to forty-eight inches, should be planned. If gastrointestinal studies are performed, a barium preparation area may be required. A floor drain and a restroom adjacent to the room are additional considerations.

The radiology room itself must be lead lined as must the control area which usually can be accommodated in a space three feet wide and two feet deep within the radiographic room. A sheet of lead one-sixteenth of an inch thick and seven feet high is sufficient in most cases. If there is occupied space below the radiographic procedure room, shielding in addition to the floor slab may be required. Traditionally, lead glass has been used for the control area, but many architects presently are using four thicknesses of ordinary glass. All requirements for X-ray shielding to be built into the facility should be verified by a qualified radiation physicist. The method of film processing chosen—automatic, manual, or a combination of the two—is an additional departmental decision which will influence the design of the radiology suite. In addition, whether films are sent out to be read, read by the ordering physician, or read by radiologists located in-house (centrally or decentrally) will determine many of the final design considerations for the radiology department.

When a centralized film reading and dictating area is planned, consideration should be given to the flooring in that area. Most radiologists stand to read film and to dictate reports, moving from one viewbox or strip to the next. Carpeting or cushioned linoleum, as opposed to a concrete slab or tile, provides a more comfortable floor covering in this area. The filing of film and medical records in a common room is found in small group practices, while separate film and medical record file rooms are more prevalent in larger groups. Usually, the radiologist will review a patient's film file, if one exists, for comparison with the film that he currently is reading. In planning for future expansion, a room intended as a second radiographic room can be used initially as a dark room or can provide convenient space for storing current film. Filing can be relocated to a new area when the second radiographic room is activated.

The laboratory area must provide space for two functions—specimen collection and laboratory analysis. Laboratory size, configuration, and equipment will vary depending upon the activities to be performed by the group practice lab and the volume of tests. Generally, the functions performed in the laboratory include hematology, biochemistry, serology, bacteriology, urinalysis, histology, and parasitology. When blood samples are collected outside the laboratory proper, they can be transported via lifts and/or conveyors to the laboratory for processing and results. If the group has a pediatrics specialty, a separate area for children's venapuncture should be considered. A minimum of two blood drawing stations should be planned and designed so that the patients cannot observe one another. Such an arrangement can be facilitated by placing two student-desk-type chairs side by side and 12 inches apart, with a curtain between them. It also may be desirable to provide a small, one- to four-seat waiting space off of the corridor adjacent to the specimen collection area.

For the small group, one urine collection room with a pass-through directly into the lab may suffice. In terms of convenience, efficiency, and future expansion, however, a minimum of two such rooms should be planned. It is desirable to shield the doors of urine collection rooms from the venapuncture stations both visually and acoustically.

While specific counter and equipment requirements for the working laboratory are dependent on the types and numbers of procedures to be performed, a working lab area of 240 square feet would appear to be the minimum for most small but growing groups who are performing usual blood and urine tests. Shortcomings commonly found in laboratory work space are a result of shortage of electrical outlets and a failure to plan for reasonably economical future expansion. A single outlet for every eighteen inches of countertop or continuous plug strips with a separate circuit every four to six feet of counter space is a reasonable rule to follow. After the lab's electrical requirements have been determined, consideration could be given to placing the entire laboratory on circuits separate from the balance of the facility, thus protecting instrument calibration, refrigeration, and timed tests while facilitating cost accounting. Acid resistant sinks, waste traps, and waste pipes usually are required in all laboratories. While a number of acid resistant countertops are available for a reasonable cost, standard plastic-laminate tops of good quality offer the greatest versatility for the price.

In developing a general design for a group practice laboratory, a check list of important areas includes:

1. Location of space for expansion
2. Electrical requirements and circuitry
3. Work counters thirty to thirty-six inches in height
4. Knee space for seated technicians carrying out hematology and microscopic procedures
5. Natural gas outlets
6. Refrigeration for the storing and possible freezing of specimens
7. Noise isolation of centrifuges
8. Fume hood or exhaust fan for areas such as biochemistry
9. An area in which to wash and sterilize glassware
10. A compressed air and/or vacuum source to dry pipettes
11. Shower or wash area for possible emergencies resulting from test accidents.

Because hot and cold water, waste, gas, compressed air, and vacuum plumbing facilities are required in the usual laboratory, color coding the plumbing by type facilitates identification of pipes when maintenance must be performed or modifications made to the system. Leaving pipes exposed in order to determine their function usually is not practical. The laboratory area should have a good ventilation and exhaust air system which generally keeps the lab under a slight negative pressure, thus preventing lab odors from drifting into other areas of the facility. From an environmental and safety standpoint, a lab exhaust to the outside of the building must not pose a hazard to neighbors and should not allow exhaust fumes to be drawn back into the clinic's ventilation system.

ADMINISTRATION-BUSINESS OFFICE AREA

In the small group setting, administrative and business office space should be versatile and flexible and, similar to medical space, may be designed either in modules or specifically to house each activity. If modular medical space is used, modular administrative space would provide functionally interchangeable areas. The administrator should be accessible to the physician as well as to the patient, and in the small group practice, the administrator often is chief accountant, credit manager, recruiter and personnel director, complaints recipient, purchasing agent, chamber of commerce representative, and building engineer.

The business office in the small medical group practice may house such nonbusiness office functions as the switchboard and the records room. No matter how small the group, however, activities such as accounting, typing, records filing, and switchboard should be shielded from the public space. Ideally, only reception, registration, cashiering, and appointments should be within the patients' view. Depending upon the operational mode of the group, the insurance department and patient accounts activities may or may not be accessible to the public. In a very small group, all patient-related functions may be the responsibility of one or two persons at the single control desk position. As the group grows, patient-related administrative functions can be separated from the medical control desk. The registration desk, for example, can become easily identifiable and accessible to patients as they enter the facility. The close system interface between registration and credit, however, would necessitate that the two activities remain in close proximity to one another. In most cases, the cashiering area should be obviously visible to patients as they leave the building.

If a central appointment system is to be used and the central appointment desk is to be available to the public, it should be located in close proximity to the registration desk, with the business office work area and administrative offices located behind the registration and cashiering areas. Typical administrative/business office space is shown in figure 26-10. As the group grows, administrative functions not directly related to the public could be relocated to more remote space, thus allowing for expansion of those functions related to the public. If sections of the administration and business office are to be separated and on different floors, it is desirable to consider connecting them with a document transport system. Sections often located in remote areas of the facility are administration (except for the credit manager), data processing, and certain insurance and bookkeeping functions. Adequate storage space should be provided for administration and for the business office, primarily for files such as administrative, personnel, accounts receivable, aging reports, accounting and budgeting transactions, etc. Off-site storage is a possibility for alternative storage space for such files; however, such a decision should be based on issues such as dollars saved, accessibility, and convenience.

MEDICAL RECORD STORAGE

Activities usually associated with the medical records department are:

1. Receiving, processing, and retrieving charts
2. Initiating charge tickets
3. Records storage
4. Records maintenance—posting hospital reports, lab and X-ray reports, etc.
5. Release of information
6. Preparation of new charts.

The degree to which some of these functions are performed by other departments, such as the preparation of new charts by registration personnel or the inserting of hospital, lab, and other reports into the chart by nurses, will affect space requirements. The system of filing records—file cabinets, vertical or circular shelves, or tracked shelves—will influence the amount of file space required. For example, an open shelf unit which is three feet long and has six shelves can accommodate approximately the same number of charts as can ten file drawers (two cabinets, four feet in width). Both file cabinets and open shelf files can be placed on tracks or wheels so that an aisle can be formed only when and where needed. There are available even more elaborate and automated methods of file storage and retrieval which require no aisle access space.

Appointment and registration procedures can have a significant influence on design of the medical records area. For example, if a requisition slip is used to obtain the medical record, its transportation to the record room must be planned. Assuming record files are on floor zero of a multistory building, a gravity chute similar to a mail drop in office buildings may be used. By including the chute initially, the cost would be relatively low. To decide later upon a chute may result in a ten-fold increase in expense. A lift or pneumatic tube also can be used to transport records to the requestor. In a small, one-story facility the record room may be placed adjacent to the medical control desk, but in larger groups with multiple control desks, the record room should be connected to the desks by a record conveyance system. These systems are available with capacity for both horizontal and vertical movement, but horizontal conveyance increases the cost of the system. In multistory facilities in which the medical record room is located directly above or below the stacked control desks, relatively inexpensive record conveyance systems can be used.

Internal system procedures within the medical records department also influence the internal design. As seen in the diagram below, initial space allocation may be six modules around the registration or control activity, with modules three through six housing active medical record files and modules one and two, inactive files:

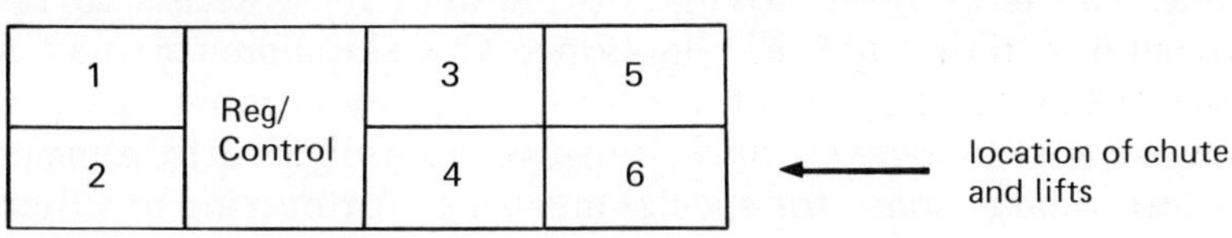

Record procedures may necessitate a conveyor using production type techniques. In this case, space might better be allocated and planned according to the second diagram:

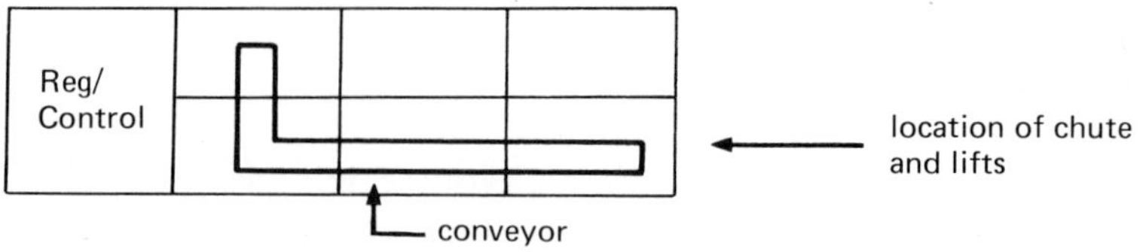

If appointments are centralized with a direct, in-house telephone line access for patient use, the central appointments area may be located within or adjacent to medical record areas.

The medical record room should be planned with a capacity for several years of growth, plus future expansion. While at some time computerization may eliminate the need for a large medical record room, presently the best method for limiting the need for record room growth appears to be the microfilming of inactive records. Off-site storage is another alternative for the storage of inactive files, but when supposedly inactive patients arrive and the record is not accessible, inefficiencies, delays, and inconvenience to both physician and patient occur.

Because medical records represent a substantial and irretrievable investment by the group physicians, adequate protection should be provided for the records. Many existing groups employ a sprinkling system in the records department (wet records often can be salvaged), along with a two- or three-hour fire resistant vault for fires occurring adjacent to the records space. Other activities closely associated with the medical records, such as insurance processing, record abstracting, or transcription, may be located in space adjacent to the records department, and acoustical shielding may be installed between different areas.

LIBRARY AND PHYSICIANS' LOUNGE

Many groups conbine the library and physicians' lounge into one dual-purpose space. Library shelving may be located along one or more walls or may be arranged as a small stack area. One end of the room often is designed for informal lounge seating while the other may be furnished with a conference table and chairs. A chalkboard and projection screen can be included for presentations and continuing education sessions, and provisions for X-ray viewing also should be included. Within the small group setting, lounge space also may be used as the radiology consultant's reading area. A small restroom area could be provided adjacent to the room, but should not open directly off of the lounge. A small kitchenette area may also be incorporated either in or adjacent to the lounge area. The employees' lounge also should have access to restrooms, a small kitchenette unit, and a telephone. One kitchenette may serve both lounges. Several existing groups have found that by combining the employees' and the physicians' lounges in one elongated area divided by a movable acoustical partition, a large space for special meetings, for nursing or other employee training, or for patient education classes is available when needed. In developing a long-range master plan, the lounges may be thought of as "soft" spaces which can be relocated to make room for those areas which must expand in place. Lounge areas should relate primarily to medical space rather than to public space. With easy access, lounges can be best utilized with minimum loss of staff time.

RECEIVING, STORAGE, AND MAINTENANCE

The receiving and refuse pickup area should be located so that site congestion is kept at a minimum. The refuse area should be visually shielded and must be monitored for refuse odor. The receiving area should be sufficient in size for short-term holding storage prior to transfer to the general storage area which may be a soft shell area planned for the future expansion of adjacent functions. This arrangement would necessitate the continuous regeneration of the storage area. Another solution is to develop dedicated storage areas. While this approach is not always economically feasible, one central supply room should be provided for sterile supply and pack preparation use only. In a small group, the nurses' work area may serve as the central supply room. In larger groups, the nurses' work areas may serve as secondary central supply areas. Finally, at least one janitors' custodial closet with a service sink and storage space should be provided on each of the facility floors. When space prohibits such closets, a small storage shed on the site might provide a suitable alternative for cleaning and maintenance storage.

OUTPATIENT PHARMACY

The pharmacy is a common adjunct to many group practice clinics. It may be run by the group or by an independent pharmacy in space leased from the group. If a pharmacy is a part of the program, it should be located adjacent to and be accessible from the public entrance-exit way. This location is convenient for the patient who otherwise would have to drive out of his way, park his car, and walk to and from a pharmacy. Drive-up windows are a possibility if they do not disrupt in any way the circulation of pedestrians and patient automobiles.

The size of clinic pharmacies can vary greatly. For groups of up to forty or more physicians, pharmacies with an area of from 600 to 1200 square feet, including storage, should be sufficient. Ascertaining pharmacy volume can provide space requirement guidance. Assuming that on the average each clinic patient will receive a prescription associated with a visit to a group physician, many of the planning concepts described in Chapter 4, which relate to demand and penetration projections, also could be applied to pharmacy volume. Rosenthall, in his unpublished book, *The Design of Medical and Dental Offices*, offers the following percentage of patients seen who are served by pharmacies in various types of outpatient facilities:

Facility	*% of Patients Seen*
Group Practice	90%
Medical Office Building	75%
Medical Park Project	40%

In addition, he projects that one pharmacist can fill between forty and sixty prescriptions in an eight-hour day. This rate can be increased to seventy prescriptions per day if a pharmacy formulary is adopted and used by the ordering physicians.

For planning purposes, each pharmacist will need approximately six lineal feet of counter space for compounding and packaging and an additional four lineal feet for labeling and dispensing prescriptions. Drug storage requirements for the lone pharmacist are approximately twelve lineal feet of tall (five to eight shelves), open shelf storage. Each additional pharmacist would require an additional six lineal feet of storage space. Other arrangements for the pharmacy include an adequate narcotics and dangerous drug storage area, a sink, and a refrigerator.

OPTICAL DISPENSING

Optical dispensing is an added service to clinic patients; visits to pick up eyeglasses or contact lenses or for fitting adjustments have no relationship to the ophthalmologist. Thus, a direct connection between the dispensing area and the medical space generally is not required; however, in cases in which a patient feels his lenses are incorrect, easy access between the physician and the dispensary is helpful. If optical dispensing can be located in an area that is accessible to all clinic patients, it will be able to serve the greatest number of patients with the least interference to the total medical group practice function. The space assigned to optical dispensing varies greatly; however, an area of from 250 to 500 square feet should suffice with 50 percent to 75 percent of that space assigned to fitting and display areas and the remainder to the work room.

HEATING AND VENTILATION

Heating and ventilation systems have a definite effect on the working environment and therefore on the comfort of both staff and patients. Generally, the minimum fresh air supply should be 15 percent with a maximum velocity of 800 feet per minute. In providing adequate heating and ventilation throughout the entire facility, some of the general considerations include:

1. Controls—individual room controls or zone controls
2. Supply and return air ducts in each room
3. Balancing dampers on trunk ducts
4. Ceiling diffusers and movable dampers
5. Steel versus fiberglas ducts
6. Turning vanes at duct elbows
7. Sound transmission
8. Continuous fan operation
9. Filters.

INTERIOR FINISHES

As the group practice facility is subject to high volume traffic, certain attention must be given to durable interior finishes that will serve the aesthetic requirements of both the group and the architect. High volume traffic can affect floor covering quickly; therefore, floor maintenance and long-term cost differentials should be considered. Many medical facilities use marble, terrazzo, or tile flooring because of its durability, but such materials do require regular cleaning and polishing. The use of carpeting is a reasonable alternative although it will significantly increase the initial flooring costs. Over time, however, carpeting may prove to be more economical when compared to the maintenance costs of other floorings. Should floor carpeting be chosen for all or for some areas of the facility, preference should be given to low pile-height, commercial carpet. Carpet, however, also must be properly cleaned and maintained on a regular basis, or it will show wear and quickly become unserviceable.

The walls in the group practice facility are the second most abused interior finish. When hard surface flooring is used, baseboards of sufficient substance and height should be considered along the wall base for protection against floor buffing and polishing machines. Existing group practice facilities employ vinyl covering, enamel paint, and wood paneling as favorite wall finishings. Ceilings in modern group practice buildings are most often acoustical tile.

ELECTRICAL REQUIREMENTS

Electrical requirements for each facility component have been discussed throughout this chapter. In summary, the electrical engineer should consider coordinating the total electrical design with facility consultants: laboratory, radiology, communications, and parking consultants. Planning should include an emergency power generator as well as an emergency PBX battery pack.

HOSPITAL-BASED GROUP PRACTICE

Although the master plan has important long-term significance to all operational modes of group practice, it has particular significance to the hospital-based practice because the growth of that type of group often is linked directly to the hospital's long-range projection. The hospital-based practice may encounter limitations in the initial facility design or renovation, and the group's facility may have to be linked directly in some way to the existing hospital facility. Consequently, for the hospital-based group, some of the design latitude discussed in this chapter may have limited application.

A common expansion strategy of many health groups appears to be to plan for a selective expansion of the staff in an effort to provide for the total outpatient medical needs of the patients they serve. Success breeds success. As the number of patients increases, so must the number of physicians within the various specialties as well as the number of specialties covered. Many groups whose original goal may have been primary care or single specialty have grown to include various new specialties and subspecialties. Ironically, the development of acute and primary care and family practice appears to be a trend in many highly specialized groups. Some groups also are gradually including multiphasic screening and one-day, outpatient surgery. The continuing addition of new services and specialties soon requires evaluation of existing facilities and their expansion, renovation, etc. The differences between programming and planning a free standing facility and hospital-based facility are minimal when both facilities have their own laboratory and radiology. When a group shares laboratory and radiology facilities with a hospital, however, the design and planning of these departments and their future expansion can become complex. In terms of the economics of the operation, such sharing can have definite advantages to both organizations and to the community as long as an equitable system is established for sharing costs and income.

Chapter 27

Equipment for a New Facility

ESTABLISHING CRITERIA FOR EQUIPMENT PURCHASING

Equipment needs will vary significantly depending upon individual group mission and planning decisions, as well as upon systems' design and facility configuration. Prior to any consideration of specific need, therefore, it is advisable for the medical group to establish guidelines for use in all equipment purchase decisions. The purpose of this chapter is to present variables which may influence the establishment of such criteria. As the group practice changes, these criteria may require revision.

The proximity of the new facility to a fully equipped hospital will affect many of the group's purchasing guidelines. If, for example, the group will be located immediately adjacent to a major hospital, there are some procedures and tests of a fairly specialized nature that might be more practical to perform on an outpatient basis using hospital equipment, rather than in the physician's office with equipment supplied by the group. While any revenue generated by these ancillaries would be lost to the group, the hospital would bear equipment expenses as well as operating expenses. An analysis of specific medical facilities, their technicians, equipment resources, and locations can assist a group in determining potential advantages or disadvantages inherent in a hospital-clinic equipment sharing relationship. In addition, tax regulations affecting profit and nonprofit entities, insurance reporting requirements, and federal regulations may affect any arrangements made between the group and a hospital. It also is necessary to consider the demographic characteristics of the group's anticipated patient service area (see Parts I and II). Population, age, race, religion, avocations, occupations, etc., will play an important role in determining equipment needs. Such needs vary according to the specific nature of the practice, even within a given specialty, and it is reasonable to assume that the character of the population served also will be influential. In all probability, the medical practices and equipment needs of the same multispecialty group would vary greatly if the group were located in New York City, or in Aspen, Colorado, or in Sun City, Arizona. Although not always a primary criterion, some thought should be given to the economic benefit derived by the group from any given piece of equipment purchased. Whether or not an item under investigation will pay for itself over a given period of time should be determined. Additional consideration should be given to alternative uses of the physicians' time if tests or procedures related to specific pieces of equipment are performed at another location by other individuals. Furthermore, the use of paramedical staff and the duplication of services offered by other segments of the medical community within a given area should be analyzed according to the long-term economic effects both may have on the group. One final consideration is the loss of control associated with another organization's performing patient services which the group itself does not or cannot offer. This loss of control can range from the inability to arrange for group patients to be seen when necessary to the actual loss of patients to other organizations better equipped to perform certain services.

EQUIPMENT SHARING

The next phase in establishing equipment needs is to determine how acceptable the concept of sharing with one another is among members of the group. For example, it is less expensive initially and will reduce ongoing maintenance costs if ten people use one duplicating machine rather than each individual having his own machine. Usually, sharing enables the group to purchase a better, more flexible, and probably more efficient piece of equipment. Ten physicians plus attendant personnel using one piece of equipment may necessitate scheduling, but this inconvenience may be a small price for the benefits accruing. Obviously, equipment which relates to only one specialty or subspecialty cannot be purchased on a shared basis. The ultimate approach in sharing, however, includes not only equipment but also clinic areas such as waiting rooms, exam rooms, consultation and office areas, business and reception areas, cast rooms, special procedure rooms, lab and X-ray facilities, etc. Again, the obvious benefits are decreased cost and maximum utilization of required equipment. Sharing such areas in the clinic on a scheduled, staggered basis not only reduces the overall area required, but also reduces the number of rooms needing equipment and furnishing. In addition, the efficiency of technicians working in these areas should increase; rather than expecting one person to be a competent nurse, lab technician, receptionist, insurance clerk, and record librarian, several individuals could specialize in only one or two endeavors, and could do so with increased efficiency. The sharing concept also allows the group to purchase highly specialized equipment, which often is not practical for a single practitioner. With medical technology changing as rapidly as it has in recent years, some physicians have ordered equipment that required a substantial lead time, only to discover that when it finally was delivered, it already was somewhat outdated or functionally obsolete. Sharing equipment could increase equipment use and thereby partially close the gap between physical and technical obsolescence.

PURCHASING EQUIPMENT

With basic planning and analysis and an inventory of existing equipment accomplished, the group is ready to contact equipment suppliers and salesmen. At this point, the traditional equipment check list should be helpful and should be consulted. The Department of Health, Education and Welfare's publication entitled *Equipment Guidelines for Ambulatory Health Centers* will prove especially helpful in this area. Check lists may not help in determining need but should remind the group of any major item which may have been overlooked; initially, overbuying usually is more prevalent than overlooking. If a piece of equipment is questionable, it is probably prudent to wait until a need can be justified concretely. If a knowledgeable consultant is available who is thoroughly acquainted with the specific practice or potential practice, his assistance can be invaluable. Many consultants, however, are in fact equipment suppliers or salesmen and consequently may offer the group advice which is biased.

The final ingredient in determining what equipment is to be acquired involves the equipment budget. Need is irrelevant if acquisition is impossible. The high "start-up cost" for a new practice is generally understood; however, outright cash on delivery purchase is not the only plan available to most new groups. When discussing equipment acquisition, two basic alternatives should be considered—purchase or lease. There are, of course, almost as many subtle variations of these alternatives as there are equipment suppliers and money lenders. In its simplest terms, the decision to lease or to purchase is a choice between two methods of financing equipment necessary for the practice. As such, the conclusion must be appropriate and considered within the context of the overall financial planning for the practice. Any discussion of economic alternatives should include a consideration of the cost of the money involved. In evaluating a leasing proposal, as opposed to a sales contract, the length of the lease period as well as the amount of interest charged should be considered carefully. When comparing sale to lease over the same number of years, the difference between the outright sale price and the cost of leasing is equivalent to interest. If maintenance is included in a package price, however, it may be difficult to determine exactly how much is being paid for the principal and how much for the interest and maintenance. It is common practice for companies to use a standard interest rate applied to the sale price to determine lease charges. In a conditional sales contract, interest is deductible for tax purposes while principal is not.

Whether borrowed from an external source or generated internally from earnings, capital used for equipment purchase, down payment or deposit, or for monthly payments does have an assignable value. The cost of capital is the interest paid to a bank for money used to conduct business. Capital financing can be obtained from a wide variety of sources, and rates will vary with the type of source involved, the group's size, its earnings, and its credit rating. For comparison purposes, usually an average cost of capital is used and is expressed as a percentage. As with the purchase of any capital equipment, the purchase of medical equipment will allow for the recovery of the purchase through depreciation over the useful life of the equipment and through possible resale. Judgments may vary as to type of depreciation method used and the length of useful life of the equipment. Acceleration depreciation methods are currently permitted for tax purposes.

Medical equipment also is subject to various taxes. *Sales tax* may be levied by the state, the city, or both, and items considered taxable will vary by location. Typically, the tax is based on the purchase price or its equivalent value (total installed cost). Many districts also apply the tax to services, such as maintenance contracts and lease payments, even when title does not pass to the lessee. Actual state tax rates typically vary from 3 percent to 7 percent with an average of 5 percent in many states. The addition of a city sales tax may result in a slightly higher rate. *Personal property tax* usually is applicable to purchased medical equipment and usually is levied in terms of dollars per hundred dollars assessed valuation. While the definition of assessed valuation differs from state to state, there are two basic approaches to assessing valuation of equipment; valuation may be based on purchase price, with a possible allowance for depreciation, or may be based on replacement value. Because personal property ordinances are not always enforced uniformly, the group may need to seek interpretation of property tax laws from a qualified tax expert. It also would be wise to confer with a tax consultant concerning *federal excise tax* which may be applied to equipment in various ways.

Investment Tax Credit does not fall under the general category of tax levies, but rather is a provision for a credit against taxes due to the federal government. The tax credit is applicable to equipment which is purchased outright and distinctions are not made between equipment of domestic or of foreign origin. The tax credit also can be transferable, and in the case of leased equipment, the vendor may pass the tax credit as a gift to the lessee. In such cases, a certificate is prepared and given to the lessee as proof that the lessor will not claim the credit. The group should have its attorney or accountant make a judgment on the tax credit before it is applied to any proposal comparisons. Once determined, a tax credit is applied against any tax liability that the group may have.

The ownership of the group practice facility also may affect the financing of equipment. For example, if the group is going to occupy a new building that it will own, it may be practical to have much of the cabinet work, desks, waiting room furniture, etc. included as built-ins. Conversely, if a five-year lease on the group's new facility is the maximum commitment obtainable, it probably would be advisable to minimize built-ins and make as much of the equipment and furnishings as possible free standing and, therefore, personal property rather than attached to and part of the real estate. Obviously, the specific conditions and terms of the lease would affect these judgments substantially. If the building is owned by a clinic-related organization which does not actually render medical service, the clinic's equipment also may be owned by that organization. For example, a medical partnership may form a corporation to own and lease the equipment to the partnership. Such ownership would allow investment in the equipment corporation by individuals who by statute could not invest in the medical partnership.

Finally, whether leased or purchased, the best equipment is useless if it cannot be economically, efficiently, and promptly maintained. When all other considerations are equal, the choice among similar pieces of equipment from different manufacturers should be based on the availability of vital equipment parts and the proximity of maintenance personnel. The implications of medical equipment malfunction are much more critical than the implications of ordinary office equipment breakdown. Deciding upon what equipment is necessary and how best to acquire it are critical decisions for a viable medical group practice.

Notes

PART I—THE FORMATION AND DEVELOPMENT OF GROUP PRACTICE

Notes to Chapter 1
Historical Perspectives, Current Status, and Future Trends

1. G.A. Silver, "Group Practice—What It Is," *Medical Care* 1, 2 (April-June 1963): 95.

2. C. Rufus Rorem, *Private Group Clinics* (Chicago: University of Chicago Press, 1931), p. 16.

3. Ibid., p. 104.

4. National Advisory Commission on Health Manpower, *Report of the National Advisory Commission on Health Manpower*, II (Washington, D.C.: United States Government Printing Office, 1967), p. 186.

5. Silver, "Group Practice," p. 94.

6. Robert F. Allison, "The Role of the Medical Group Manager," *Medical Group Management* 22, 2 (January/February 1975): 30.

7. Joseph Axelrod, "AMA Congress on Socio-Economics of Health Care," *Medical Group Management* 14, 3 (March 1967): 21.

8. *Report of the National Advisory Commission on Health Manpower*, p. 432.

9. George T. Harrell, "The Relationship of the Medical School to Group Practice," *Group Practice* 16, 9 (September 1967): 624.

10. Public Health Service, "Promoting the Group Practice of Medicine," *Report of the National Conference on Group Practice* (Washington, D.C.: United States Government Printing Office, 1967), p. 22.

11. John S. Millis, "The Graduate Education of the Physician," *The Report of the Citizens Commission on Graduate Medical Education of the American Medical Association* (Chicago: American Medical Association, 1966), p. 4.

12. John E. Kralewski, "Group Practice of Medicine," *Rocky Mountain Medical Journal* 66 (February 1969): 38.

13. Rorem, *Private Group Clinics*, p. 15.

14. Anne R. Somers, "Factors Affecting Group Practice Growth," *Medical Group Management* 11, 2 (January 1964): 13.

15. Commission on Medical Care Plans, "Report of the Commission on Medical Care Plans," *Journal of the American Medical Association*, Special Edition (January 17, 1959), p. 48.

16. Axelrod, "AMA Congress," p. 20.

17. L.T. Coggeshall, "Planning for Medical Progress through Education," *Report to the Executive Council of the Association of American Medical Colleges* (Evanston, Illinois: Association of Medical Colleges, 1965), p. 29.

18. Robert J. Erickson, "The Impact of Medicare on a Group Practice Prepayment Plan," *Bulletin of the New York Academy of Medicine* 44 (November 1968): 1315.

19. Rhona L. Wetherille, Jean M. Nordby, and Robert E. Schlenker, "HMOs Today," *Medical Group Management* 22, 4 (May/June 1975): 18-19.

20. Ibid., p. 22.

21. Legislative Department, *Summary of the National Health Planning and Resources Development Act of 1974* (Chicago: American Medical Association, 1974), p. 1.

22. American Association of Medical Clinics, American Medical Association, Medical Group Management Association, *Group Practice—Guidelines to Joining or Forming a Medical Group* (Chicago: American Medical Association, 1970), p. 4.

23. Goodman, L.J.; Bennett III, E.H.; and Odem, R.J.: *Group Medical Practice in the U.S., 1975.* (Chicago: Center for Health Services Research and Development, American Medical Association) forthcoming October 1976.

24. *Report of the National Conference on Group Practice*, p. 28.

25. Goodman, Bennett and Odem, *op. cit.*

26. Ibid.

27. *Report of the National Advisory Commission on Health Manpower*, pp. 572-574.

28. Mary E. McNamara and Clifford Todd, "A Survey of Group Practice in the United States, 1969," *American Journal of Public Health*, 60, 7 (July 1970): p. 1309.

29. Rorem, *Private Group Clinics*, p. 104.

30. Committee on the Costs of Medical Care, "Medical Care for the American People," *The Final Report of the Committee on the Costs of Medical Care* (1932), reprinted by Public Health Service (Washington, D.C.: United States Government Printing Office, 1970), p. 77.

31. Public Health Service, *Medical Groups in the United States, 1959*, Publication No. 1063 (Washington, D.C.: United States Government Printing Office, 1963), p. 107.

32. Goodman and Bennett, "Survey of Group Practice,"

33. McNamara and Todd, p. 1306.

34. Austin Ross, "The Potential Impact of National Health Insurance on Group Practice," *Medical Group Management* 22, 3 (March/April 1975): 29.

35. Annis, Jere W., "How Fast Will Group Practice Grow," *Medical Economics* 47, 8 (April 13, 1970): 141.

Notes to Chapter 2 Considerations for Medical Group Formation

1. Mary E. McNamara and Clifford Todd, "A Survey of Group Practice in the United States, 1969," *American Journal of Public Health* 60, 7 (July 1970): 1308.

2. Donald R. Olson, "E.D.P. in Perspective," *Medical Group Management* 19, 3 (March 1972): 6.

3. David W. Stewart, "Insuring for Group Practice: The Role of Blue Cross," *Bulletin of the New York Academy of Medicine* 44 (November 1968): 1337.

4. Avedis Donabedian, "An Evaluation of Prepaid Group Practice," *Inquiry* 6, 3 (September 1969): 17.

5. National Advisory Commission on Health Manpower, *Report of the National Advisory Commission on Health Manpower*, Vol. 2 (Washington, D.C.: U.S. Government Printing Office, 1967).

6. C. Todd and M.E. McNamara, *Medical Groups in the United States, 1969* (Chicago: American Medical Association, 1971), p. 52.

7. R.O. Egeberg, "Multi-Specialty Group Practice and the Future of Medicine," *Group Practice* 19, 5 (May 1970): 42.

8. Fred E. Graham, "Group Versus Solo Practice: Arguments and Evidence," *Inquiry* 9, 2 (June 1972): 58.

9. G.A. Silver, "Group Practice—What It Is," *Medical Care* (April–June 1963): p. 100.

10. F.W. Wasserman and P. Wasserman, "Blueprint for Group Practice: You Can Spot a Winner at the Starting Gate," *Prism* 2, 8 (August 1975): 59.

11. Austin Ross, "Trends in Clinic Administration," *Medical Group Management* 19, 2 (January 1972): 10.

12. William D. Barry, "What To Expect from Your Clinic Manager," *Group Practice* 15, 5 (May 1966): 340.

13. Keith Davis, "The Management of Science," *Medical Group Management* 13, 6 (September 1966): 4.

14. George S. Custer, "The Role of the Administrator in Group Practice," *Medical Group Management* 19, 1 (November 1971): 5.

15. Davis, "Management of Science," p. 4.

Notes to Chapter 3
Establishment of Group Mission

1. D.M. DuBois, "Organizational Viability in Group Medical Practice," paper presented at the 94th Annual Meeting of the American Public Health Association, November 2, 1966, San Francisco, California.

2. In addition to applicable state statutes, the group practice planner should be familiar with the federal "Certificate of Need Law." Section 1122 of the Social Security Act was added by Public Law 92-603 (enacted October 30, 1972). Its purpose is to assure that federal funds appropriated under the Maternal and Child Health, Medicare, and Medicaid programs "are not used to support unnecessary capital expenditures made on behalf of health care facilities or health maintenance organizations. . . ." A recently completed study of the Section 1122 review process may be obtained from: Division of Comprehensive Health Planning, Room 11-11, Parklawn Building, 5600 Fishers Lane, Rockville, Maryland, 20852.

3. Delmar E. Caywood, "Productivity and Manpower Utilization in a Group Practice Setting," *Medical Group Management* 15, 4 (May 1968): 9–11.

4. "Unhealthy Start: Prepaid Medical Plans Run Into Difficulties As Enrollment Falters," *Wall Street Journal*, February 11, 1975, p. 1.

5. "Chapter VIII: Prepaid Group Practice Plans," *Manual on Insurance* (Denver, Colorado: Medical Group Management Association, 1974), pp. 87–89.

6. *Self-Analysis Manual for Maternity and Infant Care Projects*, Case Western Reserve University School of Medicine; Health Systems Division, Westinghouse Electric Corporation (supported in part by Grant No. MC-R-390129, U.S. Department of Health, Education, and Welfare), July 1973.

7. This approach was adapted from "Chapter I: Strategic Planning," *Financial Planning In Ambulatory Health Programs*. The Boston Consulting Group, Inc. (Developed under Contract No. HSM 110-73-53, Department of Health, Education, and Welfare), DHEW Publication No. (HSM) 73-3027, 1973.

PART II—ORGANIZATIONAL PLANNING

Notes to Chapter 4
Establishment of Planning Criteria

1. The planning process presented in this chapter is adapted from *Financial Planning in Ambulatory Health Programs*, (Washington, D.C.: National Center for Health Services Research and Development, 1973). This manual—U.S. Department of Health, Education, and Welfare Publication No. (HSM) 73-3027—was developed under contract with The Boston Consulting Group, Inc. and was written by Lawrence M. Butler.

2. Joel W. Kovner, "Measurement of Outpatient Office Visit Services," *Health Services Research*, (Summer 1969), pp. 120-21.

3. The list consists of expenditure accounts recommended in *Accounting and Cost Reporting System for Comprehensive Health Service Programs*, prepared by Wolfe and Company for the Community Health Service, Department of Health, Education, and Welfare under Contract (HSM) 110-70-391.

Notes to Chapter 5
Legal Organization

1. B.D. Hirsh, *Business Management of a Medical Practice* (St. Louis: C.V. Mosely Company, 1964), p. 27.

2. The essence of partnership law in 43 states plus the District of Columbia is the *Uniform Partnership Act* (*UPA*), which is set forth in full in Appendix 5A. The *UPA* established basic principles of law which operate regardless of any agreement between the partners, and it defines certain principles which function only in the absence of agreement between the partners. The *UPA* as enacted by various states, however, may vary considerably.

3. H.C. Cotton, *Medical Partnership Practice* (Oradell, New Jersey: Medical Economics Book Division, 1971), p. 9.

4. Ibid., p. 22.

5. Ibid., pp. 34-35.

6. Medical Group Management Association, ed., "Organization," *The Clinic Manager's Manual* (Denver: Medical Group Management Association, 1974), p. 6.

7. Cotton, p. 38.

8. "Organization," *The Clinic Manager's Manual*, p. 7.

9. *Internal Revenue Code of 1954*, Sub-section 702. Hereafter cited as *IRC*

10. *IRC*, Sub-section 704.

11. *IRC*, Sub-section 6031.

12. Cotton, p. 71.

13. American Law Institute, *Restatement (Second) of Agency* (1958), Sub-section 1.

14. American Law Institute, Sub-section 8(a).

15. E. Hyat, L.R. Hyat, and A.H. Groeschel, *Law of Hospital, Physician and Patient* (Berwyn, Illinois: Physician Record Company, 1972), p. 193.

16. Ibid., p. 191.

17. Ibid.

18. Ibid., p. 188.

19. Ibid., p. 185.

20. Hirsh, *Business Management*, p. 35.

21. Ibid., p. 34.

22. Cotton, *Medical Partnership Practice*, p. 49.

23. Hirsh, *Business Management*, p. 35.

24. Ibid.

25. Cotton, *Medical Partnership Practice*, p. 77.

26. Ibid., p. 78.

27. Ibid., p. 79.

28. Ibid.

29. H.D. Andrews, "Clinic Organization," *Professional Paper of the American College of Clinic Managers* (Denver: July 5, 1961), p. 10.

30. Chester Rohrlich, *Organizing Corporate and Other Business Enterprises* (Albany: Mathew Bender, 1968), p. 165.

31. Andrews, "Clinic Organization," p. 10.

32. Rohrlich, *Organizing Business Enterprises*, p. 166.

33. R.N. Davies and K.H. Lawrence, *Choosing a Form of Business Organization* (Durham, North Carolina: Duke University School of Law, 1963), p. 126.

34. Ibid., p. 127.

35. Ibid., p. 139.

36. Ibid., p. 135.

37. Rohrlich, *Organizing Business Enterprises*, pp. 170–71.

38. Howard O'Leck, *Non-Profit Corporations, Organizations and Associations*, 2nd ed. (Englewood Cliffs, New Jersey: Prentice-Hall, Inc., 1965), p. 1.

39. *Internal Revenue Code*, Section 501(c).

40. O'Leck, *Non-Profit Corporations*, p. 3.

41. Ibid., p. 2.

42. Ibid., p. 5.

43. Ibid., p. 7.

44. Ibid. A deed of trust is an instrument in use in many states by which real property may be conveyed to trustees for a particular purpose and not as an outright sale of land.

45. *Dartmouth College* v. *Woodward, 4 Wheat.* 518, 1819.

46. Ibid., p. 439.

47. *American Medical Association Principles of Medical Ethics*, (1971), Section 6.

48. J.M. Hannaford, "Risks and Rewards of Professional Corporations," Address given at the Medicolegal Symposium, A.B.A., (1969), p. 5.

49. Ibid.

50. *American Medical Association Principles of Medical Ethics*, (1971), Section 7.

51. *Business Organizations*, p. 387.

52. H.B. Jones, "Professional Corporations: Practical Realities," *The Professional Corporation* (Practicing Law Institute, 1971), p. 73.

53. Ibid., pp. 67-69.

54. Ibid., p. 77.

55. Ibid., p. 53. The reader may be interested in reviewing Sub-chapter B of the *Internal Revenue Code of 1954*, as amended, for further information on business expense deductions.

56. J.K. Logan, "Professional Corporations: A Current Look," *The Journal of the Kansas Bar Association*, 40 (Spring 1971), 10-11.

57. M.N. Weinberg, "What's New with Professional Corporations," *Journal of the Medical Group Management Association* 20, (November-December 1972): 26.

58. Ibid., p. 28.

59. Logan, "Professional Corporations," p. 55.

60. "Professional Corporations: A Panel Discussion," *The Tax Lawyer* 24 (Winter 1971): 226.

61. Logan, "Professional Corporations—Current," p. 54.

62. George Ray, "Professional Corporations: Factors That Go Into the Decision Whether to Operate as a Professional Corporation," *Journal of Taxation* 34 (March 1971): 130.

63. Jones, "Professional Corporations—Practical," Sub-section 3.5.

64. *Social Security Benefits, Including Medicare*, (New York: Commerce Clearing House, 1971), pp. 24-25.

65. Weinberg, "What's New," p. 19.

66. R.L. Griffith and S.L. Mukai, "Professional Corporations After the Salesmanship: A Sober View," *The Professional Corporation* (Practicing Law Institute, 1971), pp. 43–44.

67. Logan, "Professional Corporations—Current," p. 61.

68. Griffith and Mukai, "Professional Corporations—After Salesmanship," p. 44.

69. R.C. Taylor, "P.H.C. Penalty Tax: Steps that Corporations of Professionals Can Take to Sidestep It," *The Journal of Taxation* 34 (March 1971): 141.

70. Griffith and Mukai, "Professional Corporations—After Salesmanship," p. 41.

71. Weinberg, "What's New," p. 19.

72. *Business Organizations*, p. 396.

73. B.I. Bittker, "Professional Service Organizations: A Critique of the Literature," *Tax Law Review* 23 (May 1968): 430.

74. Jones, "Professional Corporations—Practical," p. 29.

75. K.M. Worthy, "I.R.S. Chief Counsel Outlines What's Ahead for Professional Corporations," *Journal of Taxation* 32 (February 1970): 90.

76. Ibid.

77. Weinberg, "What's New," p. 18.

78. Logan, "Professional Corporations—Current," p. 59.

79. Weinberg, "What's New," p. 18.

80. M.N. Weinberg, "A Brief Look at the Advantages and Disadvantages of Professional Incorporation," *Creighton Law Review* 6 (1973): 32.

81. Weinberg, "A Brief Look," p. 35.

82. *Business Organizations*, p. 410.

83. Bittker, "Professional Service Organizations," p. 445.

84. *Business Organizations*, p. 404.

85. Ibid., p. 446–449.

86. A.C. O'Neill, Jr., "Professional Service Corporations: Coping with Operations Problems," *The Journal of Taxation* 31 (August 1969): 95.

87. Jones, "Professional Corporations—Practical," p. 335.

88. Ibid., p. 332.

89. Ibid., p. 333.

90. B.C. Eaton, "Professional Corporations and Associations," *Business Organizations* (New York: Matthew Bender, 1974), pp. 17a, 1023.

91. Hannaford, "Risks and Rewards," p. 8.

92. Logan, "Professional Corporations—Current," p. 56.

93. *Business Organizations*, p. 443.

94. O'Neill, "Professional Service Corporations," p. 96.

95. "Professional Corporations: A Panel Discussion," p. 244.

96. R.O. Jacobs, "Stock Ownership Control Agreements for Professional Corporations," *The Florida Bar Journal*, 45 (June-July 1971), 416.

97. Ibid., p. 388.

98. W.A. Levinson, "What It Costs to Incorporate a Practice," *Medical Economics* (September 1970): p. 100.

99. Ibid., p. 104.

100. Ibid.

101. Jones, "Professional Corporations—Practical," p. 336.

102. Ibid., p. 135.

103. W.H. Horsley and M.S. Dray, "Compensating Officer-Shareholders of Professional Corporations: An Analysis," *Journal of Taxation* 34 (March 1971): 147.

104. "Professional Corporations: A Panel Discussion," p. 238.

105. H.B. Jones, "Is There a Dividend Requirement for Professional Corporations?" *Journal of Taxation* 34 (March 1971): 139.

106. Weinberg, "A Brief Look," p. 35.

107. Logan, "Professional Corporations—Current," p. 62.

108. *Business Organizations*, p. 445.

Notes to Chapter 6
Governance

1. Lillian Doris and Edith J. Friedman, *Corporate Meetings, Minutes and Resolution* (Englewood Cliffs, New Jersey: Prentice-Hall, 1951), p. 227.

2. Ibid., p. 420.

3. William M. Scranton, "The Layman in Group Practice," *Medical Group Management* 19, 1 (November 1971): 12.

4. Miklos S. Nicolson, *Duties and Liabilities of Corporate Officers and Directors* (Englewood Cliffs, New Jersey: Prentice-Hall, 1972), p. 40.

5. Clyde T. Hardy, Jr., "The Role of Medical Director in Group Practice," *Medical Group Management* 19, 1 (November 1971): 17.

6. Philip Selznick, "The Informal Organization," *Organizations: Structure and Behavior*, ed. Joseph A. Litterer (New York: John Wiley & Sons, 1969), pp. 146–148.

7. Eliot Freidson and Buford Rhea, "Processes of Control in a Company of Equals," *Social Problems* 11, 2 (1963): 119–132.

Notes to Chapter 7
Facility Ownership

1. Jerome S. Gross, *Encyclopedia of Real Estate Forms* (Englewood Cliffs, New Jersey: Prentice-Hall, Inc., 1973), p. 17.

2. Libby F. Jessup, *Landlord and Tenant* (Dobbs Ferry, New York: Oceana Publications, Inc., 1974), p. 42.

3. Ibid., pp. 30–32.

Notes to Chapter 8
Financial Planning

1. *1975 Cost Survey* (based on 1974 data), (Denver, Colorado: Medical Group Management Association, 1975), p. 3.

2. "Chapter Two," *The Clinic Manager's Manual*, (Denver, Colorado: Medical Group Management Association, 1974), p. 2.

Notes to Chapter 9
Staff Compensation

1. James Bakken, John McCormick, and Marcy J. Firth, "Employee Benefits: A National Survey," *Medical Group Management* 22, 2 (January/February 1975): 8–9, (unpublished portions); *1975 Cost Survey* (based on 1974 data), (Denver, Colorado: Medical Group Management Association, 1975).

2. James A. Reynolds, "Group-M.D. Fringe Benefits: Where Will They Stop?" *Medical Economics*, October 23, 1973, p. 211.

3. Bakken, McCormick, and Firth, "Employee Benefits," pp. 8–9.

4. George W. Baird, Jr., "An Overview of Compensation Strategy," *Medical Group Management* 22, 3 (March/April 1975): 14.

5. Donald A. Starr, "Equal Compensation," *Medical Group Management* 22, 3 (March/April 1975): 18.

6. William D. Barry, "Other Factors," *Medical Group Management* 22, 3 (March/April 1975): 21.

7. Starr, "Equal Compensation," p. 18.

8. Stanley N. Allen, "Productivity," *Medical Group Management* 22, 3 (March/April 1975): 20.

9. "Courtesy Discounts," *Medical Group Management Newsletter*, question #2 (December 1973).

Notes to Chapter 10
Policy Planning

1. Donald H. DuBois, "Organizational Viability in Group Medical Practice," unpublished study prepared for the ninety-fourth annual meeting of the American Public Health Association.

PART III—MEDICAL GROUP SYSTEMS DEVELOPMENT

Notes to Chapter 11
Communications Systems

1. M.R. Greenlick et al., "Determinants of Medical Care Utilization: The Role of the Telephone in Total Medical Care," *Determinants of Medical Care Utilization* (March-April 1973): 121-34.

2. Mountain Bell, *Plain Talk About Communications Proposals and How To Compare Them*, (June 1973).

3. J. Zaffarano, "The Many Advantages of Owning Your Own Phone System," *Administrative Management* (October 1973): 28-61.

4. Mountain Bell, *Plain Talk.*

Notes to Chapter 13
Patient Appointments, Scheduling, and Referral Systems

1. J.F. Rockart and P.B. Hoffman, "Physician and Patient Behavior Under Different Scheduling Systems in a Hospital Outpatient Department," *Medical Care* 7, 6 (November/December 1969): 463-470.

2. Arnold V. Hurtado, Donald K. Freeborn, John E. Myers, and Maradee A. Davis, "Unscheduled Use of Ambulatory Care Services," *Medical Care* 12, 6 (June 1974): 498-511.

3. John McCormick, "A Systematic Approach to Patient Scheduling," *Medical Group Management* 22, 4 (May/June 1975): 13-17.

Notes to Chapter 14
Medical Records Systems

1. Conrad E.H. Herr and Elaine O. Patrikas, "Keeping Track of Ambulatory Care," *Hospitals* 49, 5 (March 1, 1975): 92.

2. Walter Balfour, "Choosing the Medical History Cover," *Medical Group Management* 16, 2 (January 1969): 20.

3. Richard E. Easton, *Problem-Oriented Medical Record Concepts* (New York: Appleton-Century-Crofts, 1974), pp. 2-4.

4. James F. Fries, "Alternatives in Medical Record Formats," *Medical Care* 12, 10 (October 1974): 876.

5. *Uniform Medical Record System: Manual for Nursing Staff and Other Health Related Personnel* (Boone, Iowa: Boone County Hospital, n.d.), p. 1.

6. Herr and Patrikas, "Keeping Track of Ambulatory Care," p. 91.

Notes to Chapter 15
Charge Systems

1. C.T. Frock, *Medical Credit and Collection, a Survey of Group Practices* (Durham, North Carolina: Duke University, 1974).

2. W.L. McClure, Jr., "Your Uncollected Accounts: Aging Gracefully?" *Physicians' Management* 13, 8 (August 1973): 62P.

3. A. Owens, "Collection Agencies to Steer Clear Of," *Medical Economics* 51, 25 (November 25, 1974): 236-239.

4. *Medical Credit and Collections* (Denver, Colorado: Medical Group Management Association, 1974), pp. 94-96.

Notes to Chapter 16 Purchasing, Supply Inventory, and Maintenance

1. Walter G.D. Strothers, "Management of Clinic Resources," *Medical Group Management* 19, 2 (January 1972): 12.

2. "Prudent Buyer," *Provider Reimbursement Manual* (Department of Health, Education and Welfare, HIM-15 July 1967), Sec 2103; reprinted June 1972, p. 21.

3. Medical Group Management Association, *Accounting Committee's Report on 1974 Cost Survey, Based on 1973 Data* (Denver: Medical Group Management Association, 1974), pp. 3-4.

4. Marshall M. Baker, "The Clinic Purchase Order," *Medical Group Management* 21, 2 (January/February 1974): 24.

5. Peter F. Drucker, *Management, Tasks, Responsibilities, Practices* (New York: Harper and Row, 1973), p. 68.

6. Paul E. Widman, "Purchasing and Its Relation to Management," *Medical Group Management* 12, 5 (July 1965): 20.

7. Baker, "Clinic Purchase Order," p. 24.

8. T. Leroy Martin, *Hospital Accounting Principles and Practice* (Chicago: Physicians Record Company, 1951), pp. 188-89.

9. Horace Cotton, *Medical Practice Management* (Oradell, New Jersey: Medical Economics Company, 1967), p. 50.

10. Baker, "Clinic Purchase Order," p. 24.

Notes to Chapter 18 Systems Automation

1. Carl Hammer, *Computers in Research* (Moscow, USSR: Sperry Rand Seminar Presentation, May 30, 1974).

2. Tom L. Battisto and C. Robert Fox, "Computer Input, The Best Way," *Medical Group Management* 21, 6 (September/October 1974): 7.

3. Edward G. Harshfield, "Financing Without Peril," *Computer Decisions* 6, 3 (March 1974): 19.

4. Richard A. McLaughlin, "A Survey of 1974 Data Processing Budgets," *Datamation* 20, 2 (February 1974): 54.

5. Willis H. Ware, "Records, Computers, and the Rights of Citizens," *Datamation* 19, 9 (September 1973): 113.

6. Frederick G. Withington, "Five Generations of Computers," *Harvard Business Review* 52, 4 (July/August 1974).

7. Leslie H. Matthies, *Forms Design Applied Principles* (Colorado Springs, Colorado: Systemation, 1969), p. 41.

Notes to Chapter 19 Statistical Analysis Systems

1. *Systems Analysis Applied to Health Services*, Scientific Publication #239 (Washington, D.C.: Pan American Health Organization, 1972), p. 4.

2. *Self-Analysis Manual for Maternity and Infant Care Projects*, Case Western Reserve University School of Medicine; Health Systems Division, Westinghouse Electric Corporation (supported in part by Grant No. MC-R-390129, U.S. Department of Health, Education, and Welfare, July, 1973). See chapter on "Documenting Clinic Objectives," pp. 2-6 through 2-21.

3. *Self-Analysis Manual*, p. 2-20.

4. Gerald Giebink, "Developing a Data System for Ambulatory Care," *Community Hospitals and the Challenge of Primary Care* (New York: Center for Community Health Systems, Columbia University, January 1975), p. 234.

5. "Projections of Anticipated Data Requirements for Professional Standard Review Organizations," (prepared by the Executive Committee of the American Association of Health Data Systems, January 19, 1973), *Medical Record News* 44, 2 (April 1973): 37-38.

6. *Ambulatory Medical Care Records: Uniform Minimum Basic Data Set. A Report of the United States National Committee on Vital and Health Statistics*, U.S. DHEW Publication No. (HRA) 75-1453 (Rockville, Maryland: United States Department of Health, Education, and Welfare, August 1974).

7. The encounter form package presented here was originally developed by the author on behalf of Rhode Island Health Services Research (SEARCH) under a grant from the United States Department of Health, Education and Welfare. A fee-for-service group practice served as the setting for which the package was designed.

8. Helen V. Howerton, "First Principles of Information System Design," *Medical Record News* 44, 2 (April 1973): 66.

Bibliography

PART I—THE FORMATION AND DEVELOPMENT OF GROUP PRACTICE

Chapter 1
Historical Perspectives, Current Status, and Future Trends

Allison, Robert F. "The Role of the Medical Group Manager." *Medical Group Management* 22, 2 (January 1975): 28-38.

American Association of Medical Clinics, American Medical Association, Medical Group Management Association. *Group Practice—Guidelines to Joining or Forming a Medical Group.* Chicago: American Medical Association, 1970.

Annis, Jere W. "How Fast Will Group Practice Grow." *Medical Economics* 47, 8 (April 13, 1970): 136-137, 141-142, 146.

Axelrod, Joseph. "AMA Congress on Socio-Economics of Health Care." *Medical Group Management* 14, 3 (March 1967): 20-21, 25.

Coggeshall, L.T. *Report to the Executive Council of the Association of American Medical Colleges.* Evanston, Illinois: Association of Medical Colleges, 1965.

Commission on Medical Care Plans. "Report of the Commission on Medical Care Plans." *Journal of the American Medical Association*, Special Edition (January 17, 1959), pp. 1-96.

Committee on the Costs of Medical Care. *The Final Report of the Committee on the Costs of Medical Care* (1932), reprinted by Public Health Service. Washington, D.C.: United States Government Printing Office, 1963.

Erickson, Robert J. "The Impact of Medicare on a Group Practice Prepayment Plan." *Bulletin of the New York Academy of Medicine* 44 (November 1968): 1312-1319.

Harrell, George T. "The Relationship of the Medical School to Group Practice." *Group Practice* 16, 9 (September 1967): 623-631.

Kralewski, John E. "Group Practice of Medicine." *Rocky Mountain Medical Journal* 66 (February 1969): 35-41.

Legislative Department. *Summary of the National Health Services and Planning Act of 1974.* Chicago: American Medical Association, 1974.

McNamara, Mary E. and Clifford Todd. "A Survey of Group Practice in the United States, 1969." *American Journal of Public Health* 60, 7 (July 1970): 1303-1313.

Millis, John S. *The Report of the Citizens Commission on Graduate Medical Education of the American Medical Association.* Chicago: American Medical Association, 1966.

National Advisory Commission on Health Manpower. *Report of the National Advisory Commission on Health Manpower,* II. Washington, D.C.: United States Government Printing Office, 1967.

Public Health Service. "Promoting the Group Practice of Medicine." *Report of the National Conference on Group Practice.* Washington, D.C.: United States Government Printing Office, 1967.

Rorem, C. Rufus. *Private Group Clinics.* Chicago: University of Chicago Press, 1931.

Ross, Austin. "The Potential Impact of National Health Insurance on Group Practice." *Medical Group Management* 22, 3 (March 1975): 29-31.

Rushner, Robert F. *Medical Engineering—Projections for Health Care Delivery.* New York: Academic Press, 1972.

Silver, G.A. "Group Practice—What It Is." *Medical Care* 1, 2 (April-June 1963): 94-96 98-100, 102.

Somers, Anne R. "Factors Affecting Group Practice Growth." *Medical Group Management* 11, 2 (January 1964): 10-16.

Wetherille, Rhona L., Jean M. Nordby, and Robert E. Schlenker. "HMO's Today." *Medical Group Management* 22, 4 (May 1975): 18-20.

Chapter 2
Considerations for Medical Group Formation

Barry, William D. "What To Expect from Your Clinic Manager." *Group Practice* 15, 5 (May 1966): 339-341.

Custer, George S. "The Role of the Administrator in Group Practice." *Medical Group Management* 19, 1 (November 1971): 4-5, 22.

Davis, Keith. "The Management of Science." *Medical Group Management* 13, 6 (September 1966): 4-5.

Donabedian, Avedis. "An Evaluation of Prepaid Group Practice." *Inquiry* 6, 3 (September 1969): 3-27.

Egeberg, R.O. "Multi-Specialty Group Practice and the Future of Medicine." *Group Practice* 19, 5 (May 1970): 5, 42-43.

Graham, Fred. E. "Group Versus Solo Practice: Arguments and Evidence." *Inquiry* 9, 2 (June 1972): 49-60.

McNamara, Mary E. and Clifford Todd. "A Survey of Group Practice in the United States, 1969." *American Journal of Public Health* 60, 7 (July 1970): 1303-1313.

National Advisory Commission on Health Manpower. *Report of the National Advisory Commission on Health Manpower,* vol. 2. Washington, D.C.: U.S. Government Printing Office, 1967.

O'Donnell, Walter E., M.D. "Going Group: Have You Got What It Takes?" *Medical Economics* (January 17, 1972): 83-86.

Olson, Donald R. "E.D.P. in Perspective." *Medical Group Management* 19, 3 (March 1972): 6-7, 22.

Ross, Austin. "Trends in Clinic Administration." *Medical Group Management* 19, 2 (January 1972): 9-11, 26-27.

Silver, G.A. "Group Practice—What It Is." *Medical Care* (April-June 1963): 94-102.

Stewart, David W. "Insuring for Group Practice: The Role of Blue Cross." *Bulletin of the New York Academy of Medicine* 44 (November 1968): 1336-1338.

Todd, C. and M.E. McNamara. *Medical Groups in the United States, 1969.* Chicago: American Medical Association, 1971.

Wasserman, F.W. and Wassermen, P. "Blueprint for Group Practice: You Can Spot a Winner at the Starting Gate." *Prism* 2, 8 (August 1974): 59, 63-67.

Chapter 3
Establishment of Group Mission

Affirmative Action and Equal Employment: A Guidebook for Employers. 2 vols. Washington, D.C.: United States Equal Opportunity Commission, 1974.

"Allied Health Personnel in Group Practice Plans: Special Interest Session," Proceedings, 21st Annual Group Health Institute. Washington, D.C.: Group Health Association of America, 1971, pp. 80-111.

Barro, A.R. "Survey and Evaluation of Approaches to Physician Performance Measurement." *Journal of Medical Education* 48 (November 1973): 1047-1093.

The Boston Consulting Group. "Chapter I: Strategic Planning." *Financial Planning In Ambulatory Health Programs.* (Developed under Contract No. HSM 110-73-53, Department of Health Education, and Welfare). DHEW Publication No. (HSM) 73-3027, 1973.

Brown, Carol A. "The Division of Laborers: Allied Health Professions." *International Journal of Health Services* 3 (1973): 435-444.

Caywood, Delmar E. "Productivity and Manpower Utilization in a Group Practice Setting." *Medical Group Management* 15, 4 (May 1968): 9-11.

Dale, Martin G. "PSRO: A Primer." *Journal of the American Medical Association* 229 (July 8, 1974): 166-171.

A Digest of State Laws Affecting the Payment of Medical Care, Group Practice and HMO's. 1973 ed. Rockville, Maryland: Aspen Systems, 1973.

DuBois, D.C. "Organizational Viability in Group Medical Practice." Paper presented at the 94th Annual Meeting of the American Public Health Association, November 2, 1966, San Francisco, California.

Equal Employment Opportunities Compliance. 2nd ed. New York: Practising Law Institute, 1973.

Fisher, T.L. "Doctors in Groups Must Take Extraordinary Care With the Other Men's Patients." *Canadian Medical Association Journal* 110 (1974): 1104-1105.

Frommeyer, Jr., Walter B. "Recertification: A Status Report." *Annals of Internal Medicine* 79 (September 1973): 441-443.

Handy Reference Guide to the Fair Labor Standards Act. United States Department of Labor, Employment Standards Administration, Wage and Hour Division, WH Publication 1282.

HMO and Health Services Report. Ed. Jeffrey A. Prussin. Mt. Arlington, New Jersey: Girard Associates, Inc. This is a monthly newsletter reporting on current issues and activities relative to HMO's.

Income Distribution: An Abstract and Analysis. Alexandria, Virginia: American Association of Medical Clinics, 1974.

Korkmas, Carolyn. *Bibliography on National Health Insurance.* Denver: Library Reference Service, Medical Group Management Association, 1975.

Manual on Insurance. Denver: Medical Group Management Association, 1974.

McCain, J.R. "The Background and Development of Peer Review." *Journal of the Medical Association of Georgia* 62 (October 1973): 336-341.

Medical Group Management Association. "Training Programs for Physician Support Personnel." *Medical Group Management* 17, 6 (September 1970): 16-18.

MGMA Digest of Medical Group Employment Contracts and Income Distribution Plans. Denver: Medical Group Management Association, 1974.

"National Health Insurance: Which Way to Go?" *Consumer Reports* (February 1975): 118-124.

A bibliography on nurse practitioners, prepared by the Library Reference Service, Medical Group Management Association, appears in *Medical Group Management* 21, 5 (July/August 1974): 35.

Occupational Safety and Health Administration. *Handy Reference Guide.* Available from any OSHA office.

Patterson, Douglas. Unpublished paper on equal employment opportunity legislation, Denver, Colo., Medical Group Management Association, 1974.

"Peer Review. A Comprehensive Appraisal." *Rhode Island Medical Journal* 56 (October 1973): 405-408.

Pfeffer, R.I. "Bad, Good, Better Ways to Divide Group Income." *Medical Economics* 50, 1 (1973): 139-145.

Pinel, Patricia N. *Comprehensive Bibliography on Health Maintenance Organizations: 1970-1973.* Denver: Medical Group Management Association, 1974.

Prussin, Jeffrey A. *Health Maintenance Organization Legislation in 1973-1974.* Washington, D.C.: Science and Health Publications, 1974.

Prybil, Lawrence. "Physician Terminations in Large Multi-Specialty Groups." *Medical Group Management* 18, 6 (September 1971): 4-6.

Review and Comment Responsibilities of State and Areawide Comprehensive Health Planning Agencies. Washington, D.C.: United States Government Printing Office, 1973.

Schwarz, M. Roy. "Medical Education and Medical Care: Underserved Areas. WAMI: A Concept of Regionalized Medical Education." *Journal of Medical Education* 48 (December 1973): 116-118.

Self-Analysis Manual for Maternity and Infant Care Projects. Case Western Reserve University School of Medicine; Health Systems Division, Westinghouse Electric Corporation (supported in part by Grant No. MC-R-390129, United States Department of Health, Education and Welfare), July 1973.

Shuman, Larry J., et al. "Location of Ambulatory Care Centers in a Metropolitan Area." *Health Services Research* (Summer 1973): 121-138.

Special Report on the Occupational Safety and Health Act of 1970. Denver: Medical Group Management Association, 1973.

Task Force on Guidelines of Care of the American Medical Association Advisory Committee on PSRO. "PSRO's and Norms of Care." *Journal of the American Medical Association* 229 (July 8, 1974): 166-171.

"Unhealthy Start: Prepaid Medical Plans Run Into Difficulties As Enrollment Falters." *Wall Street Journal*, February 11, 1975, p. 1.

PART II—ORGANIZATIONAL PLANNING

Chapter 4
Establishment of Planning Criteria

The Boston Consulting Group, Inc. *Financial Planning in Ambulatory Health Programs.* U.S. Department of Health, Education and Welfare Publication No. (HSM) 73-3027, Washington, D.C.: National Center for Health Services Research and Development, 1973.

Kovner, Joel W. "Measurement of Outpatient Office Visit Services." *Health Services Research* (Summer 1969): 112-127.

Wolfe and Company. *Accounting and Cost Reporting System for Comprehensive Health Service Programs.* U.S. Department of Health, Education, and Welfare Contract No. (HSM) 110-70-391. Washington, D.C.: Community Health Service, 1970.

Chapter 5
Legal Organization

American Jurisprudence, 2nd ed. New York: Jurisprudence Publishers, Inc., 1964.

Andrew, H.D. "Clinic Organization." *A Professional Paper for the American College of Clinic Managers.* Denver, Colorado, July 5, 1961.

Bittker, B.I. "Professional Service Organizations: A Critique of the Literature." *Tax Law Review* 23 (May 1968): 429-449.

The Clinic Managers Manual. Denver, Colorado: Medical Group Management Association, 1974.

Cotton, H.C. *Medical Partnership Practice.* New Jersey: Medical Economics Book Division, 1971.

Davies, R.N. and K.H. Lawrence. *Choosing a Form of Business Organization.* Durham, North Carolina: Duke University School of Law, 1963.

Eaton, B.C. "Professional Corporations and Associations." *Business Organizations.* New York: Mathew Bender, 1973.

Griffith, R.L., and S.L. Mukai. "Professional Corporations After the Salesmanship: A Sober View." *Hawaii Bar Journal* 7 (July 1970): 37-46.

Hannaford, J.M. "Risks and Rewards of Professional Corporations." Address at the Medicolegal Symposium, A.B.A., 1969.

Hirsh, B.D. *Business Management of a Medical Practice.* St. Louis: C.V. Mosby Company, 1964.

Horsely, W.H., and M.S. Dray. "Compensating Officer-Shareholders of Professional Corporations: An Analysis." *Journal of Taxation* 34 (March 1971): 146-149.

Hyat, E., L.R. Hyat, and A.H. Groeschel. *Law of Hospital, Physician and Patient.* Berwyn, Illinois: Physician's Record Company, 1972.

Hynes, J.D. *Agency and Partnership: Cases, Materials and Problems.* Indianapolis: Bobbs-Merrill Company, Inc., 1974.

Internal Revenue Code of 1954.

Jacobs, R.O. "Stock Ownership Control Agreements for Professional Corporations." *The Florida Bar Journal* 45 (June-July 1971): 336-40 and 412-17.

Jones, H.B. "Is There A Dividend Requirement for Professional Corporations?" *Journal of Taxation* 34 (March 1971): 139-140.

——. *Professional Corporations: Practical Realities.* New York: Practising Law Institute, 1970.

Logan, J.K. "Professional Corporations: A Current Look." *Journal of the Kansas Bar Association* 40 (Spring 1971): 7-11 and 53-63.

Levinson, W.A. "What It Costs to Incorporate A Practice." *Medical Economics* 47 (September 14, 1970): 99-105.

O'Leck, H.L. *Non-Profit Corporations, Organizations and Associations.* 2nd ed., New Jersey: Prentice-Hall, Inc., 1965.

O'Neil, A.C., Jr. "Professional Service Corporations: Coping With Operational Problems." *Journal of Taxation* 31 (August 1969): 95-97.

"Professional Corporation or Association under State Law." *Business Organizations.* New York: Mathew Bender, 1974.

"Professional Corporations: A Panel Discussions." *The Tax Lawyer* 24 (Winter 1971): 223-48.

Ray, George. "Professional Corporations: Factors that Go into The Decision Whether to Operate as a Professional Corporation." *Journal of Taxation* 34 (March 1971): 130-33.

Restatement (Second) of Agency. American Law Institute, 1958.

Rohrlich, Chester. *Organizing Corporate and Other Business Enterprises.* Albany, New York: Mathew Bender, 1958.

Taylor, R.C. "P.H.C. Penalty Tax: Steps that Corporations of Professionals Can Take to Sidestep It." *Journal of Taxation* 34 (March 1971): 141-42.

Weinberg, M.N. "A Brief Look at the Advantages and Disadvantages of Professional Incorporation." *Creighton Law Review* 6 (1973): 17-38.

Worthy, K.M. "I.R.S. Chief Counsel Outlines What Lies Ahead for Professional Corporations." *Journal of Taxation* 32 (February 1970): 88-92.

Chapter 6
Governance

Doris, Lillian and Edith J. Friedman. *Corporate Meetings, Minutes and Resolutions.* 3rd ed. Englewood Cliffs, New Jersey: Prentice-Hall, 1951.

Freidson, Eliot and Buford Rhea. "Processes of Control in a Company of Equals." *Social Problems* 11, 2 (1963): 119-132.

Hardy, Clyde T., Jr. "The Role of the Medical Director in Group Practice." *Medical Group Management* 19, 1 (November 1971): 16-17, 26.

Nicolson, Miklos S. *Duties and Liabilities of Corporate Officers and Directors.* Englewood Cliffs, New Jersey: Prentice-Hall, 1972.

Scranton, William M. "The Layman in Group Practice." *Medical Group Management* 19, 1 (November 1971): 12-13.

Selznick, Philip. "The Informal Organization." *Organizations: Structure and Behavior.* Ed. Joseph A. Litterer. New York: John Wiley & Sons, 1969, pp. 146-148.

Chapter 7
Facility Ownership

Colby, Edward E. *Practical Legal Advice for Builders and Contractors.* Englewood Cliffs, New Jersey: Prentice-Hall, Inc., 1972.

Eiteman, Wilford John. Ph.D. and Charles N. Davisson, *The Lease: As a Financing and Selling Device.* Ann Arbor, Michigan: University of Michigan, 1951.

Gross, Jerome S. *Encyclopedia of Real Estate Forms.* Englewood Cliffs, New Jersey: Prentice-Hall, Inc., 1973.

Jessup, Libby F., J.D. *Landlord and Tenant.* Dobbs Ferry, New York: Oceana Publications, Inc., 1974.

Krasnowiecki, Jan. *Ownership and Development of Land: Cases and Materials:* Brooklyn, New York: Foundation Press, Inc., 1965.

Kratovil, Robert. *Real Estate Law*, 5th ed. Englewood Cliffs, New Jersey: Prentice-Hall, Inc., 1969.

Moynihan, Cornelius J. *Introduction to the Law of Real Property: An Historical Background of the Common Law of Real Property and Its Modern Application.* St. Paul, Minnesota: West Publishing Co., 1962.

Payne, John C. "Ancillary Costs in the Purchase of Homes." *Missouri Law Review* 455 (1970): 1-35.

Chapter 8
Financial Plannng

Accounting Manual for Health Maintenance Organizations. Stock #1720-00041. St. Paul, Minnesota: Group Health Plan, Inc., March 1972.

Accounting Manual for Health Maintenance Organizations. U.S. DHEW Publication No. (HSM) 73-13008. Rockville, Maryland: Health Maintenance Organization Service, March 1972.

Adams, R.M. *Capitalizing on Capital Financing.* (Professional paper) Denver, Colorado: American College of Clinic Managers, June 30, 1970.

Administrative Cost Determination Manual for Hospital Outpatient Accounting U.S. DHEW Publication No. (HSM72-3022. Rockville, Maryland: National Center for Health Services Research and Development, 1972.

Ambulatory Health Care Information System: Computer Operations Manual. U.S. DHEW Pub. No. (HSM)72-6204. Rockville, Maryland: Bio-Dynamics, March 1972.

Ambulatory Health Care Information System: Overall System Description. U.S. DHEW Pub. No. (HSM)72-6202. Rockville, Maryland: Bio-Dynamics, 1 March 1972.

Ambulatory Health Care Information System: Training and Procedures Manual. U.S. DHEW Pub. No. (HSM)72-6203. Rockville, Maryland: Bio-Dynamics, 1 March 1972.

"Annual Administrative Review." *Hospitals* 48, 1 (April 1, 1974): entire issue.

Baloff, N. *An Integrated Health Services Data System.* Research Paper #106) Stanford, California: Stanford University, Graduate School of Business, August 1972.

Baloff, N. *Management Information Systems for Medical Care Organizations.* (Research Paper #75) Stanford, California: Stanford University, Graduate School of Business, May 1972.

Berman, H.J. "How Reports Can Help You Manage Working Capital." *Hospital Financial Management* 26, 1 (January 1972): 18-21.

Black, H.A. *Accounting in Business Decisions: Theory, Method and Use.* 3rd ed. Englewood Cliffs, New Jersey: Prentice-Hall, 1973.

Blakely, D.S. *Developing a Proposal on Financing the Constuction of a Clinic Building.* (Professional paper) Denver, Colorado: American College of Clinic Managers, May 21, 1970.

Blum, M.S. et al. *Cost Containment Workshop.* Ann Arbor, Michigan: Community Systems Foundation, Ltd., 1971.

Brier, R. "Reaching the Operational Stage: A Study of HMO Financial Planning." Masters thesis, Great Neck, New York, Hofstra University, January 31, 1972.

"Budgeting: A Traditional Tool Enters the 70's, Special Issue." *Hospital Financial Management* 24, 11 (December 1970): 3-27.

Clinic Managers Manual. Denver, Colorado: Medical Group Management Association, 1973.

Cost Determination Manual for Hospital Outpatient Accounting. U.S. DHEW Publication No. (HSM)73-3022, March 1972.

Cost Finding and Reporting System Comprehensive Health Services Project, November 1971. Washington, D.C.: Office of Economic Opportunity, 1971.

1975 Cost Survey (based on 1974 data). Denver, Colorado: Medical Group Management Association, 1975. Availability is restricted.

Danielson, H.P. *Financial Reports.* (Professional paper) Denver, Colorado: American College of Clinic Managers, May 1968.

Dearden, J. *Cost Accounting and Financial Control Systems.* Reading, Massachusetts: Addison-Wesley, 1973.

Falk, I.S. "Financing for the Reorganization of Medical Services and Their Delivery." (Part 2, Medical Cure and Medical Care) *Milbank Memorial Fund Quarterly* 50, 4 (October 1972): 191-221.

Financial Planning in Ambulatory Health Programs. U.S. DHEW Publication No. (HSM)73-3027, July 1973.

Funk, D.A. *Health Data Systems: An Informational Manual.* Chicago: Blue Cross Association, 1973.

Fyke, K.J. *An Examination of the Application of Planning-Programming-Budgeting To the Health Care Field.* Edmonton, Alberta: University of Alberta, Spring 1971.

Gaus, C.R. "Information Requirements for Management of New Health Care Organizations." *Medical Care* 11, 2 (March/April 1973): 51-60.

Gooche, G.W. *Methods and Detection of Embezzlement in the Medical Office.* (Professional paper) Denver, Colorado: American College of Clinic Managers, August 15, 1966.

Goodman, S.R. *Financial Manager's Manual and Guide.* Englewood Cliffs, New Jersey: Prentice-Hall, 1973.

Guidelines for Producing Uniform Data for Health Care Plans. U.S. DHEW Publication No. (HSM)73-3005. Washington, D.C.: United States Government Printing Office, July 1972.

Health Care Data for the Medical Services. (NTIS Report #PB218-974) Burlington, Vermont: University of Vermont, June 1971.

Herbert, M.E. *A Financial Guide for HMO Planners.* Minneapolis: Institute for Interdisciplinary Studies, September 1972.

Horner, J.C. *Internal Control of Patient Source Document.* (Professional paper) Denver, Colorado: American College of Clinic Managers, July 1, 1967.

Kimbell, L.J. and J.H. Lorant. "Methods for Systematic and Efficient Classification of Medical Practice." *Health Services Research* (Spring 1973): 46-60.

Knight, W.D. "Working Capital Management—Satisfaction versus Optimization." *Financial Management* (Spring 1972): 33-40.

Lewellen, W.G. and R.W. Johnson. "Better Ways to Monitor Accounts Receivable." *Harvard Business Review* 50, 3 (May/June 1972): 101-109.

Macro Systems. *Financial Management Information System for Health Maintenance Organizations,* I-IV, Rockville, Maryland: Macro Systems/Health Maintenance Organizations Service, April 1973.

McFarlane, A.H. and G.R. Norman. "Medical Care Information System: Evaluation of Changing Patterns of Primary Care." *Medical Care* 10, 6 (November/December 1972): 481-487.

Moore, D.W. *Budgeting in Clinics.* (Professional paper) Denver, Colorado: American College of Clinic Managers, June 1, 1970.

Murnaghan, J.H. "Health Services Information Systems in the United States Today." *New England Journal of Medicine* 290, 11 (March 14, 1974): 603-610.

Neuner, J.J.W. *Cost Accounting Principles and Practice: The First Phase of Managerial Control for Attaining and Improving the Profit Objective of Business Operation.* 8th ed. Homewood, Illinois: Richard D. Irwin, Inc., 1973.

Newhouse, J.P. "Economics of Group Practice." *Journal of Human Resources* 8 (Winter 1973): 37-56.

"The Organization and Financing of Personal Health Care Services: Report of a Symposium." (Part 2, Medical Cure and Medical Care) *Milbank Memorial Fund Quarterly* 50, 4 (October 1972): 225-239.

Parsons, B.H. *Professional Services Summary, a By-product of Accounts Receivable Posting.* (Professional paper) Denver, Colorado: American College of Clinic Managers, June 1, 1969.

Pointer, D.D. "Multiple Regression Analysis: A Tool for Examining Health Care Costs." *Medical Group Management* 21, 2 (January/February 1974): 16-20.

Preservation of the Financial Management Information System for Health Maintenance Organizations. Silver Springs, Maryland: Macro Systems, December 1972.

Prussin, J.A. "Health Maintenance Organizations: Organizational and Financial Models: *Hospital Progress* vol. 55, pp. 33-5, April '74; pp. 56+, May '74; pp. 60-3, Jun. '74.

Puglisi, D.J. and R.J. Paretta. *A Model for Resource Allocation in Health Care Delivery Systems.* Paper presented at the Financial Management Association Meetings, Atlanta, Georgia, October 11-13, 1973.

Phyrr, P.A. *Zero-Base Budgeting: A Practical Management Tool for Evaluating Expenses.* New York: John Wiley and Sons, 1973.

Raatjes, R.B. "Control Personnel Costs through Manhours Budgeting." *Hospital Financial Management* 26 (March 1972): 24-25.

Rickard, J.C. "Current Computer Hardware/Software Can Give Financial Manager Instant Cost Finding." *Hospital Financial Management* 27 (June 1973): 58-61.

Robertson, R.L., et al. "Costs and Financing Policies at a Neighborhood Center." *Inquiry* 10, 3 (September 1973): 36-48.

Schultze, R. "Comparability Is the Key for Outpatient Unit Cost Measurement." *Hospital Financial Management* 26 (March 1972): 17+.

Sgontz, L.G. "Economics of Financing Medical Care: A Review of the Literature." *Inquiry* 9, 4 (December 1972): 3-19.

Thibodaux, T.T., et al. "Computer-based Information Systems Generate Comprehensive Financial Operation Reports." *Hospitals* 47, 6 (March 16, 1973): 51-56.

Towle, W.F. "Innovations in Health Care Delivery, Capital Financing." *Fund Raising Management* 4 (July/August 1972): 15+.

United States Health Services and Mental Health Administration. Health Maintenance Organization Service. *Financial Planning Manual.* Rockville, Maryland: United States Health Services and Mental Health Administration.

United States Office of Economic Opportunity. *Training and Installation Manual for Cost Finding and Reporting System, Comprehensive Health Services Projects, August 1971.* (OEO Manual 6128-1) Prepared by Wolf and Company, 1971.

Weston, J.F. *Managerial Finance.* 4th ed. New York: Holt, Rinehart and Winston, 1972.

Whitworth, G.C. "To Improve Cash Flow, Bank-Finance Private-Pay Receivables." *Hospital Financial Management* 26, 12 (December 1972): 23-24.

Chapter 9
Staff Compensation

Baird, George W., Jr., L.S. Doyle, Donald A. Starr, Stanley N. Allen, and William D. Barry. "Income Distribution in Group Practice: An Overview and Four Factors to Consider." *Medical Group Management* 22, 3 (March/April 1975): 14-22.

Bakken, James John McCormick, and Marcy J. Firth. "Employee Benefits: A National Survey." *Medical Group Management* 22, 2 (January/February 1975): 8-9.

1975 Cost Survey (based on 1974 data). Denver, Colorado: Medical Group Management Association, 1975. Availability is restricted.

"Courtesy Discounts." *Medical Group Management Newsletter*, (question #2), (December 1973).

Reynolds, James A. "Groups—M.D. Fringe Benefits: Where Will They Stop?" *Medical Economics* (October 23, 1972): 211-213, 216-218.

Rhombery, J.A. "A New Look at Pension Plans." *Medical Group Management* 22, 3 (January/February 1975): 10-11.

Shearer, W.M. *Survey: Staff Compensation*, Los Angeles, California: (1975).

Chapter 10
Policy Planning

Allison, Robert F., W.L. Dowling and F.C. Munson. "The Role of the Medical Group Manager." Unpublished paper, Denver Colorado, Medical Group Management Association, 1971.

"Boulder Medical Center Income Distribution Agreement." Unpublished paper, Boulder,

"Boulder Medical Center Income Distribution Agreement." Unpublished paper.

Campbell, Donald T. and J.C. Stanley. *Experimental and Quasi-Experimental Designs for Research.* Chicago: Rand McNally and Company, 1963.

Clinic Manager's Manual. Denver, Colorado: Medical Group Management Association, 1974.

The Denver Clinic Policy Manual. Unpublished manual. Denver, Colorado.

Drake, Jerry F. and F.I. Millar. *Marketing Research: Intelligence and Management.* Scranton, Pennsylvania: International Textbook Company, 1969.

DuBois, Donald M. *Group Medical Practice: Determinants of Success or Failure.* Doctoral Dissertation, Ann Arbor, Michigan: University Microfilms Inc., 1966.

DuBois, Donald M. Unpublished paper prepared for presentation at the 94th Annual Meeting of the American Public Health Association.

Houma Medical and Surgical Clinic Policy Manual. Unpublished manual, Houma, Louisiana;

International Directory of the Medical Group Management Association. Denver, Colorado: Medical Group Management Association, 1973.

Isaac, Stephen and W.B. Michael. *Handbook in Research and Evaluation.* San Diego, California: Robert R. Knapp. 1971.

Kaiser Permanente Employee Handbook. Unpublished manual. Oakland, California: Permanente Medical Group.

Linberg, Robert. "Policies." Unpublished paper.

"Management Review Program: Overall Hospital." Unpublished paper.

Manual on Insurance. Denver, Colorado: Medical Group Management Association, 1974.

MGMA Digest of Medical Group Employment Contracts and Income Distribution Plans. Denver, Colorado: Medical Group Management Association, 1973.

Personnel Policy for the Executive Staff of the Medical Group Management Association. Unpublished manual, Denver, Colo., Medical Group Management Association, 1974.

Policy Formulation in Health Care Institutions. Unpublished report, 1974.

Polyclinic Policy Manual. "Personnel Section." Unpublished manual.

Rokeach, Milton, *Beliefs, Attitudes and Values.* San Francisco: Josey-Ball, Inc., 1968.

Towne, Dudley P. "Developing the Goals and Objectives of a Private Medical Clinic." Unpublished paper, Denver, Colo., Medical Group Management Association.

Watson Clinic Policy Manual. Unpublished manual. Lakeland, Florida, Watson Clinic, 1972.

PART III—MEDICAL GROUP SYSTEMS DEVELOPMENT

Chapter 11 Communications Systems

"Communications." Clinic Design and Construction, St. Louis, Missouri, March 17-20, 1974. Denver, Colo., Medical Group Management Association.

Conomikes, G.S. "Practice Productivity." *Internal Medical News*, July 15, 1973.

Garrity, R.K. "Clinic Design and Related Systems." Clinic Design and Construction Educational Institute, St. Louis, Missouri, March 19, 1974. Denver, Colo., Medical Group Management Association.

Gibson, J.L., et al. *Organizations: Structure, Process, Behavior*, Dallas, Texas: Business Publications, Inc., 1973, Ch. 6.

Greenlick, M.R., et al. "Determinants of Medical Care Utilization: The Role of the Telephone in Total Medical Care." *Medical Care* (March-April 1973): 121-34.

Jacobs, S.L. "More Firms Buying Their Own Telephone Systems." *The Wall Street Journal*, July 30, 1973, p. 22.

Kinkead, F.A. "Buying Telephone Equipment Can Mean Substantial Savings." *Hospital Financial Management* (May 1973): 36-39.

Plain Talk About Communications Proposals and How To Compare Them. Mountain Bell, Denver, Colorado: June 1973.

Zaffarano, J. "The Many Advantages of Owning Your Own Phone System." *Administrative Management* (October 1973): 28-61.

Chapter 13 Patient Appointments, Scheduling, and Referral Systems

Greenlick, M.R., A.V. Hurtado, C.R. Pope, E.W. Saward, and S.S. Yoshioka, "Determinants of Medical Care Utilization." *Health Services Research* 3 (1968): 269.

Hurtado, Arnold V., Donald K.Freeborn, John E. Myers, and Maradee A. Davis. "Unscheduled Use of Ambulatory Care Services." *Medical Care* 12, 6 (1974): 498-511.

Johnson, W.L., and L. Rosenfeld. "Factors Affecting Waitng Time in Ambulatory Care Services." *Health Services Research*, (Winter 1968).

McCormick, John. "A Systematic Approach to Patient Scheduling," *Medical Group Management* 22, 4 (1975): 13-17.

Pope, C.R., S.S. Yoshioka, and M.R. Greenlick. "Determinants of Medical Care Utilization: the Use of the Telephone for Reporting Symptoms." *Journal of Health and Social Behavior* (1971): 155.

Rockart, J.F. and P.B. Hoffman. "Physician and Patient Behavior Under Different Scheduling Systems in a Hospital Outpatient Department." *Medical Care* 7, 6 (Nov./Dec. 1969): 463-470.

Torrens, P.R., and D.G. Yedvab. *The Impact of Emergency Service on Patterns of Ambulatory Care.* Washington, D.C.: U.S. Department of Health, Education and Welfare, Division of Medical Care Administration, 1969.

Villegas, E.L. "Outpatient Appointment System Saves Time for Patients and Doctors." *Journal of the American Hospital Association* 41 (1967).

Weinerman, E.R., R.S. Ratner, A. Robbins, and M.A. Lavenhar. "Yale Studies in Ambulatory Medical Care: Determinants of Use of Hospital Emergency Services." *American Journal of Public Health* 56 (1966).

Welch. J.D., N.J.J. Bailey. "Appointments Systems in Hospital Outpatient Departments." *The Lancet* (May 31, 1952): 106.

Chapter 14
Medical Records Systems

Ackerman, F.K., Jr. "Converting to Terminal Digit Filing of Medical Records." *Hospitals* 42, 21 (November 1, 1968): 63-64, 66, 70.

"Advocates Insurance Number at Birth to Provide Lifetime Medical Records." *Hospital Administration in Canada* 15 (October 1973): 94.

"Ambulatory Medical Care Data: Report of the Conference on Ambulatory Medical Care Records Held at Chicago, Illinois, April 18-22, 1973. *Medical Care* 11, 2, Supplement (March/April 1973): entire issue.

Aronson, M.D. "The Problem-Oriented Record: A Two-Column Modification." *Journal of the American Medical Association* 225, 7 (August 13, 1973): 716-717.

Balfour, Walter. "Choosing the Medical History Cover." *Medical Group Management* 16, 2 (January 1969): 20.

Bashook, Philip G., Leslie J. Sandlow, and William H. Hammett. "Education Plan Key to POMR Success." *Hospitals* 49, 8 (April 16, 1975): 54-58.

Beck, J.C. "An Administrative Record System for Ambulatory Facilities." *Medical Care* 12, 3 (March 1974): 241-250.

Beggs-Baker, Susan, et al. "Individual Privacy Considerations for Computerized Health Information Systems." *Medical Care* 12, 1 (January 1974): 75-84.

Bjorn, John C., and Harold D. Cross. *The Problem-Oriented Private Practice of Medicine (A System for Comprehensive Health Care).* Chicago: Modern Hospital Press, 1970.

Bowden, L."Social Security Numbers for Patient Identification." *Hospitals* 46, 7 (April 1, 1972): 14, 16.

——. "Social Security Numbers: Yea." *Hospitals* 48, 13 (July 1, 1974): 23, 26, 30, 34.

Brabson, M.L. "Social Security Numbers Identify Patients." *Southern Hospital* 36 (December 1968): 14.

Bragg, E.A., Jr. "Social Security Numbers in Record Filing." *Journal of the American Medical Association* 193, 3 (July 19, 1965): 250.

Buckley, J.D., et al. "Computer Based Medical Record System." *Methods of Information in Medicine* 12 (July 1973): 137-142.

Budd, M.A. and B. Reiffen. "Implications of Computer Science for Developing Ambulatory Medical Record Systems." *Medical Care* 11, 2, Supplement (March/April 1973): 132-137.

Burger, C.S. "Automating Medical Records." *Delaware Medical Journal* 43 (May 1974): 127-129.

Campbell, Bernice C. "Confidentiality of Health Records in Emergency Medical Services Systems." *Medical Record News* 46, 3 (June 1975): 16-17.

"Confidentiality of Medical Records." *The Internist* 14, 12 (December 1973): 10-11.

Converse, M.E. "Unit Record System." *Hospitals* 43, 3 (February 1, 1969): 34.

Cordle, F. "The Automation of Clinical Records: An Overview of Special Emphasis on the Automation of Office Records in the Primary Medical Care Setting." *Medical Care* 10, 6 (November/December 1972): 470-480.

Costello, Addis C. "Memorandum to Ralph F. Reinfrank, M.D. Subject: Problem-Oriented Medical Records," October 17, 1969.

Curran, W.J., et al. "Protection of Privacy and Confidentiality." *Science* 182 (November 23, 1973): 797-802.

Daechsel, W.F.O. "Problems Arising from Universal Numbering and Record Linkage Systems." *Canadian Hospital* 49 (March 1972): 23-24.

Day, P.R. "Some Questions about Privacy." *Health and Social Service Journal* (England), 83, Part 1 (March 10, 1973): 547-548.

DeLong, J.L. "Compact Medical Record System: New Forms, Folders, Filing." *Hospitals* 46, 22 (November 16, 1972): 56-58.

"Discovery of Nonmedical Data in Hospital Record Allowed: New York." *Newsletter*, American Society of Hospital Attorneys, 8 (August 1973): 6.

Donahoe, A.M. "Computer System Provides Flexible Control of Medical Records." *Hospitals* 47, 12 (June 16, 1973): 116, 118-121.

Easton, Richard E. *Problem-Oriented Medical Record Concepts.* New York: Appleton-Century-Crofts, 1974.

Esley, Carole E. "Implementing the POMR System: Guidelines for Medical Record Personnel." *Medical Record News* 44, 1 (February 1973): 33-59.

——. "The MRL and the Structure and Elements of the PRoblem Oriented Medical Record." *Medical Record News* 42, 5 (October 1971): 31-33.

Fortuine, R. "Medical Audit and the Problem-Oriented Record." *Alaska Medicine* 14 (October 1972): 115-117.

Fries, James F. "Alternatives in Medical Record Formats." *Medical Care* 12, 10 (October 1974): 871-881.

Froom, J. "Conversion to Problem-Oriented Records in an Established Practice." *Annals of Internal Medicine* 78 (February 1973): 254-257.

"Give the Patient His Medical Record, Swedish Doctor Urges." *Modern Hospital* 120 (May 1973): 44.

Grossman, J.H., et al. "Automated Medical Record System." *Journal of the American Medical Association* 244, 12 (June 18, 1973): 1616-1621.

A Guide for the Retention and Preservation of Records with Destruction Schedules. 4th Ed. Chicago: Hospital Financial Management Association, 1973.

Hager, S.A. "Soundex Filing for Medical Histories." *Medical Group Management* 10, 3 (March 1963): 8-11.

Hart, P.F. "Unit Record System" *Hospital Administration of Canada* 15 (March 1973): 75-76.

Hasard, H. "Retention of Medical Records." *California Medicine* 119 (November 1973): 76-77.

Hayt, Emanuel. *Legal Aspects of Medical Records.* Berwyn, Illinois: Physicians' Record Co., 1964.

Herr, Conrad E.H., and Elaine O. Patrikas. "Keeping Track of Ambulatory Care." *Hospitals* 49, 5 (March 1, 1975): 89-92.

Holmes, L.K. "Organization of a Medical Record Service." *Canadian Association Medical Record Librarian Bulletin* 4 (June 1972): 11-15.

Hopkins, R.T. and K. Trout. "Numeric Filing Systems." *Medical Records* (England), 10 (May 1966): 48-53.

Hospital Medical Records: Guidelines for Their Use and the Release of Medical Information. Chicago: American Hospital Association, 1972.

Huffman, E.K. *Medical Record Management.* 6th Ed. Berwyn, Illinois: Physicians' Record Co., 1972.

Hurst, J. Willis, M.D. and H. Kenneth Walker, M.D., and Mary F. Woody, R.N. *Applying the Problem-Oriented System.* New York: MEDCOM Press, 1973.

Hurst, J. Willis, M.D. and H.Kenneth Walker. *The Problem-Oriented System.* New York: MEDCOM Press, 1972.

An Instruction Guide for Organizing Health Records. Chicago: American Medical Record Association, n.d.

Laboratory of Computer Science and Harvard Community Health Plan. *COSTAR—Computer-Stored Ambulatory Record: A Progress Report.* Boston, Massachusetts: Massachusetts General Hospital and Harvard Medical School, n.d.

Lee, B.S., et al. "Introducing a Fiche System of Microfilming." *Medical Record News* 44, 5 (October 1973): 32-37.

Lennox, B. "Debate on Patient Identification." *The Lancet* (September 16, 1972): 589-591.

Lewis, E.N. "Government and Privacy: The Promise and the Peril." *American Medical News* 17, 29 (July 29, 1974): 10.

McFarlane, A.H. and G.R. Norman. "Methods of Classifying Symptoms, Complaints, and Conditions." *Medical Care* 11, 2, Supplement (March/April 1973): 101-108.

McIntire, M.S. and B.M. Clapp. "Is a Central Health Record Possible?" *Medical Record News* 43, 5 (October 1972): 19-22.

McLean, E.R., et al. "Questionnaire Becomes Preadmission Too." *Hospitals* 47, 12 (June 16, 1973): 56-59.

MacLeod V. and R. Vaughan. "To Microfilm or Not? How to Make the Decision." *Hospitals* 43, 6 (March 16, 1969): 71-76.

MacPherson, H. "Hospital Records—The Threat to Individual Freedom." *World Medicine* 8 (June 13, 1973): 22-29.

Mazure, J.L.R. *Significant Trends in Medical Records.* Chicago: American College of Hospital Administrators, 30 May 1971.

"Medical Records in Patients' Hands." *New England Journal of Medicine* 290, 5 (January 31, 1974): 287-288.

Roberta A. Monson. "The POMR and the Physician." *Hospitals* 49, 8 (April 16, 1975): 51-53.

Morehead, M.A. and D. Moore. *Medical Record Manual for Ambulatory Health Centers.* U.S. DHEW Publication No. (HSM) 73-6206. Rockville, Maryland: Community Health Service, April 1972.

Morgan, R.W. *Medical Records in Community Health Centres* (A Commissioned Paper to the Community Health Centre Project). Ottawa, Ontario: Canadian Public Health Association, 1973.

Murnaghan, J.H. and K.L. White. "Ambulatory Medical Care Records." *Medical Record News* 43, 4 (August 1972): 17-19.

Nagaprasanna, B.R. *Medical Records Systems Study.* Jamaica, New York: Mary Immaculate Hospital, June 1973.

Owens, A. "Weed Out Your Records with This Retention Guide." *Medical Economics* (June 24, 1974): 84-88.

Phillips, Donald F. "Some POMR Criticism Clearly Misdirected." *Hospitals* 49, 8 (April 16, 1975): 58-61.

"Position Statement on the Confidentiality of Medical Research Records: American Psychiatric Association." *American Journal of Psychiatry* 130 (June 1973): 739.

Price, Elizabeth. "The Letter Box. Social Security Numbers." *Medical Record News* 39, 3 (June 1968): 4-5.

"Record Retention and Microfilming." *Medical Record News* 43, 5 (October 1972): 56-62.

Reid, M.H. "Fishing through Patient Records." *Medical Care* 10, 6 (November/December 1972): 488-496.

"Responsibility in the Use of Medical Information for Research: Statement by the Medical Research Council." *British Medical Journal* 1 (January 27, 1973): 213-216.

Rockart, J.F. "Medical Record Storage: A Method for Determining Level of Activity." *Health Services Research* 7 (Winter 1972): 276-287.

Rozovsky, L.E. "Retention of Medical Records." *Dimension in Health Service* (Canada), 51 (March 1974): 8-9.

Rumsey, J.M. "Medical Records Must Remain Confidential." *American Medical News* 16 (November 12, 1973): 20.

Salvekar, A.M. "Design of a Medical Record Department." *Medical Record News* 44, 1 (February 1973): 29-32.

Sheehan, D.M. and R.C. Reinehr. "Large-Scale Computerized Clinical Records System." *Evaluation* 1, 2 (1973): 74.

Shenkin, B.N. and D.C. Warner. "Giving the Patient his Medical Record: A Proposal to Improve the System." *New England Journal of Medicine* 289, 13 (September 27, 1973): 688-692.

Sheridan, Bart. "The Alarming New Assaults on Doctor-Patient Privacy." *Medical Economics* (April 15, 1974): 31-32, 35-36, 41, 45.

Sigfried, M. "Workable Filing Systems Detailed." *Southern Hospital* 36 (December 1968): 15-16.

Sims, Thomas F. "Medical History Potpourri." An address presented to the Medical Group Management Association Western Section Conference, Lake Tahoe, Nevada, June 17, 1969.

"Single-Number System May Revolutionize Record Keeping." *Medical World News* 8, 10 (March 10, 1967): 21-22.

Smith, J.T. "Central Dictating System." *Medical Group Management* 2, 4 (July 1955): 9-10.

Springer, E.W. *Automated Medical Records and the Law.* Pittsburgh: Aspen Systems Corporation, 1971.

——. "Physician-Patient Privilege: Two Rulings For, One Against" *Hospital Topics* 51 (September 1973): 37-38.

"Statement on Preservation of Patient Medical Records in Health Care Institutions: AHA." *Hospitals* 48, 1 (January 1, 1974): 124-125.

"Statement on the Preservation of Patient Medical Records in Health Care Institutions." *Medical Record News* 44, 6 (December 1973): 31.

Tannenbaum, R.S. "Resource Guide: Introduction to Computerized Information Processing." *Medical Record News* 44, 4 (August 1973): 30-36.

Toussaint, J.L. "Central Dictation System Promoted Complete and Legible Medical Records." *Hospitals* 40, 1 (January 1, 1966): 44-45.

Uniform Medical Record System: Manual for Nursing Staff and Other Health Related Personnel. Boone, Iowa: Boone County Hospital, n.d.

Van Tassel, D. *Keeping Confidential Information Confidential.* Cleveland: Associations for Systems Management, February 1969.

Wagner, K.R. *Developing a Record Retention Schedule for a Private Medical Clinic.* (A professional paper) Denver, Colorado: American College of Clinic Managers, June 30, 1972.

Weed, Lawrence L., M.D. *Medical Records, Medical Education, and Patient Care (The*

Problem Oriented Record As a Basic Tool). Cleveland: Case Western Reserve University Press, 1971.

Willett, D.E. "Medical Records: The Patient's Right to Information." *California Medicine* 119 (November 1973): 77-79.

Yoder, R.D., et al. "Identification Codes for Medical Records." *Health Services Research* 1 (Summer 1966): 53-65.

Chapter 15
Charge Systems

Abrahamson, I.A. "How I Handle Tough Fee Situations." *Physician's Management* 11, 12 (December 1974): 37-39.

American Medical Association. *Current Medical Information and Terminology.* 3rd ed. Chicago: American Medical Association, 1973.

American Medical Association. *Current Procedural Terminology.* 3rd ed. Chicago: American Medical Association, 1973.

"Best New Views on Collecting What's Owed." *Physician's Management* 14, 3 (March 1974): 47D-58D.

Blair, V. "You and the Law." *Professional Medical Assistant* 6, 5 (September/October 1973): 10-11, 17.

The Boston Consulting Group. *Financial Planning in Ambulatory Health Programs.* (Developed under Contract No. HSM 110-73-53, Department of Health, Education, and Welfare). DHEW Publication No. (HSM) 73-3027, 1973.

Brier, R. *Reaching the Operational State: A Study of HMO Financial Planning.* (Masters thesis) Great Neck, New York: Hofstra University, January 13, 1972.

Burket, J.M. "Can Your Patients Lighten Your Insurance-Form Load? Mine Do." *Medical Economics* (October 14, 1974): 198-199.

Corless, H.C. "How to Boost Your Collections without Getting Tough." *Medical Economics* (June 25, 1973): 145-153.

Doctor's Medicare Handbook (Draft for Doctor's Office Assistants). Washington, D.C.: Blue Shield, Medical Service of D.C., October 1971.

Eisenberg, H. "Charge Interest on Overdue Accounts? These Doctors Do." *Medical Economics* (July 17, 1972): 86, 91, 95, 100, 105-106, 111.

Frock, C.T. *Medical Credit and Collection, a Survey of Group Practices.* Durham, North Carolina: Duke University, 1974.

Herbert, M.E. *A Financial Guide for HMO Planners.* Minneapolis: Institute for Interdisciplinary Studies, September 1972.

Hospital Coding Instruction Manual for the Eighth Revision of International Classification of Diseases, Adapted for Use in the United States (ICDA-8). Chicago: AHA.

H-ICDA, Hospital Adaptation of ICDA. 2nd ed. Vol. 1, Tabular List; Vol. 2, Alphabetic Index. Ann Arbor, Michigan: Commission on Professional and Hospital Activities, 1973.

Jeannotte, P.D. "Check Your Collection Agency's Effort." *Hospital Financial Management* 28, 8 (August 1974): 36.

McClure, Jr., W.L. "Your Uncollected Accounts: Aging Gracefully?" *Physician's Management* 13, 8 (August 1973): 60P-62P.

Medical Credit and Collections. Denver, Colorado: Medical Group Management Association, 1974.

Mosley, J.A. "Get Out of the Health-Insurance Business." *Physician's Management* 11, 9 (September 1974): 70-72, 74.

Owens, A. "Collection Agencies to Steer Clear Of." *Medical Economics* (November 25, 1974): 236-239.

Rosenburg, C.L. "How to Get Paid in Compensable Accident Cases." *Medical Economics* (March 18, 1974): 97-105.

Shalowitz, Mervin. "Intergroup—One Alternative: Part II, Benefits, Rates and Marketing." *Medical Group Management* 21, 1 (November/December 1973): 26-28.

The Superbill. Denver, Colorado: Medical Group Management Association, 1974.

Zachs, R. "Bills by the Cycle?" *Physician's Management* 13, 12 (December 1973): 35-40.

Chapter 16
Purchasing, Supply Inventory, and Maintenance

Anderson Carl. "The Question Box—'How do I set up a simple purchasing system?'" *Medical Group Management* 11, 1 (November 1963): 22.

Baker, Marshall M. "The Clinic Purchase Order." *Medical Group Management* 21, 2 (January/February 1974): 23-24.

Caruso, John T. "The Gray Flannel Suit." *Medical Group Management* 10, 5 (July 1963): 12-13.

Cotton, Horace. *Medical Practice Management.* Oradell, N.J.: Medical Economics Company, 1967.

Drucker, Peter F. *Management, Tasks, Responsibilities, Practices.* New York: Harper and Row, 1973.

Hirsh, Bernard D. *Business Management of a Medical Practice.* St. Louis: C.V. Mosby Company, 1964.

Layer, Raymond H. "MGMA Group Purchasing Plan: How and Why It Holds Down Costs." *Medical Group Management* 21, 2 (January/February): 26-28.

MacEachern, Malcolm T. *Hospital Organization and Management.* Chicago: Physicians Record Company, 1974.

Maloney, James. *Purchasing in Medical Groups.* Denver: American College of Clinic Managers, June 1967.

Medical Group Management Association. *Accounting Committee's Report on 1974 Cost Survey, Based on 1973 Data.* Denver: Medical Group Management Association, 1974.

Medical Group Management Association. *The Clinic Manager's Manual.* Denver: Medical Group Management Association, 1974.

Martin, T. Leroy. *Hospital Accounting Principles and Practice.* Chicago: Physicians Record Company, 1951.

"Prudent Buyer." *Provider Reimbursement Manual.* Washington, D.C.: Department of Health, Education and Welfare, HIM-15 July 1967, Sec 2103: reprinted June 1972, p. 21.

Strothers, Walter G.D. "Management of Clinic Resources." *Medical Group Management* 19, 2 (January 1972): 12-13.

Widman, Paul E. "Purchasing and its Relation to Management." *Medical Group Management* 12, 5 (July 1965): 20-24.

Chapter 17
Personnel Systems

Administrative Problems of Hospital Organization and Management. New York: United Hospital Fund of New York, 1970.

An Administrator's Survey of Systems Concept. New York: United Hospital Fund of New York, 1971).

Bass, B. and G. Barrett. *Man, Work and Organizations.* Boston: Allyn and Bacon, 1972.

Beck, L.C. "Getting Down to Personnel Basics." *Group Practice* 22, 11 (November 1973): 22-24.

Bernstein, Lewis and Richard Dana. *Interviewing and the Health Professions.* New York: Appleton-Century-Corfts, 1970.

Black, James Menzies. *How to Get Results from Interviewing.* New York: McGraw-Hill Book Co., 1970.

Chruden, H. and A. Sherman. *Readings in Personnel Management.* Cincinnati, Ohio: South-Western Publishing, 1972.

"Copy for a Model Help-Wanted Ad." *Physician's Management* 14, 7 (July 1974): 64.D.

Donabedian, Avedis. *Aspects of Medical Care Administration: Specifying Requirements for Health Care.* Cambridge, Massachusetts: Harvard University Press, 1973.

——. *A Guide to Medical Care Administration (Volume II: Medical Care Appraisal).* New York: The American Public Health Association, Inc., 1969.

Doren, M.J. "To Get Results, Tell Employees What Results You Expect." *Modern Hospital* 122, 3 (March 1974): 96–99.

Durbin, Richard L. and Herbert Springhall. *Organization and Administration of Health Care: Theory, Practice, Environment.* St. Louis: C.V. Mosby Co., 1966.

Employee Performance Appraisal Programs: Guidlines for Their Development and Implementation. Chicago: American Hospital Association, 1971.

Emshoff, J. *Analysis of Behavioral Systems.* New York: MacMillan Company, 1971.

Evolving Health Care Patterns and Issues, ed. by The Catholic Hospital Association. St. Louis: The Catholic Hospital Association, 1969.

Fear, R.A. *The Evaluation Interview.* 2nd ed. New York: McGraw-Hill, 1973.

Feinberg, M. *Effective Psychology for Managers.* Englewood Cliffs, New Jersey: Prentice-Hall, 1969.

Ford, Robert N. *Motivation Through the Work Itself.* New York: American Management Association, 1969.

Foulkes, Fred K. *Creating More Meaningful Work.* New York: American Management Association, 1969.

Garrett, Raymon D. *Hospitals—A System Approach.* Philadelphia: Auerbach Publishers, Inc., 1973.

Gellerman, S. *Management by Motivation.* New York: American Management Association, 1968.

——. *Motivation and Productivity.* New York: American Management Association, 1963.

Georgopoulos, Basil S. *Organization Research on Health Institutions.* Ann Arbor, Michigan: Institute for Social Research, University of Michigan, 1972.

The Governance of the Hospital: A Report of the 1970 National Forum on Hospital and Health Affairs. Durham, North Carolina: Duke University, Graduate Program in Hospital Administration, 1970.

Grant, Colin. *Hospital Management.* Edinburgh: Churchill Livingstone, 1973.

Greenman, R.L. et al. *Personnel Administration and the Law.* Washington, D.C.: Bureau of National Affairs, 1972.

Haas, J. Eugene and Thomas E. Drabek. *Complex Organizations: A Sociological Perspective.* New York: MacMillan Co., 1973.

Haimann, Theo. *Supervisory Management for Health Care Institutions.* St. Louis: The Catholic Hospital Association, 1973.

Hanlon, John J. *Principles of Public Health Administration.* 5th ed. St. Louis: C.V. Mosby Co., 1969.

Herzberg, Frederick. *Work and the Nature of Man.* New York: Thomas Y. Crowell, 1966.

"It Really Does Pay to Check References." *Physician's Management* 14, 5 (May 1974): 51.P–55.P.

Kach, P.A. "The How and Why of Job Descriptions." *Medical Record News* 44, 5 (October 1973): 38–40.

Letourneau, Charles U. *The Hospital Adminsitrator.* Chicago: Starling Publishers, 1969.

Mathieu, Robert P. *Hospital and Nursing Home Management.* Philadelphia: W.B. Saunders Co., 1971.

Metzger, N. and D. Pointer. *Labor-Management Relations in the Health Services Industry.* Washington, D.C.: Science and Health Publications, 1972.

Missildine, W.H. "Planned Interviews: Key to Successful Hiring." *Physician's Management* 13, 8 (August 1973): 70-77.

Neuhauser, Duncan. *The Delivery of Health Services—Teaching Cases.* Cambridge, Massachusetts: The School of Public Health and the Center for Community Health and Medical Care of Harvard University, 1972.

O'Donovan, Thomas R. *Executive Administration.* Detroit: Mount Carmel Mercy Hospital and Medical Center, 1971.

Rakich, Jonathan S. *Hospital Organization and Management.* St. Louis: The Catholic Hospital Association, 1972.

Rosengren, William R. and Mark Lefton. *Hospitals and Patients.* New York: Atherton Press, 1969.

Silber, M.B. and V.C. Sherman. *Managerial Performance.* New York: American Management Association, 1974.

Somers, Anne R. *Hospital Regulation: The Dilemma of Public Policy.* Princeton, New Jersey: Princeton Unviersity, 1969.

Stolhanski, J.G. "The Importance of Personnel Policies to Yourself and Others." *Medical Group Management* 20, 6 (September/October 1973): 10-12.

Strauss, G. and L. Sayles. *Personnel.* Englewood Cliffs, New Jersey: Prentice-Hall, 1972.

Stukaloff, D. "Better Check Those References." *Physician's Management* 14, 1 (January 1974): 86.U-90.U.

"When the Physician Is Hiring a New Employee." *Medical World News* 14, 48 (December 28, 1973): 39.

Wieland, George F. and Hilary Leigh. *Changing Hospitals: A Report on the Hospital Internal Communications Project.* New York: Harper and Row, 1971.

Chapter 18
Systems Automation

Battisto, Tom L. and C. Robert Fox. "Computer Input, The Best Way." *Medical Group Management,* 21, No. 6 (September/October 1974), 6-12.

Burnett, Gerald J. and Richard L. Nolan. "At Last, Major Roles for Mini-Computers." *Harvard Business Review,* 53, No. 3 (May/June 1975), 148-156.

Hammer, Carl, Ph.D. *Computers in Research.* Moscow, U.S.S.R.: Sperry Rand Seminar Presentation, 30 May 1974.

Harshfield, Edward G. "Financing Without Peril." *Computer Decisions,* 6, No. 3 (March 1974), 17-22.

Hospital Computer Systems, ed. Morris F. Collen. New York: Wiley Biomedical Health Publications, 1974.

Kaye, Donald. "The Systems and EDP Manager: A Profile." *Data Management,* 7, No. 6 (June 1969), 62-64.

Knauss, Leonard I. *Administering and Controlling the Company Data Processing Function.* Englewood Cliffs, New Jersey: Prentice-Hall, Inc., 1969.

Matthies, Leslie H. *Forms Design Applied Principles.* Colorado Springs, Colorado: Systemation, 1969.

McLaughlin, Richard A. "A Survey of 1974 Data Processing Budgets." *Datamation,* 20, No. 2 (February 1974), 52-56.

Ware, Willis H. "Records, Computers, and the Rights of Citizens." *Datamation,* 19, No. 9 (September 1973), 112-114.

Chapter 19
Statistical Analysis Systems

Ambulatory Health Care Information System: Overall System Description. U.S. DHEW Publication No. (HSM)72-6202. Cambridge, Massachusetts: Bio Dynamics, 1972.

"Ambulatory Medical Care Data, Report of the Conference on Ambulatory Medical Care Records." Ed. Jane H. Murnaghan. *Medical Care*, 11 No. 2 (March/April 1973), Supplement. This conference was held at Chicago, Illinois (April 18-22), and was sponsored by the National Center for Health Services Research and Development, National Center for Health Statistics, Johns Hopkins University.

Ambulatory Medical Care Records: Uniform Minimum Basic Data Set. A Report of the United States National Committee on Vital and Health Statistics. U.S. DHEW Publication No. (HRA) 75-1453. Rockville, Maryland: United States Department of Health, Education, and Welfare, August 1974.

Baldwin, J.A. "Linked Record Medical Information Systems." *Proceedings of the Royal Society of London, Series B*, 184 (December 21, 1973), 403-420.

Beggs-Baker, Susan, et al. "Individual Privacy Considerations for Computerized Health Information Systems." *Medical Care*, 12, 1 (January 1974), 75-84.

Brenner, M. Harvey and E. Richard Weinerman. "An Ambulatory Data System." *American Journal of Public Health*, 59, 7 (July 1969), 128-140.

The Design of an Information System for the Wichita Clinic Health Plan, American Association of Medical Clinics, 1972. Developed by Management Decision Systems, Inc. under contract No. (HSM) 110-71-148, Department of Health, Education, and Welfare.

Geibink, Gerald. "Developing a Data System for Ambulatory Care." *Community Hospitals and the Challenge of Primary Care.* New York: Center for Community Health Systems, Columbia University, January 1975), pp. 233-239.

Howerton, Helen V. "First Principles of Information System Design." *Medical Record News*, 44, 2 (April 1973), 64-66.

Murnaghan, Jane H. "Health Services Information Systems in the United States Today." *New England Journal of Medicine*, 290, 11 (March 14, 1974), 603-610.

"Projections of Anticipated Data Requirements for Professional Standard Review Organizations." (Prepared by the Executive Committee of the American Association of Health Data Systems, January 19, 1973.) *Medical Record News*, 44, 2 (April 1973), 22-38.

Self-Analysis Manual for Maternity and Infant Care Projects, Case Western Reserve University School of Medicine; Health Systems Division, Westinghouse Electric Corporation (supported in part by Grant No. MC-R-390129, U.S. Department of Health, Education, and Welfare), July 1973.

Systems Analysis Applied to Health Services, Scientific Publication #239. Washington, D.C.: Pan American Health Orgnaization, 1972.

Systems and Medical Care, ed. Alen Sheldon, F. Baker, and C.P. McLaughlin. Cambridge, Massachusetts: M.I.T. Press, 1970.

PART IV—FACILITY DESIGN, FINANCING, AND CONSTRUCTION

Agron, G.A. "Physical Facilities—How Do You Plan for Them? *Medical Group Management* 15, 2 (January 1968): 17-19.

"Ambulatory Care—Medical Office Building Facilitates Inpatient, Outpatient Care." *Hospitals* 48, 12 (June 16, 1974): 54-60.

Andruk, R.D. *The "Program Plan" and Hospital Construction.* Durham, North Carolina: Duke University, May 1971 (Xerox University Microfilms, Reel #592).

Arneill, B.P. "Guidelines for Design of Facilites: Ambulatory Care." *Hospitals* 49, 8 (April 16, 1975): 83-87.

"Auto Ferris Wheel: St. Joseph Mercy Hospital, Ann Arbor." *Michigan Hospital* 10 (January 1974): 13.

Babnew, D., Jr. "Vert-A-Park: A New Concept in Parking Systems." *World Hospitals* 9 (April 1973): 60-64.

Baum, A.Z. "How to Succeed in a One-Specialty Building." *Medical Economics* (March 4, 1974): 157-159.

Betts, J., et al. *Analysis of Radiology Department.* Ann Arbor, Michigan: Community Systems Foundation, 1970.

Block L. "Project Management—New Characters, New Results." *Hospital Progress* 54 (May 1973): 68-71.

Blum, M.S. "Control Technique Cuts Walking Time." *Hospitals* 47, 17 (September 1, 1973): 86-92.

Boldon, C.M. "Plan Parking for Optimum Land Use." *Buildings* 68 (May 1974): 53-57.

Bowen, B. "Cost Planning System." *Progressive Architecture* 55 (February 1974): 56-57.

"Bridgeport Invests $1 Million in Parking Deck As Part of Hospital Modernization Program." *Modern Hospital* 110 (May 1968): 126.

"Buildings for a Broad Spectrum of Health Care." *Architectural Record* 149, (March 1971): 135-150.

Burgun, J.A. "Determining the Size of Health Facility." *Architectural Engineering News* 7, 11 (November 1965): 64-68, 71.

Carner, D.C. *Planning for Hospital Expansion and Remodeling.* Long Beach, California: The Executive Letter Publishing Company, 1972.

Clibbon, S. *Innovation in the Design of Health Care Facilities: Some Influences of Systems Building.* Reprinted from Synopsis and Proceedings of the 1st International Systems Building Round Table Conference, November 17-19, 1971, pp. 121-127.

Conrad, R.B., et al. "Utilization Study Saved Hospital from Needless Expansion of Radiology Facility." *Hospital Financial Management* 27, 9 (September 1973): 40-42, 44-49.

Darby, D. *In-Depth Study of the Radiology Department.* Ann Arbor, Michigan: Community Systems Foundation, 1970.

—— and C. McCollum. *Radiology Department Study.* Ann Arbor, Michigan: Community Systems Foundation, 1971.

Davis. E.W. and L. White. "How to Avoid Construction Headaches: Construction Management." *Harvard Business Review* 51 (March/April 1973): 87-93.

"Design Portfolio of Therapy, Outpatient and Emergency Departments." *Hospitals* 43, 10 (May 16, 1969): 39-54.

Downey, G.W. "Few Rules for Parking Lot Planning Can Help Cut Costs, Irritation, and Nighttime Danger." *Modern Nursing Home* 25 (August 1970): 43-44.

Drachman, R.P. "Park Small for Big Savings." *Buildings* 68 (April 1974): 76-77.

Duquette, J.R. "Financial Planning for a Construction Program." *Medical Group Management* 13, 2 (January 1966): 18-20.

"Efficiency Intrinsic in Two Hospital Parking Facilities." *Hospitals* 48, 18 (September 16, 1974): 28, 32, 34.

ENO Foundation for Transportation, Inc. *Parking and Access at General Hospitals.* Westport, Connecticut: ENO Foundation for Transportation, 1973.

"Facing Up to Our Parking Problems." *Building Operating Management* 19 (February 1972): 13+.

Field, H.H., et al. *Hospital Design Evaluation—An Interdisciplinary Approach.* Boston: Tufts-New England Medical Center, December 1971.

"Five Points to Consider When Planning a Parking Lot." *Administrative Management* 29 (May 1968): 44.

Gottschalk, C.A. "Consortium Short Cut to Design, Bidding and Construction." *Hospital Forum* (Calif.), 16 (July 1973): 7-8.

"Great Parking Flap: Attempt to Enforce New Regulations Causes a Furor in Boston." *Investor-Owned Hospital Review* 7 (August/September 1974): 22.

Green, J.R.B. *Planning and Design of Health Services Buildings.* Kensington, NSW, Australia: University of New South Wales, School of Health Administration, March 1974.

Group Practice Facilities: A HUD Handbook. No. 4630.1. Washington, D.C.: United States Department of Housing and Urban Development, April 1973.

A Guide to Capital Financing for Hospitals. New York: Eastdil Health Care Funding, Inc., 1974.

Guide to Selecting Architects for Hospital Projects. Chicago: American Hospital Association, 1967.

Hadawi, N. and C.V. Heath. "Santa Rosa Parking Project." *Health Care Engineering* 2 (March/April 1974): 33-34.

Hamilt, M.W. "Planning the Clinic." *Medical Group Management* 13, 2 (January 1966): 12-13.

Hardy, R.C. and L. Lackey. "What to Do until the Architect Arrives." *Medical Group Management* 19, 4 (May 1972): 9-11, Part I; 19, 5 (July 1972): 10-11, Part II; 19, 6 (September 1972): 7-8, 28, Part III.

Harley, R.G. "Contracting for Your Building." *Medical Group Management* 13, 2 (January 1966): 15-18.

Harris, N.J. and L.R. Bennett. "Planning a Nuclear Medicine Service." *Hospitals* 47, 19 (October 1, 1973): 90-94.

Hayes, J.V. "One Way to Prevent Parking Lot Vandalism." *Texas Hospitals* 28 (September 1972): 24.

"Hospital Parking." *Hospital Building and Engineering* 2 (May 1969): 29-30.

"Hospital Parking Lot, Garage Held Exempt from Taxation: Maine Medical Center, Portland." *Hospitals* 48, 8 (April 16, 1974): 17.

Hospitals, Clinics and Health Centers: An Architectural Record Book. New York: McGraw-Hill, 1960.

Kirk, P.H. and E.D. Sternberg. *Doctors' Offices and Clinics, Medical and Dental.* New York: Reinhold, 1955.

Leland, G.H. "Planning for Hospital Parking." *Hospitals* 46, 6 (March 16, 1972): 119-121.

Lindheim, R. *Uncoupling the Radiology System.* Chicago: Hospital Research and Education Trust, 1973.

"Low Turnkey Cost for Dallas Parking Facility." *Hospital Management* 112 (September 1971): 10.

McCollum, C. *Radiology Department Study.* Ann Arbor, Michigan: Community Systems Foundation, 1970.

McGavin, C.T. "Asphalt Paving for Parking Areas, Driveways, and Walkways: A Report on Construction, Maintenance, Layout." *Cornell Hotel and Restaurant Administration Quarterly* 5 (February 1965): 51-94.

——. "Layout, Construction and Maintenance of Parking Areas, Driveways and Walkways." *Cornell Hotel and Restaurant Administration Quarterly* 10 (November 1969): 91-104.

Meathe, P.J. "It's a Wide Open Field: Construction Management." *AIA Journal* 59 (March 1973): 41-43.

Mencotti, J.V. "Qualified Auditors Can Help Reduce Construction Costs." *Hospital Finance Management* 28, 1 (January 1974): 40+.

Minimum Requirements of Construction and Equipment for Hospital and Medical Facilities. 6th Draft. U.S. DHEW Publication No. (HSM)73-4017. Rockville, Maryland: United States Department of Health, Education, and Welfare, March 6, 1973.

Montgomery, J.W. *Planning a Building Addition.* (Professional paper) Denver, Colorado: American College of Clinic Managers, June 1969.

Myers, K.G. "Planning—For $$ Too—Cuts Building Problems." *Hospital Financial Management* 5, 4 (April 1975): 26-30, 32-35.

Nagy, E.J., L. Witlen, and T.W. Hutchings. *Analysis of Parking Facilities.* Denver, Colorado: Midtown Hospital Association, October 1970.

——, T.W. Hutchings, and M. Weber. *Parking Facilities Study.* Denver, Colorado: Midtown Hospital Association, March 1971.

"Office Redesign, Special Issue." *Modern Office Procedures* 20, 2 (February 1975): 25-34.

O'Flaherty, C.A. "Hospital Parking." *Hospital Building and Engineering* 3 (May 1970): 9-12.

"Parking Garage at Santa Rosa Medical Center, San Antonio." *Texas Hospitals* 28 (January 1973): 13.

"Parking Lot Problems—What Hospitals Are Doing about Them." *Hospital Topics* 50 (April 1972): 20.

"Parking Lots—Self Service." *National Safety News* 95 (May 1967): 61+.

"Planning and Construction Issue: Renovation and Expansion of Health Facilities." *Hospitals* 48, 3 (February 1, 1974): entire issue.

Planning Guide for Radiologic Installations. 2nd ed. Ed. W.G. Scott. American College of Radiology, Commission on Planning of Radiologic Installations, Huntington, New York: Robert E. Kireger, 1974.

Pretsch, P.G. "Bridging the Parking Problem: 'Over the Road' Garage at Maryland General Hospital, Baltimore." *Hospitals* 47, 15 (August 1, 1973): 95-96.

Reuter, L.F., IV. "Providing Room to Care." *Hospitals* 48, 4 (February 16, 1974): 62-65.

Revesz, G., et al. "Patient Flow and Utilization of Resources in a Diagnostic Radiology Department." *Radiology* 104 (July 1972): 21-26.

Rich, R.C. "How to Solve the Hospital Parking Problem with a Deck." *Modern Hospital* 110 (May 1968): 124-126.

Ripnen, K.H. *Office Space Administration.* New York: McGraw-Hill, 1974.

Rouke, W.J. "Engineering Pointers for Parking Decks." *Architectural Record* 143 (June 1968): 169-171.

Rourke, A.J.J. "Needed for Those New Services: More Space for Parking Cars." *Modern Hospital* 114 (April 1970): 116.

Schafer, G.P. "The Role of the Architect." *Medical Group Management* 13, 2 (January 1966): 13-15.

Schedule of Rooms (Number and Size), Layout, and Design of X-Ray Diagnostic Departments. (Swedish) Stockholm, Sweden: SPRI, December 1971.

Schnarr, Sister Beatrice. *The Development of a Comprehensive Policy and Procedure for the Implementation of Projects in Hospitals.* Toronto, Ontario: University of Toronto, June 1973 (Xerox University Microfilms).

Shannon, W.R., Jr. "Architecture for Group Practice: Master Plan by Design." *Group Practice* 19, 11 (November 1970): 20-23.

——. *Medical Group Practice—Architecture, Design and Function.* New Horizons in Health Care Proceedings of the 1st International Congress on Group Medicine. Winnipeg, Manitoba, Canada, April 26-30, 1970, pp. 207-219.

Sodaro, R.S., et al. "Radiology: Inside-Out Suite Meets Patient's Needs." *Hospitals* 48, 6 (March 16, 1974): 102-107.

"Special Issue on Medical Office Construction." *Physician's Management* 11, 10 (October 1974): entire issue.

Steinle, J.G. "Space Requirements and Costs for Parking Facilities." *Hospital Topics* 50 (January 1972): 35.

Sullivan, W.G., et al. *Analysis of Optimal Radiographic Location Networks*, I-IV. Atlanta: Medical College of Georgia, 1971 (Xerox University Microfilms).

Szczechowski, W. *Radiology Room Utilization Analysis.* Ann Arbor, Michigan: Community Systems Foundation, 1971.

Taylor, S. "Building an Office the Fast Track Way." *Physician's Management* 12, 1 (January 1975): 65U, 69U, 73U.

Terry, W.G. and J.W. McLaren. *Planning a Diagnostic Radiology Department: Basic Considerations.* Philadelphia: Saunders, 1973.

"Three-Part Program for Parking Lot Security." *Safety Maintenance* 133 (April 1967): 61-62.

Tusler, W.H., Jr. "Long-Range Facility Planning." *Hospital Forum* (Calif.), 16 (February 1974): 7-8, 12.

United States Health Care Facilities Service. *Financial Feasibility Review.* Rockville, Maryland: United States Department of Housing and Urban Development, September 1972.

United States Public Health Service. *A Practitioner's Guide to the Diagnostic X-Ray Equipment Standard.* Washington, D.C.: United States Government Printing Office, 1974.

"Vital Facts on Parking for Physicians." *New York Medicine* 23 (March 1967): 119-120.

Vollmer, Roy. *Application of Modular Production Systems to Ambulatory Care Facilities.* Baltimore: United States Health Services and Mental Health Administration, Xerox University Microfilms, (1972?).

Wall, G. "Tax-Wise Way to Fix Your Building." *Physician's Management* 12, 1 (January 1975): 57D-61D.

Ward, R.M. "Proper Facility Utilization Can Reduce Demand for New Construction." *Hospital Financial Management* 4, 9 (September 1974): 14-18.

Wareing, P. "Parking Control." *Hospital Development* 1 (March/April 1973): 44-45.

"What to Know before You Build." *Group Practice* 22, 1 (January 1973): 8-13.

Wheeler, E.T. *Hospital Modernization and Expansion.* New York: McGraw-Hill, 1971.

Whieldon, D. "An Office Packed with Practice-Easing Tips." *Medical Economics* (October 14, 1974): 174-177.

Wilkins, J.G. "Advice on Hospital Parking Criteria." *Hospital Engineering Newsletter* 15 (March/April 1970): 6.

Woodworth, J. "Architectural Tips." *Medical Group Management* 19, 3 (March 1972): 14-15.

Young, B.W. "What Is a Functional Parking Structure?" *Health Care Engineering* 2 (March/April 1974): 31-32.

Zirkle, T.E. "So You're Thinking of Putting Up a Medical Building." *Physician's Management* 11, 11 (November 1971): 34-41, Part I; 11, 12 (December 1971): 38-41, Part II.

Index